Defining Jewish Medicine

Episteme in Bewegung

Beiträge zu einer transdisziplinären Wissensgeschichte

Herausgegeben von Gyburg Uhlmann
im Auftrag des Sonderforschungsbereichs 980
„Episteme in Bewegung.
Wissenstransfer von der Alten Welt
bis in die Frühe Neuzeit"

Band 8

2021
Harrassowitz Verlag · Wiesbaden

Defining Jewish Medicine

Transfer of Medical Knowledge
in Premodern Jewish Cultures and Traditions

Edited by Lennart Lehmhaus

2021

Harrassowitz Verlag · Wiesbaden

Die Reihe „Episteme in Bewegung" umfasst wissensgeschichtliche Forschungen mit einem systematischen oder historischen Schwerpunkt in der europäischen und nicht-europäischen Vormoderne. Sie fördert transdisziplinäre Beiträge, die sich mit Fragen der Genese und Dynamik von Wissensbeständen befassen, und trägt dadurch zur Etablierung vormoderner Wissensforschung als einer eigenständigen Forschungsperspektive bei.
Publiziert werden Beiträge, die im Umkreis des an der Freien Universität Berlin angesiedelten Sonderforschungsbereichs 980 „Episteme in Bewegung. Wissenstransfer von der Alten Welt bis in die Frühe Neuzeit" entstanden sind.

Herausgeberbeirat:
Anne Eusterschulte (FU Berlin)
Kristiane Hasselmann (FU Berlin)
Andrew James Johnston (FU Berlin)
Jochem Kahl (FU Berlin)

Klaus Krüger (FU Berlin)
Christoph Markschies (HU Berlin)
Tilo Renz (FU Berlin)
Wilhelm Schmidt-Biggemann (FU Berlin)

Gefördert durch die Deutsche Forschungsgemeinschaft (DFG) –
Projektnummer 191249397 – SFB 980.

Abbildung auf dem Umschlag:
Anatomical diagram explained with a diagram of a house; from Ma'aseh Tobiyah
(The Work of Tobias. In Hebrew), by Tobias Cohen; Venice: ‚Stamp Bragadina', 1708.
Wellcome Library, London (L0021883).

Bibliografische Information der Deutschen Nationalbibliothek
Die Deutsche Nationalbibliothek verzeichnet diese Publikation in der Deutschen Nationalbibliografie; detaillierte bibliografische Daten sind im Internet über https://www.dnb.de abrufbar.

Informationen zum Verlagsprogramm finden Sie unter
https://www.harrassowitz-verlag.de

© bei den Autoren
Verlegt durch Otto Harrassowitz GmbH & Co. KG, Wiesbaden 2021
Gedruckt auf alterungsbeständigem Papier.
Druck und Verarbeitung: Memminger MedienCentrum AG
Printed in Germany

ISSN 2365-5666
eISSN 2701-2522
DOI: 10.13173/2365-5666

ISBN 978-3-447-10826-3
eISBN 978-3-447-19606-2
DOI: 10.13173/9783447108263

Preface

Andrew James Johnston and Gyburg Uhlmann

Since its inception in July 2012, the Collaborative Research Centre (CRC) 980 "Epis-teme in Motion. Transfer of Knowledge from the Ancient World to the Early Modern Period", based at the Freie Universität Berlin, has been engaging with processes of knowledge change in premodern European and non-European cultures.

The project aims at a fundamentally new approach to the historiography of knowl-edge in premodern cultures. Modern scholars have frequently described premodern knowledge as static and stable, bound by tradition and highly dependent on author-ity, and this is a view that was often held within premodern cultures themselves.

More often than not, modern approaches to the history of premodern knowledge have been informed by historiographical notions such as 'rupture' or 'revolution', as well as by concepts of periodization explicitly or implicitly linked to a master narra-tive of progress.

Frequently, only a limited capacity for epistemic change and, what is more, only a limited ability to reflect on shifts in knowledge were attributed to premodern cul-tures, just as they were denied most forms of historical consciousness, and especially so with respect to knowledge change. In contrast, the CRC 980 seeks to demonstrate that premodern processes of knowledge change were characterised by constant flux, as well as by constant self-reflexion. These epistemic shifts and reflexions were subject to their very own dynamics, and played out in patterns that were much more complex than traditional accounts of knowledge change would have us believe.

In order to describe and conceptualise these processes of epistemic change, the CRC 980 has developed a notion of 'episteme' which encompasses 'knowledge' as well as 'scholarship' and 'science', defining knowledge as the 'knowledge of some-thing', and thus as knowledge which stakes a claim to validity. Such claims to validity are not necessarily expressed in terms of explicit reflexion, however – rather, they con-stitute themselves, and are reflected, in particular practices, institutions and modes of representation, as well as in specific aesthetic and performative strategies.

In addition to this, the CRC 980 deploys a specially adapted notion of 'transfer' centred on the re-contextualisation of knowledge. Here, transfer is not understood as a mere movement from A to B, but rather in terms of intricately entangled processes of exchange that stay in motion through iteration even if, at first glance, they appear to remain in a state of stasis. In fact, actions ostensibly geared towards the transmission, fixation, canonisation and codification of a certain level of knowledge prove particu-larly conducive to constant epistemic change.

In collaboration with the publishing house Harrassowitz the CRC has initiated the series "Episteme in Motion. Contributions to a Transdisciplinary History of Knowledge" with a view to showcase the project's research results and to render them accessible to a wider scholarly audience. The volumes published in this series represent the full scope of collaborating academic disciplines, ranging from ancient oriental studies to medieval studies, and from Korean studies to Arabistics. While some of the volumes are the product of interdisciplinary cooperation, other monographs and dis-cipline-specific edited collections document the findings of individual sub-projects.

What all volumes in the series have in common is the fact that they conceive of the history of premodern knowledge as a research area capable of providing insights that are of fundamental interest to scholars of modernity as well.

Contents

Part 4: Jewish Medical Episteme Around the Mediterranean
in the Medieval Period

Acknowledgments

This peer-reviewed volume combines the research of a group of international scholars, from recent PhDs to senior faculty who focus on Jewish engagement with medicine in different textual traditions, cultures and geographical realms throughout premodern times. Most articles are based on a subsection and full-day panel of the 2014 conference of the *European Association of Jewish Studies (EAJS)* at Sorbonne Université and École Normale Supérieure (ENS) in Paris. The volume owes part of its title and some other contributions to the conference "Defining Jewish Medicine" that took place just a few days after the EAJS congress at the Institute of Jewish Studies, University College London. The title also reflects the interest and approaches of the working group A03 "The Transfer of Medical Episteme in the 'Encyclopaedic' Compilations of Late Antiquity" based within the trans-disciplinary Collaborative Research Center SFB 980 "Episteme in Motion" at the Freie Universität Berlin.

The idea to this full-day panel with twelve presentations held on 24ᵗʰ July 2014 rested on three equally important pillars. First, this gathering of scholars was planned as an initial attempt to forge international links between the Talmudic part of our team, Markham J. Geller and me, and other colleagues working on Jewish medical topics in (late) antiquity. Second, in the spirit of our interdisciplinary research group, this meeting was meant to broaden the horizon by including the work of scholars who focus on Jewish medical discourse in other regions and periods. Moreover, the lively discussions during the conference provided many precious opportunities to enter into a conversation with colleagues working on similar topics (Second Temple Judaism, magic, early modern medicine) or in other fields (Assyriology, Early Christian Studies, Islamic Studies, History of Medicine/Knowledge) who attended our sessions. Third, bringing together a diverse group of then Ph.D. students, post-docs, faculty and emeriti from Europe, Israel, and North America, I sought to create a communal spirit among scholars in a still emerging subfield within Jewish studies based on our shared interest in medicine and Jewish culture. I am very happy that this attempt to foster collaboration and exchange bore fruit in the form of several international conferences that were held in Berlin but also throughout another full-day panel at the EAJS congress at Jagiellonian University Kraków in 2018, and at a seminar on late antique rabbinic knowledge culture at the AJS Annual Meeting in Washington D.C. in 2017. Moreover, many of those involved in the Paris meeting and the London conference have become valuable conversation partners and were regular contributors to the first four panels (2016–2019) of the newly founded program unit "Medicine in Bible and Talmud" at the *European Association of Biblical Studies (EABS)* Annual Meetings.

DOI: 10.13173/9783447108263.IX

The organization and accomplishment of the conference as well as the editing of this book would not have been possible without the material and intellectual support of the DFG-funded SFB 980 "Episteme in Motion". This project has benefitted from it through travel funds and sourcing of an English-speaking copy editor for several contributions. I would also like to thank the speaker of the SFB 980, Gyburg Uhlmann, and the whole board as well as the series editors for accepting this volume into the series *Episteme* at Harrassowitz. I express my sincere gratitude to the staff at Harrassowitz publishing house, specifically to Julia Guthmüller and Andrea Johari who accompanied this editing project from its inception with steady advice, purposefulness and, not to be underestimated, patience. I am equally indebted to many colleagues from global Jewish Studies and different other disciplines who volunteered for the anonymous peer review process. Their comments and suggestions helped the authors to shape their arguments and to revise their articles in multiple ways.

The one-day thematic panel would not have been such a success without the support of the EAJS program committee, specifically the former President of the EAJS, Judith Olszowy-Schlanger, and the many contributors and attendants who flocked to Paris from far and wide. First and foremost, I would like to thank the speakers and authors whose presentations triggered stimulating discussions and who have worked hard and patiently on their articles. I am grateful to colleagues such as Danielle Jacquart (Paris) or Efraim Lev (Haifa) who were willing to chair or respond to a panel of our subsection. Moreover, I appreciate the many attendants, from students to senior colleagues, who joined our panels and contributed substantially to our discussions.

My special thanks go to my colleague Matteo Martelli for his intellectual curiosity that made him leave his home territory of ancient Greek philology and the history of medicine and science in order to venture into the *terra incognita* of a major Jewish Studies conference. Our joint paper gave us a welcome opportunity to work on our theoretical and methodological approaches which we could share with a broad-minded audience. Grazie mille! I am grateful for the constant support of my other colleagues in the SFB-working group A03 on late antique medicine, Christine Salazar, Philip van der Eijk, and in particular Mark Geller who also organized the 2014 UCL conference on "Defining Jewish Medicine" and facilitated the inclusion of some contributions of this event into the present volume.

Since every event or publication is just as good as the professional infrastructure and working conditions allow, I would like to express my gratitude to various people who worked in the background but were involved directly and indirectly with this project. I thank Kristiane Hasselmann, managing director of the SFB 980, who promoted this conference subsection as an integral part of the events of the Berlin based Collaborative Research Center. I am grateful to Viktor Schmidt, student assistant in A03, who has done a very good job helping with proofreading some parts of the manuscript and aiding with researching specific bibliographical entries. My thanks go to Sara Ben-Isaac (IJS, UCL London) who was in charge of the 2014 conference mentioned above. Finally, I am indebted to my colleague Agnes Kloocke (FU Berlin) who was always eager to offer thoughtful advice regarding the conceptualization, the concrete logistic, and the outreach during the formation process of both the EAJS conference and the book.

Putting the finishing lines to this manuscript focusing on premodern medical knowledge and practice in a time, in which half of the globe (or more) is in lockdown due to the effects of the recent pandemic, adds some rather peculiar touch to this project. Despite the current situation, I still hope that the present volume will stimulate the interest in and discussion of Jewish medical knowledge which will allow for many future transfers and exchanges—may they happen in books, virtually or, most hopefully, through personal encounters.

Hattingen an der Ruhr, March 2021   Lennart Lehmhaus

Part 1:
Introduction, History of Scholarship, and Bibliography

Defining or Defying Jewish Medicine?—
Old Problems and New Questions*

Lennart Lehmhaus

I will start this introductory chapter with a full disclosure.[1] The scheme of defining "Jewish medicine" introduced in the title of this volume is as bold as it is unattainable. In light of a long history of Jewish medical knowledge in different traditions and cultures through the ages and a significant amount of scholarship on the topic, it seems pointless to strive after any conclusive definition of Jewish medicine. From the perspective of the cultural history of medicine, science and knowledge, there is a more promising take on the subject at hand. The present book, in concert with various recent research initiatives, rather explores different cases of the dynamic interaction between medical and other kinds of knowledge in premodern Jewish traditions, through which one may grasp what Jewish medicine could be about. But first, taking one step back, the following survey of popular and academic perspectives on Jewish medicine will present different theoretical and methodological approaches that have emerged over the past two centuries.

Attestations to a deep connection between medicine and Jews, or even to Judaism as a cultural-religious entity, are abundant throughout history and in various contexts, as has been noted by John Efron: "Few occupations are as immediately linked to a group as medicine is to the Jews."[2] As such, the 'Jewishness' of medicine and the almost cliché figure of the Jewish doctor has become commonplace in today's Western cultures, specifically in North America. Even in everyday culture, the Jewish contribution to healthcare and the culinary universe has crystallized in the designation 'Jewish penicillin' for a salubrious chicken soup, combining the taste of immigrants from the 'Old World' with the reputed medical wisdom of Jewish traditions.[3] Often,

---

*   I thank the anonymous readers for their remarks. I am much obliged to Mark Geller (UCL, London) who was willing to read and comment on this and the following introductory chapter and provided very valuable remarks.
1   All references in the following footnotes are in short-citation form (i.e. author, year). The corresponding bibliographic entries can be found in the third chapter of this volume (*Medical Knowledge in Premodern Jewish Cultures and Traditions: Selected Bibliography*), 57–89.
2   Efron 2001, 3.
3   By searching for "Jewish penicillin" online, one comes across an abundance of different recipes for chicken soup, often with specific family's history attached. The Jewish Museum of Maryland has played with this term for a touring exhibition on Jewish involvement with medicine, especially in North America. Cf. Alan Kraut et al., eds., *Beyond Chicken Soup: Jews and Medicine in America* (Baltimore: Jewish Museum of Maryland, 2016). The virtual tour can be found

DOI: 10.13173/9783447108263.003

personal anecdotes—some seasoned with historical accounts and references to the astonishing number of preeminent Jewish scientists in bio-medical research—would be invoked as reliable proofs of a putative Jewish vocation for medicine and sciences.[4]

However, history has proven and scholarship has analyzed how such an alleged 'natural' Jewish affinity to medicine could be easily turned against Jewish physicians, scientists or Jews in general. Similar to their important roles as cultural 'brokers' or intermediaries in the realm of trade, financing and banking, and politics, since medieval time Jews, or Jewish converts, have flourished as physicians at the Muslim and Christians courts or served to other important persons of high-standing in different regions. This proximity to power, which at times translated into actual political involvement, let them come under the suspicion or even accusation of competing political players, religious stakeholders and the wider public who engaged in shaping and fostering anti-Jewish stereotypes.[5] Access to medical education at certain universities from the pre-Enlightenment period onward did not put an end to such long-lasting anti-Semitic prejudices. Quite to the contrary, Jewish physicians (and those engaging in other scientific branches) often fell victim to political and academic struggles, slander, agitation and incitement.[6] Sometimes these reservations assumed the form of a compliment. Thus, Rudolf Virchow praised the impact of Jews and Muslim on medieval medicine and traced the achievements of Jewish physicians back to a hereditary talent that was ultimately grounded in the Jewish valorization of learning. While Virchow's remarks have to be seen as defending Jews against the increasingly nasty discourse of the völkisch movement with its anti-Semitic attacks directed towards Jewish academics and scientists, such a positive and uncritical assumption of a common Jewish appraisal of medicine is burdened with its own difficulties.[7] This is

---

online: http://chickensoupexhibit.org/virtualtour/. See also the media coverage in Vered Gutta man, "A Brief History of Chicken Soup, the 'Jewish Penicillin'," *Haaretz*, 7.10.2019.

4   An interesting combination of all three aspects can be found in the popular assemblage of historical and contemporary vignettes by Nevins 2006, who tries to delineate "Jewish medicine". Cf. also the anecdotal examples in Nevins 2006, 2–4, which seem to be based partly on the discussion in Ruderman 1995, 2–3.

5   On the apologetic discourse of Jewish thinkers and physicians, see Friedenwald 1942a, 1942b. On anti-Jewish polemics against physicians, see Münz 1922, 127–141; Muntner 1953.

6   Cf. Donaldson-Evans 2000. The contexts of the success of Jews within the emerging fields of bio-medicine and other natural sciences in the 19th and early 20th centuries is analyzed in Charpa/ Deichmann 2007. For the scientification of anti-Jewish stereotypes through race-theory and on the Jewish and non-Jewish research into illnesses, disabilities or bodily features that were deemed "Jewish", see Jütte 2016, 31–92 and 289–329; Gilman 1991, esp. 169–193; Efron 1994, esp. 1–32; Oistenau 2009, esp. 38–137. A recent exhibit (*Trail of the Magic Bullet: The Jewish Encounter with Modern Medicine, 1860–1960*) at the Yeshiva University Museum addressed the many difficulties Jews faced entering the medical profession in the US in light of their European predecessors and the intersections between Jewish tradition and modern medical practice. Cf. Rony Caryn Rabin, "Tracing the Path of Jewish Medical Pioneers," The New York Times, May 14,2012. Cited 15 June 2019. Online: https://www.nytimes.com/2012/05/15/health/exhibition-traces-the-emergence-of-jews-as-medical-innovators.html.

7   Cf. Landauer 1895, 9 who quotes Virchow's presentation from 30 March 1894 in Rome. Virchow's idea was based on a scheme of thought that is not much different from publications that

at stake also for the contemporary study of what is often hastily called "Jewish medicine", as Gad Freudenthal has called to mind:

> One may wonder whether this subject matter is at all legitimate: is there something specific about Jewish medicine and science? The Nazi proponents of "German science" railed against what they perceived as a distinctly "Jewish science" (notably the theory of relativity, quantum mechanics, formal mathematics). This historical lesson should make us cautious with respect to any intellectual project that may end up in an ethnic relativization of scientific knowledge.[8]

From a very different perspective, a growing body of publications, especially in Israel and the United States, deals with the intersection between medicine and Judaism, especially in its traditional or orthodox form. This discourse might be taken as proof that one can easily delineate the nature of "Jewish medicine". However, this scheme of thought is often not much different from a naïve naturalization of a Jewish affinity to medicine. Some books and several online sources start from a background of contemporary bio-medical sciences or botany in order to ascribe some modern natural (herbal medicine) and holistic (complementary medicine) approaches to the Jewish sages of (late) antiquity.[9]

Some authors simply bridge the gap between modern and ancient knowledge trying to emphasize the progressiveness of the ancient Jewish sages. In several instances, these texts draw on biblical and Talmudic accounts of healing, comparing the approaches in these traditional sources with modern medical strategies. Particular attention is paid to the religious underpinnings of Jewish healing practices (such as the importance of prayers and good deeds), emphasizing the medicinal use of food, herbs and other substances or the advice for successful pregnancy and childbirth.[10] Others, however, relate the existence of medical knowledge and scientific information in tradi-

---

tie the existence of medical knowledge and scientific information in traditional sources and the talent of preeminent thinkers like Maimonides, Nahmanides and others to a general Jewish superiority (even trumping modern sciences) through learnedness and the supreme legacy of the Sages.

8 Gad Freudenthal, "Review of Koroth: A Bulletin Devoted to the History of Medicine and Science," *Isis: A Journal of the History of Science Society* 82, 2 (1991): 295–296, here 295.

9 Avraham Dahan, ‏רפואה יהודית—יש דבר כזה‎, http://www.herbology.org.il/?CategoryID=250& ArticleID=419; On the Jewish (herbal) drug cabinet, see http://www.simple-natural.net/ index.php?cosmetic=695; on other dimensions of Jewish medicine until Maimonides, see http://www.simple-natural.net/index.php?cosmetic=695; As an example for the holistic approach in practice the reference to the *Rambam Institute of Jewish Medicine* in Safed shall suffice here, cf. http://www.zissil.com/topics/Rambam-Institute-of-Jewish-Medicine-Safed.

10 Cf. Theodore Brod, *Healing Practices: Insights from the Torah, Talmud and Kabbalah* (Bloomington, IN: Xlibris, 2005); Avraham Greenbaum, *The Wings of the Sun: Traditional Jewish Healing in Theory and Practice* (New York/Jerusalem: Moznaim Publishing Corporatio, 1995). Eyal Goldberger, *Human Healing—A Torah Model. 3 methods of healing: new look at spiritual strength.*; online: https://www.chabad.org/kabbalah/article_cdo/aid/380341/jewish/Human-Healing-A-Torah-Model.htm, argues for a strong correspondence between biblical or Jewish religious approaches and various Western medical concepts such as antagonistic therapies

tional sources and the talent of preeminent thinkers (like Maimonides, Nahmanides, and others) to a general Jewish superiority through learnedness and the supreme legacy of the Sages, even trumping modern science. Finally, some authors focus rather on pious ideas and explain how general Jewish observance (the dietary laws of *kashrut*, fasting, prayer etc.) might be understood as a strategy of "well-being" or medico-bodily regimen. Accordingly, Jewish religious life intersects with healing practices in a complementary, mutually enriching way. These books form a body of "*frum* medical handbooks" or self-help literature for members of different Jewish movements, ranging from ultra-orthodox and Hasidic to Conservative and Reform[11]—not always without causing controversy.[12] The very popularity of traditional medicine can be gleaned from the increase of the use of herbalist approaches as complementary and alternative medicine in Israel, which is reflected also in various TV formats and online outlets.[13]

Moreover, contemporary discussions on "Jewish medicine" are often connected with a kind of New Age Jewish spiritualism that bases itself on ideas about Kabbalistic healing and various other approaches with roots in the spiritual movements of the early 20th century.[14] This often merges with the already mentioned growth of interest

(fighting a disease or its symptoms), isopathy (immunization) or homeopathy (as focusing on spiritual dimensions and the individual patient).

11 Cf. Wally Spiegler, *Sha'arei Refuah Gates of Jewish Healing* (Morrisville, North Carolina: Lulu. com, 2006); Kerry M. Olitzky and Debbie Friedman, *Jewish Paths Toward Healing and Wholeness: A Personal Guide to Dealing with Suffering* (Woodstock, Vermont: Jewish Lights Publishing, 2000); Avraham Y. Finkel, *In My Flesh I See God: A Treasury of Rabbinic Insights about the Human Anatomy* (Northvale, NJ: Jason Aronson, 1995).

12 The growing popularity of such alternative medical practices seems to necessitate also halakhic discussions of the permissibility of such healing, as attested in Rabbi Rephoel Szmerla, *Alternative Medicine in Halachah* (Israel Book Shop, 2017), which itself became a matter of dispute when several authorities withdrew their rabbinic approbation (*haskamot*) after its publication. Hassidic approaches to the art of healing can be found at http://www.inner.org/6levels/sixlevels. htm. At times, these new approaches exhibit an idiosyncratic merging of Jewish prayers or KabK balistic rituals with meditation practices known in Buddhism. Cf. http://www.shomreitorah. org/2018/05/11/silence-and-healing/, last retrieved on 26.06.2018. A business model built on those ideas can be found at https://torahhealing.com/.

13 Cf. Eran Ben-Arye et al., "Integration of Herbal Medicine in Primary Care in Israel: A Jewish-Arab Cross-Cultural Perspective," *Evidence-Based Complementary and Alternative Medicine* 2011 (https://doi.org/10.1093/ecam/nep146). As one example for popular TV shows, see the short program "Grandma's medicine" on the Israeli channel Kaan 11.

14 Cf. Alfred Geiger Moses, *Jewish Science: Divine Healing in Judaism: with Special Reference to the Jewish Scriptures and Prayerbook* (Mobile, AL: Gill, 1916), who as a Reform rabbi sought to counter the popularity of Christian Science and psychological ideas among modern American Jews. For contemporary approaches, see Matiyahu Glazerson, *Torah, Light and Healing: Mystical Insights into Healing Based on the Hebrew Language* (Lanham, MD: Jason Aronson, 1996); Douglas Goldhamer and Peggy Bagley, *Healing with God's Love: Kabbalah's Hidden Secrets* (Burdett, NY: Larson Publications, 2015). A search on "Kabbalah healing" or "Jewish healing" will bring up an abundance of online platforms and published books. For illustrational purposes, I will mention here a discussion on the healing secrets of the Torah according to the Zohar at https://kabbalah.com/en/concepts/secrets-of-healing-revealed; Robert Zink and Rachel Haas, *Magical Energy Healing: The Ruach Healing Method,* Portland (Oregon:

in alternative "medicine of the sages" (*refu'at ḥazal*), "Hebraic Medicine" or "Traditional Jewish Medicine"—in analogy to Traditional Chinese medicine (TCM) or Indian Ayurveda medicine and sometimes even neatly intertwined with it. Such approaches favor a non-deterministic, holistic healing model of body and mind that intersects with ethical deeds and spiritual well-being.[15] These developments have been the subject of recent research in social history and contemporary cultural studies.[16]

In some cases, Jewishness looms large in publications that are specifically aimed at individuals suffering from an illness, but also aimed at rabbis, care-givers, or volunteers visiting the sick (*bikur ḥolim*) in Jewish congregations; they often have to deal with issues of illness, medical interventions and their limitations from a personal, spiritual and ethical perspective.[17] In particular, this discourse, firmly embedded in a broader Jewish healing movement, seeks to find a way to balance or supplement contemporary, techno-medical and bio-medical knowledge with spiritual approaches such as prayer, narratives and other aids drawn from religious tradition that relate to a healing of body and soul.[18]

Law of Attraction Solutions, 2014); Devi Stern, *Energy Healing with the Kabbalah: Integrating Ancient Jewish Mysticism with Modern Energetic Practices* (Woodbury, Minnesota: Llewellyn Worldwide, 2018); Jospeh H. Gelberman and Lesley Sussman, *Physician of the Soul: A Modern Kabbalist's Approach to Health and Healing* (Berkeley: Crossing Press, 2000). See also Steven J. Gold, *Om Shalom: Yoga and Judaism* (Golden Glow Productions, 2009), esp. 123–128 (ch. 9: *Jewish Healing Meditation*).

15　On "Hebraic Medicine", see Epstein 1987. Cf. http://www.traditionaljewishmedicine.com/, where the Jerusalem based Yehuda Frischman offers holistic treatment of "people, not diseases" through a dietetic therapy based on Chinese and other 'energetic' food, craniosacral therapy, acupuncture and individualized herbal biomedicine. It is not entirely clear to what degree these treatments are 'traditionally Jewish', though. However, in some of his writings, Frischman relates to fear of God, a pious lifestyle and study as the very tenets of human health, which is also based on a contemporary approach to nutrition. See also Frischman's elaboration on the principles of TJM: health as a state of divine existence; (ethical) misconduct as a reason for sickness; holistic healing; medical practitioners as "agents of HaShem" who seek the physical and spiritual balance of their patients and utilize Shabbat as a healing device; God has created the remedy to every illness. Cited on 6 January 2020. Online: https://www.breslev.co.il/articles/family/health_and_fitness/traditional_jewish_medicine.aspx?id=11565&language=germany.

16　Nicole M. Bauer, *Kabbala und religiöse Identität: Eine religionswissenschaftliche Analyse des deutschsprachigen Kabbalah Centre* (Bielefeld: transcript, 2017). For a quite interesting study that touches upon the precursors (e.g. Alfred Geiger Moses) of the contemporary surge of Jewish spiritual healing, see Ellen M. Umansky, *From Christian Science to Jewish Science: Spiritual Healing and American Jews* (Oxford University Press, 2004).

17　See Nacy Flam, *The Jewish Way of Healing* (cited 6 January 2020; online: http://kalsman.huc.edu/articles/JewishWayOfHealing.pdf), published by the Reform Kalsman Institute of Hebrew Union College. Some finely nuanced discussions can be found in Cutter 2007, 2011; or the Orthodox approach in Tsvi G. Schur, *Illness and crisis: Coping the Jewish way* (New York: NCSY/Orthodox Union, 1987). For a general introduction about providing medical care for Jewish patients, see Joseph Spitzer, *Caring for Jewish Patients* (Boca Raton: CRC Press, 2020).

18　For an analysis, see Michele F. Prince, "Judaism, Health, and Healing: How a New Jewish Communal Field Took Root and Where it Might Grow," *Journal of Jewish Communal Service* 84,3–4 (2009): 280–291. And ibid., 281: "The rediscovered heritage of Judaism, health, and healing

Similar ideas can also be found in summaries of contemporary Halakhic decisions on medical issues like, for instance, Steinberg's summary of the *responsae* (religious decisions) on medical and bio-ethical questions written by Rabbi Yehuda Waldenberg.[19] Various authors have produced surveys of rabbinic traditional thought on medicine based on texts from the Bible up to the Halakhic commentaries and codes of the early modern period, or even including more recent Halakhic authorities.[20] Topics range from more general ideas (role of the physician, visiting the sick, medical fees) to very specific aspects (e. g., sterilization, plastic surgery, genetic screening, organ transplantation, psychological treatment, HIV/AIDS etc.).[21] At times, such discussions overlap with the discourse on Jewish medical ethics and bioethics. However, this topic, which was shaped by the seminal work of Immanuel Jakobovitch, has formed a distinct academic subfield within Jewish religious, philosophical and historical studies. Various authors in North America, Israel and Europe have contributed to a substantial and growing body of publications on these matters, in which the medical ideas in premod-

---

is grounded in traditional Judaism, but it also is characterized by a new elasticity, stretched by the search for a personal and professional spirituality, demographic shifts, and the feminist movement."

19 Cf. Avraham Steinberg, *Jewish Medical Law. Compiled and edited from the 'Tzitz Eliezer'.* Translated by David B. Simons (Woodmere, N.Y.: Beit-Shamai Publications, 1989). See also Mordechai Halperin, *Medicine and Halacha: Practical Aspects. Collections of Essay for the Conference of European Rabbis Jubilee Comvention Iyar 5766, May 2006* (Jerusalem: Schlesinger Institute for Medical-Halachic Research, 2006); Debates about halakhic aspects of medical care and biomedical science can be found specifically in the journals *Tehumin—Tora, Hevra u-Medina* and ורפא ירפא—*The Journal of Torah and Medicine of the Albert Einstein College of Medicine Synagogue and Rabbi Isaac Elchanan Theological Seminary* (RIETS), New York. Several other journals feature medical topics occasionally: *Hakirah. the Flatbush Journal of Jewish Law and Thought,* Brooklyn, NY; *B'Or Ha'Torah,* Jerusalem; *CCAR Journal—a Reform Jewish Quarterly,* New York; or *Journal of Halacha and Contemporary Society* (New York); *Tradition. A Journal of Orthodox Jewish Thought* (New York), *L'Eylah. A Journal of Judaism Today* (London), *Journal of Jewish Communal Service* (New York), *Judaism; a Journal of Jewish Life and Thought* (New York).
The journal *Assia* (Jerusalem) in most issues includes a mix of contributions from the field of practical medical Halakhah, Jewish medical ethics and medical history of mandatory Palestine and Israel. Some other journals had special thematic issues like *The Reconstructionist* 49,6 (1984) on "Judaism and medicine", or *European Judaism* 19,1 (1985) on "Judaism and psychotherapy". On the latter subject (and some cultural aspects of medicine), see also the *Journal of Psychology and Judaism.*

20 Cf. Bleich 1981; Fred Rosner (ed.), *Medicine and Jewish Law. Two volumes* (Northvale, NJ: Jason Aronson, 1990–1993). Fred Rosner and Moshe D. Tendler (eds.), *Practical Medical Halachah* (Northvale, NJ: Jason Aronson, 1990). Cf. the more technically and halakhically inclined discussion in Steinberg 2003.

21 An interesting exception to most of these publications is Mordchai Halperin, ed. *Reality and Medicine in the Order Nashim (Women). Collection of essays.* (Hebr.). Jerusalem: Schlesinger Institute, 2010. The contributions to this book, coming from rabbis, medical practitioners and Wikipedia, form a kind of technical compendia or manual for understanding many of the medicinal details in the Talmudic tractates on women about anatomy, pregnancy, childbirth and menstruation. This is an excellent contemporary example of a medical *florilegium* or *vademecum* aimed at an audience of non-experts.

ern sources, philosophical ideas, contemporary sociopolitical and ethical discourse, and clinical practice intersect.[22]

Except for some of the works on bioethics and law, most of this discourse can be described as mainly non-academic, not primarily historical or philological research. Those developments in the field of Judaism, health and healing discussed above lend themselves to and have themselves become objects for sociological and anthropological research.[23] These publications give us a glimpse of what modern and contemporary rabbinic authorities or Jewish authors would put under a rubric of "Jewish medicine", and how contemporary Jews seek to navigate tradition and bio-medical science and practice.

1 "Jewish Medicine" in academic scholarship

In order to evaluate and further explore the question of the nature of "Jewish medicine", I will turn now to the perspective of those scholars who created and shaped this subfield in the first place. This is a difficult task, since most studies have focused on specific medical subjects, texts or particular figures, without sticking their necks out and tackling the thorny question of the nature of their subject.[24] Earlier scholarship, however, seems to have addressed these issues. The historian Reuven Wunderbar stated that he had no intentions either to present Talmudic knowledge as a new and unknown medical system or to defend it. Rather, he claimed that his study would aim at a true depiction of the medical principles of the Jewish people, a culture whose contributions to human civilization are abundant. In his view, Jewish traditions, like the Hebrew Bible or Talmudic texts, made important contributions to the development of medical science from which one can learn even in modern times.[25] Joseph Bergel portrayed healing as the field of knowledge that is most frequently featured in the Talmud, due to its religious and ritual relevance, mainly with regard to purity issues

---

22 Besides Jakobovits 1959, one may mention here also Dorff 1996; Feldman 1986; Bleich 1981. See further, Noam Zohar, *Alternatives in Jewish Bioethics* (Albany: SUNY Press, 1997); Louis H. Flancbaum, *"And you shall live by them": contemporary Jewish approaches to medical ethics* (Pittsburgh, PA: Mirkov Publications, 2001); David J. Bleich, "Ethico-halakhic considerations in the practice of medicine," *Diné Israel*, 7 (1976): 87–135.

23 See, for instance, Hillel Gray, "The transitioning of Jewish biomedical law: rhetorical and practical shifts in the Halakhic discourse on sex-change surgery," *Nashim* 29 (2015): 81–107; Jeff Levin and Michele F. Prince, "Judaism and Health: Reflections on an Emerging Scholarly Field," *Journal of Religion and Health* 50,4 (2011): 765–777. Susan Sered, "Healing as resistance: Reflections upon new forms of American Jewish healing," in *Religion and Healing in America* (eds. L. Barnes and S. Sered; New York: Oxford University Press, 2004), 231–252; Asaf Sharabi, "Deep healing: ritual healing in the teshuvah movement," *Anthropology and Medicine* 21,3 (2014): 277–289.

24 Ruderman 1995, 3, still pointed to the dearth of substantial academic studies into the subject: "It is all the more remarkable, then, that although the relation between Jews and science and medicine is often noticed, little scholarly analysis has been devoted to exploring this perceived relation in its historical context, and particularly to elucidating the factors in the Jewish cultural experience that might have encouraged the Jewish interest in and pursuit of the sciences."

25 Wunderbar 1850, I–IV.

and dietary laws. In his eyes, medical science exerted pressure urging Jewish scholars of Halakha to keep up with the times. Bergel saw Jewish medical erudition primarily as derived from Egypt (via Moses) and in the hand of either priests or prophets, while the rabbinic collection of medical knowledge is comparable to Pliny's encyclopaedic compilation.[26] In contrast to Bergel, Aaron Friedenwald could not find traces of Egyptian medicine in the Bible or later traditions. He stresses that the Jews developed a complex system of sanitary regulations (isolation in cases of skin diseases, dietary laws, *niddah* etc.) that won them a unique place in the history of public hygiene.[27] This notion of superiority of the Jewish tradition in matters of hygienic principles has been reiterated by scholars throughout the following century, as can be seen in the following statement:

> …Mosaic preventive medicine and public health with a series of religious laws concerning food, water, both personal and environmental sanitation and hygiene, and the purity of conjugal life. At its very origin, the most important distinguishing feature of Jewish medicine is its emphasis on prevention of disease, and Moses, the father of Judaism, may indeed also be regarded as the father of preventive medicine and public health.[28]

The study of Abraham Stern oscillates between very cautious approaches and bold, positivist assessments. He depicts the "instruments of medical research" of the Talmudic sages—namely, empiricism, experiment and dissection—as comparable to ancient and modern medical approaches. Jewish medicine is perceived not only as deeply imbued with the healing sciences of India, Egypt and Greece, but also as being more advanced in its knowledge in several ways.[29] Similar praise of ancient Jewish medical erudition and its insights surpassing Greek or even modern medicine has been voiced by other scholars.[30]

---

26 Bergel 1885, IV–VI (*Vorwort*). Cf. the same opinion in Carmoly 1844, 2. In his study on other scientific branches (Bergel 1880), he stressed that some mistaken approaches in ancient rabbinic sources can be condoned, whereas, in modern times, Halakha has to be reformed in accordance with contemporary scientific insights.

27 Friedenwald 1897, 4–7, quotes Baas *Outlines of the History of Medicine and the Medical Profession*, p. 34 who described the Jews as "creators of the science of public hygiene".

28 Sabin 1983, 195. Cf. Landau 1895, 11, who depicts Moses as a physician whose "immortal merit lies in the field of public hygiene". See also Boss 1952, who praises the Mosaic Law as the most consistent system of hygiene that putatively anticipated the modern ideas of asepsis and antiseptic measures. But against this see Stern 1909, 4f; and Preuss 1911/1992, 588–603, who both pointed out that the biblical and later Jewish laws of im/purity or *kashrut* lack any hygienic, let alone, medicinal rationale. Rather, they lend themselves to the phantasy and interpretation of later scholars who liked to provide such rational or bio-medical explanations. On Jewish public health, see the chapter by Dvorjetski in this volume.

29 Cf. Stern 1909, esp. 5–19 and 24: „Welche Wege hätte wohl die Wissenschaft genommen, wenn sie die in dieser Hinsicht und in Bezug auf pathologische Anatomie ihrer Zeit um Jahrtausende vorausgeeilten Anschauungen und Erfahrungen der Talmudisten nicht übersehen, sondern sich zu eigen gemacht hätte."

30 Cf. Silber 1932, esp. 4: „that the high regard which the Rabbis of the Talmud had: for medicine

Pointing to the relative scarceness of relevant information in the Bible and the lack of any elaborated conceptual medical system in ancient Judaism, Wilhelm Ebstein argued that the absence of evidence should not be taken as evidence of absence, since medical expertise, which may have circulated among Jews, might have been of little interest to the authors of those works.[31] In a similar vein, Cohen in his lecture on Hygiene and Medicine in the Talmud concluded:

> To the modern physician the diagnosis of a disease by some mishnaic doctor and the remedy prescribed may occasionally seem curious if not puerile; but it cannot be gainsaid that the Jews of old were in the dim light that flickered two thousand years ago, fully abreast of their contemporaries, and in many instances in advance of them.[32]

Among those earlier scholars, Steinschneider was probably the first to take a very minimalist stance. He argued that, if it existed at all, a distinct "Jewish medicine" or "medicine of the Israelites" had ceased to exist after the destruction of the Second Temple by the Romans. He critiques any attempt to foist a medical rationale on Jewish dietary and purity regulations. The Talmudic as well as the later medieval medical passages and texts should, therefore, only be studied within the greater cultural (Graeco-Roman, Muslim-Arabic or Christian-European) context of their production. Steinschneider argues that even preeminent Jewish medical authors like Maimonides were passive recipients and should be discussed rather as part of Jewish cultural history than as belonging to the history of medicine.[33] In a similar way but to a very different end, Simon Scherbel lauded the crucial role of Jewish physicians in Jewish culture, who became influential players controlling the fate of the Jewish people and leading them with a sense of their historical mission.[34]

While the title of his opus magnum (*Biblical and Talmudic Medicine*) might let one expect otherwise, Julius Preuss took also a rather skeptical stance towards his own subject. After describing the lack of any primary medical interest in Talmudic traditions, he concluded:

> There is, therefore, no "medicine of the Talmud", which might perhaps be compared to the medicine of Galen or of Susrutas. There is also no Jewish medicine in the sense that we speak of an Egyptian or a Greek medical science.[35]

---

and the high position which physicians occupied, did not make these insensible to their tremendous responsibilities and ethical obligations."

31 Ebstein 1901/1903, 3: „Jedenfalls steht fest, dass daraus ein bestimmter Rückschluss auf den damaligen Kenntnisstand bei den Israeliten in den betreffenden medizinischen Fragen nicht gemacht werden darf".

32 Cohen 1900, 15. See also the survey on *The Sages of Israel as Doctors* (Margalit 1962).

33 Cf. Steinschneider 1896, 1–3. See also Venetianer 1915–17, 1–4.

34 Scherbel 1905, 5–7.

35 Preuss 1978, 4.

Preuss conclusion is echoed in Samuel Kottek's contribution to the present volume:

> Is there, in fact, a Jewish medicine? The answer is indeed a question of defini-
> tion. Historiography can individualize Egyptian, Mesopotamian, Greco-Ro-
> man, and Arabic medicine(s), but no Jewish medicine can be documented; no
> Hebrew or Aramaic medical works from the biblical and/or Talmudic peri-
> od(s) have reached us. There was, in ancient times, apparently no specific Jew-
> ish way of medical practice.[36]

In light of this different opinions on the (non-)subject at hand and with some caveats
or caution, one might identify three different approaches within academic scholarship to be summarized as: 1) Jewish Medicine, 2) Medicine among Jews, 3) Medicine
in Jewish Traditions/Culture(s). In the following, some of their main theoretical underpinnings and methodological implications will be briefly discussed.

1.1 Jewish Medicine

As for the "Jewish Medicine" approach, its main outlines have been already discussed
in the first section on popular ideas and early scholarship. One can subdivide this
"school" into various concepts that frequently overlap and supplement each other.
One strand, in early studies and among the proponents of *Traditional Jewish Medicine*, stresses the particularities, and sometimes superiority of Jewish approaches to
healing and a healthy life. This is quite obvious in the previously mentioned praise of
dietary rules (*kashrut*), im/purity laws and other religious commandments regarding
hygiene (e. g. circumcision) that are regarded as unique features of Jewish culture.[37]
Another faction, equally to be found among early (or current) positivist scholars and
asserters of *frum* or orthodox medicine, (mis)represent scientific knowledge, especially in biblical and ancient rabbinic traditions, in order to arrive at the conclusion that,
in fact, the sages already knew (most of) what constitutes modern (Western) medicine
or they knew even better. Sometimes, this uniqueness is linked to a "collaboration between God and Man" that turn physicians into "medical menschen" practicing "val-
ue-based Jewish medicine [...] concerned with people as much as with disease, with
relationships more than with technical ability".[38] In its milder form, this exaltation

---

36 See p. 177 in the present volume.
37 See above, 9–10. Circumcision was a main subject both in the surveys (cf. Preuss 1911, 278–
   289), in monographs (cf. Brecher 1845), and in early studies collected in Glasberg 1896. On the
   hygienic and medical discourse about Jewish ritual practices, see Efron 2001; and Beth Wenger,
   "Mitzvah and Medicine: Gender, Assimilation, and the Scientific Defense of 'Family Purity',"
   Jewish Social Studies 5 (1998–99): 177–202.
38 Nevins 2006, 2, 81–97 (Part III: More Medical Menschen), and 107f. One may notice the similarity between this concept of "medical *menschlicheit*" (ibid., 108) and Yehuda Frischman's take
   on Traditional Jewish Medicine (see above, n. 13). Nevins, who focuses "upon the social history
   of medicine" (ibid., 4), regards "conventional wisdom" agreeing on the non-existence of Jewish
   medicine as "too facile" (ibid., 2). He adds that he would welcome, if his historical patchwork,
   "celebrating 'Jewish Medicine'" and triggered by his "concern that American medicine is becoming dehumanized" (ibid., x), would inspire some physicians "to embrace Jewish values at

flows into an essentialist approach that automatically equates medical information in premodern Jewish sources with "Jewish medicine" or represents Jewish physicians as "manifestations and incarnations of a particular Jewish archetype of the Eternal Doctor".[39] Such essentializing views, however, produce a "seamless" Jewish "history of medicine that is teleologically linear, Whiggish, and indeed heroic [..]", while attributing to its subjects (i.e. Jewish medical practitioners and authors) "a false Jewish consciousness".[40]

Still another version of this strand can be found in numerous shorter studies that fall back on 'Jewish medicine' as a standard topic for stock articles written mostly for the history section of journals dealing with modern bio-medicine. In this field, the discussion of X or Y in 'Jewish/Biblical/Talmudic medicine' (just as 'Persian, Iranian, Arabic, Islamic' etc. medicine) apparently appeals to scholars to fulfill the requirements of publishing enough research papers. Coming from an academic background of medical school, those studies essentialize everything medical contained in Jewish tradition, from Bible and Talmud to Maimonides, in ways similar to the positivistic approaches in early 19th century scholarship. Accordingly, they have little interest in religious, cultural or historical contexts and the complex textual history of the sources. Moreover, most studies use solely translations of source texts or rely exclusively on main works of the secondary literature (e.g. Preuss/Rosner).[41]

1.2 Medicine among Jews

Aware of the many flaws and naïve shortcomings that encumber both the idea of superiority and essentialism of "Jewish Medicine", the majority of (medical) historians adheres to a view that John Efron has summarized as follows:

> Yet despite the rich tradition that has seen the rabbis give great consideration to Jewish health and well-being and despite the fact that the physician became a role model in Jewish society, especially after the high Middle Ages, Jews never developed a particular field that can be called "Jewish" medicine, something akin to the Chinese, Galenic, Arab, or Ayurvedic medical traditions. This makes the Jewish engagement with medicine a singular one. While there is no particularly Jewish medical system and the mere thought of a Jewish acupuncture or a Jewish yoga is ludicrous, Jews are central to the history of medicine, first in the Islamic orbit and later under Christendom.[42]

---

the work place, then scholarly debate about whether or not there is or ever was an entity that could be called Jewish medicine would be irrelevant", (ibid., 4).

39 Heynick 2002, 4.

40 John M. Efron, "Review of Frank Heynick *Jews and Medicine: An Epic Saga* (Hoboken, NJ: Ktav, 2002)," *Shofar* 22,3 (2004): 140–143, here 141.

41 Due to limitations of space it should suffice here to mention Dubovsky 1989; S. Lurie and Y. Mamet, ""Yotzeh dofen": Cesarean section in the days of the Mishnah and the Talmud," *Israel Journal of Obstetrics and Gynecology* 12,3: 111–113.; Marios Loukas et al., "Surgery in Early Jewish History," *Clinical Anatomy* 24,2 (2011): 151–154;

42 Efron, "Review of Frank Heynick Jews and Medicine: An Epic Saga", 140.

Consequently, academic endeavors turned to different ways of exploring the role of medicine in Jewish history that focused predominantly on Jewish physicians, medical authors or translators, whose Jewishness was only of secondary importance.[43] This decision implied several limitations regarding the possible scope of such undertakings. Studies were largely confined to authored treatises only available from medieval times onward. In most of the earlier scholarship and into the 20th century, a predominantly biographic approach often generated a history of 'great men' that resembled the great inventors/inventions approach in the 'old history of science'.[44] Other studies used information about Jewish medical practitioners, known and less known, in non-Jewish (i.e. Muslim, Christian) sources or records in order to flesh out both the historical contexts of individual physicians or authors and the socio-political factors at play. For instance, scholars pointed to the traditional Jewish obligation and penchant for study, to strict bans from many other professions, as well as to opportunities for social mobility via polyglotism and cultural bridging functions; these made Jews receptive to medical training and practice and turned them into important transmitters and actors in this field.[45]

More recently, this approach has evolved into addressing the social contextualization and the history of texts or traditions rather than solely the biography of Jewish doctors.[46] Within these studies, medicine is often understood as part of or, at least, associated with the group of the classical sciences or liberal arts and often connected to Jewish discourse that negotiated and developed the Graeco-Roman and Arabic philosophical heritage.[47] The vivid and multifaceted transfers of knowledge through the Graeco-Arabic translation movement(s) and maybe some other (Indian, Persian?) traditions (e.g. in *Sefer Asaph* or Donnolo) stimulated research that focuses on diachronic, synchronic and cross-cultural comparison of texts and, albeit rarely, practices. The underlying "grand narrative", however, sharply distinguishes between (late) antique Jewish scientific knowledge and those medieval traditions after their encounter with Graeco-Roman sciences. As a consequence, most research concentrated, as if naturally and exclusively, on the eminent medical authorities and bulk of texts from

---

43 Cf. Ebstein 1903, 2, who mentions the preeminent Jewish doctors and their many accomplishments. In his view, however, from medieval time onward those Jewish practitioners merged as if naturally into the medical culture of their host societies.

44 One might single out the influential study by Friedenwald 1944 as the pinnacle of this approach. Cf. in the following chapter (now 25, n. 46 35f). On the 'old history of science' approach, see Lourraine Daston, "The History of Science and the History of Knowledge," *KNOW* 1,1 (2017): 131–154.

45 Some of these aspects were mentioned already by Landau 1895, 9f. For the imminent scholarly accomplishment in the field of Jewish medical history in medieval and early modern time, see the following chapter, 27–55.

46 Cf. Kozodoy 2019 on the history of Jewish medical texts and manuscripts.

47 This close relation can be witnessed in publications such as Caballero Navas 2011; Freudenthal 2018a; Freudenthal and Fontaine 2016. Besides general journals on the history of medicine, the sciences and philosophy, the most vibrant forum for pertinent studies has become *Aleph. Historical Studies in Science and Judaism.*

North Africa and Southern Europe, which inherited the Graeco-Arabic knowledge.[48] More recently, studies have begun to question the tradition-burdened binary opposition between Sephardic scientific curiosity and Ashkenazic intellectual seclusion. Scholars have pointed out that such knowledge, while possibly different from one another, thrived in both spheres and can be found in a broader pool of sources, traditionally associated with other cultural and religious aspects (e. g. mysticism, halakhic opinions, commentaries).[49]

Another objection to an historiography concentrating on individual Jewish physicians has been raised by several scholars. Already Landau stressed that in the wake of the emancipation, the field of "Jewish Medicine" and the subject of "Jewish doctors" ceased to exist, as they turned into German, French or English physicians with a Jewish background that might or might not have played any role in their professional life.[50] Recent scholarship on modern Jewish history has accepted the challenge through more nuanced analysis of the interplay between religious, ethnic, national and cultural facets of (a hybrid) identity that was of crucial importance for Jewish medical practitioners from the Haskalah onward.[51] Moreover, Jewishness, mostly as an ethnic or national denominator, remained a crucial factor for the life and career of modern Jewish physicians and scientists in the face of persisting and growing Antisemitism.[52]

---

48 Cf. the brief and rather rejecting discussion of science/medicine in Northern Europe in Freudenthal 2018a, 704.

49 Cf. Langermann 2009b; Shyovitz 2017; Visi 2014, 2019; and Tamás Visi, *On the Peripheries of Ashkenaz. Medieval Jewish Philosophers in Normandy and in the Czech Lands from the Twelfth to the Fifteenth Century* (Habilitation Thesis; Palacký University Olomouc, 2011).

50 Landau 1895, 8. Cf. Efron, "Review of Frank Heynick," 141: "And is it the job of the historian to laud those discoveries as though they are a "Jewish" invention? The identification of this scientific principle or that mathematical theorem as Jewish is a very slippery slope. So too is celebrating Nobel Prize winners in medicine who happen to be Jews.". See also Freudenthal, "Review of Koroth," 295: "[...] is it legitimate to focus on a Jewish scientist or physician because he or she was a Jew? In my view, the Jewish aspect should be allowed to have a heuristic significance: one may set out to investigate whether being Jewish influenced the scientific work of a given individual or group; after all, other cultural factors also occasionally influence science. The question whether the Jewish factor somehow went into a given piece of scientific work is then decided empirically. But it is intellectually improper, and morally perilous, to define one's object of study as consisting of individuals or groups of individuals who, by I know not what criteria, qualify as Jews."

51 Cf. Wolff 2014.

52 Efron, "Review of Frank Heynick," 141: "Some Jewish physicians did indeed possess highly developed Jewish consciousnesses and even brought that to their medical work by doing clinical work on Jewish patients, writing scholarly papers on disease among Jews, using medicine to further the cause of Jewish emancipation, acculturation, and nationalism. Even the role Jewish doctors played in the discourse and practice of antisemitism is, of course, central to the larger story." Cf. Charpa and Deichmann 2007; Efron 2001, and the remarks by David Ruderman, "Review of John M. Efron, *Medicine and the German Jews: A History*," *Jewish Quarterly Review* 92,3–4 (2002): 638–643.

1.3 Medicine in Jewish traditions and cultures

Dissociated from but also bearing relations to both previously discussed approaches, scholarship has developed several ways to avoid some pitfalls, while forging links with various adjacent disciplines. Already Walter Ebstein preferred not to speak of "Jewish Medicine" but rather of "Medicine in Bible and Talmud". These textual traditions constitute the only available sources, although none of them is a technical text and medical information serves multiple purposes to be investigated.[53] Other early scholars aimed with their studies of ancient Jewish medicine to contribute to general cultural history and anthropology.[54] Among others, these two fields of research have more recently become increasingly fruitful interlocutors.

While many studies of the first category ("Jewish Medicine") treated their subject in an extremely essentializing way, the beginnings of the second approach, at times, tended to represent medical or scientific knowledge as either something foreign (Graeco-Arabic) or as a universal domain that existed, as if detached from cultural or religious dimensions. Admittedly, during the past three decades, this direction of thought has shifted considerably towards the inclusion of cultural and socio-historical factors:

> During many historical periods Jews, although influenced by the various cultures in which they lived, maintained a cluster of cultural identities of their own, of which medical theory and practice and scientific ideas were an integral part. It seems appropriate, therefore, to define a "subdiscipline" of the history of science and medicine investigating the cultural systems of science and medicine within Jewish societies.[55]

The third way, therefore, seeks to explore the first group's idea of particular Jewish aspects of medical knowledge and practice and to reintegrate this into the second school's approaches, focusing on comparative textual studies and social history. With a deeper grounding in philology and literary studies, this group's research reflects the construed nature of our sources and their complicated, sometimes irretrievable history of transmission.[56] However, given the naïve essentialism and positivism, one has to address what has been identified as the basic questionability of "Jewish Medicine":

---

53 Cf. Ebstein 1903, 2. See also Preuss 1911, 2/ Preuss 1978, 4: "There does not exist a work from Jewish antiquity devoted exclusively to medicine; nor even a compendium of natural history, such as that of Plinius. The Torah and the Talmud are primarily law books, and medical matters are chiefly discussed only as they pertain to the law."

54 Cf. Bergel 1885. See Preuss 1911, 5/ Preuss 1978, 6: "The history of medical science is part of the history of culture. Every culture, however, has evolved: as soon as it becomes incorporated into the writings or other monuments of a nation, it has already undergone development, which is rarely purely esoteric."

55 Freudenthal, "Review of Koroth," 295.

56 Cf. *Social History of Medicine* 32,4 (2019), 659–750 ("Special Cluster Learning Practice from Texts: Jews and Medicine in the Later Middle Ages"); and the various recent editions of medieval and later medical texts mentioned in the following chapter, esp. 39–52.

But when the time came for me to prepare this lecture I faced a dilemma. Is the meaning of the words "Judaism" and "medicine" self-evident? Can I proceed to explore the existence of a special linkage between them without first exploring some of the many facets of both Judaism and medicine? The answer was no, because Judaism to me is more than the religion of different Jews as it evolved over the ages, and the full meaning of the word "medicine" is not self-evident.[57]

Being aware that "value and meaning of disease and curing could differ according to context and circumstance"[58], this strand follows the lines of inquiry and academic soundness of the second approach, while broadening its scope and making it work also for pre-medieval traditions. Accordingly, the studies tackle medical knowledge in different premodern Jewish traditions, biblical to early modern, from multiple perspectives including the history of medicine and sciences, biblical and rabbinic studies, religious studies, cultural history, (medical) anthropology, philosophy, and theology.[59] In some way, this follows Julius Preuss' rather forward-thinking research agenda of identifying the roots of Talmudic medicine and its interactions with other (medical) cultures.[60] Simultaneously, such scholarship draws on more recent approaches in network theory, transculturality or entangled history/*histoire croisée* that transcend the notion of traditions and cultures as static entities and focuses on the hybridization and the dynamics of encounter, exchange, and transfer.[61] In addition, history of science, "science studies and feminist new materialist analyses of knowledge-making and agency offer approaches that go beyond dualist framings".[62]

In earlier scholarship, such dichotomies had been particularly strong with regard to the ideas of "religion" and "medicine" (or "science") that were often depicted as diametrical opposites.[63] Instead of focusing on an often misconstrued mutual ex-

---

57 Sabin 1983, 188.
58 Kottek 1988, 25.
59 While Kottek 1988 (seconded by Bilu 1988) already formulated a program of a trans-disciplinary Jewish medical anthropology and cultural history, this approach is still emerging within a variety of more established subfields of Jewish studies (i.e. Bible, Talmud, Rabbinics, Jewish history and culture) and relevant areas (e.g. history of medicine and science, anthropology).
60 Cf. Preuss 1911, 5/Preuss 1978, 6: "Indeed, every nation has possibly at some time or other come into contact with another, and the result has certainly been an exchange of cultural elements. Such relationships between the Jews and other peoples is quite obvious [...] Which teachings in the Talmud are generally Semitic, which are exclusively the property of the Hebrews, and which were borrowed from others must in each individual case be investigated and shown. This is the question of the original sources of Talmudic medicine."
61 Cf. Margit Mersch, „Transkulturalität, Verflechtung, Hybridisierung—„Neue" epistemologische Modelle in der Mittelalterforschung," in *Transkulturelle Verflechtungsprozesse in der Vormoderne* (ed. W. Drews; Berlin: De Gruyter, 2016), 243–255; Jochen Althoff, Dominik Berrens, and Tanja Pommerening, eds., *Finding, Inheriting or Borrowing? The Construction and Transfer of Knowledge in Antiquity and the Middle Ages* (Bielefeld: transcript, 2019), esp. 13–38 (Introduction).
62 Neis 2019, 183.
63 Kottek 1988 already pointed out that, despite a dominance of theology in ancient Jewish dis-

clusiveness, the focus has shifted to the interplay and intertwining of scientific, halakhic and theological thinking, practice and materiality that form the Jewish cultural
universe.[64] Questioning the older narrative of decline from late antiquity onward,
when medical science got tainted by religious healing and superstitious practices, one
can investigate the different ways in which the interweaving of religion and medicine
in premodern Jewish traditions, among predominantly Muslim, Christian and other
cultures, "transformed constructions of the body, healing practices, medical education, and healthcare institutions in interesting and important ways".[65]

   This change of perspective also sheds new light on the relation between medical,
religious and ritual knowledge and practices. Breaking away from a focus on allegedly
irreconcilable differences reveals various overlaps between the realms of medicine and
magic, which appear as branches of ancient scientific thinking with competing but
also collaborating experts.[66] In relation to this, recent studies also attempt to rethink
the time-honored distinction between elitist or learned medicine and folk medicine.
Frequently, such categorizations reveal more about contemporary scholarly perspectives than about what happened in premodern times "on the ground", where boundaries were rather fuzzy, permeable, and the transfer of knowledge and practice developed its own dynamics. Such an approach also acknowledges that premodern medical
practitioners should not be mistaken for modern physicians. For premoderns, the
scope of pertinent experts included root-cutters, midwives, nurses, herbalists, phar-
maceutic experts, medical scribes, conjurors or surgeons.[67]

   As can be seen, this strand of research benefits from a nascent dialogue with ancient history of knowledge, science and medicine and contemporary critical science
study. These fields, which have undergone major transformations during the 20th

---

course, one cannot delineate an opposition between religion and other facets, because Jewish
(rabbinic) religion is all-encompassing and, thus, "more culture than religion", in which rabbinic law or Torah have a propaedeutic and a prophylactic function for most aspects of life. Cf.
Reed, 2014, 218: "What is assumed and asserted by such a move—I suggested— is an anachronistic understanding of "religion" and "science" as self-contained and mutually-exclusive approaches to explaining the world and human experience."

64 Cf. Fonrobert 2000; Kessler 2009; Lehmhaus 2016; Neis 2017. For further literature, see the
following chapter, 27–55.

65 Heidi Marx-Wolf and Kristi Upson-Saia, "The State of the Question: Religion, Medicine, Disability, and Health in Late Antiquity," *Journal of Late Antiquity* 8, 2 (2015): 257–272, here: 257.
Cf. also ibid., 268–270, and 272: "Just as religious people of Late Antiquity strove to grasp the
nature of health and the means by which to attain it—as a religious pursuit—scholars of Late
Antiquity are finding that the study of these pursuits enables us to better understand how reli-
giosity absorbed, reflected, and modified existing medical ideas and practices."

66 Cf. Christopher Faraone, "Magic and Medicine in the Roman Imperial Period: Two Case Studies," in *Continuity and Innovation in the Magical Tradition* (ed. G. Bohak, S. Shaked, and I.J. Yuval; Leiden: Brill, 2011), 135–157. See further Kottek 2000b, Bohak 2008, 2017; Geller 2000,
2004, 2006; Ronis 2015; Harara 2017; Levene 2003; Blasco Oranella 2011; Shoham-Steiner
2010a; Langermann 2009a; Ruderman 1988.

67 Cf. Lehmhaus and Martelli 2017, 17 (and the literature referred to in ns. 59 and 60).

century, may help to address the cultural construction of Jewish medical knowledge within its broader historical contexts:

> [...] scientific practices are both socially constructed *and* real. That is, they depend on the cultural resources at hand in a given context [...] and they capture some aspects of the world; they work. But they are neither inevitable nor metaphysically true. Rather, they are contingent to a certain time and place yet valid for certain purposes.[68]

This perspective, thus, focuses on the genuine cultural construction of complex metaphors and concepts used in Jewish (and other) medical and scientific thinking in order to investigate how these imageries rebounded in many ways on these very traditions, but also more broadly on societies and people's everyday experience.[69] Such an endeavor is multi-dimensional. On one hand it includes the sociocultural involvement of Jews in science/medicine as practiced in their respective periods and localities. This requires a trans-cultural comparison—with a broad variety of medical traditions (e.g. ancient Egyptian, Mesopotamian, Persian-Zoroastrian, Coptic, Syriac, local North African, Middle Eastern or European etc.) and their concepts—that bids farewell to an exclusive fixation on Graeco-Roman medicine.[70] On the other hand, studies simultaneously scour the medical discourse for genuine or distinctive Jewish ways of thinking about bodies, illnesses and healing, and strategies of integrating medical knowledge and practice into Jewish culture, writ large. Both strands help to explore "the political, social and gendered contexts of rabbinic content without simply going to Greco-Roman sources to fill in the gaps in the more laconic Tannaitic sources, or viewing the rabbis as 'influenced' rather than as engaged".[71] This allows us to look for the choices of literary form and framing, the authorial strategies and epistemic preferences that shaped medical discourse in premodern Jewish traditions.[72] Finally, these traditions can be understood in light of recently expanded ideas of ancient knowledge-making that con-

---

68 Lorraine Daston, "Science Studies and the History of Science," *Critical Inquiry* 35,4 (2009): 798–815, here: 813. Cf. Jürgen Renn, "From the History of Science to the History of Knowledge—and Back," *Centaurus* 57 (2015): 37–53. Exemplarily, one may refer here for the medieval period to the research of Monica H. Green or Carmen Caballero Navas or for the early Modern period to Ruderman 2010, esp. 99–133, among many others. See in the following chapter, esp. 41–49.

69 Cf. Fonrobert 2000; Baker 2002; Lehmhaus 2019 (on the female body/sexual organs as a "house"); and the contributions in John Z. Wee, ed., *The Comparable Body—Analogy and Metaphor in Ancient Mesopotamian, Egyptian, and Greco-Roman Medicine* (Leiden: Brill, 2017).

70 Cf. Geller 2006, 2004; Strauch Schick 2019, 2021; Ronis 2015; Yoeli-Tlalim 2018. See also the contributions of Kiperwasser, Dal Bo, Visi and Yoeli-Tlalim in the present volume.

71 Neis 2017, 297. Cf. Francesca Rochberg, *Before Nature. Cuneiform Knowledge and the History of Science* (Chicago: University of Chicago Press, 2016), who argues that modern, Western or Graeco-Roman concepts of 'nature' and 'science' fail to discern ancient Mesopotamian scientific interest in the world.

72 Cf. Reed 2007, and 2014, esp. 218: "To neglect of the Jewishness of Jewish engagement with ancient sciences is to skew our understanding of the richness of reflection on the stars, cosmos, and human body within the history of Judaism."

nected different fields of expertise (law, philosophy, rhetoric, religion, various sciences) and take place in a broader spectrum of genres not confined to technical texts.[73]

2 Summary of contributions

The contributions to the present volume, mostly adhering to the second and third approach outlined beforehand, accept and address important methodological and theoretical challenges for the study of premodern Jewish medical knowledge. The collection of essays opens with a group of four papers that deal with medical thinking or terminology in rabbinic texts and beyond. In their discussion, all authors apply a diachronic perspective on the internal rabbinic as well as on the transcultural transfer of medical ideas in the thorough discussion of their specific topics.

Reuven Kiperwasser's contribution opens with an inquiry into various rabbinic perceptions of human memory and the senses as one of the, or even, the most central "cultural value" in rabbinic oral tradition. Memory was interpreted in ancient times mainly as a physiological process channeling incoming information from the limbs and orifices into the inner storehouse of the heart, the center of emotions and intellect. A loss of memory was understood as a major impairment calling for a cure. Second, the careful literary and cultural history approach to the sources demonstrates how in rabbinic ideal concepts about learning intellectual development is understood as embodiment of knowledge tied to a range of bodily practices that help the student in this process or may cure him, in case of lost memory. Finally, on the level of transcultural entanglements, the study points to possible parallels in Coptic, Manichean and Irano-Persian literature that conceptualize the reception of knowledge and information through the five senses (especially hearing) as a physiological process. Kiperwasser suggests that this indicates a shared knowledge of the body and a cultural pattern that was appropriated differently in order to suit theological or other discursive purposes of the respective texts.

With a distinctive focus on diachronic and intercultural comparison, **Federico Dal Bo** aims at clarifying the Hebrew term *sandāl* used for a miscarried, deformed fetus. While usually the meaning is identified as "footwear" (lit. "sandal"), he provides possible etymologies and the rather complex ways of linguistic transfer between Hebrew, Aramaic, Persian, Arabic, and Greek. Accordingly, the meanings also include different types of "boats", "(flat-)fish" or "ox tongue (fish)". The diachronic discussion suggests that rabbinic legal decision-making was aware of ancient ideas of embryology and Greek terms, while also producing their own categories of gestational development.[74] It also traces the rabbinic usage of the *sandāl* back to ancient Mesopo-

---

73 The various formats included among others exegesis, commentaries, isagogic summaries, encyclopaedias letters, monastic writings, sermons, poems, epic and dramatic texts. Cf. Markus Asper, *Writing Science* (Berlin: De Gruyter, 2013); Liba Taub, *Science Writing in Greco-Roman Antiquity* (Cambridge: Cambridge University Press, 2017); Heidi Marx-Wolf, Jared Secord, and Christoph Markschies, eds., *Health, Medicine, and Christianity in Late Antiquity* (Studia Patristica Vol. LXXX, 2017).

74 This article can be read together with Shulamit Shinnar's contribution to this volume. Both

tamian embryology that knew connections between a fetus and a fish, as appearing in some ancient myth, which might have shaped the halakhic-legal discourse on a "fetus shaped like a *sandāl*". The contingency of the interpretation becomes evident in later commentaries of rabbinic texts (Rashi, Maimonides, Betinoro and others) whose authors drew on their contemporary medical and other knowledge to clarify the term *sandāl*. Dal Bo argues for a 'failed transfer': while some Talmudic texts might have used *sandāl* in reference to a fish and, thus, a fish-like appearance of a fetus, later texts, commentators, and scholars mistook this term for a shoe.

The diachronic development of terminology and concepts related to fever from the Bible, as well as rabbinic textual traditions into Judeo-Arabic medical writings, are the focus of **Kenneth Collin**'s contribution. Beginning with a survey of rabbinic therapies and remedies for fever, he argues that many of these earlier Jewish sources, deviating from some perceptions of fever in Hippocratic-Galenic medicine as a crisis of illness, exhibit a different understanding of the underlying physiology. Some passages deal with the phenomenon that, during an infection, feverish patients usually are anorectic, showing no appetite and reducing their consumption of food. Accordingly, rabbinic notions of such a positive, or "nourishing fever" might indicate a rabbinic awareness of the body's defenses and it self-healing powers. The second part of the paper addresses the Galenic influence on concepts of fever that prevailed within the early Judeo-Arabic medical tradition in Northern Africa. Based on Isaac Israeli's *Book of Fevers* (*Kitāb al-Ḥummayāt*) and some teachings of Maimonides, Collins aims at demonstrating that those Graeco-Roman ideas, while being certainly highly influential, cannot be considered the only transfer of medical knowledge attested in this tradition. The medical discourse cherished by Israeli and others feeds on two competing sources—the Talmudic tradition and Galenic thought—that merged in surprising ways.[75] Finally, Collins grants us a glimpse into contemporary medical findings about "nourishing fevers" and how they may enhance the effects of antibiotic therapy, thus, pointing to the reliability of ancient medical knowledge which easily has been discarded as fanciful musings.

In contrast to the previous three papers that studied a certain medical phenomenon in detail, **Aviad Recht** explores an important subfield of ancient medicine comparing the "rules for a healthy way of life" (*diaita*/ 'diet and regimen') in rabbinic traditions with those known to us from Graeco-Roman sources. Passages on regimen accumulate in the Babylonian Tamud but mainly figure as (anonymous) Hebrew aphoristic sayings. Recht understands the "rabbinic health regimen" as following a Graeco-Roman model. However, appropriated by the Talmudic redactors these teachings exhibit some substantial differences compared with Graeco-Roman *diaita*. On a socio-historical level, they reflect different backgrounds of both authors and audiences of the two traditions. Graeco-Roman texts often display detailed advice for (exotic

---

may enter into a conversation with the recently published work of R.R. Neis on species, generation, and rabbinic reproductive science (Neis 2017, 2018, and 2019).

75 On fever in rabbinic traditions, see Wandrey 2003. See also the discussion of Isaac Israeli and pertinent literature by R. Veit and others in the following chapter, 40.

or expensive) nutrition based on a complex theoretical system, as well as physical exercises and a strictly time regimen. Recht observes that such a "health regimen" was only affordable and manageable for an elite class with enough time and economic means. By contrast, rabbinic teachings about health regimen tend to make use of simple and easily available foodstuff or staples, and the advice refers rather to daily routines (walking, sitting, sleeping) than to athletic or physical exercises per se. For the astonishing predominance of this particular genre in the Babylonian Talmud (and not in the Western, Palestinian traditions), two possible ways of knowledge transfer are suggested: a Jewish, internal exchange between rabbinic elites in Palestine and Babylonia; and the Talmudic authors' cosmopolitan context of Sassanid Persia, where Graeco-Roman and Indian cultural elements had been already appropriated.[76]

The second section consists of four chapters addressing the image of the physician, rabbinic interaction with non-rabbinic or non-Jewish experts and their knowledge as well as rabbinic concepts of healthy living.

In his diachronic survey, **Samuel Kottek** asks why no particular corpus or system of "Jewish medicine" had developed until Talmudic time, although ancient Jewish ideas about healing, medicine, and the different healing experts—physicians, herbal experts, apothecaries or midwifes—are known to us from several texts. He argues that in the Bible, healing and healing personnel (often the prophets themselves) are directly connected to and dependent upon God's will to cure or even revive people. He dismisses, however, the identification of the priests as medical professionals for *ṣoraʿat* (צרעת), a skin affliction, often falsely identified as "leprosy". Kottek insists that the biblical emphasis on God as the ultimate healer and a certain bias against technical, medical intervention should be understood in accordance with a holistic, religious worldview and as admonition against learned haughtiness of medical experts. Therefore, both the New Testament narratives and Second Temple sources stressed the divine origin of medical knowledge and the continuum between religious and healing practices. In Talmudic texts, however, one finds a greater diversity of references and attitudes to physicians and healing experts—ranging from praise, professional appreciation of their expertise, to suspicion and rejection, as will be discussed in the two following papers. Kottek stresses that the Talmudic authors—with a certain sense of realism regarding the dangers involved in ancient medical practice—tried to navigate between the ethical imperative to heal and their religious concepts in order to make way for a proper rabbinic, or even "Jewish way of practicing medicine".[77]

Hierarchies of expertise play a crucial role for the (negative) knowledge transfer in **Tirzah Meacham**'s paper. Her survey on physicians in Jewish traditions resonates with Samuel Kottek's paper in pointing out the biblical role of God as the true healer and the understanding of illness in relation to sin. Talmudic texts, by contrast,

---

76 Cf. Geller 2004b.
77 On this, see the preceding discussion in this introduction and the literature referenced. Cf. also Hezser 2016; and, in particular, Reed 2014.

mention not only individual doctors but their broader terminology seems to reflect a pluralism in ancient medical systems of healthcare. However, rabbinic sources are far from displaying a consistent attitude to such healing experts. Again, the cultural (and religious) value of *piquaḥ nephesh* ('saving a life'), health, and care for the suffering is weight against the many uncertainties of medical therapies and unethical practice of some ancient physicians. The main part of the paper focuses on medical expertise and reliability in their relation to legal (halakhic) decision-making. While in most of the texts the physicians' opinions seems to stand in opposition to the sages (as in the case of intercourse with an admired woman or suckling from a living goat as a remedy), or supporting one particular view-point (as for the anatomy of cows and the number of bones), the diachronic analysis of a discussion of im/purity and unusual abortions (*Niddah*)[78] points to a change in attitude that gradually limits the value of the external experts (doctors) in favor of rabbinic expertise.

In some ways related to the previous chapter, the relevance of and anxieties towards non-Jewish discourse of knowledge in Talmudic texts are explored by **Shulamit Shinnar** in her article. Following scholars like Fonrobert, Kessler or Neis,[79] she focuses on the discussions of female bodies and im/purity, embryology, and birth in tractate *Niddah* (30b), in order to flesh out the epistemic approaches championed by the (anonymous) Talmudic authors. How did the rabbis reach any halakhic conclusion about the human body, and specifically about the rather concealed physiological processes of conception, gestation and pregnancy in women? Which sources or strategies (e.g. biblical or oral traditions, non-Jewish scientific knowledge, independent legal reasoning, observation) were utilized for their decision-making and, in fact, their engagement with the natural world? In particular, the discussion focuses on a dense cluster concerned with the stages of fetal development. The featured narratives portraying Queen Cleopatra's empirical experiments on her pregnant slaves are examined regarding their reliability and contrasted with proofs derived from Scripture. Shinnar argues that the late Talmudic authors, while remaining critical to a straightforward adoption of biblical and ritual law, used a contrast between two distinct epistemological sources—a scriptural proof and a "proof from fools" (the Cleopatra story)—to frame a severe distrust toward knowledge that was associated with non-Jews and women.[80]

The last study in this section addresses the field of public health and hygiene, a topic that was highly valued in earlier scholarship and has been singled out by numerous scholars to represent one of, if not the most outstanding Jewish contributions to medicine. Moreover, due to its neat intertwinement with questions of ritual, dietary

---

78 Purity issues related to the realm of female physiology replete with bodily fluids and flux which were at times tricky to navigate for the male rabbinic authorities and authors. The cultural implications of that discourse have been studied over the past two decades with different approaches, and Meacham has contributed significantly to this scholarly discourse herself. Cf. Meacham 1989, 1995; Fonrobert 2000; Rosen-Zvi 2013.

79 Cf. Fonrobert 2000; Kessler 2009; Neis 2017, 2018, 2019.

80 On rabbinic epistemology and the empirical approach, see Vârtejanu-Joubert 2009; Lehmhaus 2017b, 2019.

laws and rules about im/purity, the particular "Jewishness" of this field of knowledge (and practice) has been emphasized.[81] The chapter provides an exhaustive discussion of relevant theory and practice as depicted mainly in early rabbinic sources, which may contain some valuable information about these issues for the time well preceding their compilation in the early third century—i.e. the Second Temple period. **Esteé Dvorjetski** suggests that a considerable portion of the religious or ritual concepts and rules regarding purity adopted or at least showed some overlap with ancient secular knowledge about healthcare and hygiene. Her chapter, as part of a broader study of the issue, combines the material aspects of archaeological findings in Jerusalem and its surroundings with the information to be found in rabbinic texts, the New Testament, Philo, Josephus or Roman sources. This study presents a good survey of the issue at hand and might serve as a basis for future inquiries into questions of human-animal interactions and environmental history from the perspective of late antique Jewish culture(s).

The third section marks also chronologically a transfer of sorts. The texts discussed are all produced after the advent of Islam and are firmly embedded in various contexts around the Mediterranean and in the Middle East spanning from the Indus Valley in the East to the Iberian Peninsula in the West. While later, medieval works (like those studied by Langermann and Caballero Navas), written by Jews in Hebrew or (Judeo-) Arabic, clearly draw on Graeco-Roman and Arabic medical traditions and the Abassid translation movement, the *Book of Asaf* might even demonstrate more layers of cultural entanglement between Asian, Near Eastern and Western medical thinking.

In her study, **Ronit Yoeli-Tlalim**, addresses the first, exclusively medical Hebrew compendium *Sefer Asaf* (*Book of Asaf*) in light of its own narratives about the origin of the knowledge contained. The text, having circulated in various manuscripts and printed editions, has a long and at times complicated transmission history, which led to much confusion about its textual identity and coherence in early scholarship. In many witnesses the work commences with an etiological narrative about the origins of medical knowledge in the world. Overlapping in parts with the *Book of Jubilees* and *1 Enoch*, *Sefer Asaf* narrates an angelic revelation of all remedies and related information to Noah and his children who passed it on to the Jewish sages as well to the learned men of India, Babylonia, Egypt, Greece and Syria. Moreover, the text mentions a distortion of this knowledge and a rediscovery by Hippocrates and those who followed him. Yoeli-Tlalim's focus on the introduction emphasizes the importance of self-referential etiologies for these premodern discourses as well as for our own scholarship on the history of medicine in their cultural contexts.[82]

The complexity of the history of origin and transmission not only of the actual content but of the *Sefer Asaf / Book of Remedies* as a tradition is touched upon by **Tamás Visi**. He points out that this work consists of up to six different parts provid-

---

81 Cf. the preceding discussion on "Jewish Medicine" in academic scholarship, esp. 9–10.
82 For similar etiological narratives on Judaism and scientific knowledge, see Reed 2014; Syfox 2018.

ing diverse medical knowledge from Hippocratic traditions, Syriac-Persian material, *materia medica* and recipes, to various short texts and the etiological introduction, as discussed by Ronit Yoeli-Tlalim in this volume. Visi suggests a rather composite nature for the *Sefer Asaf* tradition that has grown over time, or was compiled from various textual traditions, in different periods and places. Focusing on the Hebrew rendering of Hippocratic *Aphorisms* in *Sefer Asaf,* he questions Suesmann Muntner's assumptions about an early authorship for this material, which he presented in his somewhat jumbled edition of the *Book of Remedies* almost fifty years ago. Visi argues instead that the Hippocratic material in *Sefer Asaf* exhibits not only a close proximity in style and content with, but maybe, indeed, depends on the earlier, direct translation of Greek into Hebrew produced by Shabbetai Donnolo (and his students) from Southern Italy in the tenth century. Such a relationship (or even identity of authorship) might be corroborated from a stylistic comparison of the shared Hebrew paraphrase of the Hippocratic *Aphorisms* in Donnolo's translation and *Sefer Asaf* with Donnolo's other writings. Moreover, in a preliminary comparison between the *Asaf*-version and the *Donnolo*-version of the Aphorisms, Visi is able to flesh out considerable differences. Whereas the *Donnolo*-version always features the "nucleus" of the Hippocratic Aphorisms with additional explanations, the *Asaf*-version at times foregoes the aphoristic teachings and just provides the explanations and complementing information. As such, the transfer of the Aphorisms into medieval Hebrew traditions encompassed also the use of earlier Jewish scholarly discourse and cultural appropriations.

Tzvi Langermann introduces Nuʿmān al-Isrāʾīlī, a later Jewish author who wrote in Arabic and possessed knowledge of the most important medical works of the Graeco-Arabic medical tradition. The work consists of two major parts. The first part is a commentary to the *Kitāb al-Miʾa* ("Book of the Hundred"). The second, more independent part of Nuʿmān's work provides the reader with a solid introduction to all necessary medical knowledge of his time. This type of *vademecum*, or compendium, makes heavy use of the formerly praised *Kitab al-Miʾa* but draws also on a broad variety of other sources. In the more practical chapters, Nuʿmān even seeks to supplement or substitute his base texts with contemporary knowledge or empirical findings about tested remedies. Langermann concludes his preliminary inquiry into this fascinating manuscript with a close reading of three passages that deal with the transmission history and reliability of Hippocratic and Galenic medical ideas, and with a discussion about Plato's teachings on color and the colors of the humors. This contribution does not only show the importance of Jewish authors for the transfer of Greek and Arabic-Persian medical thought but also highlights the unique tone that a writer like Nuʿmān, equipped with an impressive range of medical knowledge, was able to add. Moreover, Langermann questions Nuʿmān's assumed biographical background as a practicing physician. The preference of the overtly theoretical *Kitab al-Miʾa* as its main source and the absence of any case-stories and personal references may suggest that his transfer of medical knowledge was overtly a theoretical and intellectual project.

This section as well as the whole book will be concluded by an inquiry into the emergence of a distinct field of Hebrew gynaecology in the Middle Ages by **Carmen**

Caballero Navas. She addresses the still less studied transfer of medical knowledge, and gynaecological expertise in particular, from Graeco-Roman and Arabic traditions into Hebrew as well as the practical purposes of these endeavors. A comprehensive survey introduces the relevant texts that were produced between the late twelfth and the late thirteenth century. The translation projects from Latin were mainly pursued by *Do'eg the Edomite* in Provence and those from Arabic sources by two authors on the Iberian Peninsula. These inspired several minor works and the integration of gynaecological knowledge in general books on medicine in Hebrew. The study explains the beginnings of Hebrew gynaecological texts in medieval times with the general rise of a Hebrew medical corpus that facilitated access to this information for Jewish practitioners. In a dominantly Christian context, these readers were mostly excluded from the medical traditions transmitted in a monastic context or later on taught in universities. Still, the early incorporation of gynaecological texts may also point, according to Caballero Navas, to issues of gender biased expertise. First, the overtly theoretical nature of the Hebrew works suggests that they had no practical purpose but were rather intended for an audience of learned male physicians. Second, such a male theorization of female physiology resonates with earlier (Talmudic and Christian) attempts to delegitimate and displace the "native speakers"—female practitioners who worked as healers, midwifes or nurses. Furthermore, especially Doeg's *Sēfer hatōledet* exhibits a strategic appropriation of contemporary medical knowledge through "Judaization". Since those texts were imbued with familiar biblical characters or quotations and rabbinic teachings, terminology and concepts they could be used to establish or extend male rabbinic authority over women's bodies, while at the same time functioning as guidebooks for Jewish self-help in a period of cultural anxieties.

As the discussion of earlier scholarship on the matter has shown, it remains an open question whether we can in fact speak of a distinct "Jewish medicine". This question requires tremendous scholarly efforts, and, thus, it cannot be answered sufficiently in one collection of articles. Still, the various contributions to this volume have produced rich evidence for the diverse approaches to the body, illness and healing that prevailed among Jews in various localities and throughout different periods. They show how one may define "Jewish medicine" by way of delineating the broader web of cultural, religious and socio-historical entanglements and transfers, in which medical knowledge and practice thrived.

The Academic Quest for "Jewish Medicine"— a Survey of the Field*

Lennart Lehmhaus

Jewish medical history as a distinct field of research began to flourish in the 19th century with two different major areas of interest. On one hand, scholars turned to either the biography of Jewish physicians or to the historiography of medicine within specific Jewish communities, mostly from medieval time onward.[1] On the other hand, there was an increased interest in medical (and other scientific) knowledge in the major 'canonical' traditions of ancient Judaism, from biblical to Talmudic texts. Most of the earlier scholarship on the latter topic has often been rather biased and scholars tended to take maximalist or minimalist positions. Both strands of research on Jews and medicine entertained the rather positivistic approach prevailing within 19th century historiography and philology. Moreover, several scholars identified with the academic, ideological and political agenda of the *Wissenschaft des Judentums,* longing for a place within modern, Western academia. Both trends made scholars susceptible to a selective reading of their sources that emphasized those aspects regarded as sufficiently scientific and rational in comparison to ancient (Graeco-Roman, Arabic) traditions and modern Western culture. Propensity for a non-historical interpretation or 'retrospective diagnosis' was especially widespread among those Jewish historians of medicine who were historically trained doctors and practicing physicians. This approach, which can be also found even in some contemporary publications, focused on extracting the "pure" medical information, or what scholars conceived as such (e.g., on pharmacology, anatomy, physiology etc.) from biblical and rabbinic sources without attending carefully to philology, literary aspects, source-criticism and to historical or cultural dimensions. Julius Preuss' *opus magnum,* bearing the title *Biblisch-Talmudische Medizin,* represented the peak of this first wave of scholarly interest. He stressed the dispersed and often elliptic character of medical discussions in Biblical and Talmudic texts. Preuss was well aware of the artificial structure of his own study that mirrored, in fact, the main interest and heuristic strategies—writing

---

* For the full entries of the short references in the following notes, please consult the third chapter of this volume (*Medical Knowledge in Premodern Jewish Traditions: Select Bibliography*), 57–89.

1 The most comprehensive and very detailed survey of Jewish physicians throughout history was compiled by Steinschneider 1914. Among the major comprehensive publications are Holub 1880/84, Münz 1922; and Krauss 1930 with a focus on different localities and regions. Cf. also the literature in the medieval and early modern sections.

DOI: 10.13173/9783447108263.027

medical history according to modern medical subfields—predetermined by his training as a historian and doctor. He paid little attention, however, to the philology of his sources and the varying cultural contexts.

Well into the 21st century, the historical role of medicine was touched on in broader surveys on the topic of science in (premodern) Jewish traditions.[2] In addition to the distinct difficulty of essentialism (i.e. 'Judaism' and/vs. 'Science') straining some of those endeavors, medicine was frequently and regrettably judged in a rather cursory inspection.[3] Many shorter or longer historical reviews, and surprisingly also some more in-depth studies, generally highlight the positive value of medicine in ancient Judaism as a God-given science and refer to an ethical imperative to heal. Scholars seem troubled by contradictory opinions about the divine origin of healing and its usefulness on one hand, and some resistance to medical knowledge and the expertise of physicians on the other. While noting this ambivalence, there has been too often little interest in a more precise assessment. Consequently, studies tend to stress rather the unsystematic "eclecticism [...] not confined to theory" that turned ancient Jewish medical discourse into an "expansive magpie pluralism" or, as a kind of last resort, they impute to the rabbis an overwhelming inclination to cling to the concept of God as the ultimate healer.[4]

Other comprehensive historical surveys, such as the impressive study *Jews and Medicine* by the eminent historian Harry G. Friedenwald, largely abstained from all sources earlier than the medieval time. Friedenwald's research focused mainly on the involvement of Jewish physicians in the medicine of their time (e.g. as court physicians), while touching sometimes on the implications of medical issues for broader Jewish history (e.g., the idea of typical "Jewish diseases" or "the Jews" as carriers or sources for epidemics like the plague). However, his work did not cover biblical or rabbinic texts and he was not much interested in the particular Jewishness of their medical knowledge and practice.[5] Friedenwald's seminal studies followed earlier scholars

---

2 Ruderman 1995, 375–383 provides a brief and very useful bibliographic essay on scientific and medical interest in Jewish traditions into the early medieval period (i.e. *Sefer Asaf*).

3 One may refer to the exemplary controversy between Jacob Neusner (*Why No Science in Judaism?*; New Orleans: Jewish Studies Program of Tulane University, 1987) and Menachem Fisch (*Rational Rabbis: Science and Talmudic Culture*; Bloomington: Indiana University Press 1997), which is aptly summarized and elaborated upon in Alexander 2002, 223–229. See also Ruderman 1995, 1–13.

4 Efron 2007, 57. On Efron's book, see the review in Aleph 7 (2007), 319–322 that points to the essentialism of this survey and its lack of direct engagement with primary sources. One may add also the dearth of references to pertinent studies in the section on biblical and talmudic traditions in Efron's book. On the role or image of the physician in ancient Jewish sources, see Hezser 2016, who in some places seems to overgeneralize. See ibid., 174: "The attempts of rabbis to regulate the treatment of their fellow Jews' bodies were mainly governed by their fear of idolatry. They believed that, ultimately, only the one Jewish God could bring about healing."

5 But see his catalogue of *Jewish Luminaries in Medical History* (Friedenwald 1946) and his bibliography on earlier sources in Friedenwald 1935b as well as the additions by Kagan 1948. Cf. the comprehensive survey by his father's lecture published as Friedenwald 1897, and earlier portraits of Jewish physicians starting with the Talmudic (Mar) Samuel in Scherbel 1905.

in championing a "history of great men" approach. With a conspicuous penchant for writing a biographic study of Jewish medical practitioners, this model has persisted in the field for a long time.[6] Also, various popular, non-academic publications on the subject, often with denotive titles, followed along that very path with a blatant penchant for creating a narrative or mosaic of biographies of "medical" Jews.[7]

Besides such historical surveys, there was a growing body of scholarly editions and translations of relevant texts from various periods, which will be discussed in the following. Still, with the exception of one compilation by Judith Abrams and David Freeman, who organized their texts thematically (illness, health, healers, ethics etc.), one finds little in the way of sourcebooks for a diachronic approach to medical knowledge in Jewish traditions.[8] In a volume accompanying an exhibition, Natalia Berger has gathered brief contributions by experts who provide a profound introduction to different aspects and periods of Jewish engagement with medical issues.[9]

Besides the journal *Korot*, dedicated in its entirety to the research into Jewish medical history, and the journal *Aleph*, several academic journals have published special thematical issues addressing Jewish medical knowledge and practice in different times.[10] In addition, a series of edited volumes on the topic of medicine and Judaism with a broad thematic scope but a rather modern focus has been established.[11]

1 Biblical traditions

Not every historian of medicine has been as decent and honest as Erwin Ackerknecht, who admitted that he is not interested in medical contents within biblical and Talmudic literature, because those are primarily religious and not medical texts. While in

---

6 Cf. Kozodoy 2019. For previous surveys following this pattern, see Carmoly 1844, Landau 1895, Friedenwald 1897, and Scherbel 1905.

7 Cf. Heynick 2002; Nevins 1996, 2006; and, most recently, Eisenberg 2019.

8 See Abrams and Freeman 1999. For other editions as sourcebooks, see the publications by Bos, Ferre, and several others, in the medieval section below. See also M.J. Geller, L. Lehmhaus, E. Kiesele, and T. Hidde, *Sourcebook of Medical Passages in Talmudic Texts (Mishnah, Tosefta, Yerushalmi, Bavli). First Volume: The Medical Clusters* (Tübingen: Mohr Siebeck, 2021, forthcoming).

9 Berger 1995. Waserman and Kottek 1996 edited another diachronic volume but with a decisively local or regional focus on Palestine/Eretz Israel. Cf. also Jütte 2016 who is not primarily interested in medicine but deals with various aspects of the body, health, illness, death etc. throughout Jewish history and culture.

10 *Korot(h): The Israel Journal of the History of Medicine and Science* (Jerusalem: Magnes) has been edited for decades now by Samuel Kottek who succeeded Joshua O. Leibowitz in his role as the chief editor and as the chair for the history of medicine at the Hebrew University in Jerusalem. The journal *Aleph. Historical Studies in Science and Judaism* (Bloomington: Indiana University Press) is currently edited by Reimund Leicht and Resianne Fontaine. Cf. the special issue of the journal *Ashkenas* 29,1 (2019) on "Judaism and Illness", and *Social History of Medicine* 32,4 (2019), 659–750, with a "Special Cluster Learning Practice from Texts: Jews and Medicine in the Later Middle Ages".

11 The series *Medizin und Judentum* (Frankfurt: Mabuse Verlag), edited by Caris-Petra Heidel, comprises several thematic volumes, which are mostly based on the annual meetings held under the same title since 1994. The topics include among others: hygiene, bio-medical sciences, medical education, ethics, sexuality, the image of the Jewish physician, Zionism and medicine.

this regard he pointed to his lack of theological and philological expertise to research these traditions, he was less reticent regarding the history of Jewish physicians in their different cultural contexts from early medieval time onward.[12]

Similar to Talmudic medicine, as we will see in the following, broad surveys as well as very specific studies into medical knowledge in the Bible, in ancient Israel, or among "the Hebrews," proliferated, especially in the 18th, 19th and early 20th centuries, but were preceded only by a few dissertations. Often in a rather cursory treatment, biblical evidence from various places and in different medical subfields was then merged with later sources (New Testament, rabbinic literature etc.), or only catalogued without further discussions.[13] Even in more recent publications, one may still notice certain methodological flaws, especially the de-contextualized treatment of the sources, which produce rather strange results.[14] In some cases, they draw heavily on modern medical, bio-chemical and phytological knowledge, while displaying little or no interest in or understanding of ancient texts and their historical contexts.[15] Other studies take into account research in biblical studies but are primarily interested in skimming the texts for medical information and applying a retrospective (or retrojective) diagnosis to these traditions.[16] A different group of scholars concentrates on a socio-historical reconstruction of healthcare and medical practitioners, mostly thought to be concentrated in the hands of the priestly families, or they address the religious

---

12 Cf. Ackerknecht 1981, 27, where, bearing a bold title ("Jewish physicians as designers of world medicine") he provides a brief, kind of fast-forward survey of Jewish doctors from the 9th to the 17th centuries, mostly based on the seminal work in Friedenwald 1944, augmented by a list of brilliant Jewish scholars in 19th century Germany who contributed to the new field of bio-medical sciences.

13 The very early works were pursued by Major 1672, Antonius 1707, Colmar 1729, Schmidt 1743, Reinhard 1768, Eschenbach 1779, and Bennett 1887 (on diseases). Ebstein 1901, in his major study, proceeded from socio-historical aspects of housing, hygiene and nutrition to sexuality, diseases and death. Hempel 1958 provides an interesting combination of medical history and religious or theological aspects. Cf. also Preuss 1911/1978, and Rosner 1995 who mixed biblical and rabbinic sources. Gordon 1941 explicitly sought to avoid this "coloring" with later traditions. For pharmaceutical knowledge, see Harrison 1961. On ophtalmology, see Kotelmann 1910.

14 The special volume of the journal *Koroth* 8, 5–6 (1982) on *Medicine in the Bible* gives a good overview of the field before the recent turns in biblical studies and the history of medicine during the past 40 years. Some of the contributions still follow very conservative paradigms, while others already bridge over between different disciplines and engage new research questions.

15 Most of these studies rely on translations of the Bible and on secondary literature like the standard work by Zohary 1982. For a questionable approach to biblical pharmaceutical knowledge, see Duke 2007. Cf. Jacob and Jacob 1993, Jensen 2012 and Włodarczyk 2007 for a more nuanced approach and some critique of the naïve interpretation of biblical text.

16 Some examples that already indicate their approach in their titles should suffice here: Macht 1946 (cardiac pathology); Blondheim 1982 (obstetrics and Benjamin's birth); Meijer 1982 (maternal influence on Jewish medicine); Roth 1982 (lower back trauma in Ezechiel). For more recent examples, see Ben-Noun 2001, 2002, 2004; Friedmann and Marr 2017 (epidemiological chain reaction in Ex 10).

and theological dimension of medicine in the Bible.[17] Another group of works, mostly authored by Christian scholars, deals with the theological dimensions of illness, suffering and healing in the Old Testament.[18]

In recent years, scholarly interest has shifted away from the search for "pure" medical information and, in the wake of the cultural, body and gender studies approaches, has turned towards a more comprehensive understanding of illness, health and healing in biblical traditions as inextricably bound to its diverse religious, cultural, socio-political and textual backgrounds. Many studies now focused more on a comparison and contextualization of medical issues in the Bible within the neighboring cultures in the Mediterranean and Ancient Near East, in particular Mesopotamia and Egypt.[19] In light of findings from source criticism or archeological and historical studies, some scholars seek to question traditional concepts about medical insights to be gained from biblical texts, the role of priests and prophets in ancient Israel, and the indiscriminate translation of certain terms. This includes, at times, the reception, utilization (psalms and verses for healing) and explanation (commentaries) of biblical texts in later traditions.[20] Others have brought the literary approach in biblical studies into a fruitful conversation with the history of medicine, medical anthropology and gender studies.[21]

After a rather cursory treatment in earlier scholarship, studies in the second half of the 20th century developed keen interest in disabilities, the dis/abled body or mental health and illness in biblical traditions.[22] Over the course of the past 25 years, the cultural, anthropological, or corporeal turns in the Humanities had an impact on biblical studies, that brought forth a substantial surge of fresh research addressing these topics with new approaches that are often triggered by developments in the emerging

---

17 Cf. Wood 1920 (Mosaic law and preventive medicine); Kramer 1933 (Jewish apothecaries) and Penfield 1946 (Abraham as a transmitter of Mesopotamian and Egyptian medicine) for a slightly naïve reconstruction of the socio-historical background of medical knowledge and practice in biblical texts. For Friedenwald 1897 or Scherbel 1905 it seemed an unquestionable fact that the Israelite priests were medical experts and in charge of general healthcare. See also Preuss 1911/1992, 10–43 (on the health personnel); Kasher 1982 (prophet as healer); and new perspectives in Allan 2001 and Avalos 1995 (Temple medicine in the ancient world).

18 As few examples shall suffice here Seybold and Müller 1978 (illness and healing); Niehr 1991; Lindström 1994 (illness and sin); Oeming 1994/2003 (illness and suffering); Gaiser 2010 (healing and Christian ministry).

19 For a comprehensive comparison, see especially Stol 2000, Zucconi 2010, Avalos 1995, and Berlejung 2015. A lot of comparative reading has been done regarding king Nebuchadnezzar's (mental) affliction in Daniel 4. Cf. Henze 1999; Hays 2007; Davis Bledsoe 2012; Avalos 2014. For other comparative studies, see Bodi 2015; Vargon 2014.

20 See, for instance, Hulse 1975; Kahle 1982; Davis 1982; O'Kennedy 2001; Baden 2011; Rosenstock 2014; Cranz 2018b. On the healing of king Hezekiah, see Williams 1989, Barker 2001, Kasher 2001.

21 Cf. Bat-Adam 1982 (holistic healing); Paganini 2010 (conceptions of illness); Bledstein 1992 (female healing); Hurowitz 2004 (magico-medical healing rituals); Cranz 2018a, 2018b, 2021.

22 Cf. Gorlin 1970; Ohry and Dolev 1982; Perl and Irsai 1982; Carny 1982; Shy 1982; Bledstein 2007.

fields of disability and queer studies. Various publications discuss bodily "defects" within the priestly laws, im/purity regulations and disabilities (ṣaraʿat/skin-disease, zav/genital fluxes), gendered dimensions of disability (ugliness, bareness, sterility, eunuchs) and different other impairments (speech, hearing, seeing, walking). These works interrogate the biblical representations of disabilities and their discursive, aesthetic, theological or eschatological functions.[23]

2 Biblical Apocrypha and Second Temple traditions

For the so-called apocryphal texts, the Qumran (Dead Sea) traditions, and other texts or artifacts from the Second Temple or Hellenistic period, only a relatively small number of studies exists.[24] Although medical knowledge in these traditions and scholarly interest in them was unevenly distributed, the body of publications has substantially grown, especially over the course of the past three decades. At first, many scholars concentrated on sources that they regarded as quasi-canonical or historically more reliable, such as Philo, Josephus, (Yehoshua) Ben Sira/Sirach, and Tobit. The two former (Philo/Josephus) are mostly mined for *materia medica*, information about Jewish medical practitioners and concepts of the body.[25] Whereas scholarship on Ben Sira/Sirach focuses mostly on the role of the physician, the friction between divine and human healing, or on medical ethics.[26] Regarding Tobit, most scholars tend to focus on the link between demons and illness or angels and healing as well as on the therapeutic practices involved.[27] The research into *materia medica*, diverse healing practices, often deemed 'pure magic' in earlier studies, and relevant conceptions of health, illness and the body has constantly gained track also in Qumranic scholarship.[28] Other

---

23 A substantial discussion is provided in Abrams 1998. For other surveys of the field and a bibliography, see Avalos, Melcher, and Schipper 2007; and Moss and Schipper 2011. Other major studies include Olyan 2008; Raphael 2008; Schipper 2006, 2011. For intellectual disabilities, see Kellenberger 2011, Olyan 2008, 62–77.

24 The only attempt of a comprehensive study is Logan 1992 who covered later biblical traditions, apocrypha, pseudepigrapha, Dead Sea scrolls, Philo, Josephus, and the New Testament.

25 Based on Neuburger's earlier study (Neuburger 1919), Samuel Kottek has discussed various aspects of medicinal practice and medical knowledge in Flavius Josephus' writings. Cf. Kottek 1985, 1993, 1994, and 2011. On Philo's interest in physiognomy, see Lincicum 2013.

26 On these topics in Ben Sira, see Noorda 1979; Sulmasy 1988; Hezser 2016; and Samuel Kottek's contribution to this volume. On the cultural embeddedness and literary strategies of the medical discourse in Ben Sira, see Chrysovergi 2011, 159–202; Askin 2018, 186–231; Cranz 2018a.

27 Cf. Kollmann 1994; Chrysovergi 2011, 2011b; Stuckenbruck 2002, and 2014, esp. 124–130 (*The Medico-Magical Cures in the Book of Tobit*); Attia 2018. For an in-depth commentary on the whole Tobit tradition, see Beate Ego, *Tobit* (Stuttgart: Kohlhammer, 2021).

28 For an early survey on the 'Essenes', see Kottek 1983. On the pharmaceutical and therapeutic approaches, see Kottek 1996, esp. 2854–2860. Based on (phyto)archeological findings, Taylor 2009 has argued for the increased medical interest and expertise of groups in this area. On the connections between illness and demonology or astrology, see Fröhlich 2011, 2012, 2013, and 2017; Hamidovic 2017. Studies on special topics have been pursued by Brayer 1969 (psychology / dream interpretation); Tigay 1993 (physical examinations of virginity); Popovic 2007 (physiognomy and astrology); Feder 2012 (skin disease); van der Horst 2012 (embryology).

Second Temple traditions have also proven to be rich sources for studying Jewish ideas about medicine and other branches of scientific knowledge (e. g. calendars, astrology/ astronomy, and cosmology). This pertains in particular to *Jubilees* or the multi-lingual Enochic traditions in which one finds narrative accounts of the heavenly origin of medical, magical and other scientific knowledge. While in the Enochic texts this transfer of knowledge is seen as critical, it serves in Jubilees as a legitimation of the existence of illness and the human license to heal. This etiology of medical sciences going back to Noah and his descendants is explicitly 'Judaized', while the authors are thought to have lived in a Hellenized context.[29] In recent years, scholars have also inquired into the manifold exchanges of medical and scientific knowledge between the West (Palestine/ Mediterranean East), the Babylonia East and Central Asia, that brought about a relatively early cross-fertilization and hybridization of different systems of (medical) knowledge.[30]

3   Rabbinic literature

In contrast to Biblical and Second Temple traditions, accounts on medicine and healing are numerous in rabbinic literature, but the scholarly engagement has been rather limited.[31] As outlined above, academic interest reached its first peak with a number of published books and a surge of journal articles from the mid–19th century onwards.[32] Some of these earlier studies focused on a particular subfield (dentistry, gynaecology, ophthalmology, surgery etc.) or a specific group of illnesses, such as skin-diseases, ailments of the lung or the heart.[33] Talmudic medicine, at least those therapies understood as magico-medical, were of interest to Gideon Brecher and Wilhelm Ebstein.[34] Reuven J. Wunderbar composed a first, systematic study of medical knowledge in

---

29 Cf. Alexander 2002; Reed 2007, 2014; Syfox 2018; Chrysovergii 2011; Kottek 2000 (also on Tobit and Qumran). For an astonishingly similarly Judaized back-story, see the expanded and rather mundane history of the transmission of medical knowledge across cultures and religions in the post-Talmudic *Sefer Asaf* as analyzed in Yoeli-Tlalim 2018 and in her contribution in this volume. In general, the Babylonian or non-Hellenistic influence on these texts (esp. Enoch) is notable from their strong orientation toward the celestial sciences (astronomy / astrology).

30 For medicine and body-related exchanges, see Geller 1995, 1998; Popovic 2007. See also Reed 2007, 2014.

31 For a general survey, see Kottek 2006. Cf. also Rosner 2000. A select bibliography on general ancient and ancient Jewish medicine has been compiled by Meir Barl-Ilan. Cited 16 May 2018; online: https://faculty.biu.ac.il/~barilm/bibliography/bibmed.html. This list comprises several subcategories but it focuses mainly on works published before 2000, with some exceptions. For a survey of illness concepts and medical ideas from biblical to rabbinic traditions, see Lehmhaus 2020.

32 This surge of interest was preceded or accompanied by some dissertations on the same matter. For a survey of illness concepts and medical ideas from biblical to rabbinic traditions, see Lehmhaus 2020. Cf. Cohn 1846, Israels 1845, and the discussion of Gintzburger's dissertation from 1743 in Schiller 1988. For other earlier studies, see also the bibliographies by Steinschneider 1896; Friedenwald 1935b; and the discussion in Jütte 1999.

33 Circumcision as particular 'Jewish' field of surgery was of special interest. Cf. Brecher 1845.

34 Cf. Brecher 1850 and Ebstein 1903. The latter focused on Jesus, the apostles and the so-called 'healing miracles' in the New Testament.

the Talmud, followed by Joseph Bergel's substantial surveys on medicine and other scientific branches.[35] The scholarly efforts of the 19th century were crowned by Julius Preuss in his major oeuvre *Biblical and Talmudic Medicine*, which, as a synthesis of earlier studies covered all medical subfields, legal and socio-historical dimensions, and aimed at comparing its subject to Graeco-Roman and other ancient Mediterranean traditions.[36] Preuss's book, widely known in its English translation by Fred Rosner, has become the standard reference work in the field and is used extensively and without further questioning by many scholars outside of Jewish studies. Though not uncritical and aware of several pitfalls and challenges, most of these earlier scholars shared a positivistic approach towards the available rabbinic texts that were regarded primarily as reliable sources for (medico-)historical inquiry.[37] Assuming that Talmudic and other rabbinic texts could be skimmed primarily for medical information, these studies often disregarded or, at least, paid little attention to literary, discursive, religious and cultural dimensions of these compound traditions. A lack of philological and text-critical interest and the limited availability of textual variants, compared to present-day standards in rabbinic studies, impeded their analysis of medical terminology and historical contexts that were based on non-scholarly standard editions or translations. In many instances, scholars paid rather little attention to the different times and places of origin of various rabbinic traditions and their distinct cultural *milieux*. Information in the Western, Palestinian corpus (*Mishnah*, *Tosefta*, *Yerushalmi*) is contrasted but also conflated with contents in the Babylonian Talmud, or in some midrashic or targumic texts. Generally, led by a central question regarding medical issues, pertaining information was sometimes confounded with pre-rabbinic (Bible/ Qumran/Philo) or later sources, especially the (anachronistic) interpretations of medieval commentators like Maimonides or Rashi.[38]

In the footsteps of Preuss, research into medicine in ancient rabbinic traditions has followed largely the methodological patterns described above well into the second half of the 20th century; and a few examples can still be found today. This rather conservative orientation has been facilitated by a strict division of labor and a neat and long persisting separation between academic disciplines—history of (Jewish) medicine, Talmudic or rabbinic studies, and history of (late) ancient Jews. Besides the aspects already mentioned, some researchers were still particularly interested in isolating medical data from Talmudic texts and applying what has been critically as-

---

35 Both, Wunderbar 1850, and Bergel 1880, 1885 who discussed at length anatomy, physiology, pathology, zoology, geology, and astronomy, published their studies 50 to 30 years prior to Preuss's book that later became the standard work. Preuss, however, dismissed the works of his predecessors due to their lack of proper medical education. For other early survey studies on Talmudic (and earlier) medical knowledge, see Carmoly 1844, 1–17; Rabbinowicz 1881; Landau 1895, 14–20; Katzenelson 1928.

36 Preuss 1911. This work was translated into English by Fred Rosner (Preuss 1978) and into Hebrew by Uri Wurzburger (Preuss 2012). On Preuss's life and work, see Rosner 1977.

37 Bergel 1885, VI: sees the difficulty of identifying the many names of diseases and *materia medica* that occur in Greek, Latin, Persian, Syriac and Aramaic.

38 See the brief surveys by Cohen 1900; Stern 1909; Bergman 1951.

sessed by medical historians as "retrospective diagnosis". Such studies mainly dealt or still deal with identifying certain pathologies or syndromes or projecting knowledge from modern research in genetics or pharmacology onto rabbinic sources.[39] Accordingly, one might rather call them "retrojective diagnosis".[40] However, academic fields are dynamic and the history of medicine and the sciences underwent some major theoretical and methodological changes. Although one still may find at times anachronistic, retrospective analysis, the study of medicine in rabbinic traditions has moved away from those methods that prevailed earlier. The journal *Koroth* under the aegis of Samuel Kottek in Jerusalem has served as a bridge between the different approaches mentioned above. Owing to the persisting efforts of the editors, Jewish medical history has opened up to various comparative and inter-disciplinary perspectives, while journals and series in rabbinic studies and ancient Judaism have likewise seized upon medical topics.

For the research of the past three decades, one may identify several approaches to study medicine-related information in rabbinic texts. As in earlier years, several studies provide a thematic discussion of various subfields according to ancient or modern medical thought.[41] While some scholars tend to produce rather broad surveys, at times including biblical and medieval sources, others approach those broader fields through the more detailed study of several sample texts.[42] Similar to the first approach, several scholarly endeavors focus on a particular ailment, specific illnesses or a group of symptoms—some from a decidedly modern medical perspective[43], others with an

---

39 The following shall serve as examples: Goodman 1982 (testicular feminization syndrome); Röder 1991 (brain tumor); Eidelmann 2006; Eisenberg 2016 (hemophilia). On "retrospective diagnosis", see the critique by Leven in the following note.

40 For a critical assessment of "retrospective diagnosis", see Karl-Heinz Leven, "'At times these ancient facts seem to lie before me like a patient on a hospital bed'—Retrospective Diagnosis and Ancient Medical History," in *Magic and Rationality in Ancient Near Eastern and Graeco-roman Medicine* (eds. M. Horstmanshoff and M. Stol; Leiden: Brill, 2004), 369–386.

41 The crucial difference between modern (or rather etic) and the ancient (or rather emic) concepts underlying these approaches are indicated in the titles of Rosner 1993 (dietetics) and Geller 2004b (diet and regimen). Cf. also the social history approach championed by Kudlien 1985; Dvorjetski 2011/12, and Bar-Ilan 1999.

42 Cf. Geller 2004c (bloodletting); Lehmhaus and Martelli 2017 (pharmaceutical knowledge); Lehmhaus 2021 (pain).

43 Due to the limitations of space, it is impossible to reference those, often-brief studies in any exhaustive manner. Rosner who also specializes in medieval Judaism (Maimonides) and (modern) medical ethics, has produced a large corpus of brief articles on various medical issues. These are usually based on the respective section in Preuss' work, augmented with the quotation and translation of the actual biblical and Talmudic texts which Preuss only referenced in passing. At times, Rosner supplements these cursory diachronic surveys with midrashic texts and especially with references to later traditions, such as Maimonides, Rashi, Yehuda ha-Levi's *Kuzari*, or the *Zohar* etc. For individual references to those articles, see the survey in Rosner 1996 (esp. ns. 30–54) throughout which the author refers to his shorter discussions.

emphasis on the ancient cultural contexts.[44] Various studies deal with certain body parts, their anatomy, physiology, ailments and treatment.[45]

An approach with a long-standing tradition is the (comparative) study of medical terminology in Talmudic texts, which also draws on loanwords and calques from Greek, Latin, Akkadian and Persian. The (re)evaluation of the meaning and etymology of names of diseases and *materia medica*, often taken for granted, is still a desideratum.[46] Inextricably connected to terminology is the research into rabbinic concepts of specific diseases, healing, and in general of illness and health.[47]

Especially since the cultural turn in the Humanities from the 1990s, scholars were increasingly interested in rabbinic concepts and representations of the body, which they interpreted as a cultural construct and a powerful discursive arena that also included approaches in feminist theory and gender studies.[48] Medical ideas, especially regarding anatomy, physiology and sexuality, as part of the broader Graeco-Roman and Persian traditions, play an important role in studies into the rabbinic construction of male and female bodies or the definition of sex and gender.[49] An adjacent subfield has been formed by research into female physiology and gynecological issues in rabbinic texts. In this field, scholars of the history of medicine provided thematic surveys or specific case studies, sometimes with a comparison to Graeco-Roman sources.[50] Still, the topic lends itself also literary and cultural studies

---

44 For a broad scope from 'retrojective diagnosis' and modern medical pathology to comparative, textual and cultural approaches to illness, see the discussion on *Qordiaqos* (קורדייקוס) by Hankoff 1972; Weindling 1978; Rosner 1995, 60–64; Kottek 1996, 2924–2926; Rainbow 2008; Lehmhaus 2015. For specific skin-diseases (*ra'atan*/'leprosy'), see Ostrer 2001, 2002; for other ailments, see Kottek 2011/12; Bar-Ilan 2001 (epilepsy).

45 See for instance Rubin 1988 (soul and psyche); Kottek 1993/94 (kidneys).

46 Earlier scholarship tended to provide straightforward identifications and translations of ailments, body parts and medical ingredients that were often shaped by a modern medical understanding. Even the information in the standard dictionaries (Jastrow 1926; Sokoloff 1992, 2002) is not always reliable—since often based on Rashi and other later sources—and should be supplemented with the entries in Loew 1881, 1924–1934, and Krauss 1898–1899. On Hebrew medical terminology, see the work by Malchi 1928 and the discussion of rabbinic terms in Friedenwald 1934; Muntner 1940; Kottek 1996b. For detailed studies, see Friedheim 1990; Jacobi 1998/99; Hadas 2007.

47 Cf. Krauss 1908 (bathing and health); Amit 2020 (bodily constitution and definition of sickness); Newmyer 1984 (climate and health); Carter 1991 (disease and death); Geller 2004c (bloodletting); Lehmhaus 2017a (*materia medica*).

48 Cf. Boyarin 1993; and a discussion of his impact in Seidman 1994, Fonrobert 2005, Rosen-Zvi 2013. See also Eilberg-Schwartz 1992, 1994; and Barbara Kirshenblatt-Gimblett, "The corporeal Turn," *The Jewish Quarterly Review* 95,3 (2005): 447–461.

49 A major study on the female body in ancient Jewish thought is Baker 2002. For an anatomical and cultural discourse of sex and gender, see Levinson 2000; Marcinkowski 2002/03; Fonrobert 2007; Kiperwasser 2012; Lehmhaus 2019; and Secunda 2012 (Iranian background). Persons with a double-sex or a non-binary sex (*androgynos, aylonit, saris, tumtum*) and ambiguous gender status are discussed by Fonrobert 2006; Lev 2007, 2010, and 2018; Strassfeld 2016.

50 I will limit the references to the diachronic survey in Klein 1998/99, and the good comparative studies by Kottek 2000a and Newmyer 1996. Cf. also comparative case studies such as Reichman 2010; Reichman and Rosner 1996.

of rabbinic traditions in two main areas. First, the medical aspects of halakhic rules of im/purity regarding menstruation and genital fluxes have been studied against the backdrop of their discursive function and sociocultural contexts.[51] Second, scholars have become more and more interested in the cultural backgrounds and textual framing of rabbinic ideas of conception, gestation[52], and pregnancy or knowledge and practice of giving birth and breastfeeding, often in comparison with Hellenistic or Persian-Babylonian concepts.[53]

While the study of disabilities has not yet formed as a substantial subfield as in Biblical Studies, after rather cursory treatments in earlier publications, recently the scholarly interest has increased and a growing number of more detailed studies of particular elements has been published.[54] The ground-breaking work of Judith Abrams (z'l) has triggered a mutually enriching dialogue between rabbinics and contemporary disability studies, as in the work of Julia Watts Belser. Such research opens up multiple ways of engaging theories and methods from both fields and enter into conversations with other approaches (e.g. environmental humanities, human-animal studies).[55]

Another line of inquiry is more interested in the socio-historical and cultural background of medical practice as reflected in rabbinic texts. Some studies, among them many earlier works, seek to reconstruct the healthcare system and the main fields and practitioners known to Jews in late antiquity.[56] Other scholars deal with the conception of human medical intervention and the image of the non-rabbinic physician or the medical erudition of certain rabbinic figures. While those are sometimes understood as trained physicians or experts in a particular medical subfield, more recent scholarship questions this straightforward equation and points to different other roles of rabbis as a learned sub-elite with medical interest or as intermediaries of pertinent knowledge and practice.[57] This approach intersects in some ways with ques-

---

51 Cf. Meacham 1989, 1995; Fonrobert 2000, 2008.

52 Cf. Kessler 2009; Kiperwasser 2009; Tziraki-Segal 2009; Bar-Ilan 2009; Lepicard 2010; Hasan-Rokem 2013; Hasan-Rokem and Yuval 2017; Doruftei 2018; Strauch Schick 2017, 2019, and 2021; Walfish 2017. On rabbinic knowledge about species with regard to fetal development, see Neis 2017, 2018 and 2019.

53 The most comprehensive discussion so far, besides Preuss 1911/1992, 470–476, provides Rosenblum 2017 who aptly critiques Eidelman 2006. For the gendered, socio-economic and halakhic embeddedness of nursing in rabbinic traditions, see Laibovits 2005. On cultural and polemic dimensions, see Levinson 2000b; Kessler 2005; Bregman 2017.

54 For earlier studies, see Shifman 2002 (bad breath as disability), Kottek 1992 (insanity). Cf. recent research on particular details by Gracer 2003 (hearing impairments); Rosen-Zvi 2005 (blemishes and bodily perfection), Lehmhaus 2018 (prosthetics). Cf. Marx 2002 on halakhic-ethical discussions.

55 The path taken by Abrams 1998 has been followed and was substantially broadened by the studies of Belser 2011, 2015, 2016. Cf. also Belser and Lehmhaus 2016.

56 Cf. Preuss 1911, 10–43 and Preuss/Rosner 1978, 11–41; Bar-Ilan 1999; Dvorjetski 2007. See also the contribution of E. Dvorjetski to this volume.

57 Rabbis were perceived as trained physicians, for instance, in Friedenwald 1897, 11–13 (Ḥanina ben Ḥaniya, Rav, Shmuel); Scherbel 1905 (Shmuel, Binjamin; Gamaliel); or Rosner 1976

tions regarding legitimate and illegitimate medical practices or the permissibility and reliability of non-Jewish healers, often intertwined in complex processes of othering and identity formation.[58] Of particular interest is the discourse on female medical practitioners and the marginalized or concealed healing expertise of women, which was not limited to midwifery, obstetrics or gynaecology but also figures in various other areas, especially pharmaceutical knowledge.[59] Female medical expertise in rabbinic texts, as in other ancient cultures, was often (con)fused in modern scholarship with the realm of "folk medicine", witchcraft, magic and esoteric practices, such as healing incantations, amulets, and charms.[60] Studies have also examined the relation between Talmudic texts and contemporaneous non-rabbinic or para-rabbinic traditions, such as Babylonian 'magic bowls' (incantation bowls), ancient Mediterranean magical science, and demonology, which was, in fact, an ancient branch of expertise or even science.[61]

Whereas earlier research has always interpreted 'Talmudic medicine' against the backdrop of Graeco-Roman culture, more recent comparative studies attempt to (re)locate rabbinic medical knowledge within much more diverse contexts. These backgrounds comprise early Christian cultures in the West and the East, Akkadian and ancient Mesopotamian medical traditions, and the Irano-Persian background of the Babylonian Talmud.[62] This more comprehensive perspective is often supplemented by an increased interest in the redaction history, the literary framing and the discursive or narrative strategies (anecdotes, recipes, lists, dialogues, aphorisms, *sugyot* as structural devices) of medical discussions within rabbinic texts that may use them for various purposes (e.g. polemics, admonition, transfer of knowledge, self-fashioning).[63]

(Shmuel). For a general diachronic discussion of Jewish physician, see Hezser 2016. For ethical implications, see Teugels 2016. On non-Jewish medical experts and expertise, see Kottek 2000; Vârtejanu-Joubert 2009. See also Tirzah Meacham's and Shulamit Shinnar's contributions to this volume. On different roles of rabbis in medical discourse and practice, see Lehmhaus 2016a, 2016b, 2019; Shinnar 2019.

58 Cf. Silberman 1990; Veltri 1997, 1998/99 & 2010.

59 On the famous 'mother of Abbaye' (*em shel abbaye*), see Kottek 2010. On female healing experts, among them, Timtinis, see Ilan 2002 (190–195), 2006, Cf. also Tal Ilan, "Salome's Medicinal Recipe and Jewish Women Doctors in Antiquity," and Monika Amsler "Goats or Babies?! A Critical Evaluation of the Teachings by Abaye's Mother (bShab 134a) and the Relationship between Veterinary and Human Medicine in the Talmud," which both will appear in *Female Bodies and Female Practitioners in the Medical Traditions of the Late Antique Mediterranean World*; ed. L. Lehmhaus; Tübingen: Mohr Siebeck, 2021 (forthcoming).

60 Cf. Brecher 1850; Blau 1898; Veltri 2010; Bohak 2008, esp. 351–425; Kedar 2018.

61 Cf. Geller 2005, Bhayro 2012, 2017; Houtman 2000; Harari 2017, esp. 353–460; Kedar 2018; Levene 2003.

62 On the common comparison to Graeco-Roman medicine, see Newmyer 1980, 1996; Kottek 1996b. For ancient Babylonian or Akkadian and Sassanian-Persian parallels, see Stol 1986, 2000; Geller 2000, 2004a; Ronis 2015. For comparison with Graeco-Roman and early Christian thought, see van der Horst 2002, 2015/16; Martelli 2017; Lehmhaus 2019.

63 Cf. Noy 1988; Fonrobert 2000; Wandrey 2003; Balberg 2011, 2015; Kiperwasser 2012; Jaffe 2015; Amit 2017; Lehmhaus 2015, 2016a, 2016b, 2017a, 2017b, 2019. On the so-called „Book

4 Medieval time

In comparison to the earlier periods, medicine among Jews from the Middle Ages to the 19th century, had been a major field of scholarly inquiry from early on.[64] Much of earlier scholarship followed an approach of a history of 'great men' and concentrated on cataloguing Jewish physicians' names, their educational background and their professional life as doctors, authors and teachers in order to produce an inventory or survey of Jewish medical practitioners.[65] Other scholarly inquiry focused on identifying medical works by Jewish medieval authors.[66] Based on these seminal studies, later scholars produced research on single authors, specific diseases, their treatment and general medical contexts. These scholarly developments were facilitated by several factors, which I will elaborate upon briefly in the remainder of this section.

First, the post-Talmudic or Geonic period can be characterized by a new historical context for Jews in various localities who were (re)united under an expanding Islamic dominion that reached from Spain and North Africa to Palestine, Iraq and even Central Asia. This expansion (re)connected a political, cultural and religious diversity with their own textual and scientific traditions and practices. The new framework facilitated a surge of literary, philosophical and scientific exchanges attested by but reaching beyond the Graeco-Syriac-Persian-Arabic translation movement under the Abbasids focusing largely on Hippocratic and Galenic medicine.

Most research of early medieval Jewish medicine has concentrated on *Sefer ha-refu'ot* (*Book of Remedies*) or *Sefer Asaf ha-Rofe* (*The Book of Asaf the Physician*), which was produced between the 7th and the 9th century, somewhere between the Persian and Byzantine cultural spheres. Astonishingly, this first exclusively medical work was written in Hebrew and contains Graeco-Roman, traditional rabbinic-Talmudic and Eastern (Persian/Indian) elements.[67] This text, however, was not a complete exception of its time. A group of studies has shed light on the important work *Sefer ha-yakar/Sefer ha-Mirqahot* (on pharmaceutical mixtures) by Shabbetai Donnolo and his role as a transmitter and connector but also as inventor of Hebrew scientific knowl-

of Remedies" in b.Gittin 67b–69a, see Halperin 1982; Freeman 1998/99; Geller 2000, 2004a; Lehmhaus 2015; Amsler 2018.

64 For an updated survey of the topic, see Caballero Navas 2011; Lewicka and Freudenthal 2016; Freudenthal 2018a.

65 This is extremely obvious in the *opus magnum* (*The Jews and Medicine*) by Friedenwald 1944, 1946 (*Jewish Luminaries*). Numerous other studies also focus on surveying Jewish medical practitioners, their work and their writings. Cf. Münz 1922; Meyerhof 1938, 1977; Krauss 1930. For a biographical index of premodern Jewish physicians, see Koren 1973.

66 Cf. Steinschneider 1885; Zonta 2011.

67 For the text, see the editions by Muntner 1968/1971, 1969, and the one by Melzer 1972. Cf. also the discussion in T. Visi's contribution to this volume. On the work's multiple backgrounds in Greek, Persian, Indian and ancient Mesopotamian medical traditions, see Muntner 1951, 1957; Bar-Sela and Hoff 1965; Lieber 1984; Newmyer 1992; Yoeli-Tlalim 2018; Visi 2016a; Melzer 1972. Emunah Levy (Bar Ilan University) has worked in her PhD-research on a critical assessment of the transmission history of *Sefer Asaf*, mainly in its Ashkenazic manuscript witnesses. For an early historical take on its reception history, see also Shatzmiller 1983.

edge and technical language in the Byzantine cultural hub of Southern Italy.[68] Others have pointed to medical treatises, such as *Seder Yezirat ha-walad* (*The Order of the Formation of the Unborn*) as part of the "beginnings of Hebrew scientific literature".[69]

Simultaneous to this emergence of the first medical and scientific works in Hebrew, one finds the work of Jewish authors who, at a quite early stage, adopted Arabic and Judeo-Arabic as their language of scholarship.[70] Isaac Israeli (9th–10th c., North Africa) wrote Neoplatonic philosophical texts, ethical guides and medical treatises, most famously on fevers, dietetics and uroscopy.[71] These texts were later translated into Hebrew, Latin, and several European languages. Jewish, Muslim and Christian scholars alike held his works in high regard and the number of quotations from his writings throughout the medieval and subsequent periods outshines even those of Maimonides.[72] Moreover, one finds other Jewish physicians and medical authors in the early Islamicate world who left significantly smaller textual traces compared with Israeli's very influential work.[73]

Second, the Graeco-Syriac-Arabic scientific flourishing and the rather quick adoption of Arabic literary culture by Jews from the early medieval period onward, paved the way for new "cultural heroes" like Maimonides, Nachmanides, and Abraham ibn Ezra, among others. These prolific authors possibly initiated but definitely established the paradigmatic role model of the "rabbi-scholar" or "rabbi-physician" who was versatile in secular medicine, other sciences, and philosophy, while also thriving as a religious luminary, well versed in the particularities of halakhic thought. This ideal of a double-expertise, in religious-theological and secular traditions, prevailed among Jews and their contemporaries throughout the Islamicate world from Baghdad to the Iberian Peninsula or Southern France, and persisted until the time of Tuvia Cohen or Isaac Lampronti in early Modern Italy.

Especially Maimonides and his rich *oevre* has proven to be an invaluable source for research into medieval scientific education and Jewish thought.[74] He composed his medical writings in Arabic or Judeo-Arabic, and some of them were translated into Hebrew in later medieval time.[75] Several studies highlight the neat intertwining of

---

68 Cf. the text editions of his pharmacological work *Sefer ha-Yakar/Sefer Mirqahot* by Steinschneider 1867, Muntner 1949, and Ferre 2004. Cf. also the studies by Mancuso 2010; Putzu 2004; Rosato 2013, and the contributions in Lacerenza 2004.
69 Cf. Langermann 2002.
70 Meyerhof 1938, esp. 435–437; Chipman 2013; Langermann 2006, 2008; Ferre 2010.
71 On his work on fevers, see Latham and Isaacs 1981; Veit 2003; Paavilainen 2015/16; Ferre and Martinez Delgado 2015; cf. Kenneth Collins's chapter in this volume. On the 'book of urines', see Peine 1919; Veit 2015a; Visi 2015; Collins 1999. On Israeli's discussion of dietetics, see Veit 2015b, and Kozodoy 2015; cf. the volume by Collins, Kottek, and Paavilainen 2015.
72 For the medieval transmission, see Veit and Ferre 2009; cf. Keil 2015. Cf. Nägele 2001 for the later translations of his works.
73 Cf. Langermann 2004, 2011, 2014.
74 For biographic portraits or surveys of his live, medical and religious writings, see Münz 1895; Friedenwald 1935a; Ackermann 1986; Rosner 1969, Herst 1973.
75 For a parallel Arabic-English edition and translation, critical edition of the extant Hebrew translations and valuable commentaries, glossaries and indexes, see Bos 2001–2017, and Bos

philosophical, religious-halakhic, and scientific-medical ideas or his perspective on medical ethics.[76] While some authors focus on Maimonides' contributions to several medical subfields, such as dietetics, pharmaceutics, toxology, gynaecology, and disease taxonomy[77], other scholars stress his role as a cultural intermediary through his engagement with the Graeco-Arabic legacy, mostly Hippocratic and Galenic works, and his connection as a practicing physician with his Arabic speaking environments.[78]

Compared to Maimonides, other medical authors and practitioners produced considerably fewer works or their writings have not been transmitted.[79] An important exception was the Jewish grammarian Jonah Ibn Ganah, who composed a pharmacological dictionary in Arabic or the dietary, and pharmacological works by Ibn Biklarish.[80] Medicine, especially its astrological features, was but a small part of the abundant work in Hebrew of Abraham ibn Ezra who dealt mainly with biblical commentary, grammar, mathematics and astrology.[81] Also later authors wrote on medical astrology, the field of *melothesia*, the curative use of zodiacal signs, amulets or the influence of "critical days". Scholars have stressed the dynamics between philosophical and medical concepts in several works. Among the few known Hebrew texts we find also a gynaecological one as well as *Sefer ha-Yosher*, an encyclopaedic manual (late 13th c.).[82]

During the past three decades, the study of gynaecological texts and of ideas about generation, gestation, and the female body in its cultural contexts, has formed a veritable subfield within the topic at hand. Hebrew gynaecological works developed their own concepts and terminologies based on or in dialogue with Graeco-Arabic and Latin

---

2018–. This ongoing project will substitute the editions and translations by Muntner and Rosner. On the dissemination and reception of Maimonides' medical works, see Ferre 2009.

76 On the complementary or competing relation between sciences/medicine and religion/philosophy in his work, see Lieber 1979, 2000; Rosner 1967, 1984; Kalman 2008, Stroumsa 1993.

77 Langermann 1993; Bos 1994; Rosner 1996; Paavilainen 2013/14; Caballero Navas 2009, 2013; Ferrario 2017.

78 Wilensky 1990; Bos 2009 (Maimonides' commentary on Galen); Kottek 2009; Mesler 2018 (Maimonides' commentary on Hippocratic aphorisms). On a possible recipe by Maimonides, see Ashur 2014. On a short text on practical medicine, see Langermann and Bos 2012, 2014.

79 Judah ha-Levi remains somehow an exception, since he practiced medicine in 11th c. Toledo as a bread-and-butter job but his writing focused on poetry or philosophical and theological topics. On Nachmanides and his view of medicine, see Kottek 1996c; Langermann 1996.

80 On Ibn Ganah, see Amar and Serri 2000/2001; Fenton 2016; Bos and Käs 2016, and the new critical edition, translation and commentary of the *Kitāb Al-Talkhīṣ* by Lübke, Mensching, and Bos 2020. On Ibn Biklarish, see Levey 1971; Amar and Serri 2001; and Burnett 2008.

81 On bn Ezra's *Sefer ha-Me'orot* ("Book of Luminaries" or "Book of Lights") regarding medical astrology, see Sela 2011. Cf. Leibowitz and Marcus 1984 for other potential dealings of Ibn Ezra with medical issues.

82 On medical astrology, see Shatzmiller 1982/83; Bos, Burnett and Langermann 2005; Bos 1995a addresses the role of medicine in Moshe Narboni's oevre, while Bos and Fontaine 1999 and Amar and Buchman 2004 study Nathan b. Yoel Falaquera's *ṣori ha-guf*, a collection of therapeutic approaches based on Hippocratic and Galenic tradition as well as Averroes, Avicenna, Maimonides and the Talmud. On epistemological questions, see Fraisse 2002. On the gynaecological text (*Record of the Diseases Occurring in the Genital Organs*), see Barkai 1998, 69–76 and 109–144; on the *Sefer ha-Yosher*, see the chapter by Carmen Caballero Navas in this volume.

medical traditions.[83] The discourse on women's bodies, menstruation and the practices surrounding pregnancy, birth and nursing, were an arena of cultural or religious exchange as well as of competition and polemics.[84] Various shorter studies have explored different medical fields like dietetics, psychological aspects or medical ethics, while others addressed the issue of so called 'magical' approaches in medieval medicine.[85] Still understudied are questions of materiality (manuscripts and *materia medica*), genre and discursive strategies, which are, however, sometimes enclosed in the editorial work and philological scholarship on individual authors (e.g. Donnolo, Israeli, Maimonides).[86]

Another subfield of inquiry focuses rather on the sociocultural micro-histories of medieval Jewish involvement in medicine in various regions and localities. These inquiries covered places from the Islamic Middle East and North Africa, the Christian-Muslim Iberian Peninsula, Southern France and Italy (various Muslim Caliphats, Christian kingdoms and municipalities, French cities and regions, Italian states), to England and the Franco-German lands (Ashkenaz) or even Central Eastern Europe in a few cases.

For the Islamicate world, from Baghdad to North Africa and Al-Andalus, scholars have pointed to a high number of Jewish physicians who sometimes used their expertise in medicine and adjacent fields (sciences, poetry, philosophy, grammar, rhetorics etc.) as a door opener to the circles of the learned and political elites. From the tenth century onward, several Jewish individuals or even whole 'dynasties' of Jewish physicians were linked to courts of Muslim rulers and other elite families.[87] Besides this greater social mobility, medicine also was an area of intensive contact with few restrictions in which Jews, Muslims, and Christians became each other's masters, students,

---

83 For major studies and edition/translation of relevant texts, see Barkai 1991, 1998 (cf. the detailed review by G. Bos, "On Editing and Translating Medieval Hebrew Medical Texts," *The Jewish Quarterly Review* 89,1/2 (1998): 101–122); Caballero Navas 2004, and shorter studies, such as Caballero Navas 2006, 2008,2013, and 2014. On ideas about generation, see Fontaine 1994.

84 Cf. Koren 2004, 2009.

85 Just to mention some examples: Shy 1982; Kahana-Smilansky 2011; Einbinder 2005. On therapeutic approaches using amulets and other techniques, see Caballero Navas 2011; Blasco Orellana 2011.

86 For poetic discourse as a specific medieval medical genre, see Kottek 1984; Ferre 1994; Kozodoy 2011. For the generic aspects of medieval medical manuscripts and the importance of their circulation, see Cohen-Hanegbi 2019; Kozodoy 2019. For incorporation of medical knowledge and topics into other religious, mystical, philosophical or literary discourse, see the examples in Kozodoy 2012 and Rosen 2000; Feinsod 2013/14 (on medical themes and satirical representations of Jewish physicians).

87 For a general discussion, see Roth 1953; and Perlman 1972. One may refer to Ḥasdai ibn Shaprut as physician and political advisor to the Umayyad Caliph (10th c., Cordoba); on Abraham Ibn Muhayir (Sevilla); Meir Ibn Qamniel (physician from Sevilla), Abū ʿAlī ʿAlāʾ ibn Zuhr, and Solomon Ibn al-Muʾallim (physician and poet) at the Almoravid court of Yusuf Ibn Tashufin in Morrocco/Fez (early 12th c.), see Roth 1993/94; on Ibn Baklarish (Banu Hud court in Zaragoza,late 11th c.), see Amar and Serri 2001; on Maimonides and his links to the political elite in Egypt and beyond, see Kraemer 2008, 444–468. On medieval Jewish (court) physicians in Egypt, see Mazor 2014; Mazor and Lev 2018.

and patients.[88] The flourishing of medical works by Jews in Arabic has been noticed above and will also be discussed in the following.

The exchange between Jewish, Muslim and Christian medical experts and practitioners has been in the focus of various studies on the Iberian Peninsula and Southern France. They addressed the impact of (Judeo-)Arabic and Latin scientific and medical culture as well as the multi-religious contexts within a swiftly changing political landscape, especially in the Christian kingdoms and in Provence. Among Iberian-Provencal Jews in general, medical education, because and despite of existing on the fringes of the classic Graeco-Arabic sciences, formed an integral part of their intellectual universe. As an (religiously) accepted field of knowledge and practice and due to ubiquitous applicability and its social and economic opportunities, medicine became one of the main professions for Jews who served as (itinerant) physicians to other Jews, the Christian (and earlier Muslim) ruling classes but also to broader circles of the non-Jewish population, municipalities and private persons alike. While opposition to Jewish medical expertise was rare among halakhic authorities, such prevalence and success of Jewish doctors met the suspicion or open hostility of Christian physicians, clergy and politicians.[89]

Jewish converts to Christianity as well as migrants from Iberia to Provence played a crucial role in this transfer of knowledge, as will be discussed in relation to the translation movement in the next section.[90] Several studies inquired into the increased professionalization and academization of medicine and stressed several sociocultural aspects that impacted Jewish involvement in this field. Thus, while Jews were officially banned from universities and later in the 14th and 15th centuries faced severe anti-Jewish legislation, many still were in close contact with learned medical experts and obtained a license or training at university level (e. g. Leon Joseph of Carcassonne or Abraham Abigdor).[91] Those who practiced medicine mainly among other Jews or offered various medical services (obstetrics; small surgery; herbal medicine; production of amulets and talismans, circumcision, etc.) would not even need an official approval. Scholars have stressed the role of learned (licensed and unlicensed) Jewish women as physicians and other medical experts.[92]

Less scholarly attention has been paid so far to the development of medical knowledge and practice in Italy, a crossroads of Sephardic and Ashkenazi traditions, except for the early beginnings with Donnolo that have been described above. The protagonists (Hillel ben Samuel, Zerahya ben She'altiel Hen), sometimes even competitors to the Ital-

---

88 Cf. Seide 1954; Motzkin 1970; Lev 2003 (see the review by A. Touwaide, *Bulletin of the History of Medicine* 78 (2004): 701–702); Chipman 2010.

89 Cf. Alteras 1978; Garcia-Ballester 2001; Davidson 2004; Kozodoy 2012. On micro-histories of Jewish medicine in various Christian kingdoms and in the Midi, see the literature in Caballero Navas 2011, 337, ns. 93 and 94. Apparently, Jews made for up to thirty percent of all medical practitioners in those regions in the 14th century. On the various restrictions and polemics, see Shatzmiller 1994, 78–99.

90 Cf. Kozodoy 2015; Amasuno 1996; Robinson 2005.

91 Cf. Garcia-Ballester and Feliu 1993; Roth 1953, esp. 837–846.

92 Cf. Shatzmiller 1994; Garcia-Ballester 1996; Langermann 1996; Einbinder 2009. On women, see esp. Friedenwald 1944, 217ff.; Caballero Navas 2008; Green and Smail 2008.

ian translation movement from Latin and Arabic, lived in Rome and Northern Italy. While educated in and cultivated strong ties to the Iberian and Provencal Jewish communities, they also were familiar with North Italian university curricula. However, Jews seem to have been granted entry into university, especially in Padua and in the South, only from the early 15th century onward. Studies have focused on a rather high number of documented licenses for Jewish physicians, mainly in Southern Italy, and the relations oscillating between political and ecclesiastic protection, opposition or ignorance.[93]

For a long time, in regard to sciences and medicine, scholars have argued for great divide between Jewish communities throughout the Islamicate world, the Iberian Peninsula and Southern France on one hand and those in Ashkenaz (the Franco-German lands), North and Central Eastern Europe on the other. Such assumptions were mostly derived from observations regarding philosophy and the group of Aristotelian sciences but have recently been questioned and qualified.[94] The exceptional position of medicine as a more accepted field of knowledge among Jews and intense exchange with the non-Jewish environments, which was confirmed for Provence[95], can also be assumed for North and Eastern Europe.

Studies have found evidence, mainly in Christian documents, for a substantial number of Jewish well-educated physicians and other medical practitioners, among them many women, from at least the 14th century onward. Even earlier, one may find traces of Jewish medical practice and knowledge that might have attracted religious learned circles.[96] Regarding general exclusion from medical university training and the itinerant nature of the profession, together with the high status that allowed for social mobility, their situation was not so different from that of Jewish medical practitioners in Southern Europe. The supply of books and translations, however, took other routes. While contemporary non-Jewish works, mostly in Latin, were adapted, the Hebrew medical works from the South played a minor role, except for the *Sefer ha-refu'ot/Sefer Asaph*. Original works were composed in Hebrew, Yiddish, and German, with inter-language glossing and translations in these languages and Latin. These works mirror the Jewish and broader medical landscape in focusing mostly on practical areas such as surgery, therapeutic intervention (recipes), uroscopy or bloodletting, while only dealing *en passant* with theoretical concepts (e.g. Galenic humoral ideas) or natural philosophy.[97] One important area was astral medicine with regard to blood-

---

93 Cf. Roth 1953, esp. 840–843; Friedenwald 1922; Schwartz 2013.

94 Cf. Freudenthal 2009 and Langermann 2009, who both deal mainly with science and philosophy. Shyovitz 2017 has addressed the different but nonetheless sophisticated approach of medieval Ashkenazi Jews to nature, cosmos and bodies of animals and humans that reflected their keen interest in as well as their familiarity with scientific knowledge prevailing in the Christian majority culture. See also Visi 2014.

95 Cf. Freudenthal 2009 and 2018a.

96 Cf. Leibowitz 2009 (on the Tossafists' interest in medical ideas); Shatzmiller 1983 (Sefer Asaph/ha-Refu'ot and medical praxis); Shoham-Steiner 2006; and Efron 2001, 35f. (medical knowledge among the *Hasidei Ashkenaz*).

97 On this literature and further aspects, see the seminal article by Visi 2019 and its references to

letting or diet and regimen.[98] As in Iberia and Provence, Ashkenazi Jews wrote on medicine with regard to the various plague outbreaks —a particularly thorny realm given several anti-Jewish accusations and pogroms in the wake of the Black Death.[99]

Several studies have dealt with the reputation and social limbo of Jewish 'learned' physicians and less-learned healers, who, while being in service of Christian clergy, noblemen and the wider Christian population, often faced severe opposition, polemical accusations or even persecution.[100] Also the important role of circumcisers, midwives and wet-nurses has been recently explored more thoroughly.[101] In addition to the direct doctor-patient encounters, other studies addressed the manifold exchanges between Jews and Christians across and beyond the religious and medico-magical marketplace.[102] A similar intertwining of religious, cultural and social elements with medical discourse regarding the so-called 'madmen', the disabled or those suffering from skin-disease ('lepers') have been studied in detail.[103] Scholars with a social and cultural history approach have often focused on the micro-histories of Jewish communities in certain cities or regions, including the medical education, intra- and inter-communal relations and dimension of medical practice.[104]

Third, at least for later medieval time and through the Genizah documents even sometimes for earlier periods, scholars could tap into the greater availability of manuscripts and printed editions of relevant texts.[105] Also pertinent extra-rabbinic sources (in Hebrew, Syriac, Persian, Arabic, Latin etc.) can be used to triangulate the medical texts and inquire deeper into the intellectual and social history of Jewish medical knowledge and practice as embedded in different cultural contexts. Moreover, based on the initial efforts among the scholars of the *Wissenschaft des Judentums*, the number of critical editions, translations and commentaries of those medical texts that do not represent or intersect with the mainstream of Jewish religious or philosophical traditions has constantly grown. While critical editions and translations of the medical (and other scientific) works by Shabbetai Donnolo, Isaac Israeli, Maimonides and

---

sources and other studies. On the medical treatise by 'the Jew from Solms', see Vanková 2018. On medical education, see Roth 1953 and Shatzmiller 1994, 2016.

98 Cf. Isserles 2014, 2017.
99 Cf. Visi 2016b, 2019, 678–681; Heß 2015. On Southern Europe, see Bos 2011c; Bos and Mensching 2011; Barkai 1998b.
100 Cf. Jütte 1995, 1996; Treue 2002.
101 Cf. Baumgarten 2004, esp. 21–91, 119–153, and 2019.
102 Cf. Zier 1992; Shoham-Steiner 2010a, 2010b; Meerson 2013.
103 Cf. Shoham-Steiner 2014.
104 Cf. Treue 1999 (Frankfurt); Roth 1943 (England); Duda 2015 (Teutonic Order's state in Prussia); Efron 2001, 13–63 (survey on Ashkenaz); Taube 2010 (pre-Ashkenazic/Sephardic Eastern Europe).
105 For a preliminary survey of available sources, see Richler 1984, and the very useful and elaborated list in Zonta 2011, which is in parts based on the treasure trove of texts collected in Moritz Steinschneider, *Die hebraeischen Uebersetzungen des Mittelalters und die Juden als Dolmetscher* (Graz: Akademische Druck- u. Verlagsanstalt, 1956 [1893]).

Abraham Ibn Ezra took center stage, also some shorter treatises have been tackled, but several texts still require a comprehensive study, edition and translation.[106]

Throughout the medieval period, maybe based on similar late antique tendencies, medical education and practice enhanced the overtly oral and practical apprenticeship model with an approach of collective and individual study of texts—be it in a lecture or by reading from a written text. Consequently, medical works were produced, copied and transmitted in manuscripts for the individual use of physicians and educated Jews who often assembled them into a veritable personal medical library. These collections comprised various texts in (Judeo-)Arabic, which had, for instance, a long and productive afterlife among Castilian Jews, in Hebrew, and, sometimes, in Latin. Scholars have seen the increasing circulation of these works also as a way to gain access to the otherwise for Jews restricted learned medical knowledge at universities or as the official apprentice of a physician. Medical (and other scientific) expertise could be only obtained through direct but sanctioned personal contact with non-Jewish experts or through the study and translation of relevant texts. [107]

The foundation for these changes was laid by several broad and very active translations movements in the Provence/Midi of today's Southern France.[108] Since Jews throughout the Islamicate world had quickly adopted (Judeo-)Arabic as a language of grammar, philosophy, science, and medicine, they had no immediate need for Hebrew translations.[109] Scholars have pointed to the pioneering work, mainly in philosophy (e.g. Ibn Gabirol) and the sciences (Yehuda ben Barzilay, Abraham ibn Ezra, Abraham bar Hiyya), paving the way for a growing scientific corpus in Hebrew.[110] The northeastward movement of mostly Andalusian Jews with an (Judeo-)Arabic cultural background due to the Almohad persecutions has been singled out as the main trigger for these transcultural exchanges. The translations comprised Arabic-into-Hebrew, Arabic-into-Latin (sometimes via Hebrew or a common vernacular)[111], and

---

106 Cf. Bos 2001–2017, and 2018– (Maimonides); Sela 2011 (Ibn Ezra); Steinschneider 1867, Muntner 1949, and Ferre 2004 (Donnolo). Israeli's medical works have been only partially edited and translated within certain studies by Veit 2001; Ferre 2015; or Kozodoy 2015. See also the edition of the medico-philosophical passages in Stern 2017. A long work such as *Sefer Asaph/Sefer ha-refu'ot* still lacks a critical edition and translation, which will hopefully be amended by the future work of Ronit Yoeli-Tlalim, and the dissertation of Emunah Levy (Bar Ilan University). For editions and translations of gynaecological texts, see Barkai 1991, 1998; Caballero Navas 2004. For shorter medical treatises or partly editions/translations, see preceding and following notes.

107 On Arabic medical texts that circulated in Hebrew and Latin translations, see McVaugh, Azar, and Shatzmiller 2002; Zonta 2006. On the familiarity of Jews with Latin texts, especially in Southern France, see Iancu-Agou 2013; Einbinder and McVaugh 2013. Cf. also Carmen Caballero Navas's contribution to this volume for suggestions regarding the motivation for creating a Hebrew corpus of gynaecological texts in medieval time.

108 Cf. Freudenthal 2018b.

109 Cf. Levey 1971; Amar and Serri 2001; Burnett 2008 (on Ibn Biklarish's pharmacological work).

110 Cf. Freudenthal 2013 (cultural intermediaries).

111 For such a collaborative translation of an Arabic original by a Jewish and a Christian scholar, see McVaugh, Bos, and Shatzmiller 2019.

also Latin-into-Hebrew (and vice versa).[112] A very prominent role played the members of the Tibbonid family, beginning with the émigré and physician Judah Ibn Tibbon, who became the most prolific translators of philosophical, theological, poetic, scientific and medical texts. Their work of 150 years satisfied the newly awaken hunger for philosophical and scientific thought, probably stimulated by Maimonides' rationalism and developments in their learned Christian environment.[113] Due to the persisting familiarity of immigrant physicians with Arabic medical texts[114], medicine was a minor field of translations for the Tibbonids and others, such as Qalonymus ben Qalonymus, in Provence, but increased in 13th century Italy as a reaction to medical improvements in their Latin-speaking environment.[115]

Scholars have recently explored the role of a Jewish convert in the Midi (Provence) in the second half of the 12th century, whose importance for the history of Hebrew medical texts cannot be underestimated. Strikingly, using the pseudonym *Doeg ha-Edomi/ Doeg, the Edomite*, a character in 1 Samuel 21 and 22, he has been labelled by scholars as the "Father of the Latin-into-Hebrew Translations", Latin being known as the "tongue of Edom" (=Rome). Doeg's translations of more than twenty Latin medical works, mostly from Salerno and some translated by Constantinus Africanus, have been compared to the work of the Tibbonids. Studies pointed out that competition over patients who attended to Christian physicians, especially in or close to the centers of medical learning (e. g. Montpellier), triggered his enterprise to make this up-to-date expertise available in Hebrew.[116] Scholars have also addressed the few 13th century translations and the second substantial surge of medical translations from Latin into

---

112 For the Arabic-into-Hebrew, see Zonta 2003; Freudenthal 2012. On Latin-into-Hebrew, see the contributions in Fontaine and Freudenthal 2013. Besides the translation of scientific works, other translators, such as Yehuda al-Harizi or (13th c.) Berakhia ben Natronai ha-Naqdan (12th c.) also engaged in the Hebrew adaption of theological, literary and poetic texts. Other translators were often learned men and practicing physicians, but mainly translated philosophical and other scientific works instead of primarily medical texts (e.g. Moses Melgiuri; Shmuel ben Yehudah of Marseille, early 14th c.; Hillel of Verona, late 13th c., Italy). For some texts and translations, see Bos and Garofalo 2007; Bos, McVaugh, and Shatzmiller 2014; Bos and McVaugh 2015.

113 Cf. Robinson 2005; Kreisel 2015.

114 Up to the 16th century, Castilian Jews used and even composed medical works in Arabic, such as Solomon ben Abraham Ibn Ya'ish's commentary on Ibn Sina's *Khanun* and the anonymous *Kitāb al-ṭibb al-qasṭālī al-malūkī* (*Book of Royal Castilian Medicine*). Emigrants from the Iberian Peninsula continued with this practice even after the expulsion of 1492 in their new Ottoman environment. Cf. Garcia-Ballester 1994; Barkai 1996.

115 Cf. Ferre 1998/99; Bos 2013 (on Nathan ha-Meati). The other translator from Arabic (mainly Maimonides and Galen) and a physician was Zerahia ben She'altiel Hen from Barcelona who also worked in Rome.

116 For translations of some of Doeg's texts, see Barkai 1991, esp. 129–223 and 227–284 (Sefer ha-Toledet); Barkai 1998, esp. 22–27 (discussion), and 181–191 (*Sefer ha-Seter*), 145–180 (*Sefer ha-Em shel Galinos*). Cf. also Freudenthal 2013a; Freudenthal and Fontaine 2016. On the importance of his translations of the *Trotula* and Muscios's/Soranus' works for the emergence of Hebrew gynaecological texts, see Carmen Caballero Navas' chapter in this volume.

Hebrew, but also from vernacular languages (e.g. Catalan, Castilian, Occitan), in the 14th century, already under much more learned or even scholastic auspices.[117]

The Tibbonids, Doeg and their Italian colleagues had something in common, that they had to create, almost from scratch, a new scientific and medical vocabulary. Their multilingual erudition, their appropriations and inventions as well as the use of Latin and regional Romance vernacular (e.g. Catalan, Castilian, Occitan) have been thoroughly studied in the past two decades. The polyglot approach was particularly necessary in the realm of pharmaceutics, in which physicians collaborated with experts in herbal medicine, apothecaries and drug sellers. In some cases, this yielded the phenomenon of Judeo-Latin (Latin in Hebrew script) and accompanying Hebrew translations or writings in both Hebrew and the vernacular.[118]

The discovery and increasingly systematic study of Genizah documents has equally contributed to a better understanding of Jewish medieval medicine over the past four decades.[119] Studies utilizing this material often produced first surveys and editions of useful variants and addenda to works known from other sources or of mainly fragmentary texts. Those include Hebrew and (Judeo-)Arabic translations of famous Greek (Galen/Hippocrates) or Arabic (Avicenna, Averroes, Israeli, Maimonides etc.) medical writers but also works of less known authors and texts with a rather compilational character (lists, *pharmacopoeias*, dictionaries etc.).[120] Other research concentrates mainly on practical medicine, mining the sources for *materia medica,* recipes, medical advice (prescriptions) and other therapeutic approaches (amulets, charms, astrology).[121] At times, these technical texts can be combined with other relevant

---

117 Abraham ben Isaac translated Ibn al-Jazzar's work from its Latin version (by Constantinus Africanus) and mostly Galenic texts were adapted into Hebrew by David ben Abraham Caslari (Midi) and Hillel ben Samuel (Verona); the latter also translated Bruno da Longoburgo's *chirurgia magna* based on Abulcasis's texts in Latin. Translations of some Latin versions of Galen (by Qalonymus ben Qalonymus) and Al-Razi became available. Cf. Langermann 1998/99 and Garcia-Ballester, Ferre and Feliu 1990. For the Hebrew renderings, e.g. by Leon Joseph of Carcassonne or Moses ben Samuel of Roquemaure/ Jean of Avignon, of the works of medical experts from Montpellier (Bernard Gordon, Gerard of Solo or Arnau de Vilanova), see Einbinder 2013; McVaugh and Ferre 2000; Mesler 2013; Cohen-Hanegbi 2013, and Cohen-Hanegbi and Melammed 2013 (edition/translation of the introduction to the translation of the *Lilium Medicinae*).

118 Cf. the work on medical glossaries in works of Shem Tov ben Isaac (*Sefer ha-Shimush, Sefer Almansur*), Moshe Ibn Tibbon (*Sefer Sedat ha-Derakhim*), Nathan ha-Me'ati (commentary on Ibn Sina's *Canon*) and others by Bos 2016, 2018, and 2019; Bos and Mensching 2001, 2005, 2015; Bos, Mensching, and Hussein 2011; Bos, Mensching, and Zwink 2017. On the Hebrew-Latin-Romance "interlanguage", see Aslanov 2011a, 2011b; Iancu-Agou 2013. On Judeo-Latin, see Einbinder and McVaugh 2013; Freudenthal 2013c; Kozodoy 2019, 740–743.

119 For a survey of some sources in Genizah collections and a preliminary state of the art, see Bos 1995a and Lev 2004, 2011.

120 For a survey and discussion of the diverse material, see Fenton 1980; Isaacs 1990; Isaacs and Colin 1994; Niessen and Lev 2006;

121 Lev and Amar 2007, 2008 (on the latter, see the very detailed and critical review by Gerrit Bos in *European Journal of Jewish Studies* 2,2 (2008): 327–359; and the other reviews by S. Kottek in *Bulletin of the History of Medicine* 82 (2008): 928–929; S. Bhayro in *Medical History* 53 (2009): 455–456). Cf. also Lev 2015; Quintana Rodriguez 2015; Lev and Chipman 2012

material (personal notes, medical responsa, letters, lists of medical libraries, bills for products and medical service) to further speculate about their *Sitz im Leben* and the wider sociocultural implications of this medical knowledge.[122]

5 Early Modern period

Similar to the research on the medieval period, the last four decades have seen a constant growth of thorough studies of early modern sources and artefacts related to medicine in Jewish cultural contexts or written and practiced by Jews. This mix of social, institutional and biographical (micro-)histories focusing on Jewish medical knowledge, education and practices can be based on a relatively broad pool of sources. Besides the classical scientific languages of Arabic, Hebrew and Latin, authors also used Yiddish and Ladino with increasing use of vernaculars, such as Spanish, Portuguese, Italian, French, English or German, especially among the (returning) *conversos* and the authors of the Enlightenment period.[123] Those sources comprise personal writings (letters, notes, responsa), communal records, and medical texts in manuscripts and early printed editions. Moreover, one may access more non-Jewish official documents and other writings that attest to the Jewish engagement with medical and scientific discourse of their times.

On one hand, scholars have identified certain continuities, such as the influence of Maimonidean thought and other works important in the medieval translation movement, the continuous engagement in cross-cultural knowledge transfers via translations, (forced) migration and travel, and the importance of medicine as a rewarding profession for Jewish thinkers who primarily wrote philosophical, scientific, halakhic and theological works (e.g. Azariah de Rossi, Joseph Delmedigo). On the other hand, several studies have pointed to new developments. After the expulsions, Jewish physicians and intellectuals from the Iberian Peninsula settled all over Europe and well into the Ottoman Empire and brought with them a broad variety of Jewish and non-Jewish knowledge. This contributed to a greater diversity and allowed for long-distance economic and intellectual networks. Moreover, scholars stressed the central role of *conversos*, baptized Jews of whom many returned to Judaism after leaving Spain and Portugal, as cultural intermediaries who connected the Iberian heritage with the learned tradition of Northern Europe. They were often familiar with Christian sources and secular knowledge, and they practiced medicine and participated in the broader discourse by publishing in Latin or their respective vernacular.

Another issue addressed in several studies was the importance of medical studies of Jews for the dissemination of scientific knowledge in general and for a gradual secular-

---

(reviewed with detailed critique and lists of errata by Gerrit Bos in *Journal of the American Oriental Society* 134,4 (2014): 709–720).

122 Goitein 1963, 1967–93, pp. 240–272;

123 Cf. Lapon-Kandelshein and Baruchson-Arbib 2002, esp. 178–180. They describe an exceptional surge of works, about half of them in Yiddish, dealing with popular medicine (hygiene/diet/recipes) and medical compendia for women from the late 17th century onward. Many of those books and epitomes were probably meant as manuals for everyday medicine for a lay audience.

ization of the sciences. Still adhering to a "history of great men" scheme, studies have augmented their focus on several important figures with approaches from social, intellectual, cultural history. Most research focused on the new emerging centers in Northern Italy, in Central (Amsterdam, Hamburg, later also Berlin) and Eastern Europe (Prague, Krakow) and in the Ottoman sphere (especially Salonika, Constantinople and Palestine).[124] Particular attention has been paid to the role of the printing technology that facilitated the circulation of knowledge between and far beyond these centers.[125]

5.1 Italy

Due to changing political and cultural circumstance, the former centers in Iberia and Southern France lost their importance, while the splendid medieval medical legacy persisted well into the early modern period.[126] Among the new cultural and economic centers of Jewish life, Northern Italy and, in particular, the region between Venice, Padua, Mantua and Ferrara became a focal point of intellectual developments yielding different amalgamations of (anti-)rationalism, theology, philosophy, kabbalah and various sciences. As other Jewish thinkers, medically educated Jews strove for an ideal of the universal scholar as it was shaped by Renaissance humanism. As a hotbed of Jewish interaction with medicine and a broader Latin curriculum (liberal arts), scholars have singled out the university of Padua, which from relatively early on (late 15th c.) was open to non-Catholic students. Jews came from very different backgrounds (Iberian, Italian, Ashkenazi, Eastern European, and Ottoman), often after a propaedeutic period of study with Jewish alumni. After their graduation, they practiced medicine all over Europe and often formed a network of mutual support and intellectual exchange.[127] Among those students were several thinkers with whom scholars have dealt, but not for their medical background: the Kabbalist and scientific explorer Joseph Delmedigo (1591–1655), originally from Crete, who funded his travel to the Ottoman realm, Eastern Europe and back to Amsterdam and Prague by teaching or practicing medicine; Joseph Hamiz (died around 1676), a student of Leone Modena who graduated as a physician in 1623, became a rabbi in Venice, and turning to Kabbalah and Shabbatean ideas, he eventually moved to Palestine; David Nieto (1654–1728), from Venice who practiced medicine in Livorno (Tuscany) before he was appointed the head of the Spanish-Portuguese congregation in London.[128]

---

124 For general introductions, see Shear 2017; Ruderman 1999, 1995 (chs. 3 and 8–10), and 2010, esp. 99–132. Cf. Ravid 2004; and Levi 1998 on the secularization and tendency toward a separation of scientific, philosophical and theological discourse.

125 Cf. Fuchs and Plaut 1988; Fuchs 1990 (Jewish medical compendia).

126 Cf. Garcia-Ballester 1996b, 2001; Kimmel 2016.

127 Cf. Ruderman 1987, 1995 (ch. 3: *Padua and the Formation of a Jewish Medical Community in Italy*, 100–117); Collins 2013.

128 On Delmedigo, see Barzilay 1974. On Nieto, see Ruderman 1995, 310–331. Other students included: Judah (Leon) ben Samuel (Simon) ha-Kohen Cantarini (c. 1650–1694), an Italian physician and rabbi in Padua; his nephew, Isaac Cantarini (1644–1723) who was known as a physician, poet, preacher and rabbi in Padua also taught Isaac Lampronti; the brothers Solomon (1642–1719) and Israel Conegliano (born mid–17th c.) who practiced as physicians in Venice.

A descendant of a renowned family of doctors, Abraham Portaleone (1542–1612) studied medicine at Pavia. He, his son David and his grand-son Guglielmo (Benjamin) were practicing physicians in and around Mantua, even among Christians and in service of the local nobility (Gonzaga family) with privileges exempting them form the harsh anti-Jewish decrees of the popes.[129] Studies have focused on two aspects: first, Abraham's important encyclopaedic work *Shilte ha-Gibborim* (*Shields of Heroes*) and other discourses in which he combined scientific, medical and religious knowledge; second, Portaleone's exchange with Christian scholars on scientific and medical matters.[130] Research on his contemporary Abraham Yagel, a physician who wrote autobiographic, religious and ethical works alongside texts dealing with Kabbalah, knowledge of nature or ritualistic medicine (curing plague by praying and fasting), has been interested in his sophisticated intertwining of medical, celestial, cosmological and mystical knowledge.[131]

Scholars agree that the production of original medical writings by Italian authors was rather negligible, except for the work of three physicians, two of them with a medical degree from Padua, on which most research has focused. Jacob Zahalon (1630–1693) from Rome, served as a rabbi and teacher in Ferrara but occupied himself with medical and other natural knowledge. His comprehensive medical handbook in Hebrew (*Oṣar Ḥayim*/*Treasure of Life*) had practical purposes for a non-medical readership and its religiously attuned language was geared at rabbinic students as well.[132]

Certainly, the most studied figure is Tuviah (Tobias) Cohen (1652–1729). Heir of a family of physicians with roots in Palestine and Poland, he studied in Kraków, Frankfurt (Oder) and Padua. He practiced medicine in Poland before moving to the Ottoman Empire (Adrianople/Edirne, Constantinople, Jerusalem) where he served as a court physician. Following in the footsteps of Zahalon's handbook, his major work *Ma'asseh Tuviya*, which became very popular over the following centuries, was more encyclopaedic in nature, probably following a general trend in Italian Jewish intellectual culture.[133] Besides its main and most comprehensive sections on medicine and hygiene, it also covered celestial sciences, botanic knowledge and discourses on theol-

---

Israel Conegliano became a physician and diplomat at the Venetian embassy in Constantinople where he died (early 18th c.). Solomon taught medicine and preparatory courses for Jews enrolling at Padua, among them Tuviah Cohen. Cf. Ruderman 1995, 110–117. For another group of closely allied graduates who were known as doctors and poets, see Benayahu 1978.

129 Cf. Kottek 2009/10. Guglielmo (Benjamin) Portaleone studied medicine in Siena.
130 Cf. Berns 2011, 2012, and 2014, esp. 153–229 (chs. 4&5); Guetta 2014, 30–61 (Chapter 2: *Can Fundamentalism be Modern? The Case of Avraham Portaleone, the Repentant Scientist*).
131 Ruderman 1988.
132 Cf. Savits 1935; Altbauer-Rudnik 2013 (on *love sickness* and for biographical bibliography on Zahalon, see n. 2, p. 88). The handbook tackled general issues of hygiene and diet, specific topics (e.g. fevers or poisons and their cures), medical approaches (tongue and pulse diagnosis, uroscopy), before providing a head-to-foot discussion of symptoms, etiologies and appropriate therapies, and ending with particular ailments (women's, children's disease and mental illness). Several shorter studies have dealt with various illnesses or topics covered by this book (plague, pediatric medicine, clinical practice, hypochondria etc.).
133 The encyclopaedic character has been noticed also within the works of Yohanan Alemmano, Abraham Yagel, Joseph Delmedigo, Abraham Portaleone, David de Pomis, Isaac Lampronti.

ogy and natural philosophy. This text incorporated very recent medical and scientific insights (e.g. Paracelsian ideas, physiological chemistry), while also defending the mastery of the university-trained physician and trying to demonstrate that the learned world of the Jews kept track with that of their surrounding European cultures.[134]

Recently, more studies have focused on Isaac Lampronti (1679–1756) who served as a rabbi and head of the Talmud academy in Ferrara. Besides his duties as a religious leader, he also kept working as a physician. Scholars have stressed that in the first alphabetic encyclopaedia on Talmudic traditions, *Paḥad Yitzḥak (The Fear of Isaac)*, Lampronti linked his halakhic erudition with his medical training and broader scientific interests in manifold ways. This project transformed the organization of religious knowledge and utilized contemporary scientific knowledge, especially empiricism, for his discussion of traditional sources.[135]

The prominent role and elitist self-assessment of conversos like Amatus Lusitanus (1511–68), (Abraham) Zacutus Lusitanus (1575–1642) or Rodrigo de Castro (1550–1627) and his son Benedict (1597–1684) has been the focus of several chapter-long studies.[136] Besides those major scholarly lines of inquiry, we find some studies which mostly addressed the social history of medical practitioners in a specific city or region[137], while others with a similar focus or a more biographic approach strive to analyze Jewish medical practitioners against the backdrop of Enlightenment culture.[138] Others studies have also highlighted the necessity to look beyond the elite group of university-trained Jewish doctors and their writings in order to examine the more diverse scene of Jewish and (other) medical practitioners "on the ground".[139]

5.2 Ashkenaz and Central Eastern Europe

In contrast to medieval time, the German lands and Eastern Europe took more center stage in the research of Jewish medical practice and discourse in the early modern period. One important factor was the influx of Jews and *conversos* after the expulsions from the Iberian Peninsula. Doctors of Sephardic origin, with its longstanding medical tradition, were allowed to practice medicine in various places, such as Amsterdam, London and Hamburg, often forming whole 'dynasties' of physicians. Beyond their own community, they were also serving people of high rank, such as clergy, local

---

134 Ruderman 1995, esp. 229–255 (ch. 8: *On the Diffusion of Scientific Knowledge within the Jewish Community. The medical textbook of Tobias Cohen*); Ruderman 2001; Lepicard 2008; Zinger 2009/10. On earlier and shorter studies of Cohen's life and work, see Ruderman 1995, p. 229, n. 2.

135 Cf. Ruderman 1995, 256–272 (ch. 9: *Contemporary Science and Jewish Law in the Eyes of Isaac Lampronti and His Rabbinic Interlocutors*), and ibid., p. 256–57, n. 2 for earlier studies on Lampronti; for a fresh inquiry, see Glasberg Gail 2016, 2017.

136 Cf. Ruderman 1995, 273–309 (ch. 10: *The Community of Converso Physicians. Race, Medicine, and the Shaping of a Cultural Identity*); Gutwirth 2004; Berns 2014, 37–70; Salomon 1901; Feingold 1994.

137 Cf. Friedenwald 1922; Rothman 2013; and Ravid 2004 (Venice).

138 Cf. Dubin 2012; Bregoli 2014 (esp. ch. 4: *Jewish Physicians and the Pursuit of the Public Good*).

139 Cf. the approach of Zinger 2009/10, partly based on Zimmels 1952; and Rothman 2013.

elites, but also dukes, earls and even members of the royal family in Denmark or the Netherlands. They were also involved in other intellectual endeavors and published medical and other works in Spanish, Portuguese, Hebrew, and Latin.[140]

Similar to the situation in Northern Italy, scholars have pointed to changing socio-political circumstances and an increasing academization of Jewish medical practitioners who studied first at Padua, then at Leiden and later in different other places.[141] This is reflected in the already mentioned constant exchange of texts and ideas across the European and Ottoman spheres, facilitated through printed books and the travel of such figures as Joseph Demedigo or Tuviah Cohen. The medical (as well as the general) history of the Jews in Frankfurt am Main, where Delmedigo practiced for a while, has been the subject of several studies focusing on the local institutions and competition with several Christian groups.[142] In addition, scholars have explored the development of Jewish medical engagement in Germany from medieval to modern times or inquired into the representation and image of 'the Jewish physician'.[143]

Research regarding the new cultural centers of Central and Eastern Europe (e. g. Prague, Krakow, Vilna) have noticed that contemporary medical and scientific, especially astronomical, developments penetrated the halakhic discourse of rabbis like Moses Isserles, the Maharal of Prague, David Gans, Mordechai Jaffe, Yom-Tov Lipmann Heller, Ephraim Luntshitz, Jacob Emden or his rival Jonathan Eybeschütz. Some of those Talmudic scholars openly embraced scientific inquiry, while others at least showed a high degree of openness and interest in these matters that served to clarify questions of halakha.[144] The philological, material and literary aspects of the medical works written in these regions is still decidedly understudied. These include brief or rather comprehensive medical handbooks (*Segulot u-Refu'ot*) like those composed by Moshe ben Benjamin Ze'ev of Kalish, Abraham and Leib Wallich (*Sepher Dimyon ha-Refu'ot*) and Isaach Teller, the treatises by Eliezer Eilburg or simpler books of remedies or medical advice for women, often in Yiddish.[145] Another area of

---

140 Two such medical families were the Buenos in Amsterdam and the de Castros in Hamburg. Benjamin Musaphia, another Padua-trained Jew, served as a physician to the Danish court. Cf. Arrizabalaga 2009; and the brief biographical sketch by Weisz and Albury 2013. On Jewish physicians in the Dutch countries, see Hes 1980. Besides the already mentioned David Nieto, physician and rabbi, also other Jews or conversos flourished in early modern England. Some like Roderigo Lopez even made it into the royal court, which then as before was a particular thorny arena for Jews who faced the crudest and most sophisticated accusations. On Lopez, see Bernard 1981; Kottek 1973. Cf. also Barnett 1982 (Jacob de Castro Sarmento); Collins 2019 (Philip De la Cour).

141 Cf. Collins 2013.

142 Cf. Kottek 1979; Levi 1998; Treue 1998 (387–389 on Wallich), 1999 (46–48 on Wallich); Leibowitz 1972/73.

143 Cf. Hortzitz 1994; Efron 2001.

144 For some primary sources, see Ruderman 1995, 272, n. 58. Cf. also Ruderman 1995, 54–99 (Chapter 2: The Legitimation of Scientific Activity among Central and Eastern European Jews); Cowen 2013 (Maharal and Habad); Sariel 2018.

145 On Abraham and his son Leib Wallich, another medical student at Padua, and his family, see Treue 1998, 1999 (details above n. 146). On the genre of the medical practical handbook, see

research to be explored further looks into the role of Karaite physicians and their links to other Jews (e.g. Delmedigo) and Eastern European Christian colleagues, noblemen and royalty.[146] Most recently, several studies have begun to approach the topic with a grassroots approach that pays more attention to the voices and roles of patients, the competition between different medical practitioners, and encounters between Jews and Christians in everyday medical culture.[147] Finally, several studies have dealt with the role of medical knowledge and physicians within the period of Enlightenment. Many of the Haskalah thinkers who endorsed Jewish engagement with the new sciences and argued for a clear compartmentalized nature of science and religion were, in fact, university trained physicians who also published medical and other texts in Hebrew and in different European vernaculars. In the spirit of the Haskalah, they often stressed the pride in Jewish cultural traditions, while sharply critiquing traditional forms of living and religious customs, especially in the field of public health, sexuality, diet, and social dimensions of hygiene.[148]

5.3 Ottoman Empire

Jewish medical practitioners played also an important role in the Mediterranean East. The prominent position of Israel Conegliano and Tuviah Cohen as high-rank physicians and Jospeh Delmedigo's travels have been partly noticed by scholars as important cultural intermediaries between the Ottoman Empire and Western Europe, in particular Italy (Venice) and Eastern Europe.[149] Scholars have concentrated on Jewish interaction with aspects of Ottoman medical discourse, on the socio-medical relations between Jews and Muslims, while others studied the history and scope of medical and scientific treatises.[150]

5.4 Other places, new sources and broader questions

Besides those main geographical areas, the historical development in the early modern period brought about Jewish medical exchange with other continents. So far, a few studies have addressed new *materia medica* available from the Far East or the Americas as well as Jewish medical practitioners, mainly from or in North America.[151]

Efron 2001, esp. 80–86. Cf. also the survey in Assion 1983; and the detailed studies by Geller 2009 (Yiddish remedy books); Baumgarten 2009 (Isaach Baer Teller); and Jánošíková 2019 (Eliezer Eilburg).

146 For one recent study, see Kizilov 2011.

147 Cf. Jütte 1995, 2005; Kaspina 2006; Zinger 2009; Tuszewicki 2014.

148 Cf. Wolff 2014. On three main figures (Israel ben Moses Ha-Levi of Zamość, Aaron Solomon Gumpertz, Mordechai Gumpel Schnaber Levinson), see Ruderman 1995, 332–368 (Chapter 12: *Physico-Theology and Jewish Thought at the End of the Eighteenth Century*). Cf. also Jütte 2005, 2007; Freudenthal 2003 (Gumpertz), 2007 (Israel ben Moses Ha-Levi of Zamość).

149 Cf. Shefer 2009/10; Murphy 2002.

150 Cf. ibid.; Shemesh 2013; Erdemir 2011; Gutwirth 2001; Langermann 2007, 2009 (on *Ta'alumot Ḥokmah*).

151 Cf. Langermann 2019; Kagan 1934; Collins 2014.

Finally, one has to notice a rather new and growing field of inquiry engaging with the role of medical and other scientific knowledge in mystical, Kabbalistic and Hasidic traditions from medieval time and, in particular, from the Early Modern period onward.[152] Kabbalistic thinkers often interwove ideas of the divine, cosmological order with thoughts about the microcosmic human body, thus applying the idea of repair (*tiqun*) to body, soul, and the world.[153] While this was a crucial component of Lurianic Kabbalah as transmitted in the work of Hayim Vital and his students, scholars have shown that these works drew on contemporary technical medical knowledge.[154] Moreover, these texts contained a considerable amount of practical medicine and recipes from other fields of knowledge. The increased mobility of scholars (e.g. Moses Zacuto) and ideas contributed to a dynamic network of knowledge making spanning from Palestine and Italy to Amsterdam and Central Eastern Europe.[155] Another interesting branch of studies addresses the engagement of Hasidic rabbis, most prominently among them the *Baal Shem Tov* (R. Israel ben Eliezer), with learned medicine and so-called 'popular' medical knowledge. In Hasidic writings, often handbooks for practical medicine, herbal and pharmaceutical approaches merged with astrological and religious-spiritual therapies, sometimes including exorcisms. In addition, numerous narratives portrayed these Hasidic teachers as healers performing regular as well as miraculous healing.[156]

The discussion here and in the previous chapter has outlined the main trajectories of the broader interest in and academic scholarship of medical knowledge and discourse on bodies, health, illness, and disability in Jewish traditions from its inception in the 19th century until the very recent past. This sketch of the state of the art, necessarily confined to premodern times, demonstrated the various approaches taken and the many questions tackled by earlier and contemporary scholars. Still, it has also pointed to many sources that are still unexplored, to the rich material for diachronic and trans-disciplinary comparative work, and to the need of reexamination of known traditions with the help of new approaches. Future research will hopefully continue to explore the many ways in which Jewish medical knowledge and practices were transferred, transmitted and transformed across time, languages, and cultures.

---

152 For mystical-medical ideas in medieval religious thought (Naḥmanides, Moshe ben-Shem Tov/Moses Leon, Isaac the Blind), see Koren 2004. Preis 1928 is an early and brief study of medicine in the Zohar and other kabalistic traditions.

153 Cf. Fine 2003; Garb 2015 (also on more recent developments).

154 On the relations between Kabbalah, medicine and other sciences, see Meroz 1982; Ruderman 1988; Tamari 2016. On practical sciences and medicine and Kabbalistic epistemic texts, see Bos 1994a, 1996; Buchman and Amar 2006.

155 On this, see Petrovsky-Shtern 2011; Chajes 2003; and the ERC-funded project (2018–2023) at Freie Universität Berlin *"Patterns of Knowledge Circulation: The Transmission and Reception of Jewish Esoteric Knowledge in Manuscript and Print in Early Modern East-Central Europe"*, directed by Dr. Agata Paluch.

156 Cf. Saye 1936; Zinger 2008, 2009.

Medical Knowledge in Premodern Jewish Cultures and Traditions: Selected Bibliography

Lennart Lehmhaus

The following bibliography has two main functions. First, it serves as a long reference list for the editions and literature mentioned in the footnotes of the two preceding chapters. Second, together with the discussion in these previous chapters it shall provide an entrée for those who are interested in premodern Jewish medical discourse or in the history of and recent developments in pertinent scholarship from various ideological, theoretical and methodological angles. While it is neither comprehensive nor exhaustive, it includes surveys or sourcebooks (Preuss 1911/1978, Abrams 1998, Abrams and Freeman 1999; Friedenwald 1944, Jütte 2016) and earlier bibliographies (Friedenwald 1935b; Kagan 1948), in which one may find more references to earlier scholarship or to studies on specific topics. This preliminary bibliography also functions as a prelude and will most hopefully be augmented by a searchable bibliographic online-database with thematic subsections as part of my ongoing research project in the near future.

Abrams, Judith Z. 1998. *Judaism and Disability: Portrayals in Ancient Texts from the Tanach Through the Bavli.* Washington: Gallaudet University Press.

Abrams, Judith Z., and David L. Freeman, eds. 1999. *Illness and Health in the Jewish Tradition: Writings from the Bible to Today.* Philadelphia: The Jewish Publication Society.

Ackermann, Herrmann. 1986 "Moses Maimonides (1135–1204): Ärztliche Tätigkeit und medizinische Schriften." *Sudhoffs Archiv* 70,1: 44–63.

Ackerknecht, Erwin H. 1981. "Jüdische Ärzte als Gestalter der Weltmedizin." *Gesnerus: Swiss Journal of the history of medicine and sciences* 38: 127–133.

Aslanov, Cyrill. 2011a. "Latin in Hebrew Letters: The Transliteration/Transcription/Translation of a Compendium of Arnaldus de Villa Nova's *Speculum medicinae.*" In *Latin-into-Hebrew: Studies and Texts. Vol. 1, Studies.* Edited by Resianne Fontaine and Gad Freudenthal. Leiden: Brill. Pages 45–58.

Aslanov, Cyrill. 2011b. "From Latin into Hebrew through the Romance Vernaculars: The Creation of an Interlanguage Written in Hebrew Characters." In *Latin-into-Hebrew: Studies and Texts. Vol. 1, Studie*s. Edited by Resianne Fontaine and Gad Freudenthal. Leiden: Brill. Pages 69–84.

Alexander, Philip. 2002. "Enoch and the Beginnings of Jewish Interest in Natural Science". In *The Wisdom Texts from Qumran and the Development of the Sapiential Thought.* Edited

DOI: 10.13173/9783447108263.057

by Charlotte Hempel, Armin Lange, and Herman Lichtenberger. Leuven: Leuven University Press and Peeters. Pages 223–243.

Allan, Nigel. 2001. "The Physician in Ancient Israel: His Status and Function." *Medical History* 45: 377–394.

Altbauer-Rudnik, Michal. 2013. "Love for All: The Medical Discussion of Lovesickness in Jacob Zahalon's The Treasure of Life (Otzar ha-Ḥayyim)." In *Knowledge and Religion in Early Modern Europe. Studies in Honor of Michael Heyd*. Edited by Asaph Ben-Tov et al. Leiden: Brill. Pages 87–115.

Alteras, Isaac. 1978. "Jewish physicians in Southern France during the thirteenth and fourteenth centuries." *Jewish Quarterly Review* 68,4: 209–223.

Amar, Zohar and Yaron Serri. 2000/01. "Compilation from Jonah Ibn Ǧanāḥ's Dictionary of Medical Terms." *Leshonenu* 63: 279–291. [In Hebrew]

Amar, Zohar and Yaron Serri. 2001. "Ibn Biklarish, One of Spain's Eminent Physicians." *Koroth* 15: 79–91. [In Hebrew]

Amar, Zohar and Yael Buchman. 2004. *Nathan Joel Falaquera, Sori ha-guf.* Ramat-Gan: Bar Ilan University Press. [In Hebrew]

Amasuno, Marcelino V. 1996. "The Converso Physician in the Anti-Jewish Controversy in Fourteenth-Fifteenth Century Castile." In *Medicine and Medical Ethics in Medieval and Early Modern Spain: An Intercultural Approach.* Edited by Luis Garcia-Ballester and Samuel L. Kottek. Jerusalem: Magnes. Pages 92–118.

Amit, Aaron. 2017. "Methodological pitfalls in the identification of the כוס עיקרין: a study in talmudic pharmacology." In *Collecting Recipes; Byzantine and Jewish Pharmacology in Dialogue.* Edited by Lennart Lehmhaus and Matteo Martelli. Berlin: De Gruyter. Pages 255–271.

Amit, Aaron. 2020. "The delicacy of the rabbinic *asthenes*: sickness, weakness or self-indulgence?" In *Systems of Classification in Premodern Medical Cultures. Sickness, Health, and Local Epistemologies.* Edited by Ulrike Steinert. Abingdon: Routledge. Pages 204–218.

Amsler, Monika. 2018. *"Effective Combinations of Words and Things: The Babylonian Talmud Gittin 67b–70b and the Literary Standards of Late Antiquity."* Ph.D. Dissertation, University of Zürich.

Arrizabalaga, Jon. 2009. "Medical Ideals in the Sephardic Diaspora: Rodrigo de Castro's Portrait of the Perfect Physician in early Seventeenth-Century Hamburg." *Medical History. Supplement* 29: 107–124.

Ashur, Amir. 2014. "A newly discovered Medical Recipe written by Maimonides: Mosseri I.115.1" Cambridge University Library. Cited 23 October 2017. Online: https://www.lib.cam.ac.uk/collections/departments/taylor-schechter-genizah-research-unit/fragment-month/fragment-month–17–0.

Askin, Lindsey A. 2018. *Scribal Culture in Ben Sira.* Leiden: Brill.

Assion, Peter. 1983. "Jiddische Arzneibücher." In *Die deutsche Literatur des Mittelalters. Verfasserlexikon, vol. 4.* Edited by Wolfgang Stammler. Berlin and New York: De Gruyter. Pages 523–525.

Attia, Annie. 2018. "Disease and Healing in the Book of Tobit and in Mesopotamian Medicine." In *Mesopotamian Medicine and Magic. Studies in Honor of Markham J. Geller.* Edited by Strahil V. Panayotov and Ludek Vacin. Leiden: Brill. Pages 36–68.

Avalos, Hector. 1995. *Illness and Health Care in the Ancient Near East: The Role of the Temple in Greece, Mesopotamia and Israel.* Atlanta: Scholars Press.

Avalos, Hector, Sarah Melcher, and Jeremy Schipper, eds. 2007. *This Abled Body: Rethinking Disabilities in Biblical Studies*. Atlanta: Society of Biblical Literature.

Avalos, Hector. 2014. "Nebuchadnezzar's Affliction: New Mesopotamian Parallels for Daniel 4." *Journal of Biblical Literature* 133,3: 497–507.

Baden, Joel S. and Candida Moss. 2011. "The origin and interpretation of "ṣāraʾat" in Leviticus 13–14." *Journal of Biblical Literature* 130,4: 643–662.

Baker, Cynthia. 2002. *Re-building the House of Israel. Architectures of Gender in Jewish Antiquity*. Stanford: Stanford University Press.

Balberg, Mira. 2011. "Rabbinic Authority, Medical Rhetoric, and Body Hermeneutics in Mishnah Negaʿim." *AJS Review* 35,2: 323–346.

Balberg, Mira. 2015. "In and Out of the Body: The Significance of Intestinal Disease in Rabbinic Literature." *Journal of Late Antiquity* 8,2: 273–287.

Bar-Ilan, Meir. 1999. "Medicine in The Land of Israel in the First Centuries CE." *Cathedra* 91: 31–78. [In Hebrew]

Bar-Ilan, Meir. 2001. "On the Sacred Diseases." *Korot* 15: 20–62. [In Hebrew]

Bar-Ilan, Meir. 2009. "A Woman gives a seed: Biology and Physiology among the Jews in Antiquity." *Moʿed* 19 : 12–34. [In Hebrew]

Barkai, Ron. 1991. *Les infortunes de Dinah: Le livre de la generation. La gynécologie juive au Moyen Age*. Paris: Cerf.

Barkai, Ron. 1996. "Los mʹedicos judeo-espaˊnoles y la peste negra." In *Luces y sombras de la judería europea (siglos XI–XVII)*. Edited by Juan Carrasco. Pamplona: Gobierno de Navarra. Pages 121–132.

Barkai, Ron. 1998a. *A History of Jewish Gynaecological Texts in the Middle Ages*. Leiden: Brill.

Barkai, Ron. 1998b. "Jewish Treatises on the Black Death (1350–1500): A Preliminary Study." In *Medicine from the Black Death to the French Disease*. Edited by Roger Kenneth French. Aldershot: Ashgate. Pages 6–25.

Barker, Margaret. 2001. "Hezekiah's boil." *Journal for the Study of the Old Testament* 95: 31–42.

Barnett, Richard David. 1982. "Dr Jacob de Castro Sarmento and Sephardim in medical practice in 18th-century London." *Transactions* 27: 84–114.

Barzilay, Isaac. 1974. *Yoseph Shlomo Delmedigo, Yashar of Candia: His Life, Works and Times*. Leiden: Brill.

Bar-Sela, Ariel and Hebbel E. Hoff. 1965. "Asaf on anatomy and Physiology." *Journal of the History of Medicine* 20: 358–389.

Baumgarten, Elisheva. 2004. *Mothers and Children: Jewish Family Life in Medieval Europe*. Princeton: Princeton University Press.

Baumgarten, Elisheva. 2019. "Ask the Midwives: A Hebrew Manual on Midwifery from Medieval Germany." *Social History of Medicine* 32,4: 712–733.

Baumgarten, Jean. 2009. "Un livre de médecine en yiddish: le "Beer Mayim Hayyim" d'Issachar Ber Teller (Prague, seconde moitié du XVIIe siècle)." *Revue des Etudes Juives* 168,1–2: 103–129.

Belser, Julia Watts. 2011. "Reading Talmudic Bodies: Disability, Narrative, and the Gaze in Rabbinic Judaism." In *Disability in Judaism, Christianity and Islam: Sacred Texts, Historical Traditions and Social Analysis*. Edited by Darla Schumm and Michael Stolzfus. New York: Palgrave Macmillan. Pages 5–27.

Belser, Julia Watts. 2015. "Disability, Animality, and Enslavement in Rabbinic Narratives of Bodily Restoration and Resurrection." *Journal of Late Antiquity* 8,2: 288–305.

Belser, Julia Watts. 2016. "Brides and Blemishes: Queering Women's Disability in Rabbinic Marriage Law." *Journal of the American Academy of Religion* 84,2: 1–29.

Belser, Julia W. and Lennart Lehmhaus. 2016. "Disability in Rabbinic Jewish Sources." In *Disabilities in the Ancient World*. Edited by Christian Laes. Abingdon: Routledge. Pages 434–452.

Benayahu, Meir. 1978. "R. Abraham ha-Cohen of Zante and the Group of Doctor-Poets in Padua." *Ha-Sfiut 26*: 108–140. [In Hebrew]

Bennett, Risdon. 1887. *The Diseases of the Bible*. Oxford.

Ben-Noun, Louba. 2001. "What was the disease of the legs that afflicted King Asa?" *Gerontology* 47,2: 96–99.

Ben-Noun, Louba. 2002. "What was the disease of the bones that affected King David?" *The Journals of Gerontology. Series A, Biological sciences and medical sciences* 57,3: 152–154.

Ben-Noun, Louba. 2004. "Colorectal carcinoma that afflicted King Jehoram." *Minerva Medica* 95,6: 557–561.

Bergel, Josef. 1880. *Studien über die naturwissenschaftlichen Kenntnisse der Talmudisten*. Leipzig: Verlag Wilhelm Friedrich.

Bergel, Josef. 1885. *Die Medizin der Talmudisten*. Leipzig/Vienna: Verlag Wilhelm Friedrich.

Berger, Natalia, ed. 1995. *Jews and Medicine: Religion, Culture, Science*. Tel Aviv: Beth Hatefutsoth, The Nahum Goldmann Museum of the Jewish Diapora.

Berlejung, Angelika. 2015. "Ich bin der Herr, dein Arzt": Krankheit und Heilung im Alten Orient und im Alten Testament." *Welt und Umwelt der Bibel* 76: 26–33.

Bernard, Philippa. 1981. "Roderigo Lopez—physician to the Queen [Elizabeth I]." *European Judaism* 15,2: 3–9.

Berns, Andrew D. 2011. "Abraham Portaleone and Alessandro Magno: Jewish and Christian correspondents on a monstrous birth." *European Journal of Jewish Studies* 5,1: 53–66.

Berns, Andrew D. 2012. "Judah Moscato, Abraham Portaleone, and Biblical Incense in Late Renaissance Mantua." In *Rabbi Judah Moscato and the Jewish Intellectual World of Mantua in the 16th–17th Centuries*. Edited by Giuseppe Veltri and Gianfranco Miletto. Leiden: Brill. Pages 105–119.

Berns, Andrew D. 2014. *The Bible and Natural Philosophy in Renaissance Italy: Jewish and Christian Physicians in Search of Truth*. Cambridge: Cambridge University Press.

Bhayro, Siam. 2012. "A Judaeo-Syriac medical fragment from the Cairo Genizah." *Aramaic Studies* 10,2: 153–172.

Bhayro, Siam. 2017. "The Judeo-Syriac medical fragment from the Cairo Genizah: a new edition and analysis." In *Collecting Recipes; Byzantine and Jewish Pharmacology in Dialogue*. Edited by Lennart Lehmhaus and Matteo Martelli. Berlin: De Gruyter. Pages 273–300.

Bleich, David J. 1981. *Judaism and Healing: Halakhic Perspectives*, New York: Ktav.

Blasco Orellana, Meritxell. 2011. "Magia médica o medicina mágica en los manuscritos hebreos medievales." *El Prezente*, 5: 35–54.

Blau, Ludwig (Lajos), 1898. *Das altjüdische Zauberwesen*. Strasbourg/Budapest.

Bledstein, Adrien Janis. 1992. "Was "habbiryâ" a healing ritual performed by a woman in King David's house?" *Biblical Research* 37: 15–31.

Bledstein, Adrien Janis. 2007. "David at the Cave of Adullam, Depression and Hypergraphia." In *Text and community: essays in momory of Bruce Metzger. Vol. 1*. Edited by J. Harold Ellens. Sheffield: Phoenix Press. Pages 241–250.

Blondheim, Menahem. 1982. "The obstetrical complication of Benjamin's birth—breech delivery; the cause of Rachel's death—hemorrhage from cervical/uterine tear." *Koroth* 8,5–6: 29–34.

Bodi, Daniel. 2015. "The double current and the tree of healing in Ezekiel 47:1–12 in light of Babylonian iconography and texts." *Die Welt des Orients* 45,1: 22–37.

Bohak, Gideon. 2008. *Ancient Jewish Magic. A History.* Cambridge: Cambridge University Press.

Bohak, Gideon. 2017. "Conceptualizing Demons in Late Antique Judaism." In *Demons and Illness from Antiquity to the Early-Modern Period*. Edited by Siam Bhayro and Catherine Rider. Leiden: Brill. Pages 111–133.

Bos, Gerrit. 1994a. "Hayyim Vital's Kabbalah Macasit we-Alkhimiyah (Practical Kabbalah and Alchemy), a seventeenth-century 'Book of Secrets'." *Journal of Jewish Thought and Philosophy* 4: 55–112.

Bos, Gerrit. 1994b. "Maimonides on the Preservation of Health." *Journal of the Royal Asiatic Society* 34,2: 213–235.

Bos, Gerrit. 1995a. "R. Moshe Narboni: Philosopher and Physician, a Critical Analysis of Sefer Oraḥ Ḥayyim." *Medieval Encounters* 1,2: 219–251.

Bos, Gerrit. 1995b. "Medical and para-medical manuscripts in the Cambridge Genizah Collections." *Medical History* 39,4: 516–518.

Bos, Gerrit. 1996. "Moshe Mizrachi on Popular Science in 17th-century Palestine-Syria." *Jewish Studies Quarterly* 3,3: 250–279.

Bos, Gerrit, ed. and trans. 2001–2017. *The Medical Works of Moses Maimonides*. Provo, Utah: Brigham Young University Press.

Bos, Gerrit. 2009. "Maimonides on Medicinal Measures and Weights, from His Galenic Epitomes." *Aleph* 9,2: 255–276.

Bos, Gerrit. 2010. "Medical terminology in the Hebrew tradition: Shem Tov Ben Isaac, Sefer ha-Shimmush, book 30." *Journal of Semitic Studies* 55,1: 53–101.

Bos. Gerrit. 2011a. *Novel Medical and General Hebrew Terminology from the 13th Century. Translations by Hillel Ben Samuel of Verona, Moses Ben Samuel Ibn Tibbon, Shem Tov Ben Isaac of Tortosa, and Zeraḥyah Ben Isaac Ben She'altiel Ḥen*. Oxford: Oxford University Press.

Bos, Gerrit. 2011b. With Martina Hussein, Guido Mensching, and Frank Savelsberg. *Medical Synonym Lists from Medieval Provence: Shem Tov ben Isaac of Tortosa: Sefer ha – Shimmush. Part 1: Edition and Commentary of List 1 (Hebrew – Arabic – Romance/Latin)*. Leiden: Brill.

Bos, Gerrit. 2011c. "The Black Death in Hebrew literature: *Ha-Ma'amar be-qaddahat ha-dever* (Treatise on Pestilential Fever)." *European Journal of Jewish Studies* 5,1: 1–52.

Bos, Gerrit. 2013a. *Novel Medical and General Hebrew Terminology from the 13th Century, Volume Two*. Oxford: Oxford University Press on behalf of the University of Manchester.

Bos, Gerrit. 2013b. "Nathan ha-Me'ati, Glossary to the Hebrew Translation of Ibn Sīnā, K. al-Qānūn (Canon)." *Revue des études juives* 172,3–4: 305–321.

Bos, Gerrit. 2016. *Novel Medical and General Hebrew Terminology. Volume Three, Hippocrates' Aphorisms in the Hebrew Tradition* Oxford: Oxford University Press on behalf of the University of Manchester.

Bos, Gerrit, ed. and trans. 2018–. *The Medical Works of Moses Maimonides*. Leiden: Brill.

Bos, Gerrit. 2018. *Novel Medical and General Hebrew Terminology from the 13th Century, Vol. 4*. Leiden: Brill.

Bos, Gerrit, Charles Burnett, and Tzvi Langermann. 2005. *Hebrew Medical Astrology: David Ben Yom Tov, Kelal Qaṭan: Original Hebrew Text, Medieval Latin Translation, Modern English Translation*. Philadelphia: American Philosophical Society.

Bos, Gerrit and Ivan Garofalo. 2007. "A Pseudo-Galenic Treatise on Regimen: The Hebrew and Latin Translations from Ḥunayn Ibn Isḥāq's Arabic Version." *Aleph* 7: 43–95.

Bos, Gerrit, and Resianne Fontaine. 1999. "Medico-Philosophical Controversies in Nathan B. Yo'el Falaquera's "Sefer Ṣori Ha-Guf"." *The Jewish Quarterly Review* 90,1/2: 27–60.

Bos, Gerrit and Fabian Käs. 2016. "Arabic Pharmacognostic Literature and Its Jewish Antecedents: Marwān ibn Ǧanāḥ (Rabbi Jonah), Kitāb al-Talḫīṣ." *Aleph* 16,1: 145–229.

Bos, Gerrit, Michael McVaugh, and Jospeh Shatzmiller. 2014. *Transmitting a Text Through Three Languages: The Future History of Galen's Peri Anomalou Dyskrasias*. Philadelphia: The American Philosophical Society.

Bos, Gerrit and Michael McVaugh. 2015. *Al-Razi, On the Treatment of Small Children (De curis puerorum). The Latin and Hebrew Translations*. Leiden: Brill.

Bos, Gerrit and Guido Mensching. 2005. "The Literature of Hebrew Medical Synonyms: Romance and Latin Terms and Their Identification." *Aleph* 5: 169–211.

Bos, Gerrit and Guido Mensching. 2011. "The Black Death in Hebrew Literature: Abraham ben Solomon Hen's Tractatulus de pestilential." *Jewish Studies Quarterly* 18: 32–63.

Bos, Gerrit and Guido Mensching 2015. "Arabic-romance medico-botanical glossaries in Hebrew manuscripts from the Iberian Peninsula and Italy." *Aleph*, 15,1: 9–61.

Bos, Gerrit, Martina Hussein, and Guido Mensching. 2011. *Medical Synonym Lists from Medieval Provence: Shem Tov Ben Isaac of Tortosa: Sefer Ha—Shimmush. Book 29: Part 1: Edition and Commentary of List 1*. Leiden: Brill.

Bos, Gerrit, Guido Mensching, and Julia Zwink. 2017. *Medical Glossaries in the Hebrew Tradition: Shem Tov Ben Isaac, Sefer Almansur: With a Supplement on the Romance and Latin Terminology*. Leiden: Brill.

Boss, Seev W. 1952. *Vorschriften in Thora und Talmud im Geiste moderner medizinischer Forschung*. Zürich: Jüdischer Volksschriftenverlag.

Boyarin, Daniel. 1993. *Carnal Israel: Reading Sex in Talmudic Culture*. Berkeley: University of California Press.

Brayer, Menachem M. 1969. "Psychosomatics, Hermetic Medicine, and Dream Interpretation in the Qumran Literature (Psychological and Exegetical Considerations)." *The Jewish Quarterly Review* 60,2: 112–127.

Brecher, Gideon. 1845. *Die Beschneidung der Israeliten*. Vienna.

Brecher, Gideon 1850. *Das Transcendentale, Magie und magische Heilarten im Talmud*. Vienna: Klopf und Eurich.

Bregman, Marc. 2017. "Mordecai breastfed Esther: male lactation in Midrash, medicine, and myth." In *The Faces of Torah. Studies in the Texts and Contexts of Ancient Judaism in Honor of Steven Fraade*. Edited by Christine Hayes, Tzvi Novick, and Michal Bar-Asher Siegal. Göttingen: Vandenhoeck & Ruprecht. Pages 257–274.

Bregoli, Francesca. 2014. *Mediterranean Enlightenment: Livornese Jews, Tuscan Culture, and Eighteenth-Century Reform*. Stanford: Stanford University Press.

Buchman, Yael and Zohar Amar. 2006. *Practical Medicine of Rabbi Hayyim Vital (1543–1620), Healer in the Land of Israel and Vicinity*. Ramat-Gan: Bar-Ilan University Press. [In Hebrew]

Burnett, Charles, ed. 2008. *Ibn Baklarish's Book of Simples: Medical Remedies between Three Faiths in Twelfth-Century Spain*. Oxford: Oxford University Press.

Caballero Navas, Carmen. 2004. *"The Book of Women's Love" and Jewish Medieval Medical Literature on Women: Sefer Ahavat Nashim*. London: Kegan Paul.

Caballero Navas, Carmen. 2006. "Secrets of Women: Naming Female Sexual Difference in Medieval Hebrew Medical Literature." *Nashim: A Journal of Jewish Women's Studies and Gender Issues* 12: 39–56.

Caballero Navas, Carmen. 2008a. "Medicine and Pharmacy for Women. The Encounter of Jewish Thinking and Practices with the Arabic and Christian Medical Traditions". *European Review* 16: 249–259.

Caballero Navas, Carmen. 2008b. "The Care of Women's Health: An Experience Shared by Medieval Jewish and Christian Women." *Journal of Medieval History* 34,2: 146–163.

Caballero Navas, Carmen. 2009. "Maimonides' Contribution to Women's Healthcare and His Influence On The Hebrew Gynaecological Corpus." In *Traditions of Maimonideanism*. Edited by Carlos Fraenkel. Leiden: Brill. Pages 33–50.

Caballero Navas, Carmen. 2011. "Medicine among Medieval Jews: The Science, the Art, and the Practice". In *Science in medieval Jewish cultures*. Edited by Gad Freudenthal. Cambridge: Cambridge University Press. Pages 320–342.

Caballero Navas, Carmen. 2011. "Magia para curar : amuletos, pociones y hechizos en los textos hebreos medievales dedicados a la salud femenina." In: *De cuerpos y almas en el judaísmo hispanomedieval: entre la ciencia médica y la magia sanadora*. Edited by Ricardo Izquierdo Benito and Yolanda Moreno Koch. Cuenca: Universidad de Castilla-La Mancha. Pages 149–168.

Caballero Navas, Carmen. 2013. "Maimonides and his Practice of Gynaecology." In *Moses Maimonides and His Practice of Medicine*. Edited by Kenneth Collins, Samuel Kottek, and Fred Rosner. Haifa: Maimonides Research Institute. Pages 61–84.

Caballero Navas, Carmen. 2014. "She Will Give Birth Immediately. Pregnancy and Childbirth in Medieval Hebrew Medical Texts Produced in the Mediterranean West." *Dynamis* 34,2: 377–401.

Carmoly, Eliakim. 1844. *Histoire des médecins juifs anciens et modernes*. Brussels: Société Encyclographique des Sciences Médicales.

Carny, Pinhas. 1982. "The soul ("nephesh") in the Bible; a psychosomatic unity." *Koroth* 8,5–6: 122–133.

Carter, K. Codell. 1991. "Causes of Disease and Death in the Babylonian Talmud." *Medizinhistorisches Journal* 26,1–2: 94–104.

Chajes, Yossi. 2003. "Rabbi Moses Zacuto as Exorcist: Kabbalah, Magic and Medicine in the Early Modern Period." *Pe'amim* 96: 121–142. [In Hebrew]

Charpa, Ulrich and Ute Deichmann, eds. 2007. *Jews and Sciences in German Contexts: Case Studies from the 19th and 20th Centuries*. Tübingen: Mohr Siebeck.

Chipman, Leigh. 2010. *The World of Pharmacy and Pharmacists in Mamluk Cairo*. Leiden: Brill.

Chipman, Leigh. 2013. "The Jewish presence in Arabic writings on medicine and pharmacology during the medieval period." *Religion Compass*, 7,9: 394–401.

Chrysovergi, Maria. 2011. *"Attitudes towards the Use of Medicine in Jewish Literature from the Third and Second Centuries BCE."* PhD dissertation. Durham University. Cited on 18 October 2018. Online: http://etheses.dur.ac.uk/3568/.

Cohen, Henry. 1900. *The Hygiene and Medicine of the Talmud. A lecture Delivered at the Medical Department, University of Texas, Galveston, Texas, by Rabbi Henry Cohen*. [Reprinted from The University of Texas Record, vol. III, no. 4.] Austin.

Cohen-Hanegbi, Na'ama. 2013. "Transmitting medicine across religions: Jean of Avignon's Hebrew translation of the "Lilium medicine"." In *Latin-into-Hebrew: Studies and Texts. Vol. 1, Studies*. Edited by Resianne Fontaine and Gad Freudenthal. Leiden: Brill. Pages 121–145.

Cohen-Hanegbi, Na'ama. 2019. "Learning Practice from Texts: Jews and Medicine in the Later Middle Ages." *Social History of Medicine* 32,4: 1–11.

Cohen-Hanegbi, Na'ama and Uri Melammed. 2013. "Appendix: Jean of Avignon's Introduction to His Translation of Lilium medicine, an Annotated Critical Edition and Translation." In *Latin-into-Hebrew: Studies and Texts. Vol. 1, Studies*. Edited by Resianne Fontaine and Gad Freudenthal. Leiden: Brill. Pages 146–159.

Cohn, Sigismund. 1846. *De medicina talmudica*. Dissertation. Vratislaviae (Wrocław, Poland).

Collins, Kenneth. 1999. "Isaac Israeli and His *Book of Urine*." *Scottish Medical Journal* 44,3: 86–88.

Collins, Kenneth. 2013. "Jewish Medical Students and Graduates at the Universities of Padua and Leiden: 1617–1740." *Rambam Maimonides Medical Journal* 4,1. Cited 18 June 2019. Online: https://www.ncbi.nlm.nih.gov/pmc/articles/PMC3678911/pdf/rmmj_4-1-e0003.pdf

Collins, Kenneth. 2014. "Levi Myers (1767–1822): An eighteenth-century Glasgow medical graduate from South Carolina." *Journal of Medical Biography* 24,2: 275–280.

Collins, Kenneth. 2019. "Philip De la Cour (1710–1785), a Jewish Physician in eighteenth-century London and Bath." *Journal of Medical Biography*. Cited 3 March 2020. Online: 10.1177/0967772019886760.

Colmar, Paul. 1729. *Über die Arzneigelahrtheit der Juden, so in dem alten Testamente enthalten ist*. Gera.

Contreras Mas, Antonio. 1997. *Los medicos judios en la Mallorca bajomedieval, siglos XIV–XV*. Mallorca: Miquel Font.

Cowen, Shimon Dovid. 2013. "The Torah and the worldly sciences in the teaching of the Maharal of Prague and Chabad Chassidim." In *Rabbinic Theology and Jewish Intellectual History: The Great Rabbi Loew of Prague*. Edited by Meir Seidler. London: Routledge. Pages 162–175.

Cranz; Isabel. 2018a. "Advice for a Successful Doctor's Visit: King Asa meets Ben Sira." *Catholic Biblical Quarterly*. 80,2: 231–246.

Cranz, Isabel. 2018b. "Naaman's healing and Gehazi's affliction: the magical background of 2 Kgs 5." *Vetus Testamentum* 68,4: 540–555.

Cranz, Isabel. 2021. *Royal illness and kingship ideology in the Hebrew bible*. Cambridge: Cambridge University Press.

Cutter, William, ed. 2007. *Healing and the Jewish imagination: Spiritual and practical perspectives on Judaism and health*. Woodstock, VT: Jewish Lights Publishing.

Cutter, William, ed. 2011. *Midrash and Medicine: Healing Body and Soul in the Jewish Interpretive Tradition*. Woodstock, VT: Jewish Lights Publishing.

Davidson, H.R. 2004. *"Perceptions of Medicine and Magic within the Jewish Community of Catalonia in the 13th and 14th Centuries."* Ph.D. dissertation, Hebrew University, Jerusalem. [In Hebrew]

Davis, Eli. 1982. "Biblical inscriptions on Hebrew medical amulets." *Koroth* 8,5–6: 185–188.

Davis Bledsoe, Amanda. 2012. "The Identity of the «Mad King» of Daniel 4 in Light of Ancient Near Eastern Sources." *Christianesimo nella storia* 33: 743–758.

Donaldson-Evans, Mary. 2000. *Medical Examinations: Dissecting the Doctor in French Narrative Prose, 1857–1894.* Lincoln: University of Nebraska Press.

Dorff, Elliot N. 1996. *The Jewish tradition: Religious beliefs and health care decisions.* Chicago: The Park Ridge Center for Health, Faith, and Ethics.

Doruftei, Doru C. 2018. "When the angel infuses the Soul…Some aspects of Jewish and Christian embryology in the cultural context of Late Antiquity." *Judaica* 74,1–2: 23–68.

Dubin, Lois C. 2012. "Medicine as Enlightenment cure: Benedetto Frizzi, physician to eighteenth-century Italian Jewish society." *Jewish History,* 26,1–2: 201–221.

Dubovsky, H. 1989. "The Jewish contribution to medicine. Part I. Biblical and Talmudic times to the end of the 18th century." *South African Medical Journal* 76,1: 26–28.

Duda, Michalina. 2015. "Jewish Physicians in the Teutonic Order's Prussian State in the Late Middle Ages." In *Fear and Loathing in the North: Jews and Muslims in Medieval Scandinavia* and the Baltic Region. Edited by Cordelia Heß and Jonathan Adams. Berlin/Boston: De Gruyter. Pages 127–140.

Dvorjetski, Esteé. 2002. "The medical history of Rabbi Judah the Patriarch: a linguistic analysis." *Hebrew Studies* 43: 39–55.

Dvorjetski, Esteé. 2007. *Leisure, Pleasure and Healing. Spa Culture and Medicine in Ancient Eastern Mediterranean.* Leiden: Brill.

Dvorjetski, Esteé. 2011/12. ""A leper may as well be dead" (Babylonian Talmud, Nedarim 64b): diagnosis, prognosis and methods of treatment of "leprosy" throughout the ages." *Korot* 21: 227–254.

Ebstein, Wilhelm. 1901. *Die Medizin im Alten Testament.* Stuttgart: F. Enke.

Ebstein, Wilhelm. 1903. *Die Medizin im Neuen Testament und im Talmud.* Stuttgart: F. Enke.

Efron, John M. 1994. *Defenders of the Race: Jewish Doctors and Race Science in Fin-de-siècle Europe.* New Haven: Yale University Press.

Efron, John M. 2001. *Medicine and the German Jews: A History.* New Haven: Yale University Press.

Eidelmann, Arthur I. 2006. "The Talmud and Human Lactation: The Cultural Basis for Increased Frequency and Duration of Breastfeeding Among Orthodox Women." *Breastfeeding Medicine* 1,1: 36–40.

Eilberg-Schwartz, Howard, ed. 1992. *People of the Body: Jews and Judaism from an Embodied Perspective.* Albany: SUNY Press.

Eilberg-Schwartz, Howard. 1994. *God's Phallus: And Other Problems for Men and Monotheism.* Boston: Beacon Press.

Einbinder, Susan L. 2005. "A Proper Diet: Medicine and History in Crescas Caslari's "Esther"." *Speculum* 80,2: 437–463.

Einbinder, Susan L. 2009. "Theory and practice: a Jewish physician in Paris and Avignon." *AJS Review* 33,1: 135–153.

Einbinder, Susan L. 2013. "Latin into Hebrew—twice over!: Presenting Latin scholastic medicine to a Jewish audience." In *Latin-into-Hebrew,* Vol. I. Edited by Resianne Fontaine and Gad Freudenthal. Leiden: Brill. Pages 31–44.

Eisenberg, Daniel. 2016 "Hemophilia and circumcision: from observation to classification; connecting a Talmudic presumption to a modern diagnosis." *Assia—Jewish Medical Ethics* 8,2: 30–39.

Eisenberg, Ronald L. 2019. *Jews in Medicine: Contributions to Health and Healing Through the Ages.* Jerusalem: Urim Publications.

Epstein, Gerald. 1987. "Hebraic medicine." *Advances: The Journal of Mind-Body Medicine* 4,1: 56–66.

Erdemir, Ayşegül Demirhan. 2011. "The archives exemplifying some Jewish physicians' activities of pharmaceutical treatment and surgery in the Ottoman Empire." In *Jüdische Medizin—Jüdisches in der Medizin—Medizin der Juden?* Edited by Caris-Petra Heidel. Frankfurt: Mabuse. Pages 69–76.

Feder, Yitzhaq. 2012. "The Polemic Regarding Skin Disease in "4QMMT"." *Dead Sea Discoveries* 19,1: 55–70.

Feingold, Aaron J. 1994. *Three Jewish physicians of the Renaissance: the marriage of science and ethics.* New York: American Friends of Beth Hatefutsoth.

Feinsod, Moshe. 2013/14. "A distant reflection: the physician in the eye of the Jewish medieval satirist Kalonymus Ben Kalonymus (1287–1337?)." *Korot* 22: 239–253.

Feldman, David M. 1986. *Health and medicine in the Jewish tradition: l'Hayyim--to life.* New York: Crossroad.

Fenton, Paul. 1980. "The Importance of the Cairo Genizah for the History of Medicine," *Medical History* 24: 347–348.

Fenton, Paul B. 2016. "Jonah Ibn Ganâh's Medical dictionary, the Kitâb al-talkhîs: Lost and Found." *Aleph* 16: 343–387.

Ferrario, Gabriele. 2017. "Maimonides' Book on Poisons and the Protection Against Lethal Drugs." In *Toxicology in the Middle Ages and Renaissance.* Edited by P. Wexler. London, Elsevier.

Ferre, Lola. 1994. "Los regímenes dietéticos medievales en prosa y en verso: entre la medicina y la literature." *Espacio, Tiempo y Forma,* Serie III, *Historia Medieval* 7: 327–340.

Ferre, Lola. 1995. "The Medical Work of Hunayn ben Ishaq (Johannitius) in Hebrew Translation," *Koroth* 11: 42–53.

Ferre, Dolores (Lola). 1998/99. "Hebrew Translations from Medical Treatises of Montpellier." *Koroth* 13: 21–36.

Ferre, Dolores. 2009. "Dissemination of Maimonides' Medical Writings in the Middle Age." In *Traditions of Maimonideanism.* Edited by Carlos Fraenkel. Leiden: Brill. Pages 17–31.

Ferre Cano, Dolores. 2010. "The incorporation of foreign medical literature into the medieval Jewish corpus." In *Late Medieval Jewish Identities; Iberia and Beyond.* Edited by Carmen Caballero Navas and Esperanza Alfonso. New York: Palgrave Macmillan. Pages 171–183.

Ferre, Dolores and Jose Martinez Delgado. 2015. "Arabic into Hebrew, a case study: Isaac Israeli's "Book on Fevers"." *Medieval Encounters* 21,1: 50–80.

Fine, Lawrence. 2003. *Physician of the Soul, Healer of the Cosmos: Isaac Luria and His Kabbalistic Fellowship.* Stanford: Stanford University Press.

Fonrobert, Charlotte E. 2000. *Menstrual Purity: Rabbinic and Christian Reconstructions of Biblical Gender.* Stanford, CA: Stanford University Press.

Fonrobert, Charlotte E. 2005. "On *Carnal Israel* and the Consequences: Talmudic Studies Since Foucault." *Jewish Quarterly Review* 95,3: 462–469.

Fonrobert, Charlotte E. 2006. "The Semiotics of the Sexed Body in Early Halakhic Discourse." In *Closed and Open: Readings of Rabbinic Texts.* Edited by Matthew A. Krauss. Piscataway, NJ: Gorgias Press. Pages 69–96.

Fonrobert, Charlotte E. 2007. "Regulating the Human Body: Rabbinic Legal Discourse and the Making of Jewish Gender." In *The Cambridge Companion to the Talmud and Rabbinic*

Literature. Edited by Charlotte E. Fonrobert and Martin Jaffee. Cambridge: Cambridge University Press. Pages 270–294.

Fonrobert, Charlotte E. 2008. "Blood and Law: Uterine Fluids and Rabbinic Maps of Identity." *Henoch* 30,2: 243–266.

Fontaine, Resianne. 1994. "The facts of life: The nature of the female contribution to generation according to Judah ha-Cohen's "Midrash ha-Ḥokhma" and contemporary texts." *Medizinhistorisches Journal* 29,4: 333–362.

Fontaine, Resianne and Gad Freudenthal, eds. 2013. *Latin-into-Hebrew: Texts and Studies*. Two Volumes. Leiden: Brill.

Fraisse, Ottfried. 2012. "Moses ibn Tibbon's concept of vital heat: a reassessment of peripatetic epistemology in terms of natural science." *Jewish Philosophy: Perspectives and Retrospectives*. Edited by Raphael Jospe and Dov Schwartz. Boston: Academic Studies Press. Pages 255–278.

Freeman, David L. 1998/99. "The Gittin "book of remedies"." *Korot* 13: 151–164.

Freudenthal, Gad. 2003. "New light on the physician Aaron Salomon Gumpertz: medicine, science and early Haskalah in Berlin." *Zutot* 3: 66–77.

Freudenthal, Gad. 2007. "Hebrew Medieval Science in Zamosc, ca. 1730: The Early Years of Rabbi Israel ben Moses Halevy of Zamosc." In *Sepharad in Ashkenaz: Medieval Learning and Eighteenth-Century Enlightened Jewish Discourse*. Edited by Resianne Fontaine et al. Amsterdam: Koninklijke Nederlandse Akademie. Pages 25–67.

Freudenthal, Gad. 2009. "Introduction: Science and Philosophy in Early Modern Ashkenazic Culture: Rejection, Toleration, and Appropriation." *Simon Dubnow Institute Yearbook* 8: 17–24.

Freudenthal, Gad. 2012. "Arabic into Hebrew: The Emergence of the Translation Movement in Twelfth-Century Provence and Jewish-Christian Polemic." In *Beyond Religious Borders: Interaction and Intellectual Exchange in the Medieval Islamic World*. Edited by David Freidenreich and Miriam Goldstein. Philadelphia: University of Pennsylvania Press: Pages 124–143, 203–209.

Freudenthal, Gad. 2013a. "The Father of the Latin-into-Hebrew Translations: 'Do'eg the Edomite', the Twelfth Century Repentant Convert." In *Latin-into-Hebrew: Texts and Studies*, vol. 1. Edited by Resianne Fontaine and Gad Freudenthal. Leiden: Brill. Pages 105–120.

Freudenthal, Gad. 2013b. "Abraham Ibn Ezra and Judah Ibn Tibbon as Cultural Intermediaries." In *Exchange and Transmission Across Cultural Boundaries*. Edited by Sarah Stroumsa and Haggai Ben-Shammai. Jerusalem: Israel Academy. Pages 52–81.

Freudenthal, Gad. 2013c. "Latin-into-Hebrew in the Making: Bilingual Documents in Facing Columns and their Possible Function." In *Latin-into-Hebrew: Texts and Studies*, vol. 1. Edited by Resianne Fontaine and Gad Freudenthal. Leiden: Brill. Pages 59–67.

Freudenthal, Gad. 2018a. "Science and Medicine." In *The Cambridge History of Judaism, vol. 6—The Middle Ages: The Christian World*. Edited by Robert Chazan. Cambridge: Cambridge University Press. Pages 702–741, 899–900.

Freudenthal, Gad. 2018b. "The Brighter Side of Medieval Christian-Jewish Polemical Encounters: Transfer of Medical Knowledge in the Midi (Twelfth-Fourteenth Centuries)." *Medieval Encounters* 24: 29–61.

Freudenthal, Gad and Resianne Fontaine. 2016. "Philosophy and Medicine in Jewish Provence, anno 1199: Samuel Ibn Tibbon and Doeg the Edomite translating Galen's Tegni." *Arabic Sciences and Philosophy* 26,1: 1–26.

Friedenwald, Aaron. 1897. *Jewish Physicians and the contributions of the Jews to the science of medicine*. Philadelphia.

Friedenwald, Harry. 1922. "Jewish Physicians in Italy: Their Relation to the Papal and Italian States." *Publications of the American Jewish Historical Society* 28: 133–211.

Friedenwald, Harry. 1934. "The use of Hebrew language in medical literature." *Bulletin of the Institute of the History of Medicine* 2,2: 77–111.

Friedenwald, Harry. 1935a "Moses Maimonides The Physician." *Bulletin of the Institute of the History of Medicine* 3,7: 555–584.

Friedenwald, Harry. 1935b. "The bibliography of ancient Hebrew medicine: with an introductory note." *Bulletin of The Medical Library Association* 23,3: 124–157.

Friedenwald, Harry. 1942a. "Apologetic Works of Jewish Physicians." *The Jewish Quarterly Review* 32,3: 227–255.

Friedenwald, Harry. 1942b "Apologetic Works of Jewish Physicians (Continued)." *The Jewish Quarterly Review* 32,4: 407–26.

Friedenwald, Harry. 1944. *The Jews and Medicine*. Two Volumes. Baltimore/New York: Johns Hopkins Press and Ktav Publishing.

Friedenwald, Harry. 1946. *Jewish Luminaries in Medical History. And a catalogue of works bearing on the subject of the Jews and medicine from the private library of Harry Friedenwald.* Baltimore/New York: Johns Hopkins Press and Ktav Publishing House.

Friedheim, Emanuel. 2001. "The Real Historical Meaning of the Talmudic Expression 'A Qilor Dedicated to Idolatry'." *Tarbiz* 70: 403–415. [In Hebrew]

Friedman, Ira and John Marr. 2017. "The Exodus syndemic: the epidemiology of the tenth plague." *Jewish Bible Quarterly* 45,1: 3–12.

Fröhlich, Ida. 2011. "Medicine and magic in Genesis Apocryphon. Ideas on human conception and its hindrances." *Revue de Qumran* 25: 177–198

Fröhlich, Ida. 2012. "Healing with psalms." In *Prayer and Poetry in the Dead Sea Scrolls and Related Literature. Essays in Honor of Eileen Schuller on the Occasion of Her 65th Birthday.* Edited by Jeremy Penner, Ken Penner and Cecilia Wassen. Leiden: Brill. Pages 197–215.

Fröhlich, Ida. 2013. "Magical Healing at Qumran (11Q11) and the Question of the Calendar." In *Studies on Magic and Divination in the Biblical World*. Edited by Helen R. Jacobus, Anne Katrine de Hemmer Gudme and Philippe Guillaume. Berlin: De Gruyter. Pages 39–50.

Fröhlich, Ida. 2017. "Demons and illness in Second Temple Judaism: theory and practice." In *Demons and Illness from Antiquity to the Early-Modern Period*. Edited by Siam Bhayro and Catherine Rider. Leiden: Brill. Pages 81–96.

Fuch, James L. 1990. "Jewish medical compendia and Jewish-Christian relations in early modern Europe." *Proceedings of the World Congress of Jewish Studies 10, Division B, Volume II*: 83–90.

Fuchs, James L. and Mordecai Plaut. 1988. "Jewish Medicine and Renaissance Epistemology: Ethical and Scientific Encounters." *Koroth* 9: 218–225.

Gaiser, Frederick J. 2010. *Healing in the Bible: Theological Insight for Christian Ministry*. Grand Rapids: Baker.

Garb, Jonathan. 2015. *Yearnings of the Soul: Psychological Thought in Modern Kabbalah*. Chicago: The University of Chicago Press.

Garcia Ballester, Luis. 1991. "Dietetic and pharmacological therapy: a dilemma among fourteenth-century Jewish practitioners in the Montpellier area." *Clio Medica* 22: 22–37.

Garcia-Ballester, Luis. 1994. "A Marginal Learned Medical World: Jewish, Muslim and Christian Medical Practitioners, and the Use of Arabic Medical Sources in Late Medieval Spain." In *Practical Medicine from Salerno to the Black Death*. Edited by Luis Garcia-Ballester et al. Cambridge: Cambridge University Press. Pages 353–394.

Garcia-Ballester, Luis. 1996a. "Ethical Problems in the Relationship between Doctors and Patients in Fourteenth-Century Spain: On Christian and Jewish Practitioners." In *Medicine and Medical Ethics*. Edited by Samuel Kottek and Luis Garcia-Ballester. Jerusalem: Magnes. Pages 11–32.

Garcia-Ballester, Luis. 1996b. "Minorities and Medicine in Sixteenth-Century Spain: Judaizers, 'Moriscos' and the Inquisition." In *Medicine and Medical Ethics in Medieval Spain: an intercultural approach*. Edited by Samuel Kottek and Luis Garcia-Ballester. Jerusalem: Magnes. Pages 119–135.

Garcia-Ballester, Luis. 2001. *Medicine in a multicultural society: Christian, Jewish and Muslim practitioners in the Spanish kingdoms, 1222–1610*. Aldershot: Routledge.

Garcia-Ballester, Luis, Lola Ferre, and Eduard Feliu. 1990. "Jewish Appreciation of Fourteenth-Century Scholastic Medicine." *Osiris* 6: 85–117.

Garcia Ballester, Luis and Eduard Feliu. 1993. "Las relaciones intelectuales entre medicos judios y cristianos. La traduccion hebrea de las *Medicationis Parabole* de Arnau de Vilanova, por Abraham Abigdor (ca. 1384)." *Asclepio* 45: 55–88.

Geller, Ewa. 2009. "A new portrait of early seventeenth-century Polish Jewry in an unknown Eastern-Yiddish remedy book." *European Judaism* 42,2: 62–79.

Geller, Markham J. 1995. "The Influence of Ancient Mesopotamia on Hellenistic Judaism." In *Civilizations of the Ancient Near East*. Vol. 1. Edited by Jack M. Sasson. New York: Scribner and Sons. Pages 43–54.

Geller, Markham J. 1998. "New Documents from the Dead Sea: Babylonian Science in Aramaic." In *Boundaries of the Ancient Near Eastern World: A Tribute to Cyrus H. Gordon*. Edited by Meir Lubetski, Claire Gottlieb, and Sharon Keller. Sheffield: Sheffield Academic Press. Pages 224–229.

Geller, Markham J. 2000. "An Akkadian Vademecum in the Babylonian Talmud." In *From Athens to Jerusalem. Medicine in Hellenized Jewish Lore and in Early Christian Literature*. Edited by Samuel Kottek et al. Rotterdam: Erasmus. Pages 13–32.

Geller, Markham J. 2002. "Hippocrates, Galen and the Jews: Renal Medicine in the Talmud." *American Journal of Nephrology* 22: 101–106.

Geller, Markham J. 2004a. *Akkadian Healing Therapies in the Babylonian Talmud*. Berlin: Max Planck Institute for the History of Science.

Geller, Markham J. 2004b. "Diet and Regimen in the Babylonian Talmud." In *Food and Identity in the Ancient World*. Edited by Cristiano Grottanelli and Lucio Milano. Padua: Sargon. Pages 217–242.

Geller, Markham J. 2004c. "Bloodletting in Babylonia." In *Magic and Rationality in Ancient Near Eastern and Graeco-Roman Medicine*. Edited by H.F.J. Horstmanshoff and Marten Stol. Leiden: Brill. Pages 305–324.

Geller, Markham J. 2005. "Tablets and Magic Bowls." In *Officina Magica: Essays on the Practice of Magic in Antiquity*. Edited by Shaul Shaked. Leiden and Boston: Brill. Pages 53–72.

Geller, Markham J. 2006. "Deconstructing Talmudic Magic." In *Magic and the Classical Tradition*. Edited by Charles Burnett and W.F. Ryan. London and Turin: Warburg Institute and Nino Aragno Editore. Pages 1–18.

Glasberg, Abraham, ed. 1896. *Die Beschneidung in ihrer geschichtlichen, ethnographischen, religiösen und medicinischen Bedeutung*. Berlin: C. Boas.

Glasberg Gail, Debra. 2016. *"Scientific Authority and Jewish Law in Early Modern Italy."* PhD Dissertation, Columbia University, New York.

Glasberg Gail, Debra. 2017. "Scientific Authority and Halakhah in the Paḥad Yitzḥak." In *Nuovi Studi su Isacco Lampronti: Storia, Poesia, Scienza e Halakah*, ed. Mauro Perani. Florence: Giuntina. Pages 277–285.

Goitein, Shlomo Dov. 1963. "The medical profession in the light of the Cairo Geniza Documents." *Hebrew Union College Annual* 34: 177–194.

Goitein, Shlomo Dov. 1967–1993. *A Mediterranean Society: The Jewish Community of the Arab World as Portrayed in the Documents of the Cairo Geniza*. Berkeley: University of California Press.

Goodman, Richard Merle. 1982. "A talmudic reference to a family with probable testicular feminization syndrome." *Koroth* 8,5–6: 40–47.

Gordon, Maurice Bear. 1941. "Medicine among the Ancient Hebrews." *Isis* 33,4: 454–485.

Gorlin, M. 1970. "Mental illness in biblical literature." *Proceedings (Association of Orthodox Jewish Scientists)* 2: 43–62.

Gracer, Bonnie. 2003. "What the Rabbis Heard: Deafness in the Mishnah." *Disability Studies Quarterly* 23,2: 192–205.

Green, Monica H. and Daniel Lord Smail. 2008. "The Trial of Floreta d'Ays (1403): Jews, Christians, and Obstetrics in Later Medieval Marseille." *Journal of Medieval History* 34: 185–211.

Guetta, Alessandro. 2014. *Italian Jewry in the Early Modern Era: Essays in Intellectual History*. Boston: Academic Studies Press.

Gutwirth, Eleazar. 2001. "Language and medicine in the early modern Ottoman Empire." In *Religious Confessions and the Sciences in the Sixteenth Century*. Edited by Jürgen Helm and Annette Winkelmann. Leiden: Brill, 2001. Pages 79–95.

Gutwirth, Eleazar. 2004. "Amatus Lusitanus and the location of sixteenth-century cultures." In *Cultural Intermediaries. Jewish Intellectuals in Early Modern Italy*. Edited by David B. Ruderman and Giuseppe Veltri. Philadelphia: University of Pennsylvania Press. Pages 216–238.

Hadas, Gideon. 2007. "The Balsam 'Afarsemon' and Ein Gedi during the Roman-Byzantine period." *Revue Biblique* 114,2: 161–173.

Halperin, David J. 1982. „The Book of Remedies, the canonization of the Solomonic writings, and the riddle of Pseudo-Eusebius." *Jewish Quarterly Review* 72,4: 269–292.

Hamidovic, David. 2017. "Illness and Healing through Spell and Incantation in the Dead Sea Scrolls." In *Demons and Illness From Antiquity to the Early-Modern Period*. Edited by Siam Bhayro and Catherine Rider. Leiden: Brill. Pages 97–110.

Hankoff, L. D. 1972. "Ancient Descriptions of Organic Brain Syndrome: The 'Kordiakos' of the Talmud." *American Journal of Psychiatry* 129: 233–236.

Harari, Yuval. 2017. *Jewish Magic before the Rise of Kabbalah*. Detroit: Wayne State University Press.

Harrison, Roland Kenneth. 1961. *Healing Herbs of the Bible*. Leiden: Brill.

Ḥasan-Rokem, Galit. 2013. "Conception, Pregnancy and Birth in the Rabbinic Imagination of Leviticus Rabbah 14: Preliminary Remarks." In *Ḥut shel ḥen: Studies in Ashkenazi Culture, Women's History, and the Languages of the Jews Presented to Chava Turniansky*. Edited by Israel Bartal et al. Jerusalem: Zalman Shazar Center. Pages 393–422. [In Hebrew]

Hasan-Rokem, Galit and Israel J. Yuval. 2017. "Myth, History and Eschatology in a Rabbinic Treatise on Birth." In *Talmudic Transgressions. Engaging the Work of Daniel Boyarin*. Edited by Charlotte Fonrobert et al. Leiden: Brill. Pages 243–273.

Hays, Christopher B. 2007. "Chirps from the Dust: The Affliction of Nebuchadnezzar in Daniel 4: 30 in Its Ancient Near Eastern Context." *Journal of Biblical Literature* 126,2: 305–325.

Hempel, Johannes. 1958. *Heilung als Symbol und Wirklichkeit im biblischen Schrifttum*. Göttingen: Vandenhoeck & Ruprecht.

Henze, Matthias H. 1999. *The Madness of King Nebuchadnezzar: The Ancient Near Eastern Origins and Early History of Interpretation of Daniel 4*. Leiden: Brill.

Herst, Roger E. 1973. "Maimonides as a physician." *Judaism* 22: 84–91.

Hes, Hindle S. 1980. *Jewish physicians in the Netherlands, 1600–1940*. Assen: Van Gorcum.

Heß, Cordelia. 2015. "Jews and the Black Death in Fourteenth-Century Prussia: A Search for Traces." In *Fear and Loathing in the North: Jews and Muslims in Medieval Scandinavia and the Baltic Region*. Edited by Cordelia Heß and Jonathan Adams. Berlin/Boston: De Gruyter. Pages 109–125.

Heyd, Uriel. 1964. "An unknown Turkish treatise by a Jewish physician under Suleyman the Magnificent." *Eretz-Israel* 7: 48–53.

Heynick, Frank. 2002. *Jews and Medicine: An Epic Saga*. Hoboken, NJ: Ktav.

Hezser, Catherine. 2016. "Representations of the physician in Jewish literature from Hellenistic and Roman times." In *Popular Medicine in Graeco-Roman Antiquity: Explorations*. Edited by William V. Harris. Leiden: Brill. Pages 173–197.

Hogan, Larry P. 1992. *Healing in the Second Temple Period*. Fribourg, Switzerland and Göttingen: Universitätsverlag; Vandenhoeck & Ruprecht.

Holub, David. 1880/84. *Pardes David. Toldot Rofe Israel oder Geschichte der jüdischen Ärzte und ihrer literarischen Leistungen von den ältesten Zeiten bis auf die Gegenwart*. Vienna: G. Brög.

Horst, Pieter W. van der. 2002. „The Last Jewish Patriarch(s) and Graeco-Roman Medicine." In Idem. *Japheth in the Tents of Shem: Studies on Jewish Hellenism in Antiquity*. Leuven: Peeters. Pages 27–36.

Horst, Pieter W. van der. 2012. "Bitenosh's Orgasm (1QapGen 2:9–15)." *Journal for the Study of Judaism in the Persian, Hellenistic, and Roman Period* 43,4–5: 613–628.

Horst, Pieter W. van der. 2015/16. "Seven months' children in ancient Jewish and Christian literature." *Korot* 23: 73–98.

Hortzitz, Nadine. 1994. *Der „Judenarzt": historische und sprachliche Untersuchungen zur Diskriminierung eines Berufsstands in der frühen Neuzeit*. Heidelberg: Winter.

Houtman, Alberdina. 2000. "Sin and illness in the Targum of the Prophets." In *Purity and Holiness; the Heritage of Leviticus*. Edited by Marcel Poorthuis and Joshua Schwartz. Leiden: Brill. Pages 195–206.

Hulse, E. V. 1975. "The nature of biblical 'leprosy' and the use of alternative medical terms in modern translations of the Bible." *Palestine Exploration Quarterly* 107: 87–105.

Hurowitz, Victor Avigdor. 2004. "Healing and hissing snakes: listening to Numbers 21:4–9." *Scriptura* 87: 278–287.

Iancu-Agou, Daniele. 2013. "La pratique du latin chez les médecins juifs et néophytes de Provence médiévale (XIVe–XVIe siècles)." In *Latin-into-Hebrew: Texts and Studies. Vol. 1*. Edited by Resianne Fontaine und Gad Freudenthal. Leiden: Brill. Pages 85–102.

Ilan, Tal. 2002. "'Stolen Water is Sweet': Women and their Stories between Bavli and Yerushalmi." In *The Talmud Yerushalmi and Graeco-Roman Culture III.* Edited by Peter Schäfer. Tübingen: Mohr Siebeck. Pages 185–224.

Ilan, Tal. 2006. *Silencing the Queen. The Literary Histories of Shelamzion and Other Jewish Women.* Tübingen: Mohr Siebeck.

Isaacs, Haskell D. 1990. "Medieval Judaeo-Arabic Medicine as Described in the Cairo Geniza." *Journal of the Royal Society of Medicine* 83: 734–737.

Isaacs, Haskell D. and Colin F. Baker. 1994. *Medical and Para-Medical Manuscripts in the Cambridge Genizah Collections.* Cambridge: Cambridge University Press.

Israels, Abraham Hartog. 1845. *"Tentamen historico-medicum, exhibens collectanea gynaecologica, quae ex Talmude Babylonico depromsit."* Doctoral dissertation, Gronigen.

Isserles, Justine. 2014. "Some Hygiene and Dietary Calendars in Hebrew Manuscripts from Medieval Ashkenaz." In *Time, Astronomy, and Calendars in the Jewish Tradition.* Edited by Sacha Stern and Charles Burnett. Leiden/Boston: Brill. Pages 267–326.

Isserles, Justine. 2017. "Bloodletting and Medical Astrology in Hebrew Manuscripts from Medieval Western Europe." *Sudhoffs Archiv* 101: 2–41.

Jacob, Irene and Walter Jacob, eds. 1993. *The Healing Past: Pharmaceuticals in the Biblical and Rabbinic World: Pharmaceuticals in the Biblical and Rabbanic World.* Leiden: Brill.

Jacobi, Margaret. 1998/99. "Mai gargutani? An obscure medical term in Bava Kamma 85a." *Korot* 13: 165–170.

Jacobovits, Immanuel. 1959. *Jewish medical ethics; a comparative and historical study of the Jewish religious attitude to medicine and its practice.* New York: Bloch.

Jaffe, Dan. 2015. "Talmudic polemics and incantations in the name of Jesus: Saliva as "materia medica." *Judaica* 71,4: 334–348.

Jánošíková, Magdaléna. 2019. *"Composing Hebrew Medical Literature in the Sixteenth Century: Medicine in the Life and Work of Eliezer Eilburg."* Ph.D. Dissertation. Queen Mary's College, University of London.

Jastrow, Marcus. 1926. *A dictionary of the Targumim, the Talmud Babli and Yerushalmi, and the Midrashic literature. 2 Volumes, London and New York, 1903.* Jerusalem: Horev (Reprint of the reprint by Choreb, New York, 1926).

Jütte, Robert. 1995. "Contacts at the Bedside: Jewish Physicians and Their Christian Patients." In *In and Out of the Ghetto: Jewish–Gentile Relations in Late Medieval and Early Modern Germany.* Edited by R. Po-Chia Hsia and Hartmut Lehmann. Cambridge: Cambridge University Press. Pages 137–150.

Jütte, Robert. 1996. "Zur Funktion und sozialen Stellung jüdischer "gelehrter" Ärzte im spätmittelalterlichen und frühneuzeitlichen Deutschland." In *Gelehrte im Reich. Zur Sozial- und Wirkungsgeschichte akademischer Eliten des 14. bis 16. Jahrhunderts, Zeitschrift für historische Forschung 18.* Edited by Rainer Christoph Schwinges. Berlin: Duncker & Humblot. Pages 159–179.

Jütte, Robert. 1999. "Die jüdische Medizingeschichtsschreibung im 19. Jahrhundert und die „Wissenschaft des Judentums"." *Aschkenas* 9,2: 431–446.

Jütte, Robert. 2005. „Moses Mendelssohn und seine Ärzte." In *Jüdische Welten. Juden in Deutschland vom 18. Jahrhundert bis in die Gegenwart.* Edited by Marion Kaplan and Beate Meyer. Göttingen: Wallstein. Pages 157–176.

Jütte, Robert. 2007. "'Es müssen dem Juden seine eingerosteten Ideen benommen werden'– Anmerkungen zur Rolle jüdischer Ärzte in der Haskala." *Aschkenas* 15,2: 573–581.

Jütte, Robert. 2016. *Leib und Leben im Judentum*. Berlin: Jüdischer Verlag/Suhrkamp.

Kagan, Solomon R. 1934. *Jewish contributions to medicine in America (1656–1934). With Medical Chronology, Bibliography and Sixty-nine Illustrations*. Boston: Boston Medical Publishing Company.

Kagan, Solomon R. 1948. "The Bibliography of ancient Jewish Medicine." *Bulletin of the History of Medicine* 22,4: 480–485.

Kahana-Smilansky, Hagar. 2011. "The mental faculties and the psychology of sleep and dreams.". In *Science in Medieval Jewish Cultures*. Edited by Gad Freudenthal. Cambridge/New York: Cambridge University Press. Pages 230–254.

Kahle, Erhart. 1982. "The problem of "sara'at" in the viewpoint of Samaritan exegesis." *Koroth* 8,5–6: 48–56.

Kalman, Jason. 2008. "Job the Patient/Maimonides the Physician: A Case Study in the Unity of Maimonides' Thought." *AJS Review* 32,1: 117–140.

Kasher, Rimon. 1982. "Was the prophet a physician? On the character of healing; miracles in the Bible." *Koroth* 8,5–6: 193–201.

Kasher, Rimon. 2001. "The "Sitz im Buch" of the story of Hezekiah's illness and cure (II Reg 20,1–11; Isa 38,1–22)." *Zeitschrift für die Alttestamentliche Wissenschaft (ZAW)* 113,1: 41–55.

Kaspina, Maria. 2006. "Jewish and Slavic Folk Remedies in the Popular Medicine of Eastern Europe." In *Central and East European Jews at the Crossroads of Tradition and Modernity*. Edited by J. Siauciunaite-Verbickiene and L. Lempertiene. Vilnius: Centre for Studies of the Culture and History of East European Jews. Pages 274–283.

Katzenelson, Judah L. Benjamin. 1928. *The Talmud and the Wisdom of Medicine (התלמוד וחכמת הרפואה)*. Berlin: Ḥayim. [In Hebrew]

Kedar, Dorit. 2018. *"Who Wrote the Incantation Bowls?"* Ph.D. dissertation. Freie Universität Berlin.

Keil, Gundolf. 2015. *Die deutsche Isaak-Judäus-Rezeption vom 13. bis zum 15. Jahrhundert*. Aachen: Shaker.

Kellenberger, Edgar. 2011. *Der Schutz der Einfältigen: Menschen mit einer geistigen Behinderung in der Bibel und in weiteren Quellen*. Zürich: Theologischer Verlag.

Kessler, Gwynn. 2005. "Let's Cross That Body When We Get to It: Gender and Ethnicity in Rabbinic Literature." *Journal of the American Academy of Religion*, 73,2: 329–359.

Kessler, Gwynn. 2009. *Conceiving Israel: The Fetus in Rabbinic Narratives*. Philadelphia: University of Pennsylvania Press.

Kimmel, Seth. 2016. "Tropes of Expertise and Converso Unbelief: Huarte de San Juan's History of Medicine." In *After Conversion: Iberia and the Emergence of Modernity*. Edited by Mercedes García-Arenal et al. Leiden: Brill. Pages 336–357.

Kiperwasser, Reuven. 2009. "'Three partners in a person': the genesis and development of embryological theory in biblical and rabbinic Judaism." *Lectio difficilior* 2.

Kipperwasser, Reuven. 2012. "Body of the Whore, Body of the Story and Metaphor of the Body." In *Introduction to Seder Qodashim: A Feminist Commentary on the Babylonian Talmud V*. Edited by Tal Ilan, Monika Brockhaus, and Tanja Hidde. Tübingen: Mohr Siebeck. Pages 305–319.

Kiperwasser, Reuven. 2019. ""Three Partners in a Person", The Metamorphoses of a Tradition and the History of an Idea (edited and updated version)." *Irano-Judaica* 8: 393–438.

Kizilov, Mikhail. 2011. "Karaite Physicians at the Court of the Polish Kings: Ezra ben Nisan (1595–1666) and Avraham ben Yoshiyahu (1636–1687)." In *International Symposium on the Karaite Studies*. Ankara: Bilecik Universitesi. Pages 231–256.

Klein, Michele. 1998/99. "Obstetrics in Jewish sources." *Korot* 13: 171–188.

Kollmann, Bernd. 1994. "Göttliche Offenbarung magisch-pharmakologischer Heilkunst im Buch Tobit." *Zeitschrift für die Alttestamentliche Wissenschaft* 106: 289–299.

Koren, Nathan. 1973. *Jewish Physicians: A Biographical Index*. Jerusalem: Israel Universities Press.

Koren, Sharon F. 2004. "Kabbalistic Physiology: Isaac the Blind, Nahmanides, and Moses de Leon on Menstruation." *AJS Review* 28,2: 317–339.

Koren, Sharon F. 2009. "The Menstruant as "Other" in Medieval Judaism and Christianity." *Nashim* 17: 33–59.

Kotelman, Ludwig Wilhelm Johannes. 1910. *Die Ophthalmologie bei den alten Hebräern: Aus den alt- und neuestamenlichen Schriften unter Berücksichtigung des Talmuds dargestellt.* Hamburg/Leipzig: Leopold Voss.

Kottek, Samuel. 1973. "Doctor Roderigo Lopes. Some items of medico-historical interest." *Medical History* 17,4: 400–405.

Kottek, Samuel S. 1979. "An oath taken by Jewish community physicians at Frankfurt on Main, 1656: a contribution to Jewish medical deontology." *Koroth* 7,9/10: CCIII–CCVIII.

Kottek, Samuel S., ed. 1982. "Proceedings of the first International Symposium on Medicine in the Bible, August 1981." *Koroth* 8,5–6.

Kottek, Samuel S. 1983. "The Essenes and medicine: a comparative study of medical and para-medical items with reference to ancient Jewish lore." *Clio Medica* 18: 81–99.

Kottek, Samuel S. 1984. "Medicine in Hebrew poetry—Judah Al-Harizi." *Koroth* 8,1–2: 169–179; 299–304.

Kottek, Samuel S. 1992. "The image of the insane in ancient Jewish lore." *Medicine and Law* 11,7–8: 653–660.

Kottek, Samuel S. 1993/94. ""The kidneys give advice": some thoughts on nephrology in the Talmud and Midrash." *Koroth* 10: 44–53.

Kottek. Samuel. 1994. *Medicine and Hygiene in the Works of Flavius Josephus*. Leiden: Brill.

Kottek, Samuel S. 1996a. "Hygiene and Healing among the Jews in the Post-Biblical Period: A Partial Reconstruction." *ANRW II. 37.3.* Part 2, Principat, 37.3. Edited by Hildegard Temporini and Wolfgang Haase. New York: De Gruyter. Pages 2843–2865.

Kottek, Samuel S. 1996b. "Selected Elements of Talmudic Medical Terminology, with Special Consideration to Graeco-Latin Influences and Sources." *ANRW* II. 37.3. Part 2, Principat, 37.3. Edited by Hildegard Temporini and Wolfgang Haase. New York: De Gruyter. Pages 2912–2932.

Kottek, Samuel S. 1996c. "Medical Practice and Jewish Law: Nahmanides' Sefer Torat haAdam." In *Medicine and Medical Ethics in Medieval and Early Modern Spain: An Intercultural Approach*. Edited by Samuel S. Kottek and Luis García Ballester. Jerusalem: Magnes Press. Pages 163–172.

Kottek, Samuel S. 2000a. „Talmudic and Greco-Roman data on pregnancy: a renewed examination." In *From Athens to Jerusalem. Medicine in Hellenized Jewish Lore and in Early Christian Literature*. Edited by Samuel Kottek et al. Rotterdam: Erasmus Publishing. Pages 83–98.

Kottek, Samuel S. 2000b. "Magic and healing in Hellenistic Jewish writings." *Frankfurter Judaistische Beiträge* 27: 1–16.

Kottek, Samuel S. 2000c. "Benjamin, another talmudic physician." *Israel Medical Association Journal* 2,1: 68–69.

Kottek, Samuel S. 2006. "Medical interest in ancient rabbinic literature." In *The Literature of the Sages. Second Part.* Edited by Shmuel Safrai et al. Assen: Gorcum. Pages 485–496

Kottek, Samuel. 2009. "Critical Remarks On Medical Authorities: Maimonides' Commentary On Hippocrates' Aphorisms." In *Traditions of Maimonideanism.* Edited by Carlos Fraenkel. Leiden: Brill. Pages 1–15.

Kottek, Samuel S. 2009/10. "Guglielmo Portaleone, a scion of a dynasty of Jewish physicians in the early modern period: his "Consulti medici"." *Korot* 20: 205–219.

Kottek, Samuel S. 2010. *"Amra li em*: la transmission de la médecine populaire par les femmes dans le Talmud." *Revue des Études Juives* 169,3–4: 419–437.

Kottek, Samuel S. 2011. "Josephus on poisoning and magic cures or, on the meaning of "pharmakon"." In *Flavius Josephus; Interpretation and History.* Edited by Jack Pastor, Pnina Stern, and Menahem Mor. Leiden: Brill. Pages 247–257.

Kottek, Samuel S. 2011/12. "Epilepsy in the Babylonian Talmud and in Greco-Roman sources." *Korot* 21: 343–361.

Kozodoy, Maud. 2011. "Medieval Hebrew Medical Poetry: Uses and Context." *Aleph* 11,2: 213–288.

Kozodoy, Maud. 2012. "The Physicians in Medieval Iberia (1100–1500)." In *The Jew in Medieval Iberia 1100—1500.* Edited by Jonathan S. Ray. Boston: Academic Studies Press. Pages 102–137.

Kozodoy, Maud. 2015a. "Anonymous Introductory Verse to Isaac Israeli's Book on Particular Diets." In Isaac Israeli: The Philosopher Physician. Edited by Kenneth Collins, Samuel Kottek, and Helena Paavilainen, Jerusalem: Muriel and Philip Berman Medical Library. Pages 213–216.

Kozodoy, Maud. 2015b. *The Secret Faith of Maestre Honoratus Profayt Duran and Jewish Identity in Late Medieval Iberia.* Philadelphia: University of Pennsylvania Press.

Kozodoy, Maud. 2019. "Late Medieval Jewish Physicians and their Manuscripts." *Social History of Medicine* 32,4: 734–750.

Kramer, J. E. 1933. "The Apothecary in the Bible and Religious Lore." *American Journal of Pharmacy* 105: 554–562.

Kraemer, Joel L. 2008. *Maimonides: The Life and World of One of Civilization's Greatest Minds.* New York et al.: Doubleday.

Krauss, Samuel. 1898–1899. *Griechische und lateinische Lehnwörter im Talmud, Midrasch und Targum: preisgekrönte Lösung der Lattes'schen Preisfrage.* 2 Vols. Berlin: S. Calvary.

Krauss, Samuel. 1908. *Bad und Badewesen im Talmud.* Frankfurt: J. Kauffmann.

Krauss, Samuel. 1930. *Geschichte der jüdischen Aerzte vom frühesten Mittelalter bis zur Gleichberechtigung.* Vienna: A. S. Bettelheim-Stiftung.

Kreisel, Howard. 2015. "Moses Ibn Tibbon: Translator and Philosophical Exegete." In Idem. *Judaism as Philosophy: Studies in Maimonides and the Medieval Jewish Philosophers of Provence.* Boston: Academic Studies Press. Pages 73–115.

Kudlien, Fridolf. 1985. "Jüdische Ärzte im Römischen Reich." *Medizinhistorisches Journal* 20,1–2: 36–57.

Lacerenza, Giancarlo, ed. 2004. *Sabbetay Donnolo: scienza e cultura ebraica nell'Italia del secolo X.* Naples: Università degli studi di Napoli L'Orientale.

Langermann, Y. Tzvi. 1998/99. "Some New Medical Manuscripts from St. Petersburg." *Koroth* 13: 9–20.

Langermann, Y. Tzvi. 1993. "Maimonides on the Synochous Fever." *Israel Oriental Studies* 13: 175–198.

Langermann, Y. Tzvi. 1996. "Fixing a Cost for Medical Care." In *Medicine and Medical Ethics in Medieval and Early Modern Spain: An Intercultural Approach*. Edited by Samuel S. Kottek and Luis García Ballester. Jerusalem: Magnes. Pages 154–162.

Langermann, Y. Tzvi. 2004. "From My Notebooks: Masīḥ bin Ḥakam, a Jewish-Christian (?) Physician of the Early Ninth Century." *Aleph* 4: 283–297.

Langermann, Y. Tzvi. 2006. "Medical Israiliyyat? Ancient Islamic Medical Traditions Transcribed into the Hebrew Alphabet." *Aleph* 6: 373–398.

Langermann, Y. Tzvi. 2007. "From my Notebooks: A Compendium of Renaissance Science: *Ta'alumot Ḥokmah* by Moses Galeano." *Aleph* 7: 285–318.

Langermann, Y. Tzvi. 2009a. "Medicine, Mechanics and Magic from Moses ben Judah Galeano's "Ta'alumot Ḥokmah"." *Aleph* 9,2: 353–377.

Langermann, Y. Tzvi. 2009b. "Was There No Science in Ashkenaz? The Ashkenazic Reception of Some Early-Medieval Hebrew Scientific Texts." *Simon Dubnow Institute Yearbook* 8: 67–92.

Langermann, Y. Tzvi. 2011. "From My Notebooks: Materia Medica et Magica from Animals, including a Long, Unknown Passage from al-Mas'ūdī." *Aleph* 11,1: 169–178.

Langermann, Y. Tzvi. 2014. "From My Notebooks: On Tajriba/Nissayon ("Experience"): Texts in Hebrew, Judeo-Arabic, and Arabic." *Aleph* 14,2: 147–176.

Langermann, Y. Tzvi. 2019. "Judeo-Arabic Marginalia on New Materia Medica from the New World and China." *Aleph* 19,1: 137–156.

Langermann Y. Tzvi and Gerrit Bos. 2012. "Maimonides, Treatise on Rules Regarding the Practical Part of the Medical Art." *Iberia Judaica* IV: 241–248.

Langermann, Y. Tzvi and Gerrit Bos. 2014. *Moses Maimonides: On Rules Regarding the Practical Part of the Medical Art. A Parallel English-Arabic Edition and Translation*. Provo, UT: Brigham Young University Press.

Latham, John D. 1969. "Isaac Israeli's Kitab al-Hummayat and the Latin and Castilian Texts." *Journal of Semitic Studies* 14: 80–95.

Latham, John D. and Haskell D. Isaacs, eds. 1981. *Kitab al-hummayat li-Ishaq ibn Sulayman al-Isra'ili: al-Maqala al-thalitha : fi al-sill*. Cambridge: Cambridge Middle East Centre.

Lehmhaus, Lennart. 2015. "*Listenwissenschaft* and the Encyclopedic Hermeneutics of Knowledge in Talmud and Midrash." In *In the Wake of the Compendia: Infrastructural Contexts and the Licensing of Empiricism in Ancient and Medieval Mesopotamia*. Edited by J. Cale Johnson. Berlin: De Gruyter. Pages 59–100.

Lehmhaus, Lennart. 2016a. "Canon and Authority in Greek and Talmudic Medicine." In *Wissen in Bewegung. Institution—Iteration—Transfer*. Edited by Eva Cancik-Kirschbaum and Anita Traniger. Wiesbaden: Harrassowitz. Pages 195–221 (with M. J. Geller, Ph. J. van der Eijk, M. Martelli, C. F. Salazar).

Lehmhaus, Lennart. 2016b. "Vom Körperwissen zum Wissenskörper—rabbinische Diskurse zur menschlichen Physis im Talmud." *Paragrana—Internationale Zeitschrift für Historische Anthropologie* 25,1: 255–280.

Lehmhaus, Lennart. 2017a. "Beyond the *Dreckapotheke*/Between facts and feces—Talmudic recipes and therapies in context." In *Collecting Recipes. Byzantine and Jewish Pharmacology in Dialogue*. Edited by Lennart Lehmhaus and Matteo Martelli. Berlin: De Gruyter. Pages 221–254.

Lehmhaus, Lennart. 2017b. "'Curiosity Cures the Reb': Studying Talmudic Medical Discourses in Context." *Ancient Jew Review*. Cited 11 October 2017. Online: https://www.ancientjewreview.com/articles/2017/10/2/curiosity-cures-the-reb-studying-talmudic-medical-discourses-in-context.

Lehmhaus, Lennart. 2018. "'An Amputee May Go Out with His Wooden Aid on Shabbat': Dynamics of Prosthetic Discourse in Talmudic Traditions." In *Prostheses in Antiquity*. Edited by Jane Draycott. Abingdon: Routledge. Pages 97–124.

Lehmhaus, Lennart. 2019. "Bodies of Texts, Bodies of Tradition—medical expertise and knowledge of the body among rabbinic Jews in Late Antiquity." In *Finding, Inheriting or Borrowing? Construction and Transfer of Knowledge about Man and Nature in Antiquity and the Middle Ages*. Edited by Tanja Pommerening, Jochen Althoff, and Dominik Berrens. Bielefeld: transcript. Pages 123–166.

Lehmhaus, Lennart. 2020. "Medicine and Healing | Judaism | Rabbinic Judaism." In *Encyclopedia of the Bible and its Reception (EBR)*. Edited by Barry Dov Walfish et al.; Boston/ Berlin: De Gruyter.

Lehmhaus, Lennart. 2021. "Rabbinic Perceptions and Representations of Pain and Suffering." In *Pain and Its Representation in Biblical, Post-Biblical, and Other Texts of the Ancient Eastern Mediterranean*. Edited by Michaela Bauks und Saul Olyan. Tübingen: Mohr Siebeck. Pages 209–235.

Lehmhaus, Lennart and Matteo Martelli, eds. 2017. *Collecting Recipes. Byzantine and Jewish Pharmacology in Dialogue*. Berlin/ Boston: De Gruyter.

Leibowitz, Joshua O. 1972/73. "Town physicians in Jewish social history." In *International Symposium on Society, Medicine and Law, Jerusalem, March 1972*. Edited by Heinrich Karplus. New York/Amsterdam: Elsevier. Pages 117–124.

Leibowitz, Joshua O. and Shlomo Marcus. 1984. *The Book of Medical Experiences, attributed to Abraham Ibn Ezra: Medical Theory, Rational and Magical Therapy: A Study in Medievalism*. Jerusalem: Magnes.

Leibowitz, Aryeh. 2009. "Doctors and Medical Knowledge in Tosafist Circles." *Tradition: A Journal of Orthodox Jewish Thought* 42,2: 19–34.

Lepicard, Etienne. 2010. "The Embryo in Ancient Rabbinic Literature: Between Religious Law and Didactic Narratives: An Interpretive Essay." *History and Philosophy of the Life Sciences* 32,1: 21–41.

Lepicard, Etienne. 2008. "An Alternative to the Cosmic and Mechanic Metaphors for the Human Body? The House Illustration in Ma'aseh Tuviyah (1708)." *Medical History* 52: 93–105.

Lewicka, Paulina P. and Gad Freudenthal. 2016. "The Reception and Practice of Rationalist Medicine and Thought in Medieval Jewish Communities: East and West." In *The Routledge Handbook of Muslim-Jewish Relations*. Edited by Joseph Meri. London: Routledge. Pages 95–114.

Lev, Efraim. 2003. *Medicinal Substances in Jerusalem from Early Times to Present Day*. Oxford: Oxford University Press.

Lev, Efraim. 2004. "Work in Progress: The Research of Medical Knowledge in Cairo Genizah—Past, Present and Future." In *The Written Word Remains: The Archive and the Achievement*. Edited by Stefan Reif. Cambridge: Taylor-Schechter Genizah Research Unit. Pages 37–51.

Lev, Efraim. 2007. "Drugs held and sold by pharmacists of the Jewish community of medieval (11–14th centuries) Cairo according to lists of materia medica found at the Taylor-Schechter Genizah collection, Cambridge." *Journal of Ethnopharmacology* 110,2: 275–293.

Lev, Efraim. 2011. "A catalogue of the medical and para-medical manuscripts in the Mosseri Genizah collection." *Journal of Jewish Studies* 62,1: 121–145.

Lev, Efraim. 2015. "Botanical view of the use of plants in medieval medicine in the eastern Mediterranean according to the Cairo Genizah." *Israel Journal of Plant Sciences* 62,1–2: 122–140.

Lev, Efraim and Zohar Amar. 2006. "Reconstruction of the inventory of materia medica used by members of the Jewish community of medieval Cairo according to prescriptions found in the Taylor–Schechter Genizah collection, Cambridge." *Journal of Ethnopharmacology* 108: 428–444.

Lev, Efraim and Zohar Amar. 2007. "Practice versus Theory: Medieval *Materia Medica* according to the Cairo Genizah." *Medical History* 51: 507–526.

Lev, Ephraim and Zohar Amar. 2008. *Practical Materia Medica of the Medieval Eastern Mediterranean According to the Cairo Genizah.* Leiden: Brill.

Lev, Ephraim and Leigh Chipman. 2012. *Medical Prescriptions in the Cambridge Genizah Collections: Practical Medicine and Pharmacology in Medieval Egypt,* Leiden: Brill.

Lev, Sarra. 2007. "How the "aylonit" got her sex." *AJS Review* 31,2: 297–316.

Lev, Sarra. 2010. "They treat him as a man and see him as a woman: the tannaitic understanding of congenital eunuch." *Jewish Studies Quarterly* 17,3: 213–243.

Lev, Sarra. 2018. "The Rabbinic "Androginos" as the "Sometimes Jew": investigating a model of Jewishness." *Journal of Jewish Identities* 11,1: 75–85.

Levene, Dan. 2003. "Heal O' Israel: A Pair of Duplicate Magic Bowls from the Pergamon Museum in Berlin." *Journal of Jewish Studies* 64,1: 104–121.

Levi, Joseph. 1998. "Paracelsians versus Antiparacelsians: German Doctors against Jewish Physicians in Frankfurt am Main, 1618–1645." In *Paracelsus und seine internationale Rezeption in der frühen Neuzeit.* Edited by Heinz Schott and Ilana Zinguer. Leiden: Brill. Pages 110–130.

Levinson, Joshua. 2000. "Cultural androgyny in rabbinic literature." In *From Athens to Jerusalem. Medicine in Hellenized Jewish Lore and in Early Christian Literature.* Edited by Samuel Kottek et al. Rotterdam: Erasmus Publishing. Pages 119–140.

Levey, Martin. 1971. "The Pharmacological Table of Ibn Biklarish." *Journal of the History of Medicine and Allied Sciences* 26: 413–421.

Lieber, Elinor. 1979. "Galen: physician as philosopher; Maimonides: philosopher as physician." *Bulletin of the History of Medicine* 53,2: 268–285.

Lieber, Eleonor. 1984. "Asaf's *Book of Medicines*: a Hebrew Encyclopedia of Greek and Jewish Medicine, Possibly Compiled in Byzantium on an Indian Model." *Dumbarton Oaks Papers* 38: 233–249.

Lieber, Elinor. 2000. "Medicine versus Religion in the Works of Maimonides." *Oriente Moderno* 19,3: 577–590.

Lincicum, David. 2013. "Philo and the Physiognomic Tradition." *Journal for the Study of Judaism in the Persian, Hellenistic, and Roman Period* 44,1: 57–86.

Lindström, Frederik. 1994. *Suffering and Sin. Interpretations of Illness in the Individual Complaint Psalms.* Stockholm: Almquist&Wiksell.

Loew, Immanuel. 1881. *Aramaeische Pflanzennamen.* Leipzig. Repr., Hildesheim: Olms, 1973.

Loew, Immanuel. 1924–1934. *Die Flora der Juden*. 4 Vols. Vienna. Repr., Hildesheim: Olms, 1967.

Lübke, Maylin, Guido Mensching, and Gerrit Bos. 2020. *Marwān Ibn Janāḥ, on the Nomenclature of Medicinal Drugs (Kitāb Al-Talkhīṣ) (2 Vols): Edition, Translation and Comment*. Leiden: Brill.

Macht, David I. 1946. "Biblical references to cardiac pathology: Proverbs XXI, 4 and Psalms XXIV, 4." *Bulletin of the History of Medicine* 20,4: 513–526.

Malchi, A. 1928. *Thesaurus Medicus Hebraicus*. Jerusalem and Tel Aviv: Sifriya refuit..

Mancuso, Piergabriele. 2010. *Shabbatai Donnolo's Sefer Ḥakhmoni: Introduction, Critical Text, and Annotated English Translation*. Leiden: Brill.

Marcinkowski, Roman. 2002/03. "Kobieta i mężczyzna w ujeciu Talmudu." *Studia Judaica:* 5,2–6,1: 1–30.

Margalit, David S. 1962. *Ḥakhme Yisrael ke-rof'im (The Sages of Israel as Physicians)*. Jerusalem: Mosad ha-Rav Kook. [In Hebrew]

Martelli, Matteo. 2017. "Recipes ascribed to the scribe and prophet Ezra in the Byzantine and Syriac tradition." In *Collecting Recipes; Byzantine and Jewish Pharmacology in Dialogue*. Edited by Lennart Lehmhaus and Matteo Martelli. Berlin: De Gruyter. Pages 195–219.

Marx, Tzvi. 2002. *Disability in Jewish Law*. London: Routledge.

Mazor, Amir. 2014. "Jewish Court Physicians in the Mamluk Sultanate during the First Half of the 8th/14th century." *Medieval Encounters* 20: 38–65.

Mazor, Amir and Ephraim Lev. 2018. "Dynasties of Jewish Physicians in the Fatimid and Ayyubid Periods." *Hebrew Union College Annual* 89: 221–260.

McVaugh, Michael and Lola Ferre. 2000. *The 'Tabula Antidotarii' of Armengaud Blaise and Its Hebrew Translation*. Philadelphia: American Philosophical Society.

McVaugh, Michael, Gerrit Bos, and Joseph Shatzmiller. 2019. *The Regimen sanitatis of "Avenzoar". Stages in the Production of a Medieval Translation*. Leiden: Brill.

Meacham, Tirzah. 1989. *"Mishnah Tractate Niddah with Introduction—A Critical Edition with Notes on Variants, Commentary, Redaction and Chapters in Legal History and Realia."* Ph.D. dissertation. The Hebrew University of Jerusalem. [In Hebrew]

Meacham, Tirzah. 1995. "*Dam Himud*—Blood of Desire." *Koroth* 11: 82–89.

Meacham, Tirzah. 2000. "Halakhic Limitations on the Use of Slaves in Medical Examinations." In *From Athens to Jerusalem. Medicine in Hellenized Jewish Lore and in Early Christian Literature*. Edited by Samuel Kottek et al. Rotterdam: Erasmus Publishing. Pages 33–48.

Meerson, Michael. 2013. "Yeshu the physician and the child of stone: a glimpse of progressive medicine in Jewish-Christian polemics." *Jewish Studies Quarterly* 20,4: 297–314.

Meijer, Alexander 1982. "Matriarchal influence on ancient Jewish history; a medical-psychological study." *Koroth* 8,5–6: 240–247.

Melzer, Aviv. 1972. *"Asaph the Physician, the Man and His Book: A Historical-philological Study of the Medical Treatise, The Book of Drugs (Sefer Refu'ot)."* Ph.D. dissertation. University of Wisconsin, Madison.

Meroz, Ronit. 1982. "'Zelem' (image) and medicine in the Lurianic teaching (according to the writing of R. Hayim Vital)." *Koroth*, 8,5–6: 170–177.

Mesler, Katelyn. 2011. "The three magi and other Christian motifs in medieval Hebrew medical incantations: a study in the limits of faithful translation." In *Latin-into-Hebrew*. Vol I. Edited by Resianne Fontaine and Gad Freudenthal. Leiden: Brill. Pages 161–218.

Mesler, Katelyn. 2018. "An Unknown Iberian Manuscript from the Cairo Genizah: The Aphorisms of Hippocrates with the Commentary of Maimonides." *Ginzei Qedem* 14: 43–85.

Meyerhof, Max. 1938. "Medieval Jewish Physicians in the Near East, from Arabic Sources." *Isis* 28: 432–460.

Meyerhof, Max. 1977. "Jewish physicians contemporaries of Maimonides." *Koroth* 7,5–6: 392–400.

Moss, Candida and Jeremy Schipper, eds. 2011. *Disability Studies and Biblical Literature*. New York: Palgrave Macmillan.

Motzkin, Aryeh Leo. 1970. "A 13th century Jewish physician in Jerusalem: a Geniza portrait." *Muslim World* 60: 344–349.

Münz, Isaak. 1895. *Maimonides als medizinische Autorität*. Trier: Verlag Sigmund Mayer.

Münz, Isaak. 1922. *Die jüdischen Ärzte im Mittelalter: Ein Beitrag zur Kulturgeschichte des Mittelalters*. Frankfurt am Main: Kauffmann.

Muntner, Süssmann. 1940. *Contribution to the History of the Hebrew Language in Medical Instructions*. Jerusalem: Geniza. [In Hebrew]

Muntner, Süssmann. 1949. *Rabbi Shabbetai Donnolo (913–985): First Section: Medical Works*. Jerusalem: Mossad HaRav Kook. [In Hebrew]

Muntner, Süssmann 1951. "The Antiquity of Asaph the Physician and His Editorship of the Earliest Hebrew Book of Medicine." *Bulletin of the History of Medicine* 25: 101–131.

Muntner, Süssmann. 1953. *Accusations against Jewish Physicians in the Light of Medical History*. Jerusalem: Weiss Press. [In Hebrew]

Muntner, Süssmann. 1957. *Mavo le-Sefer Asaf ha-rofe* (Introduction to the Book of Asaf the Physician). Jerusalem: Genizah. [In Hebrew]

Muntner, Süssmann. 1968/1971. "Asaf ha-rofe, Sefer ha-refu'ot." *Koroth* 4: 389–443 and 531–573; *Koroth* 5: 435–473 and 603–649. [In Hebrew]

Muntner, Süssmann. 1969. "Be'iqvot ktav yad hadash [B. M. 12252] le-Sefer Asaf ha-rofe." *Koroth* 4: 731–736. [In Hebrew]

Murphy, Roads. 2002. "Jewish Contributions to Ottoman Medicine (15th-18th Centuries)." In *Jews, Turks, and Ottomans: A Shared History, Fifteenth to Twentieth Centuries*. Edited by Avigdor Levy. Syracuse, NY: Syracuse University Press. Pages 61–74.

Nägele, Susanne. 2001. *Valentin Schwendes „Buch von menicherhande geschlechtte kornnes und menicherley fruchtte". Der „Liber de diaetis particularibus" („Kitāb al-Aġḏiya") des Isaak Judäus in oberschwäbischer Übersetzung des 15. Jahrhunderts. Einleitung und kritische Textausgabe*. Würzburg: Königshausen & Neumann.

Neis, Rachel Rafael. 2017. "The Reproduction of Species: Humans, Animals and Species Nonconformity in Early Rabbinic Science." *Jewish Studies Quarterly* 24,4: 434–451.

Neis, Rachel Rafael. 2018. "Interspecies and Cross-species Generation: Limits and Potentialities in Tannaitic Reproductive Science." In *Strength to Strength: Essays in Honor of Shaye J. D. Cohen*. Edited by Michael S. Satlow. Providence, RI: Brown Judaic Studies. Pages 309–328.

Neis, Rachel Rafael. 2019. "Fetus, Flesh, Food: Generating Bodies of Knowledge in Rabbinic Science." *Journal of Ancient Judaism* 10,2: 181–210.

Neuburger, Max. 1919. *Die Medizin in Flavius Josephus*. Bad Reichenhall: Buchkunst.

Nevins, Michael. 1996. *The Jewish doctor: a narrative history*. Northvale, NJ: Jason Aronson.

Nevins, Michael. 2006. *Jewish Medicine. What it is and why it matters*. New York: iUniverse.

Newmyer, Stephen T. 1980. "Talmudic medicine: a classicist's perspective." *Judaism* 29,3: 360–367.

Newmyer, Stephen T. 1984. "Climate and health: classical and Talmudic perspectives." *Judaism* 33,4: 426–438.

Newmyer, Stephen T. 1992. "Asaph's 'Book of Remedies': Greek Science and Jewish Apologetics." *Sudhoffs Archiv* 76: 28–36.

Newmyer, Stephen T. 1996. "Talmudic Medicine and Greco-Roman Science. Crosscurrents and Resistance." *ANRW* II. 37.3. Part 2, Principat, 37.3. Edited by Hildegard Temporini and Wolfgang Haase. New York: De Gruyter. Pages 2895–2911.

Niehr, Herbert. 1991. "JHWH als Arzt. Herkunft und Geschichte einer alttestamentlichen Gottesprädikation." *Biblische Zeitschrift* 35,1: 3–17.

Niessen, Friedrich and Efraim Lev. 2006. "Addenda to Isaac's Medical and Para-Medical Manuscripts in the Cambridge Genizah Collections Together with the Edition of Two Medical Documents T-S 12.33 and T-S NS 297.56." *Hebrew Union College Annual* 77: 131–165.

Noorda, Sijbolt. 1979. "Illness and Sin, Forgiving and Healing. The Connection of Medical Treatment and Religious Beliefs in Ben Sira 38, 1–15." In *Studies in Hellenistic Religions*. Edited by M.J. Vermaseren. Leiden: Brill. Pages 215–224.

Noy, Dov. 1988. "The talmudic-midrashic "healing stories" as a narrative genre." *Koroth* 9: 124–146.

Oeming, Manfred. 2003. "Mein Herz ist durchbohrt in meinem Inneren" (Ps109,22)—Krankheit und Leid in alttestamentlicher Sicht." In Idem. *Verstehen und Glauben. Exegetische Bausteine zu einer Theologie des Alten Testaments*. Berlin: Philo. Pages 243–259.

Ohry, Avraham and Eran Dolev. 1982. "Disabilities and handicapped people in the Bible." *Koroth* 8,5–6: 63–67.

Oisteanu, Andrei. 2009. *Inventing the Jew. Antisemitic Stereotypes in Romanian and Other Central-East European Cultures*. Lincoln: University of Nebraska Press.

O'Kennedy, Daniël F. 2001. "Healing as/or forgiveness? The use of the term "rp'" in the Book of Hosea." *Old Testament Essays* 14,3: 458–474.

Olyan, Saul. 2008. *Disability in the Hebrew Bible: Interpreting Mental and Physical Differences*. Cambridge: Cambridge University Press, 2008.

Ostrer, Boris S. 2001. ""Ra'atan" disease in the context of Greek medicine." *Review of Rabbinic Judaism* 4,2: 234–248.

Ostrer, Boris S. 2002. "Leprosy: medical views of Leviticus Rabba." *Early Science and Medicine* 7,2: 138–154.

Paavilainen, Helena M. 2013/14. "Viper bite therapies in Maimonides' "On Poisons and the Protection against Lethal Drugs." *Korot* 22: 105–125.

Paavilainen, Helena M. 2015/16. "Isaac Israeli's diagnosis of consumptive fever." *Korot* 23: 295–321.

Palmer, Bernard, ed. 1986. *Medicine and the Bible*. Exeter: Paternoster Press.

Peine, Johannes. 1919. *"Die Harnschrift des Isaac Judaeus."* Medizinische Dissertation. Borna-Leipzig.

Penfield, Wilder. 1946. "Ur of the Chaldees and the Influence of Abraham on the History of Medicine." *Bulletin of the History of Medicine* 19,2: 133–147.

Perl, Eliezer and Oded Irsai. 1982. "Aspects in the biblical approach to mental sanity in old age." *Koroth* 8,5–6: 72–78.

Perlman, Moshe. 1972. "Notes on the Position of Jewish Physicians in Medieval Muslim Countries." *Israel Oriental Studies* 2: 315–319.

Petrovsky-Shtern, Yohanan. 2011. ""You will find it in the pharmacy": practical Kabbalah and natural medicine in the Polish-Lituanian Commonwealth, 1690–1750." In *Holy Dissent; Jewish and Christian Mystics in Eastern Europe*. Edited by Glenn Dynner. Detroit: Wayne State University Press. Pages 13–54.

Popovic, Mladen. 2007. *Reading the Human Body: Physiognomy and Astrology in the Dead Sea Scrolls in Hellenistic-Early Roman Period Judaism*. Leiden/Boston: Brill.

Preis, Karl. 1928. *Die Medizin in der Kabbala*. Frankfurt: Kaufmann.

Preuss, Julius. 1911/1992. *Biblisch Talmudische Medizin. Beiträge zur Geschichte der Heilkunde und der Kultur überhaupt*. Berlin: Karger. Repr., Wiesbaden: Fourier 1992.

Preuss, Julius. 1978. *Biblical and Talmudic Medicine*. Edited and Translated by Fred Rosner. New York: Sanhedrin Press. Repr., Lanham: Jason Aronson, 1993.

Preuss, Yizḥak (Julius). 2012. *The medicine in Bible and Talmud*. Translated into Hebrew by Uri Wurzburger. Jerusalem: Magnes. [In Hebrew]

Pummer, Reinhard. 1987. "Samaritan amulets from the Roman-Byzantine period and their wearers." *Revue Biblique* 94,2: 251–263.

Putzu, Vadim. 2004. *Shabbetai Donnolo: un sapiente ebreo nella Puglia bizantina altomedievale*. Cassano delle Murge, Bari: Messaggi.

Quintana Rodríguez, Aldina. 2015. "Cuatro fragmentos de otros tantos cuadernos inéditos con recetas de medicina y farmacologia sefardíes de la colección de la Genizah del JTS." In *Dameta leTamar. Studies in Honor of Tamar Alexander*. Edited by Eliezer Papo et al. Beer Sheva: Moshe David Gaon Center for Ladino Culture et al. Pages 161–190.

Rabbinowicz, Israel M. 1881. *Einleitung in die Gesetzgebung und die Medicin des Thalmuds*. Translated from French by Sigmund Mayer. Trier: Selbstverlag.

Rainbow, Jesse J. 2008. "The Derivation of kordiakos: A New Proposal." *Journal for the Study of Judaism* 39,2: 255–266.

Raphael, Rebecca. 2008. *Biblical Corpora: Representations of Disability in Hebrew Biblical Literature*. New York: T&T Clark.

Ravid, Benjamin. 2004. "In Defense of the Jewish Doctors of Venice, ca. 1670." In *Una Manna Bonna per Mantova*. Edited by Mauro Perani. Florence: Leo S. Olschki. Pages 479–506.

Reed, Annette Y. 2007. "Was there sciene in ancient Judaism?: Historical and cross-cultural reflections on "religion" and "science"." *Studies in Religion* 36,3–4: 461–495.

Reed, Annette Y. 2014. "Ancient Jewish Sciences and the Historiography of Judaism." In *Ancient Jewish Sciences and the History of Knowledge in Second Temple Literature*. Edited by Seth Sanders and Jonathan Ben-Dov. New York: New York University Press. Pages 197–256.

Reichman, Edward. 2010. "Anatomy and the doctrine of the seven-chamber uterus in rabbinic literature." *Hakirah; the Flatbush Journal of Jewish Law and Thought* 9: 245–265.

Reichman, Edward and Fred Rosner. 1996. "The Bone Called Luz." *Journal of the History of Medicine and Allied Sciences* 51: 52–65.

Richler, Benjamin. 1984. "Resources for the history of medicine at the Institute of Microfilmed Hebrew Manuscripts." *Koroth* 8,9–10: 407–413.

Robinson, James T. 2005. "The Ibn Tibbon Family: A Dynasty of Translators in Medieval Provence." In *Be'erot Yitzhak: Studies in Memory of Isadore Twersky*. Edited by Jay Harris. Cambridge, MA: Harvard University Press. Pages 193–224.

Röder, Friedhelm. 1991. "The Roman Emperor Titus—a victim of a tumor in the cerebello-pontile angle?" *Koroth* 9,11–12: 767–771.

Ronis, Sara A. 2015. ""*Do Not Go Out Alone at Night*": Law and Demonic Discourse in the *Babylonian Talmud*." Ph.D. dissertation. Yale University, New Haven.

Rosato, Emilio Giuseppe. 2013. "L'uomo microcosmo e la circolazione dei fluidi in Shabbetai Donnolo." In *Gli ebrei nella Calabria medievale. Studi in memoria di Cesare Colafemmina*. Edited by Giovanna de Sensi Sestito. Soveria Mannelli: Rubbettino. Pages 63–89.

Rosen, Tova. 2000. "Circumcised Cinderella: The Fantasies of a 14th Century Jewish Author." *Prooftexts* 20: 87–110.

Rosenstock, Eva. 2014. "Ringen mit dem Unsichtbaren: Zur Entstehungsgeschichte einer möglichen medizinischen Deutung von Jakobs Verletzung am Jabbok." *Sudhoffs Archiv* 98,2: 164–181.

Rosen-Zvi, Ishai. 2005. "Bodies and Temple: The List of Priestly Bodily Defects In Mishnah Bekhorot, Chapter 7." *Jewish Studies* 43: 49–87. [In Hebrew]

Rosen-Zvi, Ishay. 2013. "The Rise and Fall of Rabbinic Masculinity." *Jewish Studies—an Internet Journal (JSIJ)* 12: 1–22.

Rosner, Fred. 1967. "The Physician's Prayer attributed to Moses Maimonides." *Bulletin of the History of Medicine* 41: 440–454.

Rosner, Fred. 1969. "Maimonides the physician- a bibliography." *Bulletin of the History of Medicine* 43,3: 221–235.

Rosner, Fred. 1976. "Mar Samuel the Physician." *Proceedings (Association of Orthodox Jewish Scientists)* 3–4: 157–170.

Rosner, Fred. 1977. "Julius Preuss: father of Hebrew medical research." *Leo Baeck Institute Year Book* 22: 257–269.

Rosner, Fred. 1984. *Medicine in the 'Mishneh Torah' of Maimonides*. New York: Ktav.

Rosner, Fred. 1993. "Pharmacology and dietetics in the Bible and Talmud." In *The Healing Past; Pharmaceuticals in the Biblical and Rabbinic World*. Edited by Irene Jacob and Walter Jacob. Leiden: Brill. Pages 1–26.

Rosner, Fred. 1995. *Medicine in the Bible and Talmud. Selections from Classical Jewish Sources. Augmented Edition*. Hoboken, NJ: Ktav.

Rosner, Fred. 1996. "Moses Maimonides and Preventive Medicine." *Journal of the History of Medicine and Allied Sciences* 51,3: 313–324.

Rosner, Fred. 2000. *Encyclopedia of Medicine in the Bible and the Talmud*. Northvale, NJ: Jason Aronson.

Roth, Cecil. 1943. "Jewish Physicians in Medieval England." *Medical Leaves* 5: 42–45.

Roth, Cecil. 1953. "The Qualification of Jewish Physicians in the Middle Ages." *Speculum* 28,4: 834–843.

Roth, Norman. 1993/94. "Jewish and Muslim physicians of 'Ali Ibn Tashufin." *Korot* 10: 83–91.

Roth, Victor G. 1982. "Low back trauma; an orthopaedic case presentation (according to the prophet Ezekiel)." *Koroth* 8,5–6: 86–93.

Rothman, Leonard A. 2013. "Jewish Midwives in Late Renaissance Venice and the Transition to Modernity." *Nashim* 25: 75–88.

Rubin, Nissan. 1988. "Body and soul in talmudic and mishnaic sources." *Koroth* 9: 151–164.

Ruderman, David. 1987. "The Impact of Science on Jewish Culture and Society in Venice (With Special Reference to Graduates of Padua's Medical School)." In *Gli Ebrei e Venezia* *secoli XIV–XVII*I. Edited by Gaetano Cozzi. Milan: Edizioni Communita. Pages 417–448, and 540–542.

Ruderman, David. 1988. *Kabbalah, Magic, and Science: The Cultural Universe of a Sixteenth-century Jewish Physician*. Cambridge, Mass.: Harvard University Press.

Ruderman, David. 1995. *Jewish Thought and Scientific Discovery in Early Modern Europe*. New Haven/London: Yale University Press.

Ruderman, David. 1999. "Jewish Medicine and Science." In *The Encyclopedia of the renaissance*. Edited by Paul F. Grendler. New York: Scribner and Sons. Pages 310–312.

Ruderman, David. 2001. "Medicine and Scientific Thought in the Ghetto: The Cultural World of Tobias Cohen." In *The Jews of Venice: A Unique Renaissance Community*. Edited by Robert C. Davis and Benjamin Ravid. Baltimore: Johns Hopkins University Press. Pages 191–210.

Ruderman, David. 2010. *Early Modern Jewry. A New Cultural History*. Princeton: Princeton University Press.

Sabin, Albert B. 1983. "Judaism and Medicine." *Perspectives in Biology and Medicine* 26,2: 188–197.

Salomon, Max. 1901. *Amatus Lusitanus und seine Zeit. Ein Beitrag zur Geschichte der Medicin im 16. Jahrhundert*. Berlin: Verlag August Hirschwald.

Sariel, Eliezer. 2018. "'When the Rabbi Meets the Doctor': Differing Attitudes to Medical Diagnosis Among Halakhic Authorities in Eastern and Central Europe in the Sixteenth to Nineteenth Century." In *Jewish Medicine and Healthcare in Central Eastern Europe*. Edited by Marcin Moskalewicz, Ute Caumanns and Fritz Dross. Dordrecht: Springer. Pages 27–39.

Savits, Harry A. 1935. "Jacob Zahalon, and His Book, the Treasure of Life." *New England Journal of Medicine* 213:167–176.

Saye, Hyman. 1936. "Medical excerpts from Sefer Mifla'ot Elokim [The Book of God's Deeds], Joel Ba'al Shem, Naphtali Katz." *Bulletin of the Institute of the History of Medicine* 4,4: 299–33.

Scherbel, Simon. 1905. *Jüdische Ärzte und ihr Einfluss auf das Judentum*. Berlin: Singer& Co.

Schiller, Francis. 1988. "The earliest Western account of talmudic medicine." *Koroth* 9: 255–261.

Schmidt, Johann J. 1743. *Biblischer Medicus*. Züllichau.

Schwartz, Yossef. 2013. "Cultural Identity in Transmission: Language, Science, and the Medical Profession in Thirteenth-Century Italy." In *Entangled Histories: Knowledge, Authority, and Transmission in Thirteenth-Century Jewish Cultures*. Edited by Elisheva Baumgarten, Ruth Mazo Karras, and Katelyn Mesler. Philadelphia: University of Pennsylvania Press. Pages 181–203.

Secunda, Shai. 2012. "The Construction, Composition and Idealization of the Female Body in Rabbinic Literature and Parallel Iranian Texts: Three Excursuses." *Nashim* 23: 60–86.

Seide, Jacob. 1954. "Medicine and natural history in the Itinerary of Rabbi Benjamin of Tudela (1100–1177)." *Bulletin of the History of Medicine* 28,5: 401–407.

Sela, Shlomo. 2011. *Abraham Ibn Ezra on Elections, Interrogations, and Medical Astrology: A Parallel Hebrew-English Critical Edition of the Book of Elections (3 Versions), the Book of Interrogations (3 Versions), and the Book of the Luminaries*. Leiden: Brill.

Seybold, Klaus and Ulrich B. Müller. 1978. *Krankheit und Heilung*. Stuttgart: Kohlhammer.

Shatzmiller, Joseph. 1982/83 "In search of the "Book of Figures": medicine and astrology in Montpellier at the turn of the 14th century." *AJS Review* 7/8: 383–407.

Shatzmiller, Joseph. 1983. "Doctors and medical practices in Germany around the year 1200: the evidence of "Sefer Asaph"." *Proceedings—American Academy for Jewish Research* 50: 149–164.

Shatzmiller, Joseph. 1994. *Jews, Medicine and Medieval Society*. Berkeley, CA: University of California Press.

Shatzmiller, Joseph. 2016. "Apprenticeship or Academic Education: The Making of Jewish Doctors." In *Schüler und Meister. Disciples and Masters*. Edited by Andreas Speer and Thomas Jeschke. Berlin: De Gruyter. Pages 503–510.

Shapiro, Norman. 1988. "Rav Huna's views on medicine and public health." *Koroth* 9: 262–269.

Shear, Adam. 2017. "Science, medicine, and Jewish philosophy". In *The Cambridge History of Judaism. Vol. VII. The Early Modern World, 1500–1815*. Edited by Jonathan Karp and Adam Sutcliffe. Cambridge: Cambridge University Press. Pages 522–549.

Shefer, Miri. 2009/10. "Tobias the Ottoman: Tobias Cohen as an Ottoman Physician." *Korot* 20: 45–66.

Shemesh, Abraham-Ofir. 2013. "Medical relationships between Jews and non-Jews in the Ottoman Empire in pre-modern times according to rabbinic literature: halakhah and reality." In *Jews and Muslims in the Islamic World*. Edited by Bernard Dov Cooperman and Zvi Zohar. University Park, PA: Penn State University Press. Pages 303–320.

Shifman, Arie. 2002. "Bad breath—a major disability according to the Talmud." *The Israel Medical Association Journal* 4,10: 843–845.

Shinnar, Shulamit. 2019. ""The Best of Doctors Go to Hell": Rabbinic Medical Culture in Late Antiquity (200–600 CE)." Ph.D. dissertation. Columbia University, New York City.

Shoham-Steiner, Ephraim. 2006. "The Humble Sage and the Wandering Madman: Madness and Madmen in an Exemplum from *Sefer Hasidim*." *Jewish Quarterly Review* 96,1: 38–49.

Shoham-Steiner, Ephraim. 2010a. ""This should not be shown to a gentile": medico-magical texts in medieval Franco-German Jewish rabbinic manuscripts." In *Bodies of Knowledge; Cultural Interpretations of Illness and Medicine in Medieval Europe*. Edited by Sally Crawford and Christina Lee. Oxford: Archaeopress. Pages 53–59.

Shoham-Steiner, Ephraim. 2010b. "Jews and Healing at Medieval Saints' Shrines: Participation, Polemics, and Shared Cultures." *The Harvard Theological Review* 103,1: 111–129.

Shoham-Steiner, Ephraim. 2014. *On the Margins of a Minority: Leprosy, Madness, and Disability among the Jews of Medieval Europe*. Detroit: Wayne State University Press.

Shy, Hadassa. 1982. ""Ruah ra'a" (melancholy) as seen by medieval commentators and lexicographers." *Koroth* 8,5–6: 94–105.

Shyovitz, David. 2017. *A Remembrance of His Wonders: Nature and the Supernatural in Medieval Ashkenaz*. Philadelphia: University of Pennsylvania Press.

Silberman, Lou. 1990. "Dionysian Revellers." *Hebrew Studies* 31: 41–45.

Sokoloff, Michael. 1992. *A Dictionary of Jewish Palestinian Aramaic of the Byzantine Period*. Ramat Gan: Bar Ilan University Press.

Sokoloff, Michael. 2002. *A Dictionary of Jewish Babylonian Aramaic of the Talmudic and Geonic Periods*. Ramat Gan: Bar Ilan University Press.

Sperber, Daniel. 1994. "*Ligaturae* and amulets in talmudic times." In Idem, *Magic and Folklore in Rabbinic Literature*. Ramat-Gan: Bar-Ilan University Press. Pages 71–80.

Steinberg, Avraham. 2003. *Encyclopedia of Jewish Medical Ethics: A Compilation of Jewish Medical Law on All Topics of Medical Interest, Band 1*. Translated by Fred Rosner. Jerusalem: Feldheim Publishers.

Steinschneider, Moritz. 1867. "Donnolo: Pharmakologische Fragmente aus dem zehnten Jahrhundert, nebst Beiträgen nur Literatur der Salernitaner, hauptsächlich nach handschriftlichen hebräischen Quellen." *Virchows Archiv für pathologische Anatomie und Physiologie und für klinische Medicin* 38: 65–91; and 39: 296–336; and 40: 80–124.

Steinschneider, Moritz. 1885. "Eine medizinische hebräische Handschrift." *Magazin für die Wissenschaft des Judenthums* 12: 182–216.

Steinschneider, Moritz. 1896. *Schriften über Medicin in Bibel und Talmud und über jüdische Ärzte*. Sonderabdruck aus Wiener klinische Rundschau, Nr. 25 u. 26. Vienna.

Steinschneider, Moritz. 1914. "Jüdische Ärzte. Mit einer Vorbemerkung von A. Freimann." *Zeitschrift für Hebräische Bibliographie* 17: 63–96.

Stern, Samuel Miklos, 2017. "The Hebrew versions of Isaac Israeli's 'Book of Definitions' and 'Book on Spirit and Soul': critical editions (posthumous publication)." *Aleph* 17,1: 11–93.

Stern, Abraham. 1909. *Die Medizin im Talmud*. Frankfurt a. M.

Stol, Marten. 1986. "Blindness and Night-Blindness in Akkadian." *Journal of Near Eastern Studies* 45,4: 295–299.

Stol, Marten. 2000. *Birth in Babylonia and the Bible: Its Mediterranean Setting*. Groningen: Styx.

Strassfeld, Max. 2016. "Translating the Human: The Androginos in Tosefta Bikurim." *TSQ: Transgender Studies Quarterly* 3: 587–604.

Strauch Schick, Shana. 2017. "Depictions of childbirth in rabbinic literature: the innovation of a Genizah midrashic text." In *Mothers in the Jewish Cultural Imagination*. Edited by Marjorie Lehman, Jane L. Kanarek, and Simon J. Bronner. Liverpool, UK: The Littman Library of Jewish Civilization, in association with Liverpool University Press. Pages 285–306.

Strauch Schick, Shana. 2019. "From dungeon to haven: competing theories of gestation in Leviticus Rabbah and the Babylonian Talmud." *AJS Review* 43,1: 143–168.

Strauch Schick, Shana. 2021. "Do Women Emit Seed? Theories of Embryogenesis and the Regulation of Female Masturbation in Rabbinic Literature." In *Female Bodies and Female Practitioners in the Medical Traditions of the Ancient Mediterranean World*. Edited by Lennart Lehmhaus. Tübingen: Mohr Siebeck (forthcoming).

Stroumsa, Sarah. 1993. "Al-Farabi and Maimonides on Medicine as a Science." *Arabic Sciences and Philosophy* 3: 235–249.

Stuckenbruck, Loren T. 2002. "The Book of Tobit and the Problem of Magic." In *Jüdische Schriften in ihrem anti-jüdischen und urchristlichen Kontext*. Edited by Hermann Lichtenberger and Gerbern S. Oegema. Gütersloh: Gütersloher Verlagshaus.

Stuckenbruck, Loren T. 2014. *The Myth of Rebellious Angels: Studies in Second Temple Judaism and New Testament Texts*. Tübingen: Mohr Siebeck.

Sulmasy, Daniel P. 1988. "The Covenant Within the Covenant: Doctors and Patients in Sirach 38: 1–15." *The Linacre Quarterly* 55,4 (Article 6). Cited 17 July 2016. Online: http://epublications.marquette.edu/lnq/vol55/iss4/6.

Syfox, Chontel. 2018. "Israel's First Physician and Apothecary: Noah and the Origins of Medicine in the Book of *Jubilees*." *Journal for the Study of the Pseudepigrapha* 28,1: 3–23.

Tamari, Assaf. 2016. *"The Discourse of the Body in the Lurianic Kabbalah."* Dissertation. Ph.D. Dissertation. Ben-Gurion-University, Beer-Sheva. [In Hebrew]

Taube, Moshe. 2010. "Transmission of Scientific Texts in 15th-Century Eastern Knaan." *Aleph* 10,2:315–353.

Teugels, Lieve. 2016. "Whoever saves a soul saves an entire world"—*Pikuah Nefesh* in Rabbinic Literature". In *Religion and Illness*. Edited by Annette Weissenrieder and Gregor Etzelmüller. Eugene, Oregon: Cascade Books. Pages 235–260.

Tigay, Jeffrey H. 1993. "Examination of the accused bride in 4Q159: forensic medicine at Qumran." *Journal of the Ancient Near Eastern Society* 22: 129–134.

Treue, Wolfgang. 1999. "Lebensbedingungen jüdischer Ärzte in Frankfurt am Main während des Spätmittelalters und der Frühen Neuzeit." *Jahrbuch des Robert-Bosch-Instituts für Geschichte der Medizin* 17: 9–55.

Treue, Wolfgang. 2002. "Verehrt und ausgespien. Zur Geschichte jüdischer Ärzte in Aschkenas von den Anfängen bis zur Akademisierung." *Würzburger medizinhistorische Mitteilungen* 21: 139–203.

Tuszewicki, Marek. 2014. "Żydowska medycyna ludowa: pomiędzy swojskością i obcością." In *Polacy—Żydzi. Kontakty kulturowe i literackie*. Edited by Eugenia Prokop-Janiec. Kraków: Wydawnictwo Uniwersytetu Jagiellońskiego. Pages 25–56.

Tziraki-Segal, Chariklia. 2009. "Parental imprinting in ancient Greco-Roman and Jewish sources." *Korot* 19: 135–160.

Vanková, Lenka. 2018. „Krankheitsbezeichnungen in der Chirurgia des Juden von Salms." In *Sprachgeschichte und Medizingeschichte. Texte—Termini—Interpretationen*. Edited by Jörg Riecke. Berlin/Boston: De Gruyter. Pages 47–62.

Vargon, Shmuel. 2014. "The time of Hezekiah's illness and the visit of the Babylonian delegation." *Maarav; a Journal for the Study of the Northwest Semitic Languages and Literatures* 21,1–2: 37–56.

Vârtejanu-Joubert, Madalina. 2009. "The right type of knowledge: theory and experience in two passages of the Babylonian Talmud." *Korot* 19: 161–180.

Veit, Raphaela. 2003. *Das Buch der Fieber des Isaac Israeli und seine Bedeutung im lateinischen Westen: ein Beitrag zur Rezeption arabischer Wissenschaft im Abendland*. Stuttgart: Franz Steiner Verlag.

Veit, Raphaela. 2015a. "Isaac Israeli: His Treatise on Urine (De Urinis) and Its Reception in the Latin World." In: *Isaac Israeli—The Philosopher Physician*. Edited by Kenneth Collins, Samuel Kottek, and Helena Paavilainen. Jerusalem: Muriel and Philip Berman Medical Library. Pages 77–113.

Veit, Raphaela. 2015b. "Les Diètes universelles et particulières d'Isaac Israëli: Traduction et Réception dans le Monde Latin." *Revue d'Histoire des Textes* 10: 229–249.

Veit, Raphaela and Lola Ferre. 2009. "The different traditions in Isaac Israeli's Book on fevers in Medieval languages: Arabic, Latin, Hebrew and Spanish." *Aleph* 9,2: 309–344.

Veltri, Giuseppe. 1997. *Magie und Halakha: Ansätze zu einem empirischen Wissenschaftsbegriff im spätantiken und frühmittelalterlichen Judentum*. Tübingen: Mohr Siebeck.

Veltri, Giuseppe. 1998/99. "The "other" physicians: the Amorites of the rabbis and the magi of Pliny." *Korot* 13: 37–54.

Veltri, Giuseppe. 2010. "Magic and healing." In *The Oxford Handbook of Jewish Daily Life in Roman Palestine*. Edited by Catherine Hezser. Oxford: Oxford Unversity Press. Pages 587–602.

Venetianer, Ludwig. 1915–17. *Asaf Judaeus, der Aelteste Medizinische Schriftsteller in Hebraeischer Sprache*. Budapest: Alkalay.

Visi, Tamás. 2014. "Berechiah ben Natronai ha- Nakdan's Dodi ve- Nekdi and the Transfer of Scientific Knowledge from Latin to Hebrew in the Twelfth Century." *Aleph* 14: 9–75.

Visi, Tamás. 2015. "Tradition and Innovation: Isaac Israeli's Classification of Colors." In *Isaac Israeli: The Philosopher Physician*. Edited by Kenneth Collins, Samuel Kottek, and Helena Paavilainen, Jerusalem: Muriel and Philip Berman Medical Library. Pages 39–66.

Visi, Tamás. 2016a "Medieval Hebrew Uroscopic Texts: The Reception of Greek Uroscopic Texts in the Hebrew Book of Remedies Attributed to Asaf." In *Texts in Transit in the Medieval Mediterranean*. Edited by Y. Tzvi Langermann and Robert G. Morrison. Philadelphia: University of Pennsylvania Press. Pages 162–197.

Visi, Tamás. 2016b. "Plague, Persecution, and Philosophy: Avigdor Kara and the consequences of the Black Death." In *Intricate Interfaith Networks in the Middle Ages*. Edited by Ephraim Shoham-Steiner. Turnhout: Brepols. Pages 85–117.

Visi, Tamás. 2019. "Jewish Physicians in Late Medieval Ashkenaz." *Social History of Medicine* 32,4: 670–690.

Walfish, Miriam S. 2017. "Upending the Curse of Eve: A Reframing of Maternal Breastfeeding in BT Ketubot." In *Mothers in the Jewish Cultural Imagination*. Edited by Marjorie Lehman, Jane L. Kanarek, and Simon J. Bronner. Liverpool: Liverpool University Press. Pages 307–326.

Wandrey, Irina. 2003. "Fever and malaria "for real" or as a magical-literary topos?" In *Jewish Studies Between the Disciplines / Judaistik zwischen den Disziplinen. Papers in Honor of Peter Schäfer on the Occasion of His 60th Birthday*. Edited by Klaus Herrmann, Margaret Schlüter, and Giuseppe Veltri. Leiden: Brill. Pages 257–266.

Wasermann, Manfred and Samuel Kottek, Eds. 1996. *Health and Disease in the Holy Land: Ancient to Present*. Lewinston: Edwin Mellen Press.

Weindling, Gérard. 1978. "Le „Kordiacos" dans le Talmud: une des premières descriptions d'un delirium tremens." *Revue d'Histoire de la Médecine Hébraïque* 124: 13–16.

Weisz, George M. and William R. Albury. 2013. "Rembrandt's Jewish Physician—Dr Ephraim Bueno (1599–1665): A Brief Medical History." *Rambam Maimonides Medical Journal* 4,2. Cited 15 August 2017. Online: 10.5041/RMMJ.10110.

Wilensky, Mordechai L. 1990. "Health Conduct in Intercourse taken from Rabbi Moshe Maimon." *Proceedings of the American Academy for Jewish Research* 56: 101–110.

Williams, David Tudor. 1989. "The dial and the boil: some remarks on the healing of Hezekiah." *Old Testament Essays* 2,2: 29–45.

Wolff, Eberhard. 2014. *Medizin und Ärzte im deutschen Judentum der Reformära. Die Architektur einer modernen jüdischen Identität*. Göttingen: Vandenhoeck & Ruprecht.

Wood, Percival. 1920. *Moses: The Founder of Preventive Medicine*. New York: Macmillian.

Wunderbar, Reuben J. 1850. *Biblisch-talmudische Medicin. Erste Abtheilung. Allgemeine Einleitung, mit Einschluss der Geschichte und Literatur der Israelitischen Heilkunde. Materia medica und Pharmacologie der alten Israeliten*. Riga and Leipzig.

Yoeli-Tlalim, Ronit. 2018. "Exploring Persian lore in the Hebrew *Book of Asaf*." *Aleph* 18,1: 123–146.

Zier, Mark. 1992. "The Healing Power of the Hebrew Tongue. An Example from Late Thirteenth-Century England." In *Health, Disease and Healing in Medieval Culture*. Edited by Sheila Cambell et al. New York: St. Martin's Press. Pages 103–118.

Zimmels, Hirsch J. 1952. *Magicians, Theologians and Doctors: Studies in Folk-Medicine and Folk-Lore as Reflected in the Rabbinical Responsa (12th–19th Centuries)*. London: Edward Goldston & Son.

Zinger, Nimrod. 2008. "'Who Knows What the Cause is?': 'Natural' and 'Unnatural' Causes for Illness in the Writings of Ba'alei Shem, Doctors and Patients among German Jews in the Eighteenth Century." In *The Jewish Body: Corporeality, Society, and Identity in the*

Renaissance and Early Modern Period. Edited by Maria Diemling and Giuseppe Veltri. Leiden: Brill. Pages 127–55.

Zinger, Nimrod. 2009. ""Our Hearts and Spirits were Broken": The Medical World from the Perspective of German Jewish Patients in the Seventeenth and Eighteenth Centuries." *Leo Baeck Institute Year Book* 54: 59–91.

Zinger, Nimrod. 2009/10. ""Unto their Assembly, mine Honor, be not thou united": Doctor Tuviyah Cohen and the Medical Marketplace in the Early Modern Period." *Korot* 20: 67–95.

Zonta, Mauro. 2003. "A Hebrew Translation of Hippocrates' "De superfoetatione": Historical Introduction and Critical Edition." *Aleph* 3: 97–143.

Zonta, Mauro. 2011. "Medieval Hebrew Translations of Philosophical and Scientific Texts: A Chronological Table." In *Science in Medieval Jewish Cultures*. Edited by Gad Freudenthal. Cambridge: Cambridge University Press. Pages 17–73.

Zucconi, Laura M. 2010. *Can No Physician be Found? The Influence of Religion on Medical Pluralism in Ancient Egypt, Mesopotamia and Israel*. Piscataway, NJ: Gorgias Press.

Part 2:
Ancient Jewish Medical Discourses
in Comparative Perspective

A Foetus Shaped Like a Sandal:
Birth Anomalies in Talmudic Tractate Niddah

*Federico Dal Bo**

The talmudic tractate Niddah mainly deals with menstruation, as well as with a number of collateral cases, such as abnormal genital discharges, doubtful childbirths, and miscarriages. The assumption that underlies the connection between menstruation and miscarriage is that each of these issues can be formalized as a "discharge"—regardless of what is actually expelled from the woman's body.

Among these collateral issues, the case of a foetus shaped like a "sandal" is particularly interesting for the semantic difficulty it presents as well as for its juridical importance.

1 Etymology and semantics of the term סנדל/*sandāl*

First of all, the Hebrew term סנדל/*sandāl* is not difficult to interpret, for it is rather obvious. It is clearly modelled on the morphology and semantics of two almost homographic terms: the Greek term σάνδαλον /*sandalon* and the Persian term سندل /*sandal* (that is also reflected in the later Arabic صندل /*ṣandal*); accordingly, the Hebrew term סנדל/*sandāl* designates a very common open type of footwear: a "sandal."[1] Yet the linguistic *Sitz im Leben* is actually more complex when examined accurately. It is mostly complicated by the unclear, complex transmission of several morphologically related terms—mostly from the Persian and Arabic milieus—that indeed exhibit a quite diverse semantics. Indeed, there are several linguistic formations deriving from a common root, **sandal*, that are disseminated in several Eastern as well as Middle Eastern ancient languages: Sanskrit, Persian, Aramaic, Hebrew, Greek, and Arabic. These different lexemes appear to catalyze around a number of semantically discrete terms that are morphologically very close but that designate four different entities: a type of footwear, a plant, a boat, and a fish.

---

[*] A first draft of this paper was delivered, in an abridged form, as a conference paper at the European Association for Jewish Studies congress in Paris in July 2014 and then, in a longer, more elaborated form, as a workshop paper at the "Contemporary Bioethics and the History of the Unborn in Islam" (COBHUNI) at the University of Hamburg in April 2016. I would like to thank Prof. Tal Ilan (Freie Universität Berlin), Prof. Thomas Eich (University of Hamburg), Prof. Tirzah Meacham (University of Toronto), Dr. Doru Constantin Doroftei (University of Hamburg), and Dr. Lennart Lehmhaus (Freie Universität Berlin) as well as the two anonymous reviewers for reading and taking part in the discussion on my paper.

[1] See Marcus Jastrow, *A Dictionary of the Targumim, the Talmud Bavli, and Yerushalmi, and the Midrashic Literature* (London: Druglin, 1903), 1004.

DOI: 10.13173/9783447108263.093

A rapid summary of these semantic interferences might be useful in order to appreciate the complexity of the lexical issues. (See the chart in the appendix.)

First, we should clarify that the dependence of the Greek σάνδαλον/*sandalon* on the Persian سندل (lit. "sandal") is commonly accepted in Modern Greek lexicography. Yet the origins of the Persian term سندل/*sandal* are relatively obscure, due to its connections with morphologically similar terms and successive substitutions with the Arabic-based orthographic variant صندل/*ṣandal*, as it is the case in modern New Persian.[2] Semantic and morphological confusions were historically further aggravated especially by the necessity of transcribing these terms into different, poorly compatible alphabetical systems, such as the Syrian, the Hebrew, and the Greek. For instance, one should mention the interference with the Middle Persian, almost homographic and phonetically related term چندل/*čandal*, "sandalwood." This latter term was probably influenced in turn by the Sanskrit *candana* that is used to designate the plant *Santalum Album*, commonly known as "sandalwood."[3] Interestingly enough, the Persian term چندل/*čandal* ("sandalwood") also penetrated Aramaic-based Middle Iranian orthography with the variant צנדל/*ṣandāl*.[4] It might be useful to also briefly treat the dissemination of the Greek term σάνδαλον/*sandalon* in Jewish and Christian religious literature: namely, in the Septuagint and in the Greek patristic literature.

On the one hand, it can be noted that the term σάνδαλον/*sandalon* never occurs in the Septuagint and seems to suffer from the concurrence with its diminutive, the strictly correlated term σανδάλιον/*sandalion*, already occurring in Classical Greek.[5] The term σανδάλιον/*sandalion* is used four times to render the Hebrew term נעל/*naʿal* (in Josh 9:5; Isa 20:2; Jdt 10:4; 16:9); it also appears to suffer from the use of the concurrent Greek term πέδιλον/*pedilon* that twice renders the Hebrew term רגל/*regel* (in Hab 3:5; Od 4:5). This latter use of the term πέδιλον/*pedilon* is clearly related to πούς/*pous* already in Classical Greek[6] and manifests the "mimetic" intention of overlapping both semantically and morphologically with the Hebrew רגל/*regel* on account of its two fundamental meanings: "foot" and, by metonymy, "footwear." Intriguingly, the disambiguation of the Hebrew term נעל/*naʿal* with "sandal" rather

---

2 Arthur N. Wollaston, *An English-Persian Dictionary Compiled from the Original Sources* (London: Allen, 1882), 314. The same lexicon also reports the term نعلين/*niʿilin* to designate a "sandal."

3 Manfred Mayrhofer, *Kurzgefasstes Etymologisches Wörerbuch des Alindischen* (Heidelberg: Carl Winter Verlag, 1976), 373. For the complex dissemination of the Sanskrit term *candana* in India and Indonesia, see Robin Dorkin, *Between East and West: The Moluccas and the Traffic in Spices up to the Arrival of Europeans* (Philadelphia: American Philosophical Society, 2003), 23–35.

4 Carl Brockeann, *Lexicon Syriacum* (Berlin: Reuther & Reichard, 1895), 633; Claudia Ciancaglini, *Iranian Loanwords in Syriac* (Wiesbaden: Ludwig Reichert, 2008), 245, and also Leonid Kogan, "Proto-Semitic Phonetic and Phonology," in *The Semitic Languages: An International Handbook* (ed. Stefan Weininger; Berlin: De Gruyter, 2011), 64.

5 Johan Lust, Erik Eynikel and Karin Hauspie, *A Greek-English Lexicon of the Septuagint* (Stuttgart: Deutsche Bibelgesellschaft, 2002), 934, 1055; cf. Henry Liddell and Robert Scott, *A Greek-English Lexicon*, revised by H. S. Jones (Oxford: Clarendon, 1996), 1582.

6 Liddell and Scott, *A Greek-English Lexicon*, 1456–1457.

than with "shoe," as one would expect in Modern Hebrew,[7] is reflected also in Arabic and in the Arabic-speaking Syrian milieu, where the term نعآل/*na'āl* may be used to designate either a "sandal" or a "sole," when one does not want to recur to the Persian-based term صندل/*ṣandal*.[8] Finally, it should also be mentioned that both the New Testament and New Testament-related literature reflect the same obsolescence of the Greek term σάνδαλον/*sandalon* in favor of its diminutive: the strictly correlated term σανδάλιον/*sandalion*, which is used twice (in Mark 6:9; Acts 12:8) and which possibly reflects a Semitic נעל/*na'al*.[9] Not surprisingly, the neutral term σάνδαλον/*sandalon* also disappeared from Patristic Greek and, obviously under the influence of the New Testament, was substituted by the already mentioned diminutive: the related term σανδάλιον/*sandalion*.[10] In addition, it should also be noted that Patristic Greek introduced the use of the masculine term σάνδαλος/*sandalos*, which is unknown to Classical Greek, in order to designate "a boat."[11] Interestingly enough, this latter definition seems to reflect the Persian-Arabic lexeme صندل/*ṣandal* that would also designate "a narrow, double-master boat used on the Nile and the Barbary coast."[12] Finally, it also seems that the Classical Greek term σανδάλιον/*sandalion* was used to designate a kind of flatfish, apparently identical with another kind of fish—an "ox tongue"—designated either with the neutral term βούγλωσσον/*bouglōsson* in Classical Greek[13] or with the masculine term βούγλωσσος/*bouglōssos* in Later Patristic Greek.[14] This further meaning of the term σανδάλιον/*sandalion* as a kind of a flatfish will be examined below, due to the supplementary linguistic issues that it raises. Provided this assessment of the periphery of the semantic field, it is then possible to return to the Hebrew term in question: סנדל/*sandāl*. This term exhibits a rich semantics; indeed, it is used sixteen times in talmudic literature in order to designate a fatal birth defect that produces a miscarriage.[15] Despite its apparently transparent origin from its cognate Greek and Persian terms, it is very difficult to determine whether the Hebrew term סנדל/*sandāl* provides either a literal or a metaphoric description for the foetus's abnormal morphology. In other words, is the foetus actually shaped like a sandal or does it show a different, more complex morphology? In the latter case, should it also exhibit some similarity with the homonymous footwear or not?

These semantic difficulties depend both on the linguistic and on the semantic history of the term, as already anticipated. On the one hand, the Hebrew term סנדל/*sandāl* possibly has a Persian origin (سندل/*sandal*) and designates footwear. On

---

7 Avbraham Even-Shoshan, *Hamilon hehadash*, vol. 4. (Jerusalem: Kiryat Sefer, 1979), 1691.

8 Louis Costaz, *Dictionnaire Syriaque-Français* (Beirut: Dar el-Machreq, 2002), 128.

9 Lust, Eynikel and Hauspie, *Greek-English Lexicon of the Septuagint*, 1055.

10 G. W. H. Lampe, *A Patristic Greek Lexicon* (Oxford: Clarendon, 1961), 1222.

11 Ibid., 1222.

12 Garland Cannon and Alan S. Kaye, *The Persian Contributions to the English Language: An Historical Dictionary* (Wiesbaden: Harrassowitz, 2011), 126.

13 Liddell and Scott, *Greek-English Lexicon*, 324.

14 Lampe, *Patristic Greek Lexicon*, 301.

15 Julius Preuss, *Biblical and Talmudic Medicine* (trans. Fred Rosner; Lanham: Rowman & Littlefield, 2004), 417–418.

the other hand, the Hebrew term סנדל / *sandāl* might reflect some of the other associated, morphologically closed terms, such as footwear, a plant, a boat, or a fish. Consequently, the Hebrew term סנדל / *sandāl* may also be associated with the Greek term σάνδαλον/*sandalon*, which exhibits a rich semantic field, too; indeed, it designates two realities: a "sandal"[16] and a flatfish,[17] which is also called σάνδαλον/*sandalon* and apparently is identical with another kind of fish called βούγλωσσον/*bouglōsson* "ox-tongue," which is eventually to be identified with the generic class called σέλαχος/ *selachos*.[18] It should further be noted that the latter, neutral Greek term βούγλωσσον/ *bouglōsson* is etymologically related to a plant designated by the masculine Greek term βούγλωσσος/*bouglōssos*, "bugloss," probably identifiable with the *Anchusa Italica*.[19] The Hebrew fully reflects this complex semantics in the Greek term through either transcriptions or translations. On the one hand, the Hebrew term סנדל / *sandāl* transcribes the Greek term σάνδαλον/*sandalon*; on the other hand, the Hebrew expression לשון של שור/*lāšôn šĕl šûr* translates literally both the Greek terms βούγλωσσον/*bouglōsson* (as reflected in the Tosefta and in the Gemara) and βούγλωσσος/*bouglōssos* (as reflected in some medieval texts on medicinal plants).[20] Thus, it is unclear whether the Hebrew expression לשון של שור/*lāšôn šĕl šûr* intends to designate a *fish* or a *plant*, because it does not reflect the gender difference between a neutral (βούγλωσσον/*bouglōsson* = fish) and masculine (βούγλωσσος/*bouglōssos* = plant) Greek. The same semantic difficulty will arise again while treating the Hebrew sources from the Babylonian Talmud. There is no need to say that a supplementary meaning of the term βούγλωσσον/ *bouglōsson* as a surgical

---

16 Liddell and Scott, *Greek-English Lexicon*, 1582.

17 Ibid. Cf. also Preuss, *Biblical and Talmudic Medicine*, 418. Interestingly enough, neither the morphologically related Aramaic term סנדלא / *sandāla'* (or *sandĕlā'*) nor its homographic Jewish Palestinian Aramaic term are ever used to designate a flatfish. See Jastrow, *Dictionary*, 1004–1005 and Michael Sokoloff, *A Dictionary of Jewish Palestinian Aramaic of the Byzantine Period* (Ramat Gan: Bar-Ilan University Press, 1992), 383.

18 Liddell and Scott, *Greek-English Lexicon*, 324. The identification of the fish called βούγλωσσος/ *bouglōssos* with the σέλαχος is established on the basis of later Greek writers who classed the "bugloss" with the species described by Aristotle (Arist. *Fragmenta varia* 280). See Liddell and Scott, *Greek-English Lexicon*, 1589.

19 Liddell and Scott, *Greek-English Lexicon*, 324. See also: Max C. P. Schmidt, *Paulys Realencyclopädie der classischen Altertumswissenschaft* (ed. G. Wissowa, vol 3/1; Stuttgart: Metzler, 1897), 993.

20 In these cases, the Greek term *bouglōssos* is usually rendered with a transliteration that is unable to reflect the neutral or masculine ending of the term: either the variants בוגלוסא or בוגלוסה/*bûglôsa'* or *bûglôsah* are attested in recent rabbinic medical texts. Interestingly enough, Tobias Kohn's 18th-century encyclopedic work *Ma'ase Toviyah* uses the Hebrew terms *bûglôsah* and *bûr'agah* to designate two different plants from the same genera of the common Borage family (*Boraginaceae*): the Hebrew term *bûglôsah* designates, in Judeo-Arabic, *lisā'n šîwwîr yā'bā'n*, "a Japanese ox-tongue," modernly corresponding to an Asian plant called "purple gromwell" (*Lithospermum erythrorhizon*) from the genus *Lithospermum*, belonging to the Borage family; the Hebrew term *bûglôsah* designates, in Judeo-Arabic, *lisā'n šîwwîr*, an "ox-tongue," modernly corresponding to the Mediterranean plant, known by the common name *massed alkane* (*Hormuzakia aggregate*), also belonging to the Borage family. See Tobja Rofe Cohen, *Ma'aseh Tovayah kolel ha-Arba'ah 'Olamot* (part 3; Venice: Stamparia Bragadina, 1708), 134.

instrument used as tongue depressor[21] can obviously be ruled out from the present analysis due to its evident semantic incompatibility. One should also take into account two supplementary issues: on the one hand, the Mishnah frequently has difficulties providing a reliable embryology, possibly due to scarcity of medical data;[22] on the other hand, it exhibits a rich semantics to designate an embryo in the several phases of its development. Indeed, rabbinic literature usually distinguishes between six progressive phases in the formation of a "human being": 1) גולם/ *gôlem* or a "formless rolled-up thing" (between 0–1.5 months); 2) שפיר מרקם/ *sapîr merûqān* or an "embroidered foetus"; 3) עוֹבר/ *'ôver* or "[something] carried" or "foetus" (between 1.5–4 months); 4) ולד/ *wālād* or "child" (between 4–7 months); 5) ולד של קיימא/ *wālād šĕl qaîyama'* or "viable child" (between 7–9 months); and 6) בן שכלו חדשיו/ *ben šĕ-kālû lô ḥŏdāšāyw* or "a son who competed his [nine] months."[23] In the present case, the Hebrew term ולד/ *wālād* will always be rendered as a "childbirth" in order to designate—in its most literal and neutral sense—an offspring that is neither a "foetus" nor necessarily exhibits a "human shape" (צורת אדם/ *ṣûrat 'ādām*). This *neutral* stance is particularly important in order to treat a number of rabbinic texts that deal with the issue of סנדל/ *sandāl*. More specifically, it is particularly important not to strictly suggest that ולד/ *wālād* shall unequivocally be identified with a "foetus of human shape," especially because the anomaly of סנדל/ *sandāl* appears to put this identification in danger. Besides, this identification is overtly maintained only in two specific passages from Palestinian literature—namely from tractate Niddah both in the Mishnah and in the Tosefta[24]— and yet is not necessarily valid for any strata of rabbinic literature.[25] On the contrary, the Hebrew term עיבור/ *îbûr* will always be rendered as "foetus," in order to designate an embryo that is in the later phase of its development but does not necessarily exhibit a "human shape." The emphasis on this lexical distinction should also evidence that the term סנדל/ *sandāl* does not only exhibit a complex semantics but also applies to several stages of embryonic development; therefore, it might possibly designate a series of similar, when not correlated, medical issues. Aside from this, it should also be noted that there are other languages from the ancient Near East that designate both a sandal and a flatfish with the same common term: see for instance, the Sumerian *e-sir/sír* and the Akkadian *šēnu* in ancient Mesopotamian

---

21 Liddell and Scott, *Greek-English Lexicon,* 324.

22 On this see Federico Dal Bo, *Massekhet Keritot: Text, Translation, and Commentary* (Tübingen: Mohr Siebeck, 2013), 78–79.

23 Joseph Needham and Arthur Hughes, *A History of Embryology* (Cambridge: Cambridge University Press, 2015), 77.

24 Namely: m. Niddah 3:2 and t. Niddah 4:6. More specifically, the assumption that a ולד/ *wālād* has to exhibit a "human shape" (צורת אדם/ *ṣûrat 'ādām*) is implicitly maintained in the form of a negative assertion: "the sages say: each one that has no human shape is not a childbirth." (וחכמים אומרים כל שאין בו מצורת אדם אינו ולד). This locus is usually mentioned by commentators in order to reinforce a restrictive definition of ולד/ *wālād* in other talmudic passages, as in the case of Rashi on b. Hul. 77b. See also the following discussion.

25 See the following relevant discussion.

literature.[26] Although there is no documentation for a direct influence of Old Babylonian terms on Greek terms, in the present case it cannot be excluded that σάνδαλον/*sandalon*, designating both a sandal and a fish, is not a Greek lexical innovation but might reflect a (spontaneous?) linguistic habit in the ancient Near East, possibly on account of morphological similarities between a footwear's sole and a flatfish. If this hypothesis is legitimate, other kinds of cultural influence cannot be ruled out and it can be assumed that Old Babylonian themes might be reflected in more recent Jewish-Greek literature. In order to verify this hypothesis, it is necessary to proceed with a detailed textual analysis of some important occurrences of this term in Jewish literature and to compare them with some of its occurrences in Old Babylonian texts.

2 A Textual analysis of Hebrew sources mentioning a סנדל/*sandāl*

Rabbinic literature employs סנדל/*sandāl* as a *terminus technicus* for a miscarriage, as is evident from the standard expression in the Mishnah: המפלת סנדל/*ha-mappelet sandāl* (m. Ker. 1:3 and m. Nid. 3:4). As the Mishnah uses it, the Hebrew term סנדל/*sandāl* is unproblematic and it is employed without any further explanation in a detailed casuistic of miscarriages. The Tosefta to tractate Niddah, however, disambiguates the term:

And [the rabbis] say that a *sandāl* is similar to *sandāl*, a fish in the sea; Rabbi Shimon ben Gamliel says: [a *sandāl*] is similar to a "tongue of an ox." (t. Nid. 4:7)[27]	וסנדל שאמרו דומה לסנדל דג שבים ר"ש בן גמליאל אומר דומה ללשון של שור (ת' נדה ד ז)

It is particularly noteworthy that the Tosefta provides two concurrent explanations for the Hebrew term סנדל/*sandāl*: on the one hand, the Tosefta identifies the סנדל/*sandāl* with an homonymous sea fish called σάνδαλον/*sandalon*, according to the majority of the rabbis; on the other hand, it identifies the סנדל/*sandāl* with a לשון של שור/*lāšôn šel šûr*, a "tongue of an ox," according to the minority opinion of Rabban Shimon ben Gamliel, a Palestinian Tanna of the first century.[28] In so arranging these different opinions, the rabbis assume that there is a contradiction or at least a meaningful difference between these two species of fish. Therefore, if it is correct to assume that the Hebrew expression לשון של שור/*lāšôn šel šûr* literally translates the Greek term βούγλωσσον/*bouglōsson*, then the Tosefta maintains that there is a difference between the fishes to which the miscarried foetus is to be compared. The textual material occurring in the Tosefta is also reported in the Gemara to the Babylonian tractate Niddah with some noteworthy differences:

---

26 Erica Reiner, ed., *The Assyrian Dictionary of the Oriental Institute of the University of Chicago*, vol. 17/2 (Chicago: The Oriental Institute, 1992), 290–292.

27 All primary Jewish sources are quoted from *Bar-Ilan University. The Responsa Project. [Ramat Gan, Israel]: Bar-Ilan University, Version 23, 2018*. All translations are my own.

28 Günter Stemberger, *Introduction to the Talmud and the Midrash* (trans. M. Brockmuehl; Minneapolis, MN: Fortress, 1992), 67.

Our rabbis taught: a *sandāl* is similar to a fish of the sea. At its beginning it is a [normal] childbirth but [then] it is crushed. Rabbi Shimon ben Gamliel says: a *sandāl* is similar to a "tongue of a big ox." In the name of our rabbis it was testified that a *sandāl* needs to have a human face. Rav Yehudah said in the name of Shmuel: the [common] rule [is that] a *sandāl* needs to have a human face. Rav Ada said in the name of Rav Yosef in the name of Rav Yitshaq: a *sandāl* needs to have a human face even at its back, for instance just like someone who has slapped his fellow and made his face backward.
(b. Niddah 25b)

ות״ר סנדל דומה לדג של ים מתחלתו ולד הוא אלא שנרצף רשב״ג אומר סנדל דומה ללשון של שור הגדול משום רבותינו העידו סנדל צריך צורת פנים א״ר יהודה אמר שמואל הלכה סנדל צריך צורת פנים א״ר אדא א״ר יוסף א״ר יצחק סנדל צריך צורת פנים ואפילו מאחוריו משל לאדם שסטר את חבירו והחזיר פניו לאחוריו
(ב׳ נדה כה ע״ב)

It is evident that the Bavli agrees with the Tosefta in considering the סנדל/*sandāl* a kind of sea fish to be identified either with the homonymous σάνδαλον/*sandalon* or with a βούγλωσσον/*bouglōsson*, as Rabban Shimon ben Gamliel maintained. Yet, some important differences may be noted:

1. The Bavli provides a supplementary explanation for this anomaly; it maintains that a foetus shaped like a סנדל/*sandāl* would manifest a mixed morphology, initially normal and then abnormal—that is: the foetus's head and the upper torso would morphologically be normal but the rest of the body (possibly from the lower torso down) would be morphologically abnormal;

2. The reason for this supplementary explanation is implicit and possibly depends on a tiny, yet striking difference between the Mishnah's and the Tosefta's general casuistic of miscarriages:

Whoever miscarries a piece [...] whoever miscarries [something] like a kind of membrane, like a kind of a hair, like a kind of dust, like a kind of red flies, [...] whoever miscarries something like a kind of fishes, locusts, insects, or rodents [...] whoever miscarries a kind like a [domesticated] animal, a beast, or a fowl [...] and the sages say: anything that does not have a human shape is not [considered to be] a childbirth.
(m. Niddah 3:2)

המפלת חתיכה [...] המפלת כמין קליפה כמין שערה כמין עפר כמין יבחושין אדומים [...] המפלת כמין דגים חגבים שקצים ורמשים [...] המפלת מין בהמה חיה ועוף [...] וחכמים אומרים כל שאין בו מצורת אדם אינו ולד
(מ׳ נדה ג ב)

Whoever miscarries a piece [...] whoever miscarries [something] like a kind of
membrane, like a kind of a hair, like a
kind of dust, like a kind of red flies, [...]
whoever miscarries a kind like a [domes-
ticated] animal, a beast, or a fowl [...] and
the sages say: anything that does not have
a human shape is not [considered to be] a
childbirth.
(t. Niddah 4:2)

המפלת חתיכה [...] המפלת מין קליפה מין
שעורה מין עפר מין יבחושין אדומים [...]
המפלת כמין בהמה חיה ועוף [...] ואמרו כל
שאין בו מצורת אדם אינו ולד
(ת' נדה ד ב)

A comparison of these two Palestinian sources is of particular importance for the
treatment of the later strata of rabbinic literature and requires detailed consideration.
First of all, aside from other irrelevant differences, it is quite evident that the Mishnah *does* provide the case of a woman miscarrying something "like a kind of fishes"
(כמין דגים / *kĕ-mîn dāgim*), as is also reflected in other Palestinian sources,[29] whereas the Tosefta overtly *does not*. This difference in the sources impacts the definition
of a סנדל / *sandāl* especially because of the assumption that a legitimate "childbirth"
(ולד / *wālād*) has to exhibit "human shape" (צורת אדם / *ṣûrat ʾādām*), as maintained
both in the Tosefta and the Mishnah.[30] In other words, the Tosefta maintains
both that a "childbirth" has to exhibit a "human shape" (t. Nid. 4:6) and that the
סנדל / *sandāl* is a fish (t. Nid. 4:7) but does not explicitly treat the case of a woman
miscarrying something "like a kind of fishes" (cf. m. Nid. 3:2); conversely, the Mishnah both maintains that a "childbirth" has to exhibit a "human shape" (m. Nid. 3:2)
and treats the case of a woman who "miscarries like a kind of a fish" (m. Nid. 3:2) but
does not mention that the סנדל / *sandāl* is a fish (cf. t. Nid. 4:7). This varied constella-
tion of concepts is reflected in the corresponding page from the Babylonian Talmud
(b. Nid. 25b) that tries to harmonize them all together. Accordingly, the Bavli accepts
the Tosefta's assumption that the סנדל / *sandāl* is a fish (t. Nid. 4:7) as well as the Mishnah's and Tosefta's assumption that a "childbirth" has to exhibit a "human shape"
(m. Nid. 3:2 and t. Nid. 4:6); but it also has to face the Mishnah's indisputable case of
a woman miscarrying something "like a kind of fishes" (m. Nid. 3:2) that is discussed
at its proper place (b. Nid. 21a). As a result, the Bavli seems to offer a compromise: on
the one hand, it accepts the idea that a סנדל / *sandāl* is a fish (t. Nid. 4:7) and yet also
elaborates on it; on the other hand, it implicitly accepts the idea that a סנדל / *sandāl*
would fall into the major case of a woman miscarrying something "like a kind of
fishes" (m. Nid. 3:2) and yet it avoids the conclusion that a סנדל / *sandāl* would not
a "childbirth" (ולד / *wālād*) while not exhibiting a "human shape" (צורת אדם / *ṣûrat
ʾādām*) (m. Nid. 3:2), exactly by maintaining that a סנדל / *sandāl* would affect only
half of the body of a childbirth (b. Nid. 25b). The Bavli's complex treatment of the

---

29 Cf. Sifra, *Tazriaʿ*, *parashah* 1, *perek* 4, and y. Nid. 3:2, 9b.
30 Cf. m. Nid. 3:2 and t. Nid. 4:6. See also footnote n. 25.

tannaitic sources has an important impact on the issue of סנדל / *sandāl* and possible facial anomalies, as will be discussed further below;

3. The Bavli apparently accepts Rabban Shimon ben Gamliel's opinion from the Tosefta that identifies the סנדל / *sandāl* with a "tongue of an ox," לשון של שור / *lāšôn šĕl šûr*, but introduces a small, yet possibly important correction: a foetus shaped like a סנדל / *sandāl* shall be identified with a "bigger" variety of the former, a "large tongue of an ox," לשון של שור הגדול / *lāšôn šĕl šûr ha-gādôl*. It is evident that the Hebrew expression לשון של שור / *lāšôn šĕl šûr* reflects a possible Greek substratum (either the term βούγλωσσον / *bouglōsson* or βούγλωσσος / *bouglōssos*) but it is difficult to determine whether the Hebrew expression intends to describe a foetus (metaphorically?) shaped as a "fish" or a "plant," as specified above. Indeed, the mention of a לשון של שור הגדול / *lāšôn šĕl šûr ha-gādôl* calls for some supplementary remarks. At first, this Hebrew denomination possibly reflects a Greek expression: probably a hypothetical βούγλωσσον μέγαλον / *bouglōsson megalon* or a historical βούγλωσσον μέγα / *bouglōsson mega*. Indeed, the latter expression is actually documented by modern lexicographers and would designate a κρίσσιον / *krission*: that is, a particular plant identifiable with a *Carduus pycnocephalus*.[31] The identification of the Hebrew לשון של שור הגדול / *lāšôn šĕl šûr ha-gādôl* with a plant called after the Greek name βούγλωσσον μέγα / *bouglōsson mega* might suggest, by implication, that the rabbis use the term סנדל / *sandāl* to refer to the homonymous plant called "sandalwood" (چندل / the Persian *čandal* rather than the Persian سندل / *sandal* or Arabic صندل / *ṣandal*). Yet it is more likely that these semantic difficulties derive both from a complex linguistic-semantic condition and the conflation of four fundamental meanings of the term *sandal*: footwear, a plant, a boat, and a fish. Therefore, it is not implausible that these lexical uncertainties might have caused some confusion also in the rabbinic treatment of these terms and of the Hebrew term סנדל / *sandāl* itself;

4. It cannot be excluded that Rabban Shimon ben Gamliel did not intend to produce an ontological rather a lexicological distinction between a סנדל / *sandāl* and a לשון של שור / *lāšôn šĕl šûr*. Rabban Shimon ben Gamliel was indeed educated in Greek culture and might then have suggested calling the very same fish with the Hebrew name לשון של שור / *lāšôn šĕl šûr* rather than with the non-Hebrew name סנדל / *sandāl*. In this case, Rabban Shimon ben Gamliel would here be treating a lexicological issue, i. e., the designation of a specific kind of fish, as the occasion for making a theological-political statement;[32] 5. Besides, it is evident that the Hebrew expression לשון של שור / *lāšôn šĕl šûr* (also extant in later rabbinic literature as לשון השור / *lāšôn ha-šûr*) is neither understood as the translation of a Greek term nor perceived as idiomatic; rather it simply designates, almost literally, "the tongue of an ox," as reflected also in some later commentaries;

---

31 Liddell and Scott, *Greek-English Lexicon*, 324, 997. The identification of a βούγλωσσον μέγα / *bouglōsson mega* with a κρίσσιον / *krission* is established on the basis of the first-century Greek physician, pharmacologist, and botanist Dioscorides Pedanius (*De Materia Medica* 4, 118).

32 I owe this remark to Prof. Tirzah Meacham (University of Toronto). For a treatment of the relationship between Judaism and Greek culture, see for instance Lee I. Levine, *Judaism and Hellenism in Antiquity: Conflict or Confluence?* (Washington: University of Washington Press, 2012).

6. The Bavli also maintains that the morphology of a foetus shaped like a
סנדל / *sandāl* should also be endowed with a human face. It should be noted that this
supplementary issue stands in contrast with the previous assumption that a foetus
shaped like a סנדל / *sandāl* would "initially" exhibit a normal morphology and then
an abnormal one;

7. Finally, the Bavli provides some additional information about this anomaly and
the peculiar position of the foetus's head, i. e., oriented backwards. The Bavli does not
provide any medical reason for this but it is plausible that its remarks could be integrated into some anatomical descriptions that are extant in the Palestinian Gemara to
tractate Niddah:

"Whoever miscarried a *sandāl* or a
placenta" (m. Nid. 3:4). Rabbi Abba in
the name of Rab Yehudah [says]: there is
no *sandāl* but one which a living [foetus]
weighed down and it does not comes
out together with the living [foetus] but
rather with a dead [foetus].
(y. Niddah 4:4–5, 50d)

המפלת סנדל או שילייא (מ' נדה ג ד) רבי בא
בשם רב יהודה אין סנדל אלא שרצמו חי ואינו
יוצא עם החי אלא עם המת
(י' נדה ד ד-ה כה נ ע"ד)

Just like the Mishnah, so does the Yerushalmi provide no explanation for the meaning of the Hebrew term סנדל / *sandāl*. Yet, unlike the rest of the textual evidence, the
Yerushalmi provides a possible aetiology for this morphological anomaly and maintains that a סנדל / *sandāl* would be the major consequence of a problematic pregnancy
involving two foetuses.

3 Traditional and modern rabbinic interpretations of סנדל / *sandāl*

The textual analysis of the major occurrences of the term סנדל / *sandāl* in rabbinic
sources manifests complex semantics and some conceptual tensions between potentially divergent interpretations of this anomaly. These conceptual tensions are treated
differently in traditional and modern rabbinic interpretations.

On the one hand, traditional rabbinic interpretations—especially those stemming
from the French-German milieu, thus culturally and geographically distant from
the original Babylonian setting—usually provide a generic definition for the foetal
anomaly called סנדל / *sandāl* but do not necessarily conform to the lexical explanation
provided both by the Tosefta and the baraita in the Babylonian Gemara to tractate
Niddah. For instance, the German authority Rabbenu Gershom ben Yehudah [33] provides a rather generic explanation for the term:

---

33 Rabbenu Gershom ben Yehudah of Mainz (960–1028), called also מאור הגולה / *Me'or Hagolah*,
was the leading halakic authority for Askhenazic Jewry. One of his most famous rulings is the
prohibition of polygamy and of divorcing a woman against her will. His disciple Rabbi Jacob
ben Yaqar (d. 1064) will be the teacher of Rabbi Shlomo ben Yitshaq, better known as Rashi
(1040–1105), who refers to him as "the Elder." See Andreas Lehnardt, "Mainz und seine Tal-

"Whoever miscarried a *sandāl*" (m. Keritot 1:3): a childbirth whose form is corrupted. (Rabbenu Gershom on Keritot, chap. 1)

המפלת סנדל (מ' כריתות א ג): ולד שנתקלקלה צורתו
(רבינו גרשום מסכת כריתות פרק א)

Rashi,[34] who usually conforms to the Bavli's self-explanatory comments, while reading another talmudic passage, interprets סנדל / *sandāl* as a metaphor for an anomaly but provides very little insight and rather contradicts the above-mentioned passage from tractate Niddah:

Sandal: a childbirth that has no human face. (Rashi on b. Yebam. 12b)

סנדל: ולד שאין לו צורת פנים
(רש"י על ב' יבמות יב ע"ב)

A later commentator like Rabbi Ovadiah of Bertinoro[35] provides some more detailed explanation with different effects and discusses this term at least in two relevant occasions that I shall treat together:

Sandāl: it is a childbirth whose form is diminished and the expression *sandāl* [means]: hated childbirth.[36] So I found that most of its commentaries [maintain] that it is a piece of flesh made in the form of a sandal and normally accompanies childbirth. (Bertinoro on m. Ker. 1:3)

סנדל: ולד הוא אלא שנפחתה צורתו ולשון סנדל שנאוי ולד. כך מצאתי ורבותי פרשו שהיא חתיכת בשר עשויה כצורת סנדל ורגילה לבוא עם ולד
(ברטנורא על מ' כריתות י ג)

Sandāl: a piece of flesh made in the likeness of a "tongue of an ox" and since it has the form of a sandal it is called *sandāl*. It normally accompanies childbirth and there is who say: *sandāl* [that is:] hated childbirth.[37] (Bertinoro on m. Nid. 3:4)

סנדל: חתיכת בשר עשויה כדמות לשון של שור ומפני שיש לה צורת סנדל קורין לה סנדל.והוא רגיל לבא עם ולד וי"מ סנדל שנאוי ולד
(ברטנורא על מ' נדה ג ד)

---

mudgelehrten im Mittelalter," in *Mainz im Mittelalter* (ed. Mechtild Dreyer; Mainz: Zabern, 2009), 87–102.

34 Rashi is probably the most famous and celebrated commentator on the Bible and the Babylonian Talmud. Scholarship about him is extensive. See, for instance, Esra Shereshevsky, *Rashi, the Man and his World* (Northvale, NJ: J. Aronson), 1996; see also the new bibliography on Rashi commentary in Pinchus Krieger, *Parshan-Data* (Monsey, NY: Krieger, 2005), 41–46.

35 Rabbi Ovadia of Bertinoro, known also as Bartenura (1455–1516), was a famous Italian scholar whose commentary on the entire Mishnah is now included in every Hebrew edition. He also wrote a supercommentary on Rashi's commentary on Scripture. See, for instance, Bruno Chiesa, "Il supercommentario di Ovadya a Rasi," in *Ovadiah Yare da Bertinoro e la presenza ebraica in Romagna nel Quattrocento* (ed. G. Busi; Torino: Zamorani, 1989), 35–46; Rabbi Luciano Caro, "Rabbi Ovadyà da Bertinoro e il suo supercommentario a Rashi," *Hebraica* (1998): 165–168.

36 This is a provisory translation. See the following discussion.

37 This is a provisory translation. See the following discussion.

As far as they manifest a generic consistency, these two explanations of the term סנדל/ *sandāl* differ in many aspects and present some lexical difficulties. I will treat each of them separately for clarity's sake:

1. While commenting on tractate Keritot, Bertinoro interprets the Hebrew term סנדל/ *sandāl* according to its common literal sense: as a designation for a type of open footwear. Accordingly, he maintains that the miscarried childbirth called סנדל/ *sandāl* manifests the same morphology (צורה/*ṣûrah*) of an actual "sandal";

2. In contrast, while commenting on tractate Niddah, Bertinoro himself does not conform to his own explanation in tractate Keritot but rather tries to harmonize the conflicting talmudic opinions about the term, providing a slightly confusing interpretation. More specifically, he assumes that the term סנדל/ *sandāl* is a sort of "metaphor" that describes a miscarried childbirth whose aspect manifests "similarity" (דמות/*dĕmût*) with a—not better specified—"tongue of an ox," possibly here interpreted either in its literal (i. e., the muscular organ present in that specific animal) or metaphorical sense (i. e., the name of a fish from the sea).

3. Aside from these differences in treating סנדל/ *sandāl* either literally or metaphorically, in both cases Bertinoro notably provides a supplementary gloss that presents a number of lexical uncertainties: שנאוי ולד/ *ś(š)-n-'-w-y-w-d-l*. This expression is a *hapax* in rabbinic literature, possibly an innovation of Bertinoro himself, and presents a particularly difficult semantics. As such, the possibly corrupted expression שנאוי ולד/ *ś(š)-n-'-w-y-w-d-l* offers three conflicting disambiguations, at least, and can therefore be rendered in three different ways: (i) at first, as "a hated childbirth," (ii) traditionally, as "a hated and poor [childbirth]," (iii) in modern philological terms, as "a misshaped childbirth."

i) At first, when considering Bertinoro's wording valid and legitimate, one could vocalize the expression שנאוי ולד/ *ś(š)-n-'-w-y-w-d-l* as follows: *śan'uy/śan'ûî wālād*; therefore, one would render it literally as: "a hated childbirth." The sense of the expression would still be not particularly clear and might possibly mean that the miscarried childbirth manifests a repugnant morphology—therefore it is "hated," because it is "loathsome."

ii) Traditional commentators already acknowledged the problematic nature of the expression שנאוי ולד/ *ś(š)-n-'-w-y-w-d-l* in Bertinoro's commentary. This lexical difficulty was traditionally resolved by emending the contextually legitimate term ולד/ *wālād* "childbirth" with the quite less expected term ודל/ *wĕ-dal* "and poor" by simple metathesis.[38] As a result, the difficult expression שנאוי ולד/ *ś(š)-n-'-w-y-w-l-d* would

---

38 See Rabbi Yom Tov Lipmann ben Nathan ha-Levi Heller, *Tosfot Yom Tov*, on m. Nid. 3. This emendation has usually impacted on the modern edition (and vocalization) of Bertinoro's commentary on the Mishnah. This emendation is usually provided either directly with the resulting expression שנאוי ולד/ *ś(š)-n-'-w-y-w-l-d* or with a semiphilological correction after Bertinoro's original wording in the pertinent passages, such as: "*ś(š)-n-'-w-y-w-l-d:* one have to read childbirth (*wālād*)." שנאוי צריך ולד לקרוא ולד. See Bertinoro on m. Bekh. 8:1, m. Ker. 1:3, and m. Nid. 3:5; cf. again *Tosfot Yom Tov* on m. Nid. 3:5; cf. also *Bi'ur ḥadash* 10:12. Rabbi Yom Tov Lipmann ben Nathan ha-Levi Heller (1579–1654) was a Bohemian talmudist who wrote the aforementioned commentary on the Mishnah called *Tosfot Yom Tov* (1614–1617 and then 1643–1644) that was formally intended as a "supplement" to Bertinoro's commentary. On his

then be emended with the no less unique expression שנאוי ודל / ś-n-'-w-y-w-d-l; the latter would then be vocalised as śan'ûî wĕ-dal and consequently be rendered as "a hated and poor [childbirth]." As far as this emendation does not actually provide a clearer understanding of the text, one should also note that that vocalization śan'ûî wĕ-dal manifests a sort of phonetic similarity with the reading of sandāl; therefore, it is not implausible that Bertinoro is here simply providing a mnemotechnical tool or a sort of acronym for the term סנדל / sandāl, although this explanation is hardly convincing.[39]

iii) Yet, as anticipated, the expression שנאוי ולד / ś(š)-n-'-w-y-w-d-l is quite atypical when not idiosyncratic of Bertinoro. It is then not implausible to suggest that the term שנאוי / ś(š)-n-'-w-y shall be vocalised not as śan'ûî, "hated," rather as the slightly corrupted form šan'ûî and therefore be corrected—by lectio difficilior—with the proper form שנוי / š-n-w-y to be read finally as šinûî, "changed." Consequently, the problematic expression שנאוי ולד / ś(š)-n-'-w-y-w-l-d/ could be emended with the more valid expression שנוי ולד / š-n-w-y-w-l-d/, vocalized as šinûî wālād, and rendered as "a changed childbirth," by implication "a childbirth [whose form has] changed" and finally, by extension, a "misshaped childbirth."[40] By means of this textual emendation, Bertinoro's difficult expression would lexically be harmonized with the rest of the mishnaic passage and would also support the suggestion that the use of the term סנדל / sandāl, i. e. a "flatfish," was intended also to be descriptive of a process of transformation that the foetus undergoes—just exactly as a sole progressively changes from a "normal" into a "flatfish."[41] Remarkably,

---

life and work, see Joseph Davis, *Yom Tov Lipmann Heller: Portrait of a Seventeenth-Century Rabbi* (Oxford: Littman Library, 2004).

39 A supplementary yet possibly negligible difficulty would also be the manifest confusion between the letter *śin* and the letter *samekh*, together with the unclear meaning of the expression "hated and poor."

40 I owe this suggestion to Dr. Doru Constantin Doroftei (University of Hamburg). Unfortunately, I could not substantiate this interesting hypothesis philologically, as I was unable to consult the manuscript MS Paris, Alliance Israelite Universelle III B 173 bis, foll. 1–15, where Bertinoro's commentary on tractate Keritot is extant in a fragmentary form (see Moïse Schwab, *Les Manuscrits et les Incunables Hebreux de la Bibliotheque de l'Alliance Israelite* (Paris: Durlacher, 1904), 74–88 and 270–296). Yet it is notable that the Israeli-based Rabbi Ya'akov Shulevitz has recently commented online on the same passage from tractate Niddah and has spontaneously emended (Bertinoro's) difficult expression שנאוי ולד / ś(š)-n-'-w-y-w-l-d with שנוי ולד / š-n-w-y-w-l-d; he has specifically commented on it as follows: "the name *sandāl* does not teach about the shape of the childbirth rather on its substance and a sandal is an abridgment for 'changed childbirth,' since its shape has changed in a corrupted way" (*Havruta Niddah*, on m. Nid 3:4, § 152, quoted from: http://http://www.toratemetfreeware.com/online/f_02375.html?hc_location=ufi#HtmpReportNum0002_L5/, accessed on line: September 19, 2019.

41 I owe this remark to Prof. Dr. Tirzah Meacham (University of Toronto). In a private communication to me, Prof. Meacham has also argued that the Talmud might have used the adjective גדול / gādôl in this context especially with the purpose to signalize that "flatfishes" usually undergo morphological changes in their development—specifically, the eyes migrate to be on the same side—so that they ostensibly look "big" (גדול / gādôl) or bigger. See also several interesting remarks in Tirzah Meacham, "Fetal Death in the Palestinian Talmud. Murder in the Chamber," in *Death and taxes in the ancient Near East* (ed. Sara E. Orel; Lewiston: Mellen Press, 1992), 145–156.

it is already Maimonides,[42] possibly Bertinoro's primary source, who tries to provide a harmonizing interpretation of the term סנדל / *sandāl* and gives a long and articulate explanation for the term, on account of his education both as a Talmud scholar and as a physician:

Sometimes from the remainder of the bloods from which a man [i.e., a foetus] is formed will congeal a piece [of flesh] in the likeness of the "tongue of an ox" and [this piece] is wound around a portion of the childbirth and it is called a *sandāl*. A *sandāl* will never be formed but with a childbirth. Yet, if a similar mass is formed without a childbirth, it is not called a *sandāl*. Most foetuses will not have a *sandāl* with them. Sometimes a pregnant woman receives a blow on her belly and the foetus will be damaged and will become like this *sandāl*. Sometimes [the foetus] will keep its facial features and sometimes the childbirth will dry up and change [in form] and the bloods will congeal until it won't keep facial features. (Maimonides, *Mishneh Torah, Sefer Kedushah, 'Issurey Bi'ah* 10:12)	פעמים יקפה משאר הדמים שנוצר מהם האדם חתיכה כמו לשון השור ותהיה כרוכה על מקצת הוולד; והיא הנקראת סנדל. ולעולם לא ייעשה סנדל זה, אלא עם ולד; אבל חתיכה שנוצרה לבדה בלא ולד, אינה נקראת סנדל. ורוב העוברים, לא יהיה עימהם סנדל. ופעמים יכה המעוברת דבר על בטנה, וייפסד העובר וייעשה כסנדל זה; ופעמים יישאר בו היכר פנים, ופעמים ייבש הוולד וישתנה ויקפאו עליו הדמים עד שלא יישאר בו היכר פנים רמב״ם משנה תורה, ספר קדושה, הלכות איסורי) (ביאה, פרק י הלכה יב

As compared with Rashi's self-evident explanation and Bertinoro's inconsistency, Maimonides tries to harmonize the Talmud's different opinions on the Hebrew term סנדל / *sandāl* and also provides a list of possible causes for it, physiological as well as traumatic. Despite his efforts, Maimonides too fails to supply a comprehensive "theory" on this fatal syndrome and his coherent description is only tentative.

On the other hand, some modern commentators are not satisfied with a generic definition of the term סנדל / *sandāl* and rather prefer to harmonize the conflicting opinions on this anomaly, probably referring to Maimonides's explanation and its lexical choices. For instance, while commenting on tractate Niddah of the Bavli, the ear-

---

42 The famous Rabbi Mosheh ben Maimon, or Musa Ibn Maymun, known as Rambam or Maimonides (1135–1204), was one of the great figures of medieval Judaism for his contributions to Jewish law and Jewish philosophy. He commented on the entire Mishnah and also wrote the famous comprehensive code *Mishneh Torah*, as well as several medical works, now available in English: Fred Rosner, *Maimonides' Medical Writings*, 7 vols. (Haifa: Maimonides Institute, 1984–94). See also: Josè Faur, "Maimonides' Discovery of a Saboraitic Version of Tractate Niddah", *Tarbiz* 55,4 (1995): 721–728. [In Hebrew].

ly nineteenth-century Polish rabbi Israel Lipschitz[43] implicitly relies on the aetiology reported in tractate Niddah of the Yerushalmi and explains the expression as follows:

"Whoever miscarried a *sandāl*" (m. Ker. 1:3): it is a long piece of wounded flesh, sometimes wrapped around the child-birth, and this piece [of flesh] itself was a childbirth, only that it was mashed in his mother's belly, pressed by his brother. (Rabbi Israel Lipschitz, *Tiferet Israel*, tractate Keritot, chap. 1)	המפלת סנדל (מ' כריתות א ג) הוא כעין חתיכת בשר ארוך וכרוך לפעמים סביב להולד וגם החתיכה ההיא ולד היה רק שנתמעך בבטן אמו מדדחקו אחיו (תפארת ישראל, יכין מסכת כריתות פרק א)

The most comprehensive interpretation for this phenomenon is provided by the later eighteenth-century Italian rabbi David Pardo,[44] who comments on the Tosefta to tractate Niddah and provides a systematic analysis for the anomaly called סנדל / *sandāl* by referring to most of the relevant sources considered here. Following Maimonides's assumptions, Rabbi Pardo states that the Hebrew term סנדל / *sandāl* does not really designate a single syndrome, but rather a collection of possible anomalies that may occur quite apart one from the other, depending on specific developments during pregnancy:

Yes, indeed it is so as it is explained by the rabbis above referring to a mere piece [of flesh] without blood and [according to] Rashbag while referring to the *sandāl* which is formed in the beginning [i.e., in its upper body] as an childbirth and then [it is similar to] a "tongue of an ox" and wrapped around the [normal] child-birth—therefore the meaning is that,	הא"נ דיסבור כרבנן דלעיל בחתיכה בעלמא בלא דם ורשב"ג איירי בסנדל הנוצר מתחלה עם הולד וזהו הדומה ללשון השור וכרוכה על מקצת הולד ומשמע שזה נעשה כשמתעברת תאומים ואחד מהם נקפה ונעשה סנדל וזה מוכרח שיבא כרוך על הולד [...] ורבותינו אמרו דסנדל אם בא לבדו צריך צורת פנים שאז אמרים שהוא הולד שנרצף אבל אם אין לו צורת פנים לא חיישין

---

43 Rabbi Israel Lipschitz, alias Israel ben Gedaliah Lipschutz (1782–1860), was a prominent Polish rabbi active in Danzig. He wrote the well-known commentary on the Mishnah titled *Tiferet Isra-el*. See Shalom b. Rosenbaum, Forgotten Manuscripts of the Lipschutz Family. *Da'at* 61 (1972): 97–112; André Neher, "Cabale, science et philosophie dans le commentaire sur la Mishna de Tiferet Israel," in *'Ale Shefer: Studies in the Literature of Jewish Thought: Presented to Rabbi Dr. Alexandre Safran* (ed. Moshe Ḥallamish; Ramat Gan: Bar-Ilan University Press, 1990), 127–132.

44 Rabbi David Pardo (1718–1790) was an outstanding Italian scholar whose commentary on the Tosefta, titled *Ḥaside David*, and his commentary on the halakic midrash *Sifre*, titled *Sifre devei Rav*, are considered classics of late rabbinic thought ("Aḥaronim"). See Stemberger, *Introduction to the Talmud and Midrash*, 162; Zvi Zohar, "Sephardic Jurisprudence in the Recent Half-Millennium," in *Sephardic and Mizrahi Jewry: From the Golden Age of Spain to Modern Times* (ed. Zvi Zohar; New York: New York University Press, 2005), 167–196.

when she begets twins, one of them is
congealed and turned into a *sandāl* [...]
and our rabbis said that a *sandāl*, if it
comes alone, requires facial features, and
they say about it that it is a childbirth
that is crushed but if it does not have facial features, they do not consider him a
childbirth but rather maintain that she
miscarried a piece [of flesh] [...] and even
more so[45] if he is wrapped on a [normal]
childbirth and similar to a "tongue of an
ox" that is the *sandāl* [of which] Rashbag
[speaks] but without blood, [the rabbis]
do not consider him [a *sandāl*] unless he
has facial features [...] but if he is without
facial features, they consider him a mere
piece [of flesh] [...]
(Rabbi David Pardo, *Ḥaside David*, on
the Tosefta to Niddah, § 84, n. 7)

לולד אלא דינו כדלעיל במפלת חתיכה [...] וכ״ש
אם הוא כרוך על הולד ודומה ללשון השור דהיינו
סנדל דרשב״ג אבל בלא ולד לא מחמירין אא״כ
יש לו היכר פנים [...] אבל בלא היכר פנים אמרין
חתיכה בעלמא היא [...]
(ר׳ דוד פארדו, חסדי דוד על תוספתא נדה, פ״ד ז)

Rabbi David Pardo seems to maintain that the Hebrew term סנדל / *sandāl* designates a
potentially morbid syndrome that can develop into four different anomalies, possibly
on account of an increasing period of time, either alone or in the presence of a multiple
pregnancy. Indeed, Rabbi David Pardo focuses mostly on the central issue at stake:
that is, whether a miscarried childbirth has facial features (צורת פנים / *ṣûrat pānîm*) or
not. Notably, he does not mention any different period in the casuistic provided in his
commentary on the Tosefta. Yet in providing the following summary, I maintain that
Pardo's four distinct anomalies would also reflect four different stages of foetal compression, as is evidenced by modern medical observations, and thus would correspond
to four increasingly longer periods of time. Besides, the supposition that these four
anomalies collectively called סנדל / *sandāl* correspondingly occur in longer periods of
compression seems to be implicitly stated in the talmudic prescription to pray that the
mother will not deliver a *sandāl* "from the fortieth day to three months" (מארבעים יום
ועד שלשה חדשים) (b. Ber. 60a): this obviously evidences that the rabbis were aware that
this syndrome might manifest in longer periods of time during gestation.

I can accordingly distinguish between four different issues:
1. A deformity of the lower body morphology if the foetus is alone, since, in the case
   of facial issues, the foetus should not be treated as a סנדל / *sandāl* but rather as a
   different kind of miscarriage;

---

45 Here Rabbi David Pardo relies on an *a fortiori* argument. On this rhetorical device, see Stemberger, *Introduction to the Talmud and Midrash*, 21.

2. A deformity of the face, if the miscarried twin was pressed by his brother (possibly, for a shorter period of time) before being expelled from his mother's uterus;

3. A more severe deformity resulting in a compressed foetus, if the aborted twin was pressed by his brother (possibly, for a longer period of time) before being miscarried;

4. The most severe deformity, resulting in a formless "piece of flesh," if the aborted twin was pressed by his brother (possibly, for a very long period) before being miscarried.

Rabbi David Pardo has probably provided the most coherent and pertinent interpretation of the Hebrew term סנדל / *sandāl* with respect to its difficult treatments both in Jewish sources and their traditional commentaries. He suggests that, whatever literal or metaphorical meaning this term might have had, the Hebrew term סנדל / *sandāl* does not designate a specific single anomaly but rather a number of different issues that modern medicine classifies differently. Following his suggestion, the general use of the Hebrew term סנדל / *sandāl* and its metaphors becomes increasingly clear and can be explained in terms of modern medicine.

4   סנדל / *Sandāl* as an umbrella term for medical issues

My assumption is that the Hebrew term סנדל / *sandāl* does not designate a specific anomaly but rather serves as an umbrella term for a number of different issues: that is, anomalies that were believed either to have a common aetiology or to present the same morphological defects.

The use of a generic term to designate a larger number of medical issues is not uncommon in rabbinic literature and is justified for several reasons, such as false diagnosis, different expectations from medical classifications, and lexical economy. One should also note that medical observations from antiquity until very recent times were limited to the human senses and did not necessarily imply "medical incompetence"—at least when not abruptly contrasted with modern Western medical textbooks. Nevertheless, the system of diagnosis and prognosis implicitly adopted in the Babylonian Talmud was most possibly influenced by medical lore from Babylonia rather than from Greek sources. Thus, the medical system employed by the Babylonian Talmud would have refrained from providing a "case history," as opposed to the practice in Greece.[46] As a result, the Babylonian Talmud tends to provide anecdotes and commonly fails to provide an accurate, systematic description of symptoms. It is then not implausible to assume that the term סנדל / *sandāl* would hardly describe only a single and very specific pathology rather than a number of different medical issues whose aetiology might be common. Therefore, I assume that the סנדל / *sandāl* is employed as *terminus technicus* in rabbinic literature to designate four different pathologies. Three of them are presumably fatal pathologies—according to modern medicine—and thus usually resulting in a miscarriage, while another one is neither necessarily fatal nor the primary cause of miscarriage. I would like to anticipate that the identification of

---

46 Here I am following Markham J. Geller, *Akkadian Healing Therapies in the Babylonian Talmud*, Berlin: Max Planck Institute for the History of Science, 2004; *Preprint-series* 259: 14–15. Also accessible online: https://www.mpiwg-berlin.mpg.de/Preprints/P259.PDF.

the first three pathologies seems quite founded on textual sources, whereas the fourth one is rather less likely:

1. The modern syndrome called *Fetus Papyraceus*: that is, the fatal loss of hydration and body fluids during pregnancy, possibly caused by a mechanical trauma, as Maimonides maintains, and resulting in a compressed tissue of organic origin, sometimes preserving human physiognomy. This syndrome is probably described in the end of the quotation from the Bavli, while referring to a foetus whose head is oriented backwards. In this respect, the Hebrew term סנדל/*sandāl* would designate a flatfish and thus, metaphorically, a foetus that resembles such a flatfish as a result of intrauterine compression;

2. The modern syndrome called *Foetus Compressus*, usually associated with the former, but specifically produced by "superfoetation": that is, the uncommon pregnancy of two foetuses, which were conceived at two different times as a result of two distinct intercourses and which predate each other.[47] The Yerushalmi to tractate Niddah explicitly suggests this aetiology, as already remarked. In addition, it should be mentioned that the Babylonian Talmud's discussion on tractate Niddah is aware of this possible event, suggesting the use of birth control even during pregnancy to avoid such an occurrence.[48] Just like the previous case, the Hebrew term סנדל/*sandāl* designates a flatfish and thus, metaphorically, a foetus that resembles such a flatfish as a result of intrauterine compression;

3. The modern syndrome called *Sirenomelia* (or mermaid syndrome): a very rare congenital deformity in which the legs are fused together and give the appearance of a mermaid's tail—i.e., this applies to the references to a deformation of the lower

---

47 "Superfoetation" as the simultaneous occurrence of more than one stage of developing childbirths in the same female individual is believed to be relatively common in some species of animals (typically in fishes, rodents, rabbits, farm animals, and marsupials) but is extremely rare in humans, among whom it occurs as a dizygotic twin pregnancy. See Rabbi Edward Reichman, "Is There Life after Life? Superfetation in Rabbinic Literature,"in: *And You Shall Surely Heal* (Edited by J. Wiesen; New York: Yeshiva University Press, 2009), 39–55. The rabbis' need to treat such a rare issue like "superfoetation" shall then be judged carefully, without ruling out the possibility that this would reflect their ignorance about the physiology of human body. On the one hand, one might presume that ancient medicine, as already remarked, would mostly rely on empirical observation limited to human senses and therefore might have persuaded the rabbis that "superfoetation" might represent an actual risk in humans so that is necessary to take precautions, such as using tampons (see next footnote). On the other hand, one should also keep in mind that the rabbis are not alien to treating "extreme cases" in talmudic discussion, regardless of their actual, theoretical, or radical nature (on the use of ad absurdum cases in talmudic literature, see also Dal Bo, *Massekhet Keritot*, 253); therefore, especially because of its exceptionality, the case of "superfoetation" could then be one of them. In addition, one should also consider that the rabbis manifest the tendency to derive legal cases from the animal realm and apply them to the human world. This overlapping of animal and human world, especially with respect to bodily and medical issues, is not uncommon in rabbinic literature. On this, see Dal Bo, *Massekhet Keritot*, 346–347.

48 The use of a "tampon" (מוך/*môk*) as a contraceptive method is encouraged in some passages both from rabbinic literature and the Babylonian Talmud (t. Nid. 2:6; b. Ketub. 39a; b. Yebam. 12b; b. Ned. 35b) but is especially encouraged during pregnancy, in order to avoid "superfoetation" exactly in tractate Niddah 45a. On this, see Preuss, *Biblical and Talmudic Medicine*, 387.

body. Julius Preuss already proposed the identification of סנדל/*sandāl* with this syndrome[49] and it is also supported by the *baraita* quoted in the Bavli that mentions a foetus that is "crushed."

4. The modern syndrome called cleft lip:[50] the abnormal formation of mouth and palate resulting in a severe facial anomaly and usually concomitant with an anomaly of another severe pathology, possibly the same "superfoetation" or the intrauterine compression discussed above. Unlike the previous three fatal pathologies, the cleft lip syndrome is neither necessarily fatal nor the primary cause of miscarriage, but rather a morbid condition within a more severe pathology. Accordingly, the term סנדל/*sandāl* would be used quite exceptionally in the present case and would designate the homonymous flatfish *sandāl*, whose mouth—when observed from above—would actually recall the very same mouth defect in a childbirth affected by a cleft lip.[51]

As evident, this suggestive interpretation is mostly based on the *morphological similarity* between a flatfish's mouth and a cleft lip observed from above, but presents two major exegetical difficulties. I will discuss them separately without necessarily ruling out the validity of this hypothesis. First, one should note that a cleft lip affects the development of a more mature foetus that is usually designated with the term עיבור/*'ibûr*, as mentioned above, and can also impact live foetuses. It is argued that this horrifying deformity was apparently thought to be fatal and babies were allowed to die as nonviable.[52] Second, there is no real evidence that the term סנדל/*sandāl* explicitly refers to specific mouth anomalies. Yet the rabbinic sources mentioned above are clearly concerned with the issue that the miscarriage presents a "human face" (צורת פנים/*sûrat pānîm*), although the frequent comparison to an "ox tongue" (לשון של שור/*lāšôn šĕl šûr*) strongly suggests that the real issue at stake is the "flatness" of the childbirth rather than the shape of the mouth.

Each of these possible identifications with a modern medical syndrome relies on the Tosefta's self-explanation of the Hebrew term סנדל/*sandāl* as related to a homonymous sea fish. This assumption implicitly rejects the hypothesis that סנדל/*sandāl* designates a kind of footwear, despite its most transparent etymology. On the contrary, Jewish sources apparently suggest a sort of *lectio difficilior*: a reading of textual evidence that contrasts with some expectations on the basis of the etymology of the term. In other words, although the Hebrew term סנדל/*sandāl* suggests that the corresponding syndrome described the foetus as footwear, Jewish sources tend to understand this term rather as the name of a sea fish and thus designating a foetus shaped like a fish. Yet, Jewish sources and later commentators appear to misunderstand the Hebrew expression לשון של שור/*lāšôn šĕl šûr* as a designation of a fish, as its Greek etymology (βούγλωσσον/*bouglōsson*) evidences. This failure to understand the gloss of Rabbi Shimon ben Gamliel produces, as noted, some confusion regarding this medical anomaly.

---

49 Preuss, *Biblical and Talmudic Medicine*, 417–418.

50 William G. Holdsworth, *Cleft Lip and Palate* (New York: Grune & Statton, 1963), 22.

51 Mark Westreich and Steve Segal, "Cleft Lip in the Talmud," *Annual of Plastic Surgery* 2 (2000): 229–327.

52 Ibid., v.i.

Both this semantic consistency and the implicit rejection of a more familiar interpretation of the Hebrew term סנדל/*sandāl* as a common type of footwear suggest that Jewish sources are not producing a lexical innovation but that they are possibly relying on some ancient themes associated with creation.

5 סנדל / *Sandāl* as the secularization of Mesopotamian scholarly texts

My assumption is that the סנדל/*sandāl* as a *terminus technicus* should not be interpreted either as a Greek or a Hebrew lexical innovation but rather as a secularization (or rationalization) of an older Babylonian tradition, specifically associated with childbirth.

This correlation with older Babylonian traditions seems supported by a minor but important lexical correction introduced by the Bavli that quotes from a baraita particularly close to the same text occurring in the Tosefta: identifying the *sandāl* as not a simple לשון של שור/*lāšôn šĕl šûr* but rather a probably "bigger" one, לשון של שור הגדול/*lāšôn šĕl šûr ha-gādôl*. It is indeed interesting that it is a *Babylonian* source that corrects a most likely earlier Palestinian source emphasizing the large dimensions of the foetus shaped like a fish. This correction, which is completely misinterpreted by classic rabbinic commentators, might have been introduced on account of some familiarity with ancient scholarly Mesopotamian texts from the second and first millennium BCE that identify the foetus with a fish, regardless of whether it is a regular childbirth or a miscarriage. There are indeed two occurrences, in older Sumerian and Akkadian medical-mythical literature, which support the identification of a foetus with a fish, regardless of whether it is well formed or abnormal:

1. The first identification of a child with a fish is provided by some Sumerian and Akkadian incantations dedicated to a pregnant woman who eats a special "sweet herb" (*ú-làl*) that is typically eaten by a certain fish called either (in Sumerian) *suḫur* or (in Akkadian) *purādu*. The identification of this fish with a specific species is of particular importance, especially while treating ancient texts that deal with miscarriages and largely use the image of a "fish" as a metaphor for designating a (either normal or abnormal) childbirth. The authoritative *Assyrian Dictionary of the Oriental Institute of the University of Chicago* (CAD) maintains that a *purādu* shall unequivocally be identified with a "carp."[53] Nevertheless, this identification has not always been exclusive. On the contrary, some scholars in the past had suggested a different identification that would have an important impact on the present treatment of Old Mesopotamian sources together with later rabbinic sources. Namely, Harri Holma and William Radcliffe maintained that a *purādu* could also be identified with a kind of a flatfish that exhibits the same typical "beard" of a carp, such as a "skate" or a "ray."[54] The possibility of identifying the *purādu* with a flatfish would be important, especially when ex-

---

53 Erica Reiner, ed., *The Assyrian Dictionary of the Oriental Institute of the University of Chicago*, vol. 12 (Chicago: The Oriental Institute, 2005), 516.

54 Harri Holma, *Kleine Beiträge zum Assyrischen Lexicon* (Helsinki: Finnischen Literaturgesellschaft, 1912), 96, quoted in William Radcliffe, *Fishing from the Earliest Times* (London: Murray, 1921), 376.

amining some Old Mesopotamian texts that explicitly compare the foetus to a "fish" swimming in uterus.In his detailed investigation *Birth in Babylonia and the Bible*,[55] Marten Stol proved that a woman eats this "sweet herb" because she wishes to please the very special kind of "fish" living in her belly—that is, the foetus with which she is pregnant, as reported in an Akkadian incantation for a woman in labour:[56]

1. i-na me-e na-a-ki-im	1. From the waters of intercourse,
2. ib-ba-ni e-ṣé-em-tum	2. bone was created,
3. i-na ši-i-ir [ši]-ir-ha-ni-im	3. from the muscular tissue,
4. ib-ba-ni li-il-li-du-um	4. the baby was created
[...]	[...]
25. [li]-im-ha-as [...]	25. Let him strike [...]
26. ki-ma da-di-[im]	26. Like a *dādu*-fish
27. šu-sí ra-ma-an-ka	27. bring yourself out
(YBC 4603/YOS 11 86, ll. 1–4 and 25–27)	

Interestingly, as Stol remarks, this text does not overtly describe the foetus as a *suḫur*, as other texts do, but rather with the Akkadian term *dādum* (literally "darling") that is also employed for designating a Sumerian-Akkadian female deity of creation as well as for forming some Akkadian proper names.[57] This Semitic root occurs for instance in the Hebrew term דוד/*dôd*, "friend" or in the Hebrew name דוד/*Dawid*, "David."[58] It would then designate something that is particularly "dear" to the speaker. Therefore, the choice of describing a foetus as a *dādum* would well support a tender wordplay between a "fish" in his mother's belly and a "beloved" child.[59]

---

55 Marten Stol, *Birth in Babylonia and the Bible: Its Mediterranean Setting* (Groningen: Styx, 2000), 9–10.

56 For the (here slightly modified) translation, see Ibid., 11. For the original Akkadian text and the transcription, see Claudia D. Bergmann, *Childbirth as a Metaphor for Crisis: Evidence from the Ancient Near East, the Hebrew Bible, and 1QH XI, 1–18* (Leiden: Brill, 2000), 32, on the basis of Jja van Dijk, "Une incantation accompagnant la naissance de l'homme," *Or* 42 (1973): 502–507; see also Niek Veldhuis, "The Poetry of Magic," in *Mesopotamian Magic: Textual, Historical, and Interpretative Perspectives* (ed. Tzvi Abusch and Karel van der Toorn; Groningen: Styx, 1999), 36–48.

57 Erica Reiner, ed., *The Assyrian Dictionary of the Oriental Institute of the University of Chicago*, vol. 3 (Chicago: The Oriental Institute, 2004), 20–21. The use of *dādum* as "childbirth" follows the previous major connotations as "love-making" and "object of love." Interestingly enough the term *dādum* as "child" is a homograph to the term *dādum* that also designates an "aquatic animal." It is possible that the author intended to suggest a subtle wordplay between the "child," who is "beloved" and craves for "sweet herb" like a "fish"—or an "aquatic animal" (*dādum*).

58 For a discussion on the interferences between the Akkadian *dādum* and the Hebrew דוד, see Jaquin Sanmartin-Ascaso, "Dôdh," in *Theological Dictionary of the Old Testament* (ed. G. Johannes Botterweck and Helmer Ringgren; trans. John T. Willis, G. W. Bromiley and D. E. Green; vol. 3; Grand Rapids, MI: Eerdmans, 1997), 143–156.

59 Stol, *Birth in Babylonia and the Bible*, 11.

2. The second identification of a foetus with a fish is quite consistent with the rich imagery of the uterus filled with amniotic fluid and thus similar to an aquatic environment. More specifically, this identification is provided in a very different context: the collection of the teratological omen series called *Šumma Izbu*. This collection was transcribed (sometimes incompletely), commented on, and translated in the 1970s by Erle Leichty,[60] and has recently been re-edited in a much more exhaustive way by Nicla De Zorzi.[61] This collection provides a number of birth omens in case of miscarriage both of a child and of an animal, designated with the common Akkadian term *izbu*. Among a long list of horrible child defects, the *Šumma Izbu* reports also the case of a woman delivering a very special child. This is originally reported in an almost laconic line of text that De Zorzi has recently completed thanks to a newly published fragment:[62]

BE *iz-bu ki-ma* SUḪUR[ku6] *ù* [muš *qú-lip-ta,*] *ha-li-ip uz-za-at* [d]30 lú *ep-qa* d[ir] (*Šumma Izbu* XVII 54′)

If an *izbu* is covered with scales like a *purādu*-carp or a snake, anger of the god Sîn: a/the man will be full of *epqu*-lesions[63]

Interestingly, the Akkadian text employs the Sumerian logogram SUḪUR to designate the very same "fish" that is fond of the "sweet herb," mentioned in the Sumerian incantation reported above, and corresponding to the Akkadian term *purādu*. At this point it can be useful to resume the small semantic dispute on the meaning of this term. If one accepts the CAD's identification of the *purādu* with a "carp," the present comparison between the Old Mesopotamian and rabbinic corpora is not necessarily disqualified but mostly relies on a specific thematic congruence: the assumption that a childbirth can be compared to a fish, regardless of its normal or abnormal nature. In this respect, this thematic congruence could be justified in an anthropological perspective and would reflect the almost spontaneous acknowledgment that foetuses live in the amniotic liquid. On the contrary, if one recovers Holma's and Radcliffe's iden-

60 On the rendering of this term, see Erle Leichty, *The Omen Series Šumma Izbu* (Locust Valley, NY: Augustin, 1970), 63. For a lexicographic description, see Erica Reiner, ed., *The Assyrian Dictionary of the Oriental Institute of the University of Chicago*, vol. 7 (Chicago: The Oriental Institute, 2004), 317–318.

61 Nicla De Zorzi, *La Serie Teratomantica Šumma Izbu: Testo, Tradizione, Orizzonti Culturali* (Padova: S.A.R.G.O.N., 2014). See also Nicla De Zorzi, "The Omen Series *Šumma Izbu*: Internal Structure and Hermeneutic Strategies," *KASKAL. Rivista di Storia, Ambienti, e Culture del Vicino Oriente* 8 (2011): 43–75.

62 For the text, transcription, translation, and commentary, see De Zorzi, *La Serie Teratomantica*, ad loc. Cf. also the previous, fragmentary transcription: "if an anomaly is like a carp and a …" (BE *iz-bu ki-ma* SUḪUR.KU6 *ù* […]) (Leichty, *The Omen Series Šumma Izbu*, 171–172). De Zorzi has integrated this fragmentary source with a Neo-Assyrian and late Babylonian manuscripts as well as with the later Babylonian commentary: Uruk, SBTU 2 38 (= E. von Weiher, *Spätbabylonische Texte aus Uruk* 2), recto ll. 21–22.

63 For the identification of *ep-qa* with "lesions," see Marten Stol, "Leprosy: New Light from Greek and Babylonian Sources," *Jaarbericht van het Vooraziatisch-Egyptisch Gezelschap Ex Oriente Lux* 30 (1999): 22–31, and JoAnn A. Scurlock and Brill R. Andersen, *Diagnoses in Assyrian and Babylonian Medicine* (Chicago: Urbana, 2005).

tification of *purādu* with a flatfish (that might still be similar to a carp), it is possible to substantiate the previous analysis also on account of specific philological congruencies.

It is in this light that it might be interesting to take into account a supplementary source that is textually and thematically connected to the former one. There is indeed a well-preserved tablet containing an early Hellenistic "commentary" (*malsûtu*)[64] on this passage. This text apparently disambiguates the sense of the omen and aligns this incantation with a tentative description of a foetal monstrosity:[65]

BE *iz-bu* GIM SUḪUR.MAŠ$_2$^{ku6} *u$_3$* MUŠ
qu$_2$-lip-tu$_2$ sa-ḫi-ip/uz-za-at d SUEN^{Lu2}
ep-qa SA$_5$
(CCP 3.6.3.B—*Izbu* commentary 17 B,
lines 21–22)

If an *izbu* is covered in a skin of scales like a goatfish or a snake: anger of Sin; the man will be afflicted with *epqu*-lesions

This later commentary is particularly important. It provides a better understanding of the original Akkadian omen and also offers a relevant comparative perspective about child anomalies in the present context. In particular, the author of this commentary compares the "anomaly" (*izbu*) to a fish—or, more specifically, a mythical "goatfish" (*suhurmāšī*)—especially because it resembles some morphological aspects of an aquatic animal: possibly its "skin" that presents "scales" (*quliptu*). In addition, it should be noted that the mention of "scales" apparently resonates with the case of a woman miscarrying something "like a kind of membrane" (קליפה/*qĕlipāh*) mentioned both in the Mishnah and in the Tosefta (m. Nid. 3:2 and t. Nid. 4:2), especially on account of the ruling about a woman miscarrying "like a kind of fishes," both reported in the Mishnah (m. Nid. 3:2) and the corresponding page from the Bavli (b. Nid. 21a). It is not implausible that these congruencies are not coincidental and reflect a thematic if not textual proximity between the corpora.[66]

These textual witnesses allow us to maintain that Mesopotamian literature between the second and first millennium BCE sustained the identity between a foetus and a fish, regardless of whether it was well formed or abnormal, and that this identity was maintained both as a poetical and as a mythical-medical truth. On account of this, it would be interesting to revaluate the choice of strictly identifying the Sumeri-

---

64 On Mesopotamian scholarly commentaries, cf. Markham J. Geller, *Ancient Babylonian Medicine: Theory and Praxis* (Chichester: Wiley-Blackwell, 2010), especially 141–160. See also Eckart Frahm, *Babylonian and Assyrian Commentaries: Origins of Interpretation* (Münster: Ugarit, 2011).

65 For the text, the transcription, the (here slightly modified) translation, and commentary, see Enrique Jiménez, "Commentary on Izbu 17 (*CCP* 3.6.3.B)," *Cuneiform Commentaries Project* (E. Frahm—E. Jiménez—M. Frazer—K. Wagensonner), 2013–2019; accessed September 19, 2019, at https://ccp.yale.edu/P348643.

66 The dissemination of the Akkadian term *quliptu* through several languages of the Near East is indisputable, as is easily reflected, for instance, both in Aramaic and Syriac. The Akkadian term mostly refers to reptiles, fishes, and plants, as well as to human skin, especially in a medical context, designating a "flake of skin." See Erica Reiner, ed., *The Assyrian Dictionary of the Oriental Institute of the University of Chicago*, vol. 13 (Chicago: The Oriental Institute, 1995), 296–298.

an term *suḫur* and its correlated Akkadian term *purādu* with "a carp" and rather taking into account Holma's and Radcliffe's suggestion that a *purādu* could also designate
a *flatfish* that is not too dissimilar from a "carp." In this latter case, one could argue that
there are possibly some textual-historical connections between these corpora. As a result, the Hebrew term סנדל / *sandāl* would then represent the secularization or rationalization, even Hellenization, of these previous Old Babylonian themes and their transformation into an abstract juridical-medical concept. This concept would eventually
mobilize a number of collateral ritual issues, such as delivering a specific sacrifice in in
case of miscarriage, especially with respect to the very morphology of the foetus. In
this perspective it would then be important to distinguish both juridically and ritually
between the miscarriage of an ordinary (normal) foetus, a *sandāl*, or a "piece of flesh."

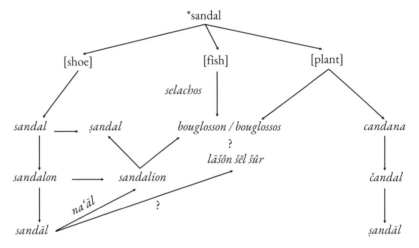

Bibliography

Literature

Bergmann, Claudia D. *Childbirth as a Metaphor for Crisis: Evidence from the Ancient Near
    East, the Hebrew Bible, and 1QH XI, 1–18.* Leiden: Brill, 2000.
Brockelmann, Carl. *Lexicon Syriacum.* Berlin: Reuther & Reichard, 1895.
Cannon, Garland and Alan S. Kaye. *The Persian Contributions to the English Language: An
    Historical Dictionary.* Wiesbaden: Harrassowitz, 2011.
Caro, Rabbi Luciano. "Rabbi Ovadyà da Bertinoro e il suo supercommentario a Rashi." *He-
    braica* (1998): 165–168.
Chiesa, Bruno. "Il supercommentario di Ovadya a Rasi." In *Ovadiah Yare da Bertinoro e la
    presenza ebraica in Romagna nel Quattrocento.* Edited by Giulio Busi. Torino: Zamorani,
    1989. Pages 35–46.
Ciancaglini, Claudia. *Iranian Loanwords in Syriac.* Wiesbaden: Ludwig Reichert, 2008.
Cohen, Tobias (Tuviah). *Ma'aseh Tovayah kolel ha-Arba'ah 'Olamot.* Venice: Stamparia Braga-
    dina, 1708.

Costaz, Louis. *Dictionnaire Syraique-Français*. Beirut: Dar el-Machreq, 2002.

Dal Bo, Federico. *Massekhet Keritot: Text, Translation, and Commentary*. Tübingen: Mohr Siebeck, 2013.

Davis, Joseph. *Yom Tov Lipmann Heller: Portrait of a Seventeenth-Century Rabbi*. Oxford: Littman Library, 2004.

De Zorzi, Nicla. "The Omen Series *Šumma Izbu*: Internal Structure and Hermeneutic Strategies," *KASKAL. Rivista di Storia, Ambienti, e Culture del Vicino Oriente* 8 (2011): 43–75.

—. *La Serie Teratomantica Šumma Izbu. Testo, Tradizione, Orizzonti Culturali*. Padova: S.A.R.G.O.N., 2014.

van Dijk, Jja. "Une incantation accompagnant la naissance de l'homme." *Or* 42 (1973): 502–507.

Dorkin, Robin. *Between East and West: The Moluccas and the Traffic in Spices up to the Arrival of Europeans*. Philadelphia: American Philosophical Society, 2003.

Even-Shoshan, Avraham. *Hamilon heḥadash*. Vol. 4. Jerusalem: Kiryat Sefer, 1979.

Faur, Josè. "Maimonides' Discovery of a Saboraitic Version of Tractate Niddah". *Tarbiz* 55/4 (1995): 721–728. [In Hebrew]

Frahm, Eckart. *Babylonian and Assyrian Commentaries: Origins of Interpretation*. Münster: Ugarit, 2011.

Geller, Markham J. *Akkadian Healing Therapies in the Babylonian Talmud*. Preprint Series 259. Berlin: Max-Planck Institut für Wissenschaftsgeschichte, 2004. Cited 19 September 2019: https://www.mpiwg-berlin.mpg.de/Preprints/P259.PDF

—. *Ancient Babylonian Medicine: Theory and Praxis*. Chichester: Wiley-Blackwell, 2010.

Holdsworth, William G. *Cleft Lip and Palate*. New York: Grune & Statton, 1963.

Holma, Harri. *Kleine Beiträge zum Assyrischen Lexicon*. Helsinki: Finnischen Literaturgesellschaft, 1912.

Jastrow, Marcus. *A Dictionary of the Targumim, the Talmud Bavli, and Yerushalmi, and the Midrashic Literature*. London: Druglin, 1903.

Kogan, Leonid. "Proto-Semitic Phonetic and Phonology." In *The Semitic Languages: An International Handbook*. Edited by Stefan Weininger. Berlin: De Gruyter, 2011. Pages 54–151.

Krieger, Pinchus. *Parshan-Data*. Monsey, NY: Krieger, 2005.

Jiménez, Enrique. "Commentary on Izbu 17 (*CCP* 3.6.3.B)," *Cuneiform Commentaries Project* (E. Frahm—E. Jiménez—M. Frazer – K. Wagensonner), 2013–2019. Cited 19 September 2019, at https://ccp.yale.edu/P348643.

Lampe, Geoffrey W. H. *A Patristic Greek Lexicon*. Oxford: Clarendon, 1961.

Lehnardt, Andreas. "Mainz und seine Talmudgelehrten im Mittelalter." In *Mainz im Mittelalter*. Edited by Mechtild Dreyer. Mainz: Zabern, 2009. Pages 87–102.

Leichty, Erle. *The Omen Series Šumma Izbu*. Locust Valley, NY: Augustin, 1970.

Levine, Lee I. *Judaism and Hellenism in Antiquity: Conflict or Confluence?* Washington: University of Washington Press, 2012.

Liddell, Henry and Robert Scott. *A Greek-English Lexicon*. Revised by H. S. Jones. Oxford: Clarendon, 1996.

Lust, Johan, Erik Eynikel and Karin Hauspie. *A Greek-English Lexicon of the Septuagint*. Stuttgart: Deutsche Bibelgesellschaft, 2002.

Mayrhofer, Manfred. *Kurzgefasstes Etymologisches Wörterbuch des Altindischen*. Heidelberg: Carl Winter Verlag, 1976.

Meacham, Tirzah. "Fetal Death in the Palestinian Talmud. Murder in the Chamber." In *Death and taxes in the ancient Near East*. Edited by Sara E. Orel. Lewiston: Mellen, 1992. Pages 145–156.

Needham, Joseph and Arthur Hughes. *A History of Embryology*. Cambridge: Cambridge University Press, 2015.

Neher, André. "Cabale, science et philosophie dans le commentaire sur la Mishna de Tiferet Israel." In *'Ale Shefer: Studies in the Literature of Jewish Thought: Presented to Rabbi Dr. Alexandre Safran*. Edited by Moshe Ḥallamish. Ramat Gan: Bar-Ilan University Press, 1990. Pages 127–132.

Orel, Sara E., ed. *Death and taxes in the ancient Near East*. Lewiston: Mellen, 1992.

Preuss, Julius. *Biblical and Talmudic Medicine*. Translated by Fred Rosner. Lanham: Rowman & Littlefield, 2004.

Radcliffe, William. *Fishing from the Earliest Times*. London: Murray, 1921.

Reichman, Edward. "Is There Life after Life? Superfetation in Rabbinic Literature." In *Shalom Rav. And You Shall Surely Heal*. Edited by Jonathan Wiesen. New York: Yeshiva University Press, 2009. Pages 39–55.

Reiner, Erica, ed., *The Assyrian Dictionary of the Oriental Institute of the University of Chicago*. 21 vols. Chicago: The Oriental Institute, 1956–2011.

Rosenbaum, Shalom B. "Forgotten Manuscripts of the Lipschutz Family." *Da'at* 61 (1972): 97–112. [In Hebrew]

Rosner, Fred. *Maimonides' Medical Writings*. 7 vols. Haifa: Maimonides Institute, 1984–1994.

Sanmartin-Ascaso, Jaquin. "Dôdh." In *Theological Dictionary of the Old Testament*. Edited by G. Johannes Botterweck and Helmer Ringgren. Translated by John T. Willis, G. W. Bromiley and D. E. Green. Vol. 3. Grand Rapids, MI: Eerdmans, 1997. Pages 143–156.

Schmidt, Max C. P. *Paulys Realencyclopädie der classischen Altertumswissenschaft*. Vol. 3/1. Edited by G. Wissowa. Stuttgart: Metzler, 1897.

Schwab, Moïse. *Les Manuscrits et les Incunables Hebreux de la Bibliotheque de l'Alliance Israelite*. Paris: Durlacher, 1904.

Scurlock, Joann A. and Brill R. Andersen. *Diagnoses in Assyrian and Babylonian Medicine*. Chicago: Urbana, 2005.

Shereshevsky, Esra. *Rashi, the Man and His World*. Northvale, NJ: J. Aronson, 1996.

Sokoloff, Michael. *A Dictionary of Jewish Palestinian Aramaic of the Byzantine Period*. Ramat Gan: Bar-Ilan University Press, 1992.

Stemberger, Günter. *Introduction to the Talmud and the Midrash*. Translated by M. Brockmuehl. Minneapolis, MN: Fortress, 1992.

Stol, Marten. "Leprosy: New Light from Greek and Babylonian Sources." *Jahrbericht ex Oriente Lux* 30 (1999): 22–31.

—. *Birth in Babylonia and the Bible: Its Mediterranean Setting*. Groningen: Styx, 2000.

Veldhuis, Niek. "The Poetry of Magic." In *Mesopotamian Magic: Textual, Historical, and Interpretative Perspectives*. Edited by Tzvi Abusch and Karel van der Toorn. Groningen: Styx, 1999. Pages 36–48.

Westreich, Mark and Steve Segal. "Cleft Lip in the Talmud." *Annual of Plastic Surgery* 2 (2000): 229–327.

Wollaston, Arthur N. *An English-Persian Dictionary Compiled from the Original Sources*. London: Allen, 1882.

Zohar, Zvi. "Sephardic Jurisprudence in the Recent Half-Millennium." In *Sephardic and Mizrahi Jewry: From the Golden Age of Spain to Modern Times*. Edited by Zvi Zohar. New York: New York University Press, 2005. Pages 167–196.

The Cure of Amnesia and *Ars Memoria* in Rabbinic Texts

Reuven Kiperwasser

1 Preliminary remarks[1]

This paper aims to discuss an aspect of classical rabbinic culture that deserves more scholarly attention: memory. Though there has been a good deal of debate about orality in rabbinic literature,[2] the systematic study of orality in relation to memorization has begun only recently.[3] In his book, Michael Swartz proposes "a brief outline of the issue, sketching in fairly broad strokes the methodological and historical significance of memory for the study of Rabbinic Judaism and indicating some ancient Jewish strategies for harnessing it for the sake of Torah,"[4] a task that he then expertly achieved.[5] In this paper, I want to add a few new observations regarding the value of memory and forgetfulness, and propose an explanation for the mechanisms of these processes as understood in rabbinic thought.

According to the typical rabbinic approach, knowledge must be accompanied by understanding. However, the learning process at the rabbinic academy involved

---

1   A preliminary version of the first part of this paper was presented at the 16th Biennial Conference of the International Society for Religion, Literature and Culture at the Faculty of Theology, University of Copenhagen, Denmark, October 19–21, 2012. The second part of this paper, on "Jewish Medicine" was presented at a one-day panel at the 10th EAJS Congress at Paris, July 24, 2014. I am grateful to Lennart Lehmhaus for proposing that I publish this paper. The paper was finished during my stay in Berlin, as a Alexander von Humboldt Fellow at the Institute of Judaic Studies at the Freie Universität. I am thankful to these institutions for their support.

2   I will mention here only a few remarkable works, such as Gerhardsson 1961, for a critique of this work's historical argument; cf. Smith 1963, 169–176; see as well Lieberman 1962, 83–99; Neusner 1979; Jaffee 1992; Jaffee 1998, Jaffee 1999; Sussman 2006, 294–384.

3   Naeh 2005, 570–582, esp. 564–566, and idem 2001, 851–875, esp. 858–875.

4   Swartz 1996, 35.

5   Michael Swartz opens his discussion with the statement that in traditional rabbinic education, the basic texts were to be memorized before they were understood and discussed (b. 'Abod. Zar. 19a). Based on the statement attributed to Rava, Swartz proposes that this statement presupposes two stages of learning: the first in which the text is learned and memorized and the second in which the act of analytic review of the learned text takes place, because this statement stresses that the student should memorize even if he does not understand what he is reciting. However, it should be mentioned that only in the Babylonian Talmud can we find such admiration for learning without deep understanding of the content of the material, though there is some mocking of this way of learning (see for example b. Soṭah 22a, where learning without understanding is defined by the term *ratin magosha*, which means "the mumbling of Zoroastrian priests"). See Greenfield 1974, 63–69; see also Rosenthal 1982, 1:48–49 and 71–72. Nevertheless, the importance of memory for the rabbinic curriculum is quite evident here.

DOI: 10.13173/9783447108263.119

the cultivation of memory training; loss of memory was perceived as a disaster and a serious problem for the rabbinic career. [6] Societies that make a distinction between knowledge *as understanding* and knowledge *as memorization* acknowledge, in a way, that memorization and knowledge are not the same thing. Nevertheless, the role of a person who can remember many texts was usually quite important in these societies.[7]

In antiquity, memory was thought to have a physiological basis. While the theories underlying this conception ranged from Aristotelian psychology to practical medicine, it was understood that memory was directly related to the makeup and composition of the body and physical mind.[8] In rabbinic culture memory is a link between the body and the mind: it has roots in the body, and it is a crucially important component of the mind, as I will show further.

In this paper, I will analyze stories from rabbinic literature about rabbis who forgot their knowledge under certain circumstances and then used certain techniques for getting it back. Talmudic literature was created by rabbis for their students and is, accordingly, characterized by a strong didactic orientation. Talmudic sages shared the view of the ancient Greeks that memory is an integral part of wisdom. Therefore, the loss of memory leads to wisdom becoming flawed. Narrators of tales about sages who forgot their knowledge, usually tend to see the loss of memory as the consequence of something untoward in the sage's behavior. Nevertheless, after that divine punishment was meted out and the delinquent scholar had lost his wisdom, the question arises: Can his pitiful condition be cured? And if so, can this be done by merely invoking mercy, or by some other kind of cure? In other words, should the cure rely on the mind, or on the body, or on both of them? This will bring us to the next question: What actually is the substrate of memory in rabbinic culture? Is it some sort of bodily function or is it a part of the mind? Through analyzing texts dealing with memory, memorization, and memory loss, I seek to reconstruct the concept of the physiology of memory that lies beneath these texts.

2 Forgotten and successfully recalled

One of the foundational narratives of rabbinic culture is the story of Hillel the Elder's appointment as patriarch.[9] This story appears in rabbinic literature in three different versions: in the Tosefta, in the Palestinian Talmud, and in the Babylonian Talmud (henceforth also called 'Bavli').[10] However, the significant motif of the loss of memory appears only in the version recorded in both Talmuds. According to the plot,[11] it hap-

---

6 See Sussman 2006, 41–42 n.30. See as well recently published Balberg 2020.
7 Carruthers 1990, 20.
8 Ibid., 47–71.
9 Cf. t. Pesaḥim 4:13–14. Cf. y. Pesaḥim 6:1, 33a, b. Pesaḥim 66a. For an analysis of the different versions of this story, see Frenkel 2001, 22–39, and Katz 2011, 81–116.
10 See also t. Temurot 1:17, Zuckermandel 1970. 552, and b. Yoma 51a, and see Lieberman 1992, 566–567.
11 I am summarizing here and below the version of the Palestinian Talmud, though on the point of memory loss this version does not differ from the Babylonian one. For comparative analyses of the Palestinian and Babylonian versions, see Frenkel, and Katz above, n. 9.

pened that one time the fourteenth of Nisan, the day on which the Passover sacrifices are performed, fell on a Sabbath. The rabbis were preoccupied with the question of what takes precedence: the Sabbath (in which slaughter, let alone roasting, is prohibited) or the festival. Should the sacrifice be postponed until after the Sabbath, or should the Sabbath be violated for the sake of the sacrifice? It seems that the proper solution for the problem was known to the learned community in the past, but unfortunately was forgotten by the present leaders. Unexpectedly, one previously unknown scholar,[12] after trying to resolve the problem with his scholastic arguments, claims after a while that he possesses an ancient tradition from the famous masters of the past on how to act in this situation. After Hillel extracts from his own memory the teachings forgotten by the sages, immediately the branch of forgetful scholars from the Batira family feel obliged to give up their seat of honor in favor of the Babylonian with the good memory.

At the end of that celebrated story we learn that after Hillel's election, the former outsider and stranger began to mock his former masters, the Batira family's sages who forgot their learning, for laziness in serving their masters. But after Hillel ascends to the position of head of sages, when faced with his first halakhic decision, for which the answer is simple enough, he forgets the tradition that would provide the answer. Salvation comes to the former outsider from outside—he sees the pilgrims coming to the temple, and their behavior according to the halakhic rule, which he had forgotten, helps him to remember the forgotten law and maintain his position. Scholars rightly interpret this story as an etiological story explaining the ascendance of the Hillel dynasty, produced by admirers of Rabbi Judah the Patriarch, the most admirable scion of this dynasty.[13] However, it is also a story about divine manipulation of memory. Memory here is a kind of charisma in the primary sense of this word—a gift from God. Knowledge fallen into oblivion is punishment for misconduct, as, for example, in this story about Hillel offending his colleagues. The story portrays memory as not only an ability to repeat things without mistake, but also an ability to recollect things. Recollection is a rational procedure, involving conceptual sequences with a variety of components, from which one can devise a new notion based on the information stored in memory.[14] The halakhic rules Hillel received from his masters were hidden in the space of his memory, and then he successfully found the relevant rule at the moment of his controversy with the Batira family. Other rules were completely lost to Hillel, but they were found with the help of an external factor; the new notion, based on something hidden in memory, was constructed.

3   Forgotten and lost

In the story discussed above, Hillel's pride led him to lose his memory. However, this is not the only reason for the loss of memory: we will now analyze a few cases of rabbinic amnesiacs and try to understand their cultural context.

---

12 He was a Babylonian immigrant to the land of Israel. I deal with this theme in another study regarding Babylonians in the land of Israel in my ongoing project. Meanwhile see Kiperwasser 2019
13 Katz 2011, 114.
14 Caruthers 2009, 2.

3.1 Rabbi Joshua ben Levi's story

In *Ecclesiastes Rabbah* 7:7 and Tanḥuma, *Vaʿeraʾeh* 5:5 we find a short story about Rabbi Joshua ben Levi, who forgot the halakhic learning he had acquired from Rabbi Judah bar Pedayah because he had been too involved in providing for community needs.[15]

Ecclesiastes Rabbah 7:7[16]

"Surely oppression turns a wise man into a fool (Eccl 7:7) ...
R. Joshua b. Levi said: Eighty halakhot did I learn from Judah b. Pedayah concerning a grave that has been ploughed over, but through being occupied with the needs of the community, I forgot them all.

כי העושק יהולל חכם (קהלת ז, ז).
...
אמר ר' יהושע בן לוי שמ[ו]נים הלכות למדתי
מיהודה בן פדיה בחורש את הקבר, ועל ידי
שעסקתי בצרכי רבים, שכחתים.

Here knowledge was lost because the rabbinic student preferred the public realm of active deeds to the quiet solitude of academia. We do not know what kind of community needs (literally "needs of the majority") this socially active rabbi attended to, but clearly his behavior was not entirely admirable for a rabbinic student, according to the narrator's perspective. No mishnaic treatise includes such a large number of laws concerning a grave. Seemingly this knowledge was lost forever. The narrator intends to tell us a didactic story in which the borders of appropriate and inappropriate behavior of sages are represented with their outcomes. The ideal sage is therefore someone not overly involved in the political life of his city and loyal and respectful to members of his class.

3.2 R. Eleazar ben Arakh's story

The loss of memory as a punishment for some inexcusable deed is evidenced by the sad story about the legendary Tanna R. Eleazar b. Arakh.[17] This is perhaps the best example of wisdom forgotten and lost forever. The sage, by the bad advice of his wife, decided not to follow his students, but to live in solitude, far from the academic center of his brethren, and waited for his students to visit him. But when they finally arrived, he completely forgot all his knowledge. This story appears in the Palestinian work *Ecclesiastes Rabbah*. The parallel to this story, which is preserved in the Babylonian Talmud (Shabbat 147b), depends on a different tradition, and there the sage's wisdom is not lost forever. Interestingly, as we shall see below, in the Bavli Rabbi Eleazar ben Arakh was cured

---

15 The story per the Tanḥuma is the same as in *Ecclesiastes Rabbah*, only with minor changes: "R. Yohanan the son of Levi said: R. Judah the son of Pedayah taught me sixty laws concerning a grave which has been ploughed over, and I have forgotten all of them because I occupied myself with the needs of the community."

16 On this passage from *Ecclesiastes Rabbah*, see Kiperwasser 2010 and recently Kister 2017.

17 For the literary portrait of this sage in rabbinic literature, see Goshen-Gottstein 2000, 233–238, and see also Levine 2002, 278–289 and recently Marienberg-Milikowsky 2015, 1–25. For a comparison of the different versions of this story, see Kiperwasser 2010, 264–271.

from his forgetfulness by the prayer of his colleagues—here the wisdom of the sage becomes the property of the community of sages and can be restored by their intervention.

Ecclesiastes Rabbah 7:7

... R. Yoḥanan b. Zakkai,[18] for as long as he lived did they sit before him. When he died, they went to Yavneh. R. Eleazar b. Arakh, however, joined his wife at Emmaus, a place of good water and lovely in every aspect. He waited for them to come to him, but they did not. As they failed to do so, he wanted to go to them, but his wife would not let him. She said, "Who needs whom?" He answered, "They need me." She said to him, "In the case of a vessel [containing food] and mice, which goes to which? Do the mice go to the vessel or does the vessel come to the mice?" He listened to her and remained there until he had forgotten his learning. After a while, they came to him and asked: "Which is better to eat along with a spread, bread made of wheat or bread made of barley?" But he was unable to answer.[19]

(ר׳ אלעזר בן ערך) [רבן יוחנן בן זכאי] כל זמן שהיה קיים, היו יושבין לפניו, וכשנפטר הלכו ליבנה. והלך ר׳ אלעז בן ערך אצל אשתו לאמאוס, מקום מים יפים ונוי יפה. המתין להן שיבאו אצלו ולא באו. כיון שלא באו, בקש לילך אצלן ולא הניחה אותו אשתו. אמרה לו: מי צריך למאן? אמ׳ לה: הם צריכים לי. חמת ועכברים, מי דרכן לילך לדבר? שיבקש העכברים אצל החמת או החמת אצל עכברים? שמע לה וישב לו, עד ששכח תלמודו. לאחר זמן באו אצלו. שאלו: פת חטין או פת שעורין מסב ואוכל בליפתן? ולא ידע מה להשיבן.

The redactor of *Ecclesiastes Rabbah* included the story in the paragraph interpreting the verse Ecclesiastes 7:7: הָעֹשֶׁק יְהוֹלֵל חָכָם וִיאַבֵּד אֶת לֵב מַתָּנָה, the translation of which is not a simple task. The plain meaning of the verse is as follows: "The fool's provocation can disable the wise man's faculties and destroy his understanding." Destruction of understanding is what is meant by the idiom "losing the heart," which our homilist takes as a reference to losing the knowledge of the Torah, or as in the verse, God's gift, מתנה to the heart of the sage. A noteworthy paronomasia (a wordplay) makes its appearance in the story about Rabbi Eleazar: חמת (vessel), the object aimed at by the mice, is paralleled by אמאוס (Emmaus)—the well-known location referred to in Hebrew as חמת—that is the destination of Rabbi Eleazar's students. When the students

---

18 I have emended the text here in order to reconstruct the correct reading. For the recent discussion about the corruptions in this fragment, see Kiperwasser 2010, 264–265.

19 I think that the original story ends here, and the line that follows, which is omitted here, is a gloss added by a later transmitter. For the detailed explanation, see Kiperwasser 2010, 269–270. This explanation was enthusiastically attacked by Marienberg-Milikowsky 2015, 17 n. 62 (though the author relied on my dissertation from 2005 and not on the abovementioned paper), who tried to find some meaning for the presence of this line in the body of the story. However, I haven't been convinced by his argument. My point of view was recently supported by Kister, 2017, 20–21.

finally arrive, the master had already forgotten his learning. According to Ecclesiastes Rabbah the purpose of the students' visit is to stage an examination for the master—a test of his halakhic learning. Their question is simple:

Wheaten bread or barley bread, which is better to eat along with a spread?	פת חטין או פת שעורים מיסב ואוכל בלפתן?

However, the master does not know the answer. In order to understand the question's halakhic background, let us look at a passage in Mishnah *Nega'im* 13:9: [20]

If a man entered a house afflicted with leprosy, bearing his garments on his shoulder and his sandals and rings in his hands, he and they forthwith become unclean; but if he was clothed with his garments and had his sandals on his feet and his rings on his hand, he forthwith becomes unclean but they remain clean, unless he stayed there time enough to eat a half-loaf of bread—wheaten bread and not barley bread, and while in a reclining position and eating the bread with spread.[21]	מי שנכנס לבית המנוגע וכליו על כתפו וסנדליו וטבעותיו בידיו והוא והן טמאין מיד היה לבוש בכליו וסנדליו ברגליו וטבעותיו בידיו הוא טמא מיד והן טהורין עד שישהא כדי אכילת פרס פת חטין ולא פת שעורים מיסב ואוכלן בלפתן.

The mishnahic passage contains discussions about the amount of time needed to eat half a loaf of bread; one source attempts to define this time unit by specifying that half a loaf's weight is equivalent to eight eggs. However, our source defines it as the time sufficient for eating wheaten bread with spread, לפתן, while reclining on a couch, as was the custom at feasts in late antiquity; this means eating slowly and without haste. In Mishnah *Nega'im* the redactor makes a point to specify that the mishnaic passage does not refer to the time it takes to eat barley bread, but rather bread made of wheat, which is normally eaten quickly because it is soft, likely polemicizing against attempts to define the amount of time in question as the time it takes to eat half a loaf of barley bread. If so, the students' question is: In light of the two ways of defining the time required to eat half a loaf of bread, which of the two definitions is to be preferred? Presumably, Rabbi Eleazar ben Arakh would opt for one of the meanings and provide arguments for his choice, but instead he gives no answer at all, because he has forgotten all of his mishnaic and extramishnaic learning. Here amnesia is punishment for the scholar's pridefulness, for being unwilling to follow the students to the new locus of learning, and for his confidence that his students must follow him. The sage's

---

20 See Danby 1938, 694 with some changes.
21 See also t. Neg. 7:10 (Zuckermandel 1970, 627): "Its half is called *pras*; to eat in the afflicted house, he reclines and eats it with a *liftan*"

inability to lower his own self-regard inevitably led to a situation where the one who owns all the wisdom (namely God) takes away memory from him.

Loss of memory, however, is not something beyond repair; as we already saw in the case of Hillel, it is curable. The repentance of the amnesiac and his newly found humility helped him to reconstruct new knowledge from the small details of everyday life, which reverses the situation of forgotten knowledge. On the other hand, in the Palestinian version of the story about R. Eleazar ben Arakh, he is incurable, probably because he was unable to recognize his fall, and, from the point of view of redaction criticism, as an explanation why, in the entire rabbinic corpus, we do not find one single tradition attributed to this most famous sage of the first generation of Tannaim.

The parallel to this story preserved in the Babylonian Talmud is dependent on a different tradition and there the wisdom of the sage is not lost forever.

B. Shabbat 147b

R. Eleazar b. Arakh visited that place.[22] He was attracted to them, and [in consequence] his learning vanished. When he returned, he arose to read in the scroll [of the Torah]. He wished to read, "Hae hodesh hazeh lakem ..." (this month is to you) (Exod 12:2) [but instead] he read "haharesh hayah libbam?" ('was their heart deaf?') Nevertheless, the scholars prayed for him, and his learning returned.

רבי אליעזר בן ערך איקלע להתם אימשיך
בתרייהו איעקר תלמודיה כי הדר את' קם למיקרי
בסיפרא בעא למיקרי החדש הזה לכם אמר החרש
היה לבם בעו רבנן רחמי עליה והדר תלמודי.

Rabbi Eleazar's amnesia is the element common to both traditions cited above, but while according to the Babylonian Talmud, the rabbi's forgetfulness is exposed by coincidence when he is called on to read the Torah during a public reading, in the Palestinian source it is discovered through a deliberate test to which the rabbi is put. Another point of difference is that in the Bavli the wisdom of the sage becomes the property of the community of sages and can be restored by their intervention, through prayer. In this version of the story, as he reads the verse wrong, without remembering the proper formulation of the verses, the Rabbi Eleazar also misreads the consonants, which are almost graphical-identical, and so the read words got a new meaning: "their

---

22 Which place was visited by the sage is not completely clear from the story itself, but the fact that a few lines earlier a short discussion mentions the "water of Diamsit" (ימיא של דיומסת) suggests that the Babylonian narrator shares the Palestinian's notion about the dwelling place of the amnesiac rabbi. *Diamsit* is probably a Babylonian substitute for Emmaus. This toponym is very often spelled in rabbinic literature as *maus*, which is a phonetic transcription of Emmaus. Therefore, it seems that the original version was ימיא דמאוס and it was later corrupted to the present from. For a similar formation in the parallel story in Avot of Rabbi Nathan, see Kiperwasser 2010, 266, n. 28. The proposition raised by Marienberg-Milikowsky 2015, 4 n. 15, that the place is the city of Damascus does not make any sense.

heart is deaf," meaning "the mind of [the audience?] was deaf." Some sort of sub-
versive message is expressed through this wordplay manipulation, which adds some
ironic element to the situation.

3.3 One student's story

Ecclesiastes Rabbah 10:10[23]

Another interpretation: "If the iron is
blunt" (Eccl 10:10). If your learning is
hard as iron to you. "And he does not
whet"—you cannot understand it by
yourself, "the edge" [kalkol]—you should
raise your voice on it.

One of the students of Rabbi Shimon bar
Yohai forgot his studies. He went crying
to the cemetery and wept at (his teacher's) resting place. He cried much. [Rabbi
Shimon] appeared to him in a dream. He
said to him: once you throw three parched
grains at me [רמי ביה ג קליא] I will come.
That student went to a dream interpreter
and related the story to him. [The dream
interpreter] told him: Go recite your lesson
three times in sequence[24] and it will come
to you. And so he did, and so it happened.

ד"א. אם קהה הברזל (קהלת י, י). אם נקהה תל-
מודך עליו כברזל והוא לא פנים קלקל (שם), אינו
בא לידך להסבירו בפניך.קלקל (שם): קלקל עליו
בקלך. חד מן תלמידוי דר' שמעון בן יוחאי אנשי
אולפניה אזל ליה בכי לבי עלמיה [בכי מדמכיה].
בכי סגי אתחמי ליה בחלמיה, וא"ל: כד תהי רמי
ביה ג' קליא, אנא אתי. אזל ההוא תלמידא לגבי
מפתר חלמא ותני ליה עובדא. א"ל: זיל אמור
פירקך מן ג' זמנין והוא אתי לך. ועבד ליה כן וכן
הוה ליה.

The memory of an individual as a divine device, which is subject to the management
of rabbinic society, appears in the following passage from *Ecclesiastes Rabbah* based
on Ecclesiastes 10:10: אִם קֵהָה הַבַּרְזֶל וְהוּא לֹא פָנִים קִלְקַל וַחֲיָלִים יְגַבֵּר וְיִתְרוֹן הַכְשֵׁיר חָכְמָה.

"If the iron is blunt, and he does not whet the edge, then must he use more strength:
but wisdom is profitable to direct." This verse is interpreted in *Ecclesiastes Rabbah*
as an allegorical depiction of the master/disciple relationship. Iron is the "talmud,"
namely the learning process of the student, which became blunt as iron. In such a
case of deterioration in the study process, the exegete advises that more strength be
applied. The words "he does not whet the edge" could be understood as a description
of poorly performed learning, but the rabbinic interpreter, in a deconstructive manner, proposes to see it as a kind of remedy to the damaged memory. "If your learning
is hard as iron to you. 'and he does not whet'—you cannot understand it by yourself,
'the edge' [kalkol]—you should raise your voice on it." The words "not whet," *kalkol*

---

23 This story was briefly mentioned by Sussman 2006: 48 n.42.
24 The textual version is a little bit strange here. It could be understood as "repeat every three
    chapters three times" or "repeat every third chapter three times".

in Hebrew, are accepted as a *haplogramma* of the word *kol*, "voice," twice repeated. If the student would raise his voice again and again his strength will come back to him. The following story is an illustration of the reconstructed memory of the student.

The order to throw parched grains on the grave of the master horrifies the student—in fact, the action seems to him like the parody on halakhic stoning of the grave of an outcast. Information obtained from the other world turns out to be useless. However, properly interpreted by a member of the academic society, it turns out to be useful and even linked to a biblical verse. Three parched grains are not really parched grains—they are voices of students. This interpretation is based on a wordplay—the word *kola* in Aramaic is a parched grain, but in Hebrew *kol* (or its Aramaized derivate in Mishnaic Hebrew—*kola*) is a voice. The recipe is very simple and quite traditional, based on the common practice of rabbinic instruction—you should recite your lesson repeatedly, three times at least, while speaking up, and the forgotten learning will come back to you. However, behind this story lies certainly a quasi-scientific conception of memory loss and its cure. The physiology of memory and the cure of its loss should take into consideration the audio abilities of the person.

Therefore, on the margins of rabbinic literature one can find opinions according to which forgetting is a benefit, because if you forgot your learning, it will induce you to come back to your Torah repeatedly.[25] These stories regarding forgetting and remembrance, reveal the self-reflective mode of Talmudic culture, debating what is allowed to its members, and what is forbidden, and permanently concerned with the definition of its own borders. Some of the stories discussed above are from relatively later layers of rabbinic literature. They point to the participation of certain sensitive organs, the ears, in the processes of memory.

The main cultural pattern that lies behind these texts is that removing memory skills is some sort of a divine punishment and a frequent punishing rod in relationships between the sage and God. Noticeably, memory here is not simple rote memory, but the ability to recollect information received from the master.

4   The cure of amnesia and the physiology of memory

What was the material basis of the perception of memory loss? Where and how is information stored and how does it disappear from the storage place? The perception that a certain storage place for wisdom exists in the human body was common in many ancient cultures. In ancient Israel, in biblical Judaism, the heart is a storage place for wisdom, emotions, the soul, and almost everything, because it is a central locus of the body.[26] To explore these issues in rabbinic literature, I will discuss two

---

25 These traditions I am analyzing in Kiperwasser 2020.

26 Fraade 2015, 113–128. Fraade suggests that "although we should be careful not to presume that their linkage is direct in any genetic sense. In other words, distinctive elements of the later version need not necessarily reflect direct reworking of the earlier one, since they could just as easily reflect dependence on other versions that are no longer extant." It is of course quite possible that before the editor of the Bavli was the other version of the Tannaitic tradition, but it is clear that it belonged to the same tradition represented in Tosefta; therefore, the additions to

passages, one early, Tannaitic, from the Tosefta (t), and one late, Amoraic, from the Bavli (b), that are clearly linked to one another.[27] The Tannaitic passage, appears as the third of three homiletical interpretations of different scriptural verses that are narratively framed as having been delivered on a single occasion at Yavneh by Rabbi Eleazar ben Azariah.[28] I will concentrate only on the end of this sermon, based on the words "masters of assemblies" from Ecclesiastes 12:11.[29]

t. Soṭah 7:12[30]

"Masters of assemblies":
[This refers to] those who enter and sit in multiple assemblies, declaring what is impure [to be] impure, and what is pure [to be] pure; what is impure [to be] in its place, and what is pure [to be] in its place. Should a person ['adam] think to himself, "Since the house of Shammai declares impure and the house of Hillel declares pure, so-and-so prohibits and so-and-so permits, why should I henceforth learn Torah?" Scripture teaches, "Words," "the words," "these are the words" (Exod 19:6). Therefore, you should make of your heart chambers of chambers,[31] and bring into it the words of the house of Shammai and the words of the house
of Hillel, the words of those who declare impure and the words of those who declare pure.

בעלי אסופות אילו שנכנסין ויושבין אסופות
אסופות ואומ' על טמא טמא ועל טהור טהור על
טמא במקומו ועל טהור במקומו.
שמא יאמר אדם בדעתו הואיל ובית שמיי מטמין
ובית הלל מטהרין איש פל' אוסר ואיש פל' מתיר
למה אני למד תורה מעתה ת"ל דברים הדברים
אלה הדברים כל הדברים נתנו מרועה אחד אל
אחד בראן פרנס אחד נתנן רבון כל המעשים
ברוך הוא אמרו אף אתה עשה לבך חדרי חדרים
והכניס בה דברי בית שמיי ודברי בית הלל דברי
המטמאין ודברי המטהרין אמ' להם אין דור יתום
שר' ליעזר שרוי בתוכו.

---

the Babylonian tradition are most likely products of the Babylonian compiler. In other words, I do claim a direct link between the ancient and late tradition.

27 It is not a simple task to translate the verse. Fraade proposed that the rabbis read this verse as follows: "The words of the wise/sages are like goads, like nails firmly planted; [taught by] masters of assemblies, they were given by one shepherd," p. 115. Most modern translations (and the Masoretic pointing) understand "firmly planted" to belong with what follows rather than with what precedes. On the difficulties of translating this verse, see Fox 2004, 83–84.

28 This passage has attracted scholarly attention; see Boyarin 2004, 151–201, esp. 159; Fraade 2007, 31–37; Naeh 2005, 570–582 and idem 2001, 858–875. To this list can be added Shapira and Fisch 1999, 91–490. Most recently, see Rubenstein 2010, 106–111; and Hidary 2010, 21–22.

29 Translation adopted from Fraade 2007, t. Soṭah 7:11–12 (Lieberman 1995, 4:194–95), who based his discussion on MS Erfurt, printed by Lieberman (194) alongside MS Vienna. For a preference for MS Erfurt here, see Brody 2014, 83–84. However, see Fraade's arguments in his article (Fraade 2007). For later parallels, which cannot be considered in any detail here, see Num. Rab. 14.4; Abot R. Nat. A18 (Schechter 1979, 68); and Tanḥuma Beha'alotekha 15.

30 See Lieberman 1995, 156.

We have here a powerful image of the activity of the mind. "Heart" in the anthropological terminology of the rabbis is synchronically "mind" and "intellect."[32] Rabbinic Judaism inherited the perception of the heart as the emotional and mental center of the human being from biblical Judaism, but the concept was significantly transformed. "Heart" has preserved its cognitive function from biblical to Talmudic Judaism, and maintained its role as the dwelling place of emotions. In this passage, the main role of the heart is cognitive; moreover, it is memory storage. Here I will embrace Shlomo Naeh's explanation that the Tosefta's image of a multichambered "heart" (that is, mind) is that of a "memory palace," in which the many discordant teachings of the houses of Hillel and Shammai can be sorted and arranged according to their form and content, thereby satisfying the critical need of rabbinic disciples to acquire and hone the mental tools required to both store and access the many contradictory teachings of the sages who preceded them.[33] As is further related by Steven Fraade, the single, multichambered "heart" that can absorb and arrange such a mass of dissimilar teachings is a fitting vehicle for the transmission of a multivocal revelation that originates with a single divine creator and a single human law giver.[34] Now let us compare the toseftan passage with its Babylonian parallel.

b. Ḥagigah 3b[35]

Therefore, you should make your ear like the hopper[43] and acquire a [perceptive] heart to understand the words of those who declare impure and the words of those who declare pure, the words of those who prohibit and the words of those who permit, the words of those who declare unfit and the words of those who declare fit.

אַף אתה עשה אזניך כאפרכסת, וקנה לך לב מבין
לשמוע את דברי מטמאים ואת דברי מטהרים,
את דברי אוסרין ואת דברי מתירין, את דברי
פוסלין ואת דברי מכשירין.

A key difference between the Babylonian and the ancient Palestinian versions of this tradition is that the Babylonia version describes the process of learning as preparing the ear and afterwards transferring the information into the heart, while in the Palestinian tradition the role of the ear is not so prominent. This difference attracted Fraade's attention and he explains it as follows:

> In either case, the address is instructed either to transform his heart into one of many "chambers" (Tosefta), or his ear into something like a funnel-shaped

---

31 Meaning, "many chambers." See Naeh 2005, 575 n. 149.
32 On the rabbinic identification of the heart, see Kiperwasser 2013, 43–59; about more ancient material see Stuckenbruck 2011.
33 Naeh 2005, 563–570.
34 Fraade 2015, 123.
35 Translation adopted from Stern 1998, 19.

"grain hopper" (Bavli), in both cases so as to better receive and internalize the multitude of contradictory legal pronouncements. While the toseftan metaphor emphasizes more the mental sorting of all such pronouncements for purposes of better storage (memorization), and, presumably, retrieval, the talmudic metaphor stresses the hopper-like ear, which is widest at its upper (or outer) opening so as to maximize its intake. It is only then the role of the "heart" (intellect) to "hear" (understand) them all, regardless of their diversity of form, content, and attribution. These are two distinct expressions, with different emphases, of the shared insistence on absorbing *all* of the contradictory rabbinic pronouncements into the singular "heart" and "ear" just as they originated from the singular divine source via his singular human transmitter.[36]

Critically scrutinizing the differences between the two versions of the midrash to Ecclesiastes 12:11 found in the Tosefta and the Babylonian Talmud, Fraade insists on "our inability to know whether the later Talmudic version is a direct descendent of the earlier toseftan one."[37] However, because of the extensive use of the image of the ear as a tool for the learning process in Babylonian traditions, I prefer to accept Shlomo Naeh's approach. Naeh argues that the Tosefta contains two independent exegetical traditions based on verses of Ecclesiastes. The Bavli, however, integrates these sections with the others to form one longer, more complex homily, which is clearly a feature of the diachronic process of the late redaction. It seems that Naeh properly concludes that the Bavli's version is not an independent tradition but a reworking of the Tosefta.

As Fraade mentioned, the metaphor is of a funnel-shaped receptacle into which grain is poured prior to its being ground into flour. The image of the funnel-shaped "grain hopper" originates in the vocabulary of the Palestinian sages. It appears at first in the Palestinian Talmud, Qiddushin 1:9 (10), 61d: "Said R. Yohanan, 'If you hear a teaching of R. Eliezer, son of R. Yose the Galilean, perforate your ear like a hopper and listen carefully.'"[38] The expression is idiomatic, meaning "to open the ear widely for absorbing learning. However, it's not only in the tradition above that the ear is more than just a tool for hearing, but for understanding as well:

Exodus Rabbah 27:9[39]

"Hear ye, the words of the Lord!" (Jer 2:4) It is written "Hear and your soul shall live" (Isa 45:3). See how beloved Israel are, that He entices them! He told to them	שמעו דבר ה' הה"ד (ישעיה נה) שמעו ותחי נפשכם, היאך חביבים ישראל שהוא מפתה אותם, אמר להם אם יפול אדם מראש הגג כל גופו לוקה והרופא נכנס אצלו ונותן לו רטייה

---

36 Fraade 2015, 126.

37 Fraade 2015, 127.

38 Actually, all the uses of this expression are part of the tradition advising the listener to open his ear to the words of aggadah of R. Eliezer, son of R. Yose the Galilean; see b. Ḥulin 89a; and Pesiqta Rabbati. 10 (ed. Friedman, 38b). The abovementioned tradition in Bavli is therefore unique.

39 Translation: Lehrman 1951, 330 with minor changes.

"When a man falls from the roof, his whole body is bruised, and when the physician visits him, he applies bandages to his head, hands and feet, and all his limbs are covered with bandages. With Me, however, the case is not so. Man has two hundred and forty-eight parts, and the ear is but one of them: yet even though his whole body be stained with transgressions, as long as his ear hearkens, the whole body is vivified"—for it says "Hear and your soul shall live" (Isa 45:3), for this reason does it say "Hear ye, the words of the Lord, O house of Israel!" (Jer 2:4).

בראשו וכן בידיו וכן ברגליו ובכל אבריו נמצא
כולו רטיות, אני איני כך אלא רמ״ח אברים באדם
הזה והאוזן אחד מהם וכל הגוף מלוכלך בעבירות
והאוזן שומעת וכל הגוף מקבל חיים שמעו ותחי
נפשכם, לכך אמר שמעו דבר ה׳ בית יעקב,
וכן אתה מוצא ביתרו שע״י שמיעה זכה לחיים
ששמע ונתגייר שנאמר וישמע יתרו את כל אשר
עשה אלהים למשה ולישראל עמו וגו

In this exegetical exercise, which enacts a dialogue between Isaiah 45:3 and Jeremiah 2:4, God compares himself to an earthly physician. The human doctor wishing to heal the person fallen from the roof applies compresses to each of the members of his damaged body. God, wishing to heal people from the consequences of their sinful behavior, does not have to treat every one of the sinning body parts separately, but only to put his divine word in human ears, and its healing power will reach the sinful body parts. The interpreter uses the image of the 248 body parts known from the context of ritual purity laws (See m. Ohalot 1:6.) in order to emphasize that all of the body can be involved in sin.[40]

We see further evidence of a physiology of hearing and learning in a story about the famous Beruria and a certain student, if we look past the trivial reading of this source. The story must be read in the context of the chain of stories in which it appears.

b. 'Eruvin 53b–54a

Beruria met a student who was studying whispering. She kicked him and said to him: "Is it not written: 'ordered in all things and secure' (2 Sam 23:5)? If [the Torah] is ordered in all of your two hundred and forty-eight parts it is secured; but if it is not, it is not secured."

ברוריה אשכחתיה לההוא תלמידא דהוה קא גריס
בלחישה. בטשה ביה, אמרה ליה: לא כך כתוב
ערוכה בכל ושמרה, אם ערוכה ברמ״ח אברים
שלך—משתמרת, ואם לאו—אינה משתמרת.

---

40 An ear is not mentioned as one of the 248 body parts in this mishnaic statement, but, as I explained elsewhere (Kiperwasser 1999, 47–48), in late rabbinic texts, the term "248 parts" stands for the "whole body," and it is obvious that ears are to be found among the 248 parts.

Tannaitic teaching: R. Eliezer had a disciple who studied while whispering. After three years he forgot his learning.

Tannaitic teaching: R. Eliezer had a student who deserved burning [for an offense] against the Omnipresent—"Leave him alone," the Rabbis pleaded, "he attended on a great man."

Samuel said to Rav Judah, "Shinena, open your mouth and read the Scriptures, open your mouth and learn the Talmud, that your studies may be retained and that you may live long, since it is stated: 'For they are life unto those that find them, and a healing to all their flesh'; read not 'To those that find them' (Prov 4:22) but 'To him who utters them with his mouth.'"

תנא: תלמיד אחד היה לרבי אליעזר שהיה שונה בלחש, לאחר שלש שנים שכח תלמודו.

תנא: תלמיד אחד היה לו לרבי אליעזר שנתחייב בשריפה למקום. אמרו: הניחו לו, אדם גדול שמש.

אמר ליה שמואל לרב יהודה: שיננא, פתח פומיך קרי, פתח פומיך תני, כי היכי דתתקיים ביך ותוריך חיי, שנאמר כי חיים הם למצאיהם ולכל בשרו מרפא (משלי ד, כב), אל תקרי למצאיהם אלא למוציאיהם בפה.

All the stories in this chain of short exempla-type stories, except the last one, are presented here as Palestinian traditions. However, even these stories are the works of the Babylonian narrator. As is well known, the famous intellectual woman Beruria referred to in the first story is frequently employed by narrators of the Babylonian Talmud.[41] The historicity of her image in the Bavli is doubtful, but the significance of her presence is beyond doubt. It is noticeable that aside from a halakhic statement in the Tosefta, she is never mentioned in the Palestinian corpora, and certainly not as the wife of R. Meir, with whom the Babylonian Talmud has a special relationship. This story is told in order to warn against the manner of learning in a low voice and advocate the demand to speak up while expounding learning. We already know from the story about R. Shimon bar Yohai's disciple that the sages believed loud recitation was the means by which to preserve one's memory. Similarly, the story about R. Eliezer's student who forgot all his learning in three years because he was learning in a low voice aims to correct this faulty custom. Clearly, the last story in this chain is also directed against this practice, and it includes praise and reward for loud recitation by students, promised by the most prominent of the Babylonian sages—Samuel. This entire chain of stories is Babylonian, and the doubtfully Palestinian attributions serve the purpose of the last text.

To return to the Beruria story: An unknown student, whose custom it is to learn his lesson whispering, rather than loudly, is honored by Beruria's attention. She is eager to teach the student a lesson, because, as it is evident from the unspoken convention shared by the narrator and his heroine, to expound a lesson in a whisper and

41 Cf. Goodblatt 1975, 68–85; Adler 1988, 28–32, 102–105; Boyarin 1993, 167–196, Ilan 1997, 3–8.

not loudly is a bad thing. We are not told that the student was unsuccessful in his learning, but it seems that it is obvious to the narrator that such a student could not be any good. Therefore, Beruria finds herself compelled to use drastic measures to curb the student's bad habits by bashing him or kicking him, while graciously interpreting the verse from the book of Samuel: "Is it not written: 'ordered in all things and secure' (2 Sam 23:5)? If [the Torah] is ordered in all your two hundred and forty-eight parts it is secured; but if it is not, it is not secured." The new meaning of the interpreted verse is about knowledge. Learning should be ordered in all the parts of a human body, but to achieve the ability to recite, one must learn loudly! Indeed, during the long history of the formation of rabbinic culture the heart lost its status as the one and only storehouse of knowledge, as it was in biblical tradition, and a few new centres in which the intellect dwells were enlisted. The idea of the dispersion of wisdom throughout the entire body is thus consistent with rabbinic thought. If knowledge is distributed equally among all 248 body parts,[42] it then is important to learn loudly, or to make your ears listen to your voice. However, is this indeed the concept underlying this text? Before returning to this fascinating text, let us examine another no less puzzling Babylonian narrative tradition, in which ear, learning, and violence meet each other again.

Ecclesiastes Rabbah 7:8 [43]

"Better a patient spirit than a haughty spirit" (Eccl 7:8). A Persian [חד פרסי] came to Rav and said to him, "Teach me the Torah!" He told him, "Say [on this] *aleph*." He told him, "Who says that this is *aleph*? Others would say it is not!" "Say [on that] *bet*." He said to him, "Who says that this is *bet*?" Rav rebuked him and drove him out in anger [גער בו והוציאו בנזיפה]. He went to Samuel and told him, "Teach me the Torah." He said to him, "Say *aleph*." He told him, "Who says that this is *aleph*?" He told him, "Say [on that] *bet*." He said to him, "Who says this is *bet*?" He took hold of his ear and the man exclaimed, "Oh my ear! Oh my ear!" Samuel asked him, "Who says that this is your ear?" He answered, "Everyone knows that this is my ear." He said to him, "In the same way, everyone knows

טוב ארך רוח (קהלת ז, ח)
חד פרסי אתא גבי רב. א"ל: אלפני אוריא. א"ל:
אמור א'. א"ל. א"ל: מאן יימר דהוא א'?
(דאמרין אנן כן) [ואמרון דאינו כן]. א"ל: אמור ב'.
א"ל: מאן יימר דהוא ב'? גער בו והוציאו בנזיפה.
אזל לגבי שמואל. א"ל: אלפני אוריא. א"ל: אמור
א'. א"ל. א"ל: מאן יימר דהוא א'? א"ל: אמור ב'. א"ל:
מאן יימר דהוא ב'? צורמיה באודניה וצווח. ואמ':
אודני, אודני! א"ל שמואל: מאן[יימר] דהוא
אודנך? א"ל: כולי עלמא [ידעין] דהוא אדני. א"ל
אוף הכא כולי עלמא ידעין דהאי א' והאי ב'.
הוי (מישנשתק) [מיד נשתתק] הפרסי וקביל עלוי
טובה היא האריכה שהאריך שמואל עם הפרסי
מהקפדה שהקפיד עליו רב. אלולי כן חזר הפרסי
לסיאורו וקרא עליו: טוב ארך רוח מגבה רוח
(שם).

---

42 See above, n. 40. Cf. also Kiperwasser 2012, 305–319.
43 For analyses of this text in detail, see Kiperwasser and Ruzer 2014, 91–127.

that this is *aleph* and that is *bet*." The
Persian was immediately silenced and accepted that. Hence, "better a patient spirit than a haughty spirit" (Eccl 7:8). Better
is the forbearance that Samuel displayed
with the Persian than the impatience
that Rav showed towards him, for otherwise the Persian might have returned to
his heathenism [חזר הפרסי לסיאורו]. It is
thus about him that Scripture said, "Better a patient spirit than a haughty spirit."

This somewhat elliptic short story is part of a larger section referring to Ecclesiastes
7:8. One may reasonably suppose that by calling the protagonist "Persian" the narrator marks him as a potential convert from Zoroastrianism, since both Iranians and
Jews seem to have perceived adherence to their religion as tantamount to fealty to
their ethnicity.[44] But why is the Persian having doubts about the letters, and why do
the sages react in so violent a fashion? Moreover, what causes the Persian to ultimately
accept the second sage's teaching? Even if humor was intended, what exactly is the
object of the humor?

While Ecclesiastes Rabbah is a Palestinian midrash, the tradition is purely Babylonian.[45] In this context, it appears to be important that the protagonists of our story
are two Jewish Babylonian sages, Rav and Samuel, and one Iranian would-be convert. This narrative unit may thus bear witness to the broader phenomenon referred
to above: the redactor of Ecclesiastes Rabbah seems to have been familiar enough
with traditions brought to the land of Israel by Babylonian tradents.[46] In *Ecclesiastes
Rabbah*, the attempt to teach the Persian the Hebrew letter *aleph* encountered opposition from the potential convert. He asks a question that could sound rude or ironic,
but might have had something to do with his cultural background. His doubts concerning the lack of certitude with regard to the meaning and/or pronunciation of the
letters might have reflected a characteristic of his native culture.[47] Or alternatively,
coming from a culture with a strong emphasis on orality, he might have been inclined
to focus on the study of word units rather than letters: while the former are crucial
for the transmission of a culture's religious content, the latter are mainly of interest to scribes, who need to properly write contracts. Indeed, until the Islamic period
Iranians retained strong reservations about putting things into writing, as attested

---

44 Broadly speaking, Persia (or Iran) in Arsacid and Sassanian times was a region lying to the West
    and the East of the Tigris River, thus including today's Iraq, Azerbaijan, and parts of Afghani-
    stan. The protagonists of the stories discussed below are perceived there as representing Iranian
    culture/religion.
45 See Kiperwasser and Ruzer 2014, 96–97.
46 Ibid.
47 Ibid., 102.

in their literary sources. Thus, one learns from Denkard V 24.13 (c. ninth century): "The legitimacy of [the] oral tradition is thus in many respects greater than that of writing. And it is logical, for many other reasons as well, to consider the living and oral Word as more essential than the written one."[48] Whatever the case, the intention of the Persian in the story seems clear: If everything you know about your religion is gleaned from a written text, how can you be sure that your understanding is right and not conditioned by the wrong ways of reciting the Holy Writ? The Persian thus aims to clarify a crucial issue: Is the sacral tradition of the Jews based on a trustworthy oral tradition, or do they have to rely only on an unreliable written text? The rabbinic sage, then, seeking to respond appropriately to this issue, wants to emphasize that language belongs to the public sphere of common knowledge and not to the personal fancy of an individual. Just as the Persian had once trusted the teachers from whom he received his native education, so, too, should he now trust a "native" Hebrew speaker teaching him a new language? However, why cause the Persian pain? Why torture his ear? In an article I coauthored with Serge Ruzer, we suggested that the pain in the ear of the Persian proselyte was intended to illustrate the relation of the Torah letters to the Torah itself—the letters are the organs of the body of Scripture. We explained this act as a body-oriented argument that should teach the student a lesson. "Samuel's use of a common, albeit mildly violent, method of instruction aims at drawing the student's attention to the undeniable certainty of his own body. Unlike the external social context, prone to change, the body is intrinsically a person's own and the pain comes from within."[49] I would now like to emphasize more the patterns that I saw then as secondary. The ear may have been chosen as the target because it is the organ used for hearing and, thus, learning.[50] Moreover, perhaps behind this motif in the story about Beruria's violent treatment of the student, lies the same idea, which serves an apologist of corporal punishment that contact with the body of a disciple can help regulate the transfer of information into and out of the inner storehouses of his body. By torturing the ear of the convert, the sage prepares his mind, his wisdom, and his storehouses for knowledge of new materials.

That use of the ear in metaphors of learning in Babylonian traditions has a physiological background can be proven by literary parallels outside of rabbinic literature, which shed light on the cultural nexus of these texts. *The Kephalaia of the Teacher*, a Coptic Manichean work,[51] provides the perfect explanation for the physiology of learning and memory. According to this text, since limbs are connected to the inner storehouse of the body, they are involved in the process of the intake of knowledge. Everything external to the body is absorbed by the limbs and transmitted to the internal storehouses. The Teacher counts eyes, ears, scent, taste, and touch as the main producers of knowledge, which is consequently deposited in five internal storehouses of the body, and all of them are connected to the heart, which is like a king, a media-

---

48 The citation is per Huyse 2008, 143. See Cereti 2001, 41–78.
49 See Kiperwasser and Ruzer 2014, 103.
50 As proposed by Amram Tropper in a personal communication.
51 Gardner 1995, 90–91. See also Smagina 1998, 166–167.

tor of all these sorts of depositories of knowledge. Five "faculties"[52] deriving from the five sensoria lead to their storehouses and from there to the heart and vice versa. All these mechanisms have a role in channelling different kinds of knowledge. The eyes have their storehouse, a repository where images of love and hate are collected and can easily be reproduced for certain purposes. Similarly, ears have their storehouse, which is used for the storage of every kind of audio information.

Kephalaia of the Teacher 139:15[53]

The faculty of the ears has its own storehouse also. Every sound it might receive, whether good or evil, shall be taken in and placed in its houses and inner repositories and it is guarded in its [storehouses]... for a thousand days. After a thousand days, if someone comes and asks that faculty about the sound that it heard at this time and took into its storehouses. Immediately it shall go into its repositories and seek and review and search after this word, and send it out from where it was first put, the place in which it was kept.

Interestingly, per the explanation proposed in this text, the storage of the information received by the ears is different from the visual information received by the eyes. Its storage in the storehouse connected directly with the ears is temporary—only for a thousand days—and afterwards it is transferred to a more distant repository, and from there the information could be requisitioned by the faculties if requested by the thinking abilities of the person. This puzzling explanation is very similar to the modern conception of long-term memory and short-term memory, though the latter, of course, does not involve the intervention the divine power.

To return to the chain of Bavli stories praising loudly voiced learning: the text about Beruria, who corporally punished her unsuccessful student, uses a physiology of memory as described in the *Kephalaia*. The violent contact with the student's body is meant to evoke chains of interaction between the body, as the target point of instruction, and the inner storehouses of knowledge. Her advice to speak up, so that the ears can accept knowledge, is intended to fill the inner storehouses of the ears. There is no contradiction between kicking the body of the student and demanding that he open his ears. The main storehouse of knowledge is the heart, and all the data from the limbs are collected there. Moreover, even the short story about the student of R. Eliezer can be corroborated by the *Kephalaia*. The student, who was not diligent enough to recall the knowledge stored in his inner storehouses, lost it because the information there could be kept only a thousand days, which is more or less three years. The Babylonian tradition from Ecclesiastes Rabbah can also be explained by the

---

52 Five is an important typological number in Manichean anthropology. There are five attributes of mind or thought, five beings evoked by the living spirit, five light elements, etc. See also Pettipiece 2009, 3–5 and 42–44.

53 See Gardner 1995, 90–91, n. 38. About this passage from the Kephalaia and the reception of this tradition in the writings of Augustine, see van Oort 2013, 168–170. Many thanks to Prof. van Oort for a very useful conversation on the topic during the international conference to mark the fiftieth Anniversary of AIEP/IAPS, Jerusalem, June 25–27, 2013.

Kephalaia's model. The rabbi says to the new convert that the storehouses of knowledge connected to his ears could now be ready to accept the new learning embodied in the sounds of the Hebrew alphabet. In Manichean teachings this entire metaphorical structure entailing five faculties of memory and their storage places and repositories has theological significance, because, as witnessed by the former Manichean Augustine, God reveals himself in these five senses and, therefore, in the faculties of memory.[54] It turns out, however, that the Babylonian rabbis shared with the Manicheans the concept of the importance of the senses and the audio regulation of memory, but not the theological background of their speculation. It is likely that in this case, we have evidence of a sort of quasi-scientific knowledge of the ancient Near East, shared by Manicheans and rabbis; but if the former built this knowledge on their theological speculations, in rabbinic storytelling culture it remained a trope for didactic stories. Manichean doctrine is a mixture of different traditions, among them Iranian and ancient Aramaic formulations. While I am not prepared to determine whether the model of the learning process as preserved in the *Kephalaia* is mostly Iranian or mostly Aramaic,[55] it is interesting to consider some late Persian anthropological concepts. P. O. Skjærvø mentioned that the Avestan and Old Persian term *ushi* may have originally meant "ear," and consequently something like the ability to hear, but in Pahlavi *osh (ush)* appears to mean "intelligence" or "memory." For example, according to Avestan text Yasna 9, a person who was in contact with a sinner has to "cover his inner hearing (*ushi*) and shatter his thought,"[56] namely to do something opposite to the demand of b. Ḥagigah 3b,[57] and then the infidel's words would not dwell in his internal storehouse of knowledge. Therefore, it may be that the identification between the ear, memory, and intellect was a common cultural pattern in Sassanian Babylonia.

To conclude, memory is the cornerstone of intelligence in rabbinic thought; a divine gift to the sage, placed in his heart by the divine patron of scholars, it can be taken away if the sage's behavior does not comply with rabbinic ethics. Tales about wise men losing their memory appear in rabbinic literature much more frequently than in all other cultures that I am aware of. And these stories reflect one of the characteristic features of this culture—orality as a marker of its identity. In rabbinic culture, memory relates to the peculiarities of the rabbis' perception of the body. The body is not only a physical shell, but has features of a subject, of a self. It, or rather, its significant part, is synonymous with mental patterns, like mind, soul, and ratio. Memory is a function of the heart and ears, which are in delicate physiological interactions with one another, similar to the relationship expounded in the Manichean *Kephalaia of the Teacher*. Thus, orality in Talmudic culture and the perception of the body as the abode of thinking and memory were complementary, and these conceptions are reflected in the stories analyzed in this article.

---

54 Cf. van Oort 2013.
55 On Zoroastrian elements in Manichean lore, see Skjærvø 2009, 269–286.
56 Cf. Skjaervo 2011, 176 and compare with the text of the Darius inscription there.
57 See above p. 14.

Bibliography

Sources

Danby, Herbert. 1933, *The Mishnah translated from the Hebrew with introduction and brief explanatory notes*, Oxford : Clarendon Press.

Friedmann, Meir. 1880. *Pesiqta Rabbati*. Vienna: Kaiser.

Gardner, Iain. 1995. *The Kephalaia of the Teacher: The Edited Coptic Manichaean Texts in Translation with Commentary*. Leiden: Brill.

Lehrman, Simon M. 1951. *Midrash Rabbah: Exodus*. London: Soncino.

Lieberman, Saul. 1995. *The Tosefta: According to Codex Vienna: The Order of Nashim, with Variants*, New-York: The Jewish Theological Seminary of America.[2]

Schechter, Solomon. 1979, *Masekhet Aboth de-rabbi Nathan*, Vienna: C. D. Lippe, 1887. (repr. Hildesheim/New York: Olms).

Smagina, Eugenia B. 1998. *Kefalaĭa = "Glavy": koptskiĭmanikheĭskiĭtraktat / perevod s koptskogo, issledovanie, kommentariĭ, glossariĭiukazatel*.(Kefalaia: Chapters, Coptic Manichean Tractate: Translation, Studies, Commentary, Glossary and Index). Moscow: Vostochnaia literatura.

Ulmer, Rivka 1997. *Pesiqta Rabbati—A Synoptic Edition of Pesiqta Rabbati Based upon All Extant Manuscripts and the Editio Princeps*, Atlanta: Scholars Press.

Zuckermandel, Moses S. 1970. *Tosephta. Based on the Erfurt and Vienna Codices*. Jerusalem: Wahrman Books[2] (= *Die Tosefta nach den Erfurter und Wiener Handschriften*, 1880–1882).

Literature

Adler, Rachel. 1998. "The Virgin in the Brothel and Other Anomalies: Character and Context in the Legend of Beruriah." *Tikkun: A Quarterly Jewish Critique of Politics, Culture and Society* 3,6: 28–32, 102–105.

Balberg, Mira. 2020. "The Subject Supposed to Forget: Rabbinic Formations of the Legal Self." In *Self, Self-fashioning, and Individuality in the Roman Empire*. Edited by Maren R. Niehoff and Joshua Levinson. Tübingen: Mohr Siebeck. Pages 445–469.

Boyarin, Daniel. 1993. *Carnal Israel: Reading Sex in Talmudic Culture*. Berkeley: University of California Press.

—. 2004. *Border Lines: The Partition of Judaeo-Christianity*. Divinations: Rereading Late Ancient Religion. Philadelphia: University of Pennsylvania Press.

Brody, Robert. 2014. *Mishnah and Tosefta Studies*. Jerusalem: Magnes.

Carruthers, Mary. 1990. *The Book of Memory: A Study of Memory in Medieval Culture*. Cambridge: Cambridge University Press.

—. 2009. "Ars oblivionalis, ars inveniendi: The Cherub Figure and the Arts of Memory." *Gesta* 48: 1–19.

Cereti, Carlo. 2001. *La Letteratura Pahlavi: Introduzione ai testi con riferimenti alla storia degli studi e alla tradizione manoscritta*. Milan: Associazione Culturale Mimesis.

Fox, Michael V. 2004. *The JPS Bible Commentary: Ecclesiastes*. Philadelphia: Jewish Publication Society.

Fraade, Steven D. 2007. "Rabbinic Polysemy and Pluralism Revisited." *AJS Review* 31,1: 1–40.

—. 2015. "'A Heart of Many Chambers': The Theological Hermeneutics of Legal Multivocality." *Harvard Theological Review* 108: 113–128.

Frankel, Jonah. 2001. *The Aggadic Narrative Harmony of Form and Content*. Tel Aviv: Hakibbutz Hameuḥad. [In Hebrew]

Gerhardsson, Birger. 1961. *Memory and Manuscript: Oral Tradition and Written Transmission in Rabbinic Judaism and Early Christianity*. Lund: C. WE. K. Gleerup, and Copenhagen: Ejnar Munksgaard.

Goodblatt, David. 1975. "The Beruriah Traditions." *Journal of Jewish Studies* 26: 68–85.

Goshen-Gottstein, Alon. 2000. *The Sinner and the Amnesiac: The Rabbinic Invention of Elisha ben Abuya and Eleazar ben Arach*. Stanford, CA: Stanford University Press.

Greenfield, Jonah. 1974. "Ratin Magosha." In *Joshua Finkel Festschrift*. Edited by Sidney B. Hoenig and Leon D. Stitskin. New York: Yeshiva University Press. Pages 63–69.

Hidary, Richard. 2010. *Dispute for the Sake of Heaven: Legal Pluralism in the Talmud*. Providence, RI: Brown Judaic Studies.

Huyse, Philip. 2008. "Late Sasanian Society between Orality and Literacy." In *The Sasanian Era*. Edited by Vesta S. Curtis and Sarah Stewart. The Idea of Iran 3. London: I. B. Tauris.

Ilan, Tal. 1997. "The Quest for the Historical Beruriah, Rachel, and Imma Shalom." *AJS Review* 22,1: 1–17.

Jaffee, Martin S. 1992. "How Much Orality in 'Oral Torah'? New Perspectives on the Composition and Transmission of Early Rabbinic Tradition." *Shofar* 10: 53–72.

—. 1998. "The Oral-Cultural Context of the Talmud Yerushalmi, Greco-Roman Rhetorical Paideia, Discipleship, and the Concept of Oral Torah." In *The Talmud Yerushalmi and Graeco-Roman Culture*. Vol. 1. Edited by Peter Schäfer. Tübingen: Mohr Siebeck. Pages 27–63.

—. 1999. "Oral Tradition in the Writings of Rabbinic Oral Torah: On Theorizing Rabbinic Orality." *Oral Tradition* 14,1: 3–32.

Katz, Menachem. 2011. "The Stories of Hillel's Appointment as *Nasi* in the Talmudic Literature: A Foundation Legend of the Jewish Scholar's World." *Sidra* 26: 81–116. [In Hebrew]

Kiperwasser, Reuven. 1999. "The 248 Parts—a Study of the Mishna Oholot 1:8." *'BDD': Journal of Torah and Scholarship* 8: 29–64. [In Hebrew]

—. 2010. "Towards the Redaction History of Kohelet Rabbah." *Journal of Jewish Studies* 61: 257–277.

—. 2012. "Body of the Whore, Body of the Story and Metaphor of the Body." In *Introduction to Seder Qodashim. A Feminist Commentary on the Babylonian Talmud*. Volume 5. Edited by Tal Ilan, Monika Brockhaus and Tanja Hidde. Tübingen: Mohr Siebeck. Pages 305–319.

—. 2013. "Matters of the Heart: The Metamorphosis of the Monolithic in the Bible to the Fragmented in Rabbinic Thought." In *Judaism and Emotion: Texts, Performance, Experience*. Edited by Sarah Ross, Gabriel Levy, and Soham Al-Suadi. New York: Lang. Pages 43–59.

—. 2019. "Going West: Migrating Babylonians and the Question of Identity." *A Question of Identity: Social, Political, and Historical Aspects of the Formation, Transition, and Negotiation of Identity in Jewish and Related Contexts*. Edited by Dikla Rivlin-Katz, Noach Hacham, Geoffrey Herman and Lilah Sagiv. Oldenbourg: De Gruyter. Pages 111–130.

—. 2020. "The Art of Forgetting in Rabbinic Narrative", In *Rabbinic Study Circles: Jewish Learning in its Late Antique Context*. Edited by Mark Hirshman and David Satran with the assistance of Anita Reisler. Tübingen: Mohr Siebeck. Pages 67–85.

Kiperwasser, Reuven, and Serge Ruzer. 2014. "To Convert a Persian and to Teach Him the Holy Scriptures: A Zoroastrian Proselyte in Rabbinic and Syriac Christian Narratives." In *Jews, Christians and Zoroastrians: Religious Dynamics in a Sasanian Context*. Edited by Geoffrey Herman. Piscataway, NJ: Gorgias. Pages 91–127.

Kister, Menachem. 2017. "Interaction of Text and Vocabulary in Rabbinic Literature and the Bible: A Case Study (Ecclesiastes Rabbah / Zuta 7:7)." *Lěšonénu: A Journal for the Study of the Hebrew Language and Cognate Subjects* 79: 7–43. [In Hebrew]

Levine, Nachman. 2002. "R. Elazar b. Arach: The 'Overflowing Spring,' the Emmaus Hot Spring, and Intertextual Irony." *Journal for the Study of Judaism* 33,3: 278–289.

Lieberman, Saul. 1968. *Hellenism in Jewish Palestine*. New York: The Jewish Theological Seminary of America.

— 1992. *Tosefta Ki-fshutah: A Comprehensive Commentary on the Tosefta*. Vol. 4. Jerusalem: The Jewish Theological Seminary of America.

Marienberg-Milikowsky, Itay. 2015. "'Exile Yourself to a Place of Torah'? Independence, Marginality and the Study of Torah in the Literary Image of Rabbi Elazar ben Arach." *Jewish Studies, an Internet Journal* 13: 1–25. [In Hebrew]. Cited 4 September 2018. Online: http://www.biu.ac.il/JS/JSIJ/13-2015/Marienberg.pdf

Naeh, Shlomo. 2001. "Make Your Heart Chambers of Chambers: More on the Rabbinic Sages on Argument." In *Renewing Jewish Commitment: The Work and Thought of David Hartman*. Edited by Avi Sagi and Zvi Zohar. Tel Aviv: Hakibbutz Hameuḥad. Pages 851–875. [In Hebrew]

—. 2005. "The Craft of Memory: Constructions of Memory and Patterns of Text in Rabbinic Literature." In *Meḥkerei Talmud 3: Talmudic Studies Dedicated to the Memory of Professor Ephraim E. Urbach*. Edited by Yaakov Sussman and David Rosenthal. Jerusalem: Magnes. Pages 570–582. [In Hebrew]

Neusner, Jacob. 1979. "Oral Torah and Oral Tradition: Defining the Problematic." In Jacob Neusner. *Method and Meaning in Ancient Judaism*. Chico, CA: Scholars Press. Pages 59–75.

van Oort, Johannes. 2013. "God, Memory and Beauty: A 'Manichaean' Analysis of Augustine's Confessions, Book 10:1–38." In *Augustine and Manichaean Christianity: Selected Papers from the First South African Conference on Augustine of Hippo*. Edited by Johannes Ort. Leiden: Brill. Pages 155–175.

Pettipiece, Timothy. 2009. *Pentadic Redaction in the Manichaean Kephalaia*. Leiden: Brill.

Rosenthal, Eliezer-Shimshon. 1982. "For the Talmudic Dictionary—Talmudica Iranica." In *Irano-Judaica: Studies Relating to Jewish Contacts with Persian Culture throughout the Ages*. Edited by Shaul Shaked and Amnon Netzer. Jerusalem: Yad Ben-Zvi. Pages 38–134.

Rubenstein, Jeffrey L. 2010. *Stories of the Babylonian Talmud*. Baltimore, MD: Johns Hopkins University Press.

Shapira, Haim and Menachem Fisch. 1999. "The Debates between the Houses of Shammai and Hillel: The Meta-Halakhic Issue." *Tel-Aviv University Law Review* 22: 91–490. [In Hebrew]

Skjærvø, P. Oktor. 2009. "Reflexes of Iranian Oral Traditions in Manichean Literature." In *Literarische Stoffe und ihre Gestaltung in mitteliranischer Zeit. Ehrencolloquium anlässlich des 70. Geburtstages von Prof. Dr. Werner Sundermann 30./31. März 2006,* Wiesbaden: Reichert. Pages 269–286.

—. 2011. *The Spirit of Zoroastrianism*. New Haven, CT: Yale University Press and Sacred Literature Trust.

Small, Jocelyn Penny. 1997. *Wax Tablets of the Mind: Cognitive Studies of Memory and Literacy in Classical Antiquity*. London: Routledge.

Smith, Morton. 1963. "A Comparison of Early Christian and Early Rabbinic Traditions." *Journal of Biblical Literature* 82: 169–176.

Stern, David. 1998. *Midrash and Theory: Ancient Jewish Exegesis and Contemporary Literary Studies*. Evanston, IL: Northwestern University Press.

Stuckenbruck, Loren. 2011. "The Heart in the Dead Sea Scrolls: Negotiating between the Problem of Hypocrisy and Conflict within the Human Being." In *The Dead Sea Scrolls in Context: Integrating the Dead Sea Scrolls in the Study of Ancient Texts, Languages, and Cul-*

tures. Edited by Armin Lange, Emanuel Tov, and Matthias Weigold, in association with Bennie H. Reynolds. Leiden: Brill. Pages 437–453.

Swartz, Michael D. 1996. *Scholastic Magic: Ritual and Revelation in Early Jewish Mysticism*. Princeton, NJ: Princeton University Press.

Sussman, Yaakov. 2006. 'Oral Torah' Literally—The Power of the Tip of Yod", In *Meḥkerei Talmud 3: Talmudic Studies Dedicated to the Memory of Professor Ephraim E. Urbach*. Edited by Yaakov Sussman and David Rosenthal. Jerusalem: Magnes. Pages 209–384. [In Hebrew]

The Fever that Nourishes:
Early Rabbinic Concepts on the Purpose of Fever

Kenneth Collins

Introduction

This paper examines the concept of the fever that nourishes in Talmudic and early rabbinic literature.[1] Indeed, the relationship of fever and food has a long history in many cultures and some of its mythology has survived even in western cultures into modern times. During a short lasting fever suppression of the demanding task of maintaining digestion might seem understandable as long as the body's need for a basic fluid balance is met. With the milder systemic upset of a cold it is less likely that the body's major metabolic processes will be challenged and consequently the ingestion of easily consumed foodstuffs may continue. The rabbis understood that some fevers were relatively benign and might even prove to be beneficial to the body possibly indicating an understanding that body defence mechanisms were involved.

These ideas are echoed in the old English saying, first recorded over four hundred years ago, that one "feeds a cold and starves a fever".[2] This simple adage remains a popular part of the traditional lay attitude to common illness despite the inexorable advance of scientific medicine. Attempts to relate the meaning of this saying to modern therapeutics have only served to enhance its reputation and there may be some shared ideas with the nourishing fever. Its simple meaning may be that the lay identification with cold implies that energy is needed for recovery and that feeding is important.[3] Conversely, the presence of a fever might indicate an excess of body heat, or energy, and thus starving is required. Another rationale would seem to be that a cold is a minor ailment with a minimum of systemic upset although the symptoms may persist for several days. Consequently, there is little to be gained by any significant change in regular nutrition. However, a fever suggests some more significant, though

---

1   All biblical verses quoted are derived from *TANAKH: A New Translation of the Holy Scriptures According to the Traditional Hebrew Texts* (Philadelphia: Jewish Publication Society of America, 1985). All translations from the Babylonian Talmud are taken from the Soncino translation: *The Babylonian Talmud* (trans. and ed. Isidore Epstein; London: Soncino, 1961). Online available: www.halakhah.org. Quotations from midrashic texts come from *Midrash Rabbah* (eds. H. Freedman, M. Simon and J. J. Slotki; London/Jerusalem: Soncino, 1977).

2   John Withals, *Shorte Dictionarie for Yonge Begynners* (London: Lewis Evans, 1553), nowadays known as *Dictionary for Young Boys,* notes that "fasting is a great remedie of fever".

3   See, for instance, Stuart A Gallacher, "Stuff a cold and feed a fever," *History of Medicine* 11 (1942): 576–581.

DOI: 10.13173/9783447108263.143

possible shorter lasting, ailment with a greater likelihood of metabolic upset. In that case fluids would seem to be more important than food given that in a fevered patient appetite is likely to be suppressed.

Fever in the Bible

Fever was clearly seen as a Divine affliction. It was said in the name of Rabbi Hiyya bar Abba that the miracle of men cast in to the furnace in the *Book of Daniel* was lesser than the recovery of a man with a fever, literally a Heavenly fire, as the furnace was kindled by man while "…a Heavenly fire, who can extinguish that?"[4] The existence of different biblical names for fever raises the possibility that it was understood that fever could be a symptom of different illnesses. *Ḥarḥur* (חרחור) referred to in *Deuteronomy* is held by scholars to be malaria. *Qadachat* (קדחת), mentioned in *Leviticus* 26:16 was thought to refer to daily fever while *daleqet* (דלקת), normally understood today to be inflammation, is tertian or quartan fever.

In the warnings to the Israelites "if you do not observe to do all (God's) commandments" notice is given of the curses, including dread diseases, which will befall them. Thus, in *Deuteronomy* 28:22:

> The Lord will smite you with consumption, and with fever and with inflammation and with fiery heat…[5]

In *Numbers* 11:4–13 the Israelites crave meat, looking for food other than manna to quell their hunger. A fire broke out and was only quelled with Moses' prayers, but the resulting surfeit of quail meat produced a severe plague. Fire, heat and plague seem to be related and the unreasonable desire for food leads to illness and death.

ויהי העם כמתאננים רע באזני יהוה וישמע יהוה ויחר אפו ותבער־בם אש יהוה ותאכל בקצה המחנה

> Now the people complained about their hardships in the hearing of the LORD, and when he heard them his anger was aroused. Then fire from the LORD burned among them and consumed some of the outskirts of the camp. (Numbers 11:1)

ויקם העם כל־היום ההוא וכל־הלילה וכל יום המחרת ויאספו את־השלו הממעיט אסף עשרה חמרים וישטחו להם שטוח סביבות המחנה:
הבשר עודנו בין שניהם טרם יכרת ואף יהוה חרה בעם ויך יהוה בעם מכה רבה מאד

> All that day and night and all the next day the people went out and gathered quail. No one gathered less than ten homers. Then they spread them out all around the camp. But while the meat was still between their teeth and before it could be consumed, the anger of the LORD burned against the people, and he struck them with a severe plague. (Numbers 11:32–33)

---

4   *B Nedarim* 41a, *Daniel* 3:19–27.
5   The whole verse reads: *The Lord will smite you with consumption, and with fever and with inflammation and with fiery heat, and with drought1 and with blight and with mildew. They shall pursue you until you perish* (יככה יהוה בשחפת ובקדחת ובדלקת ובחרחר ובחרב ובשדפון ובירקון ורדפוך עד אבדך).

The Bible mentions different types of fever. The prophet Jeremiah, in his lament for Jerusalem after the destruction of the Temple in 587BCE compares its loss with human fever:

> From on high He has sent fire into my bones and it prevails against them…He has made me desolate and faint all the day.[6]

Fever in the Talmud

The Babylonian Talmud, the corpus of Jewish oral law and tradition, was finally redacted around 500CE but is based on much older texts and traditions dating back many centuries. It contains extensive rabbinic literary material on every aspect of the historic and contemporary Jewish experience both legal and legendary and within its many weighty volumes are the discussions of the rabbis on the possible causes of fever and its treatments.

Geller reminds us that with the classical Greek approach to healing, which involved the theory of humours, treatments often consisted of the removal of the unwanted humour, whether by diet, purging or even bloodletting.[7] Babylonian medicine considered disease to result from external factors for which oral medication was the preferred remedy. Hence, one can distinguish rather clearly between the approaches of Greek and Babylonian medicine, in any particular Talmudic passage.

The rabbis knew of fevers that occurred daily or less frequently and described the symptoms of rigors. They knew that "as long as the earth exists, frost and heat from fever will not cease" (Gen. 8:22). They considered that a fever in the winter was more serious than that in the summer, noting that the warming of body temperature must be more powerful in the winter cold than in the summer heat.[8] An uncommon form of fever, designated as *aḥilu* (אחילו), was described in *Lamentations* 1:13 as "fire in the bones" which the rabbis felt to be milder than pains throughout the whole body though treatment for this condition would last until cure rather than for just around a week for other illnesses. The rabbis had other names for fever such as *ḥamah* (חמה) and *shimshah* (שימשה) both of which normally refer to the sun.[9]

The sage, Raba, noted that fever, were it not linked inevitably with death would be seen as having a protective, that is purging and purifying, effect on the body, like the noted therapy, theriac, while his colleague Nahman ben Yitzchak said he wished neither the fever nor the treatment. Preuss infers from this an approval of the notion that

---

6 *Lamentations* 1:13: *From on high He has sent fire into my bones and it prevails against them. He spread a net for my feet and turned me back. He has made me desolate and faint all the day* (ממרום שלח־אש בעצמתי וירדנה פרש רשת לרגלי השיבני אחור נתנני שממה כל־היום דוה).

7 Cf. Markham J. Geller, *Akkadian Healing Therapies in the Babylonian Talmud* (Preprint Series 259; Berlin: Max Planck Institute for the History of Science, 2004), [cited 25 May 2014]. Online: http://www.mpiwg-berlin.mpg.de/Preprints/P259.PDF

8 Cf. Genesis Rabbah, 34:11 (drawing on Genesis, 8:22), and b. Yoma 29a.

9 See Julius Preuss, *Biblical and Talmudic Medicine*, (trans. and ed. Fred Rosner; New York: Sanhedrin Press, 1978), 160–164.

the fever is an expression of the self-defence of the body against illness.[10] The Sages taught that there are six kinds of fire based on the kinds of materials consumed in the burning. One of these is the "fire that consumes liquids and does not consume solids" which is the fever "of the sick" that dehydrates the body but does not consume flesh.[11]

> ת״ר שש אשות הן יש אוכלת ואינה שותה ויש שותה ואינה אוכלת ויש אוכלת ושותה ויש אוכלת לחין כיבשין ויש אש דוחה אש ויש אש אש יש אש אוכלת ואינה שותה הא דידן שותה ואינה אוכלת דחולין אוכלת ושותה

> Our Rabbis taught: There are six different kinds of fire: Fire which eats but does not drink; fire which drinks but does not eat; fire which eats and drinks; fire which consumes dry matter as well as moist matter; and fire which pushes fire away; fire which eats fire. 'Fire which eats but does not drink': that is our fire [water quenches it]; 'which drinks but does not eat': the fever of the sick; 'eats and drinks'. (b. Yoma 21b)

Dehydration of course could simply be corrected by fluid replacement as the Midrash in *Genesis Rabba* recounts of a feverish Ishmael exhausting Hagar's supply of water.[12]

There are a number of simple remedies to be found in the rabbinic literature for different forms of fever. The following extracts indicate both the theories of the causes of fever and their treatment, involving simple remedies with olives and radishes as well as more complex folk treatments.

> מר בר רב אשי אשכחיה לרבינא דשייף לה לברתיה בגוהרקי דערלה אמר ליה אימור דאמור רבנן בשעת הסכנה שלא בשעת הסכנה מי אמור א״ל האי אישתא צמירתא נמי כשעת הסכנה דמיא

> Mar bar Rav Ashi found Ravina rubbing his daughter with unripe olives of *orla* (normally a prohibited item and thus only permitted at a time of danger) ... (Ravina) said to him: A high fever is also deemed a time of danger. (b. Pesachim 25b)

> Said Rav Judah: the sting of a wasp, the prick of a thorn, an abscess, a sore eye or an inflammation—for all these a bath-house is dangerous. Radishes are good for fever, and beets for cold shivers: the reverse is dangerous. (b. Avoda Zara 28b)

> אמר רב יהודה זיבורא ודחרזיה סילוא וסמטא ודכאיב ליה עינא ואתי עילויה אישתא כולהו בי בני סכנתא חמה לחמה וסילקא לצינא וחילופא סכנתא חמימי לעקרבא וקרירי לזיבורא וחילופא סכנתא חמימי לסילוא וקרירי לחספניתא וחילופא סכנתא

---

10 Julius Preuss, *Biblical and Talmudic Medicine*, 161.
11 See commentary in Koren Steinsaltz Hebrew/English Talmud, (Jerusalem, 2013), 91.
12 Cf. *Genesis Rabbah* 53:13. The midrashic text fills out the Biblical narrative by saying that Sarah had cast an 'evil eye' on Ishmael, producing a fever. Thus, Ishmael's water bottle became empty as a sick person drinks frequently.

One of the Talmud sages, Abbaye, frequently quoted a woman, *Em*, sometimes considered to be his adoptive mother, but increasingly regarded as an authoritative female figure, who lived in Babylonia around the fourth century and provided advice on health issues and child care.[13]

אמר אביי אמרה לי אם לשימשא בת יומא כוזא דמיא בת תרי יומי סיכורי
בת תלתא יומי בשרא סומקא אגומרי וחמרא מרקא

לשימשא עתיקתא ליתי תרנגולתא אוכמתי וליקרעה שתי וערב וליגלחיה למציעתא דרישיה
ולותביה עילויה ונחניה עילויה עד דמיסרך

Abaye said: My 'mother' told me that for a sun-stroke [fever] the remedy is on the first day to take a jug of water, [if it lasts] two days to let blood, [if] three days to take red meat broiled on the coals and highly diluted wine. For a chronic heat stroke, he should bring a black hen and tear it lengthwise and crosswise and shave the middle of his head and put the bird on it and leave it there till it sticks fast, and then he should go down [to the river] and stand in water up to his neck till he is quite faint, and then he should swim out and sit down. If he cannot do this, he should eat leeks and go down and stand in water up to his neck till he is faint and then swim out and sit down. For sunstroke one should eat red meat broiled on the coals with wine much diluted. For a chill one should eat fat meat broiled on the coals with undiluted wine. (b. Gittin 67b)

רב עמרם חסידא כי הוה מצערין ליה בי ריש גלותא הוו מגנו ליה אתלגא למחר אמרו
ליה מאי ניחא ליה למר דלייתו ליה מר אמר הני כל דאמינא להו מיפך אפכי אמר להו
בישרא סומקא אגומרי וחמרא מרקא אייתו ליה אינהו בישרא שמינא אגומרי וחמרא חייא
שמעה ילתא ומעיילא ליה לבי מסותא ומוקמי ליה במיא דבי מסותא עד דמהפכי מיא דבי
מסותא והוו כדמא וקאי בישריה פשיטי פשיט
רב יוסף איעסק בריחיא
רב ששת איעסק בכשורי אמר גדולה מלאכה שמחממת את בעליה

When the household of the Exilarch wanted to annoy R. Amram the Pious, they made him lie down in the snow. On the next day they said, What would your honour like us to bring you? He knew that whatever he told them they would do the reverse, so he said to them, Lean meat broiled on the coals and wine much diluted. They brought him fat meat broiled on the coals and undiluted wine. Yaltha heard and took him in to the bath, and they kept him there till the water turned to the colour of blood and his flesh was covered with bright spots. R. Joseph used to cure the shivers by working at the mill, R. Shesheth by carrying heavy beams. He said: Work is a splendid thing to make one warm. (b. Gittin 67b)

---

13 Cf. Tal Ilan, "Female Personalities in the Babylonian Talmud," *Jewish Women's Archive* [cited 3 August 2016]; Online: http://jwa.org/encyclopedia/article/female-personalities-in-babylonian-talmud

For a fever lasting three days, she (*Em*) recommended eating red meat and dilute wine while on the first day fluids were to be preferred and blood could be let on the second day. For a chill, literally 'snow', the treatment was fat meat broiled on the coals with undiluted wine indicating a lighter diet for the fevered patient. Not all fevered patients were given food or drink as treatment as it was recorded that the fever of a sage could be cured by incantation.[14] Naturally, the Talmud records a remarkable number of folk remedies that appear strange to the modern eye. We have just noted the remedy in b. Gittin 67b using a black hen which should be torn and applied to the shorn head of the patient, who then immerses himself in the river.

An example of an incantation for treating fever can be found in the Talmud (b. Shabbat 67a):

אמ״ר יוחנן לאשתא צמירתא לישקל סכינא דכולא פרזלא וליזל להיכא דאיכא
וורדינא וליקטר ביה נירא ברקא

Rabbi Yochanan said, For a burning fever let him take an all-iron knife, go to where thorn hedges are to be found and tie a white twisted thread to it. (b. Shabbat 67a)

After making notches and reciting various verses[15] he pulls the bush down and says:

הסנה הסנה לאו משום דגביהת מכל אילני אשרי הקב״ה שכינתיה עלך אלא משום דמייכת
מכל אילני אשרי קודשא בריך הוא שכינתיה עלך
וכי היכי דחמיתיה אשתא לחנניה מישאל ועזריה ועריקת מן קדמוהי כן תחמיניה אשתא
לפלוני בר פלונית ותיערוק מן קדמוהי

O thorn, O thorn, not because you are higher than all other trees did the Holy One, bless be He, cause his *Shechinah to* rest upon you, but because you are lower than all other trees did He cause his *Shechinah* to rest upon you. And even as you saw the fire (kindled) for Hananiah, Mishael and fled from before them, so look on the fever (lit. fire) of 'so and so' and flee from him. (b. Shabbat 67a)

Preuss notes these remedies and points out that a glance at the writings of the Roman writer Pliny indicates that 'Talmudic folk medicine abundantly found its match in the Roman medicine of its time, as far as superstition is concerned'.[16]

---

14 *Shir HaShirim Rabbah* 2:16 records the healing incantation recited by Rabbi Chanina over a febrile Rabbi Yochanan.

15 The verses to recite over a sequence of three days are Exodus 3:2–4: *(2) And the angel of the Lord appeared to him in a flame of fire out of the midst of a bush. He looked, and behold, the bush was burning, yet it was not consumed* (וירא מלאך יהוה אליו בלבת־אש מתוך הסנה וירא והנה הסנה בער באש) *(3) And Moses said, "I will turn aside to see this great sight, why the bush is not burned (4).* (והסנה איננו אכל). *When the Lord saw* (ויאמר משה אסרה־נא ואראה את־המראה הגדל הזה מדוע לא־יבער הסנה). *that he turned aside to see, God called to him out of the bush, "Moses, Moses!" And he said, "Here I am"* (וירא יהוה כי סר לראות ויקרא אליו אלהים מתוך הסנה ויאמר משה משה ויאמר הנני)."

16 Julius Preuss, *Biblical and Talmudic Medicine*, 162. While Pliny the Elder described many treatments with a medical value and opposed the many contemporary, purely magical folk reme-

The Fever that nourishes

Hippocrates ruled that body heat was important for digestion, thus the analogy that the 'cooking' of digestion matched the cooking of food on a fire, and thus could contribute to the nourishment of the body.[17] As Aramaic does not distinguish between the heat of fire and fever one can see how this notion might take hold.[18]

In the Talmudic tractate of *Sanhedrin* the rabbis consider this situation by way of examining the practicalities of life in Noah's Ark. Working from the premise that the lion, which would have normally attempted to eat most of the other animals, would have had to have its appetite curbed during the Flood, the rabbis concluded that it must have suffered from a fever, which would have sustained it, and thus the other creatures were spared. There is a Talmudic view that as febrile patients have a reduced food intake there must be something in the fever that provides the missing nourishment. The lion was, accordingly, nourished by a fever:

אכלה אריא אישתא זינתיה דאמר רב לא בציר משיתא ולא טפי מתריסר זינא אישתא

The lion was nourished by a fever, for Rav said: "Fever sustains for not less than six (days and) nor more than twelve. (b. Sanhedrin 108b)

This was assumed, as people were aware that a patient could survive a febrile illness even excreting urine and faeces during this period. Is this the origin of starving a fever? Or, does the story of the lion in the Ark underline the concept that the febrile patient has less requirement of nutrition during his illness as with a fever the inclination to eat falls away and the patient starves?

Rav's comment was that a fever can sustain its victim for no less than six days but no more than twelve. Thus, the suggestion was that the lion did not require feeding, as it had developed a fever which enabled it to go not just some days but obviously for some months without eating. This is based on the belief that some animals can survive extreme conditions without food for extended periods sustained by the fat and nutrients stored in their bodies. In humans they believed, using the analogy of the lion in the Ark, that the fever would reduce the patient's appetite and thus sustain the patient through the consumption of the body's excess of stored fat.

In another Talmudic debate, related to paternal obligations at the time of the Passover sacrifices in the time of the Temple, the Rabbis consider the case of a baby boy, who has been partially born but cannot be circumcised which devolves an additional religious responsibility onto the father:

---

edies in his *Natural Histories*, he did, for example, advocate raw veal or she-goat dung placed over the wound caused by the bite of a rabid dog, for four days, while the patient takes only lime and pig fat internally.

17 Cf. Mark Shiefsky, *Hippocrates on Ancient Medicine* (Leiden: Brill, 2005), 216–217.

18 M. J. Geller, *Akkadian Healing*, op. cit.

ומי חיי והתניא כיון שיצא העולם לאויר נפתח הסתום ונסתם הפתוח שאלמלא כן אין יכול
לחיות אפילו שעה אחת

> Can (the child) live like this? Is it not taught that once (a baby) comes into the
> air of the world, what was closed (i. e. mouth and nostrils) open, and what was
> open (i. e. the umbilical cord) closes, as if this did not occur, it could not live
> even for one hour. (b. Yevamot 71b)

The child in this unusual situation is unable to feed and is described as surviving as
he is sustained by the presence of a fever, some say in the mother but others consider
a fever, or heat, in the crying baby. If there was a delay in the circumcision, normally
carried out on the eighth day, because of the need to give the baby time to recover
from the fever, this implies that the fever has been in the child as the alternative is that
if the fever is in the mother then the child does not require any recovery time before
circumcision.

הכא במאי עסקינן כגון דזנתיה אישתא אישתא דמאן
אילימא אישתא דידיה אי הכי כל שבעה בעי אלא דזנתיה אישתא אישתא דאימיה

> With what case are we dealing with here? It is, for example, a case where he was
> sustained by (the heat) of a fever. Whose fever? If we say it is his own fever, if
> so (it is necessary) to wait a full seven days (for the circumcision). Rather, he
> (must have been) sustained by his mother's fever. (b. Yevamot 71b)

The further possibility considered by the rabbis is that the nourishing warmth is not
provided by the fever of illness but by the fever of the baby's crying which generates
the heat required and permits the baby's circumcision at the correct time. Conversely,
it was understood that the child who did not cry would not survive. In any case, the
rabbis clearly accept here that fever nourishes in the absence of food.

Israeli and Maimonides on the 'nourishing fever'

Fevers feature in the writings of the great mediaeval Jewish physicians. Many of these
discuss therapeutic approaches while others describe, often carefully and with much
attention to detail the course of a febrile illness, noting which fevers are benign and
which carry a serious threat to life.[19] One of the key Jewish medical texts of the early
period was the *Book of Fevers*, *Kitāb al-Ḥummayāt*, composed in Arabic by Isaac Israeli (855–955), known also in the Latin world as Isaac Judaeus, in Kairouan in present
day Tunisia. Based on Hippocratic traditions, it was a key medical text in its Latin
translation, by Constantinus Africanus, in the early European medical schools as was

---

19 While we examine here the opinions of the *Rambam* (Maimonides) and of Isaac Israeli, there is an
extensive literature on the subject. See for example H. J. Zimmels, *Magicians, Theologians and Doctors: Studies in Folk-medicine and Folklore as reflected in the Rabbinical Reponsa (12ᵗʰ–19ᵗʰ centuries)*
(London: Edward Goldston, 1952); Joshua Trachtenberg, *Jewish Magic and Superstition: A Study
in Folk Religion* (New York: Atheneum, 1970); J. O. Leibowitz and S. Marcus, *Sefer Hanisyonot:
The Book of Medical Experiences attributed to Abraham Ibn Ezra* (Jerusalem: Magnes Press 1984).

his influential text on urine.[20] Thus, his works were studied for some centuries in European universities that were not prepared to admit Jews as students. Indeed, Charles Singer considered it to be one of the best medical works available in the Middle Ages.[21]

The popularity of Isaac's *Book on Fevers* among physicians in the Middle Ages is confirmed by the number of translations, the number of surviving manuscripts and editions, and its use in several universities. The translators saw the work as a living text and did not merely transfer it from one language to another, but also sought to improve it and bring it closer to their readers, making definitive texts hard to establish.[22]

Isaac showed himself capable of fresh thinking and the clarity in his detailed writings shows how he moved on from some classical beliefs to create an emphasis on therapeutics.[23] In his *Book on Fevers,* Isaac combined medical concepts and philosophy in a single work, making it clear that medicine was a skill rooted in philosophy and based on philosophy.[24] Thus, he aimed to control the fever by cooling the patient and treatments, both medical and dietary, which would aid the patient's comfort by producing the nourishment the body requires.[25] However, he indicates the complexity of fevers because of their different causes and outcomes:

> I personally have yet to discover any predecessor of mine who has already made any recommendation about the management of this [hectic] fever when compounded with any form of putrid fever. That is because [any attempt at] such a recommendation presents very difficult problems owing to the fact that management of the one fever is incompatible with and dissimilar to that applicable to the other; for, whereas putrid fever requires treatment that will cleanse and purify the putridity and desiccate the moistures, hectic fever requires treatment that will abate the heat and curb its vehemence and at the same time impart moisture to the body, remove its dryness and aridity, and provide it with wholesome moisture. It is clear, then, that the two kinds of treatment widely diverge from, and contrast and conflict with, one another.[26]

---

20 Samuel Kottek, Helena Paavilainen, Kenneth Collins, eds., *Isaac Israeli: the Philosopher Physician* (Jerusalem: Muriel & Philiip Berman Medical Library, 2015), tells Isaac's story and the content of his medicine and thought, while indicating the transmission of his writings, often in Latin.

21 Charles Singer, *Short History of Scientific Ideas to 1900* (Oxford: Oxford University Press, 1959), 148.

22 Cf. Lola Ferre and Raphaela Veit, "The Textual Traditions of Isaac Israeli's Book on Fevers in Arabic, Latin, Hebrew, and Spanish," *Aleph: Historical Studies in Science and Judaism* 9,2 (2009): 309–334.

23 Cf. J. D. Latham, "Isaac Israeli's *Kitāb al-Ḥummayāt* and the Latin and Castilian Texts," *Journal of Semitic Studies* 14 (1969): 80–95, here: 83.

24 Cf. Lola Ferre, "Medicine through a Philosophical Lens: Treatise I of Isaac Israeli's Book on Fevers," in *Isaac Israeli: the Philosopher Physician* (ed. Samuel Kottek, Helena Paavilainen, and Kenneth Collins; Jerusalem: Muriel & Philiip Berman Medical Library, 2015), 115–136.

25 J. D. Latham, "Isaac Israeli's 'Kitāb al-Ḥummayāt,'" 92–95.

26 Cf. J. D. Latham, *Isaac Judaeus On fevers. the Third discourse, On consumption.* (Cambridge: Pembroke Arabic Texts, 1981), xiv and xxiv, 21.

Moses Maimonides (1138–1204) also wrote on fevers in his *Treatises on Health* and *Asthma* as well as his own *Aphorisms* and in his *Commentary on the Aphorisms of Hippocrates*. Hippocrates had pointed out: "As the soil is to trees, so is the stomach to animals. It nourishes, it warms, it cools; as it empties it cools, as it fills it warms".[27] In parallel with this, he indicates that it is important to eat well in the winter to keep warm and to eat lightly in the summer to keep cool. Thus, as we noted at the outset, feeding will warm the cold while starving will cool the fevered.

Maimonides was aware that fever was a symptom of illness and that both symptom and cause should be treated. However, he was careful to make a diagnosis before commencing treatment, even preferring to delay the start of rehydration.[28] Indeed, he notes that for some patients fluid will provide the cure while it may be harmful in other cases and he considers this to be a real dilemma for the skilled physician.[29] In his day, the prevalence of the theory of the red and black bile precluded the opportunity of accurate therapy in the modern sense yet his description of symptoms remains of much interest. In the Third Treatise, he notes that there are two types of warmth in the body. One derives from blood while the other is fever which can be called 'unnatural heat'.[30] In the next aphorism, he comments that during the crisis of an illness when there is severe hunger that purified blood, that is to say venous blood, will return to nourish the stomach, an indication of a possible mechanism for the nourishing fever. In the *Tenth Treatise* Maimonides enumerates a series of aphorisms related to fevers. In some instances, he seems to support the notion of starving a fever concluding that one should not give a quantity of cold water to a fevered patient without careful consideration[31] and feeding should only be considered when the fever subsides.[32] At other times, especially during emotion upsets, the lack of food may be more harmful and the patient may be fed.

Maimonides quotes Galen that "he who is naturally hot and dry because his constitution is naturally unbalanced, his fever will be increased by food…(he) should be given food…which is not of much nourishing value". Thus, while the fever may nourish, a more balanced judgment is required of the patient's nutritional needs. In his *Commentary on the Aphorisms of Hippocrates* Maimonides is critical of Galen's views on managing fever preferring to follow Hippocrates in continuing to use warming medicine as long as the signs indicate that this is the best therapy.[33] Further, he indicates that this warming might be done by alternating warming medicine as the body may have become accustomed to the original treatment.

---

27 Hippocrates, *Heracleitus 'On the Universe'* (trans. W. H. S. Jones; London: Heinemann, 1931), 82.

28 Fred Rosner and Suessman Muntner, eds. and trans., *The Medical Aphorisms of Moses Maimonides* (New York: Bloch, 1970/71), 203.

29 Maimonides, *On Asthma* (trans. and ed. Gerrit Bos; Provo, Utah: Brigham Young University Press, 2002), 87.

30 Rosner and Muntner, *Medical Aphorisms of Moses Maimonides*, 66 (Third Treatise 49, 1).

31 Uriel S. Barzel, ed. and trans., *The Art of Cure: Extracts from Galen: Maimonides' Medical Writings* (Haifa: Maimonides Research Institute, 1992), 99.

32 Rosner and Muntner, *Medical Aphorisms of Moses Maimonides*, 66, 1 (p. 222).

33 Fred Rosner, ed. and trans., *Maimonides' Commentary on the Aphorisms of Hippocrates* (Haifa: The Maimonides Research Institute, 1987), 66–68.

The 'fever that nourishes' in contemporary medicine

On a purely superficial level, it would seem unlikely that the body would have developed an anorexic response to infection if there was not some physical gain to be obtained from the process. Contemporary physicians have attempted to identify the mechanisms controlling appetite suppression and the role of fever in illness. They note that many stereotypical responses follow acute infection regardless of their cause and the fever is accompanied by some easily measurable responses such as *granulocytosis* and changes in insulin and C reactive protein.[34] They remark that is seems paradoxical that at a time when the body's metabolic rate rises by over 10% for each degree rise in temperature that food intake should be voluntarily suppressed. However, these same researchers noted that it was not the fever itself which reduced appetite as blocking the fever with salicylates does not restore appetite.[35] Some researchers have concluded that anorexia during infection may reduce the nutrients essential for the pathogenic organisms and as such may be part of the acute phase response.

Others report that fasting stimulates the response that tackles the bacterial infections responsible for most fevers while eating boosts the type of immune response that destroys cold viruses.[36] In a small study on healthy volunteers, researchers in Amsterdam found that after a liquid meal gamma interferon levels, a hallmark of the cell mediated immune response, quadrupled giving the body the ability to deal with viral infections. When the same volunteers took only water this increased the levels of *interleukin* 4, characteristic of the humoral immune response, in which B cells produce antibodies that attack the pathogens producing bacterial infections. These findings support other studies in which intensive care patients given the amino acid glutamine, found in milk, meat and some nuts, have an enhanced cell mediated immune response and greater ability to handle infection.[37] Further studies have indicated that fever can enhance the clinical effect of antibiotics.[38]

---

34 Donna O. McCarthy, Matthew J. Kluger, and Arthur J. Vander, "Suppression of food intake during infection: is interleukin–1 involved?" *American Journal of Clinical Nutrition* 42:6 (1985): 1179–1182.

35 Donna O. McCarthy, Matthew J. Kluger, and Arthur J. Vander, "The role of fever in appetite suppression after endotoxin administration," *American Journal of Clinical Nutrition* 40:2 (1984): 310–316. There have been recent suggestions that fever reducing medications may actually help to spread influenza; see a study from McMasterUniversity in Canada: http://dailynews.mcmaster. ca/article/fever-reducing-meds-may-help-spread-the-flu; accessed 27th January 2014. The study indicated that fever suppression actually increases the expected number of influenza cases and deaths. David J. D. Earn, Paul W. Andrews, and Benjamin M. Bolker, "Population-level effects of suppressing fever," *Proceedings of the Royal Society B: Biological Sciences* 281 : 20132570 (2014): 1–5.

36 Cf. http://www.newscientist.com/article/dn1777-feed-a-cold-starve-a-fever-might-be-right.html; cited 6 September 2009.

37 Richard D. Griffiths, Karen D. Allen, Francis J. Andrews, and Christina Jones, "Infection, multiple organ failure, and survival in the intensive care unit: influence of glutamine-supplemented parenteral nutrition on acquired infection," *Nutrition* 18:7–8 (2002): 546–552.

38 P.A. Mackowiak, M. Marling-Cason, and R.L. Cohen, "Effects of temperature on anti-microbial susceptibility of bacteria," *Journal of Infectious Diseases* 135 (1982): 550–553.

Conclusion

During a cold, it is easier to maintain nutritional levels while the illness runs its course. With a fever, appetite is suppressed and the body has to survive on its reserves though obviously this has to be supplemented by careful attention to fluid balance and energy requirements. While the old adage that one should feed a cold but starve a fever does not contain the whole story nevertheless it does possess some important core truths. As for the fever that nourishes we can understand the rabbinic logic which gave rise to it and through its association with the starving fever, and the modern understanding of its defence mechanisms, it may yet reclaim its place in the modern imagination.

Bibliography

Sources

TANAKH: A New Translation of the Holy Scriptures According to the Traditional Hebrew Texts. Philadelphia: Jewish Publication Society of America, 1985.

The Babylonian Talmud. Edited and Translated by Isidore Epstein. 18 vols. London: Soncino, 1961.

The Midrash Rabbah. Edited and translated by H. Freedman, Maurice Simon and Judah J. Slotki. 5 vols. London: Soncino, 1977.

Hippocrates. *Heracleitus on the Universe.* Translated by W. H. S. Jones. London: Heinemann, 1931.

Barzel, Uriel S., ed. and trans. *The Art of Cure: Extracts from Galen: Maimonides' Medical Writings,* Haifa: Maimonides Research Inst., 1992.

Bos, Gerrit, ed. and trans. *Maimonides On Asthma.* Provo, Utah: Brigham Young University Press, 2002.

Rosner, Fred, ed. and trans. *Maimonides' Commentary on the Aphorisms of Hippocrates.* Haifa: The Maimonides Research Institute, 1987.

Rosner Fred and Suessman Muntner, ed. and trans. *The Medical Aphorism of Moses Maimonides.* Vol. 2. New York: Yeshiva University Press, 1971.

Literature

Leibowitz, Joshua. "The Problem of Medical Licence in Hebrew Sources." *Koroth* 7, 5–6 (1977): 47–53.

Earn, David, Paul W. Andrews, and Benjamin M. Bolker. "Population-level effects of suppressing fever." *Proceedings of the Royal Society B: Biological Sciences* 22 (2014): 281.

Elman, Yaakov. "Orality and the Redaction of the Babylonian Talmud." *Oral Tradition* 14,1 (1999): 52–99.

Gallacher, Stuart A. "Stuff a cold and feed a fever." *History of Medicine* 11 (1942): 576–581.

Geller, Markham J. *Akkadian Healing Therapies in the Babylonian Talmud.* Berlin: Max Planck Institute for the History of Science, 2004. Preprint Series 259. Cited 25 May 2014. Online: http://www.mpiwg-berlin.mpg.de/Preprints/P259.PDF

Griffiths, Richard D. et al. "Infection, multiple organ failure, and survival in the intensive care unit: influence of glutamine-supplemented parenteral nutrition on acquired infection." *Nutrition* 18, 7–8 (2002): 546–552.

Halivni, David Weiss. *The Formation of the Babylonian Talmud*. Translated by Jeffrey L. Rubenstein. Oxford: Oxford University Press, 2013.

Ilan, Tal. "Female Personalities in the Babylonian Talmud." *Jewish Women's Archive*. Cited 3 August 2016. Online: http://jwa.org/encyclopedia/article/female-personalities-in-babylonian-talmud.

Latham, John D. "Isaac Israeli's 'Kitab Al-Hummayat' and the Latin and Castilian Texts." *Journal of Semitic Studies* 14 (1969): 82–96.

Latham John D. and Haskell D. Isaacs, eds. and transl. *Kitāb al-Ḥummayāt li-Isḥāq ibn Sulaymān al-Isrā'īlī. al-maqālah al-thālithah, Fī al-sill = Isaac Judaeus On fevers. the Third discourse, On consumption*. Cambridge: Cambridge Middle East Centre and Pembroke Arabic Texts, 1981.

Leibowitz, Joshua O. "The Problem of Medical Licence in Hebrew Sources." *Koroth* 5,6–7 (1977): 47–53.

Leibowitz, Joshua O. and S. Marcus, eds. and transl. *Sefer Hanisyonot: The Book of Medical Experiences attributed to Abraham ibn Ezra*. Jerusalem: Magnes Press, 1984.

Mackowiak, P.A., M. Marling-Cason, and R.L. Cohen. "Effects of temperature on anti-microbial susceptibility of bacteria." *Journal of Infectious Diseases* 135 (1982): 550–553.

McCarthy, Donna O., Matthew J. Kluger, and Arthur J. Vander. "The role of fever in appetite suppression after endotoxin administration." *American Journal of Clinical Nutrition* 40:2 (1984): 310–316.

—. "Suppression of food intake during infection: is interleukin-1 involved?" *American Journal of Clinical Nutrition* 42:6 (1985): 1179–1182.

Preuss, Julius. *Biblical-Talmudic Medicine*. Translated by Fred Rosner. New York: Sanhedrin Press, 1978.

Shiefsky, Mark. *Hippocrates on Ancient Medicine*. Leiden: Brill, 2005.

Singer, Charles. *Short History of Scientific Ideas to 1900*. Oxford: Clarendon, 1966.

Trachtenberg, Joshua. *Jewish Magic and Superstition: A Study in Folk Religion*. New York: Atheneum, 1970.

Withals, John. *Shorte Dictionarie of Yonge Beginners*. London: Lewis Evans, 1553.

Zimmels, Hirsch J. *Magicians, Theologians and Doctors: Studies in Folk-medicine and Folk-lore as reflected in the Rabbinical Responsa (12–19th centuries)*. London: Goldston, 1952.

The Rabbinic Health Regimen:
A Greek Genre Adapted by the Sages

Aviad Recht

Among all of the medical material appearing in rabbinic literature, a distinct literary genre of "health regimen" (*hanhagat ha-beri'ut*) can be identified. This literary genre is characterized by the content of its medical teachings, by the *materia medica* mentioned therein, and by the audience to whom these medical teachings are addressed. The contents of the medical teachings in this genre evince a pronounced affinity to Greek medical literature, which developed regimens into a defined field of medicine. At the same time, other characteristics of the rabbinic health regimen indicate cultural processing of the original Greek genre and its adaption for its target audience—the rabbis' communities. In order to properly discuss the characteristics of the rabbinic health regimen genre, we begin to sketch its borders in relation to the totality of medical material in the Babylonian Talmud.

Direct and indirect

The classic opening of discussions on the topic of medicine in the Talmud is typically as follows: the Talmud is a religious text with halakhic and moral motivations. It is not a medical corpus, and therefore one should not expect to find systematic medical writings in it. Nonetheless, medical content can be extracted from the text, which may illuminate the world of medicine among Jews in the era of the sages.[1] Yet within the halakhic and aggadic *sugyot*, purely medical texts do appear, with no halakhic or aggadic context. These medical texts are used within the *sugya* in a number of ways: as proof, elaboration, associative deviation, and more. The phrasing of these statements makes it clear that the medical references were initially written (or spoken)[2] separately, and were later integrated within various *sugyot*. I will refer to medical texts intend-

---

1 Julius Preuss, *Biblical and Talmudic Medicine* (trans. and ed. Fred Rosner; Northvale, NJ: J. Aronson, 1993), 4 (it should be noted that Preuss himself notes the medical list found in Gittin 68b–69a); Solomon R. Kagan, *Jewish Medicine* (Boston/Mass.: Medico-Historical Press, 1952), 27; Avraham Steinberg, *Chapters in the Pathology of the Talmud* (Jerusalem: Hamakhon Leheqer Harefu'ah 'al pi Hatorah [= Dr. Falk Schlesinger Institute for Medical-Halachic Research], 1975), 5.
2 For the written versus the oral Talmud, see Yaakov Sussmann, "The Oral Torah Literally Speaking: The Power of Every Jot and Tittle," in *Mehqere Talmud: Talmudic Studies*, vol. 3, a, (ed. Yaakov Sussmann and David Rosenthal; Jerusalem: Magnes, 2005), 209–384, who suggests that the entire Talmud, from the first rabbinic 'pairs' (*Zugot*) to the last editors (*Savoraim*), was all transmitted orally.

DOI: 10.13173/9783447108263.157

ed to transmit medical information as "direct medical content" (that is, "a medical teaching"), whereas I will refer to medical texts serving a different purpose, whether religious, halakhic, or moral, as "indirect medical content."

For instance, the Mishnah (Shabbat) discussed actions that are required for circumcising a baby on the Sabbath, even though generally these actions are restricted during the day of rest:

> We perform all the requirements of circumcision on the Sabbath. We circumcise, uncover [the corona], suck [the wound], and place a compress and cumin upon it. If one did not crush [the cumin] on the eve of the Sabbath, he must chew [it] with his teeth and apply [it to the wound]; if he did not beat up wine and oil on the eve of the Sabbath, each must be applied separately ... (m. Shabbat 19:2).

עושין כל צרכי מילה בשבת מוהלין ופורעין ומוצצין ונותנין עליה איספלנית וכמון אם לא שחק מערב[3] שבת לועס בשיניו ונותן אם לא טרף יין ושמן מערב שבת ינתן זה בעצמו וזה בעצמו ...

(משנה שבת יט, ב)

From the Mishnah we can learn that cumin was used for healing the circumcision wound. Refraining from using it may be dangerous, and therefore the Mishnah allows its use on the Sabbath even though there are restrictions on medicine during Sabbath (but it is not a life-threatening situation, and therefore the cumin must be chewed, not crushed in a bowl).[4] It seems that wine and oil too are mentioned in the Mishnah because of their medical uses.[5] This is a classic example of extracting medical information from halakhic content. From the mention of the cumin, wine, and oil as allowed for use during the Sabbath for the purposes of circumcision, we learn of their medical properties. Yet it is clear that the text's intention is to transmit halakhic

---

3 All translations from the Babylonian Talmud are taken from the Soncino translation: *The Babylonian Talmud* (trans. and ed. Isidore Epstein; London: Soncino, 1961). Online: www.halakhah.org

4 It seems that *cumin* was used in the effort to stop the bleeding. Perhaps this is its use in the prescription for gonorrhea, in b. Shabbat 110b, and in the prescription for blood that comes from the mouth in b. Gittin 69a. Dioscorides depicts the attribute of *cumin* as keeping in check flux and nose bleedings (see Pedanius Dioscorides, *De materia medica* (trans. Lily Y. Beck; Hildesheim: Olms-Weidmann, 2005), 207). According to Osbaldeston's translation *cumin* is used by chewing and applying, as it is in the above mentioned m. Shabbat 19:2, see Dioscorides, *De materia medica* (trans. and ed. T. A. Osbaldeston and R. P. A. Wood; Johannesburg: IBIDIS, 2000), 443. Pliny the Elder describes a mixture of dried and crushed cumin and honey as useful in treatment of swollen circumcision wounds. Cf. Pliny, *Natural History* (trans. D. E. Eichholz; London: W. Heinemann, 1968), Vol. 20, 57.

5 Preuss, *Biblical and Talmudic Medicine*, 4, remains doubtful regarding its usage for bandages or other uses. Cf. also in the Talmudic traditions: "Shmuel taught: we shall always refrain from oil and hot water on a wound during Shabbat" (y. Shabbat 89c); "Mar 'Ukba also said: If one knocks his hand or foot, he may reduce the swelling with wine, and need have no fear" (b. Shabbat 109a).

information, and therefore the medical information derived from the text is "indirect medical content." The purpose of the following statement is completely different:

> Ten things bring a man's sickness on again in a severe form, namely, to eat beef, fat meat, roast meat, poultry and roasted egg, shaving, and eating garden cress, milk or cheese, and bathing. Some add, also nuts; and some add further, also chate melons.[6] (b. Berakhot 57b)

עשרה דברים מחזירין את החולה לחליו וחליו קשה, אלו הן: בשר שור, בשר שמן, בשר צלי, בשר צפרים, וביצה צלויה, ותגלחת, ושחלים, והחלב, והגבינה והמרחץ. ויש אומרים: אף אגוזים, ויש אומרים: אף קשואים. (ברכות נז ע"ב)

This anonymous statement appears within a broader *sugya* that deals with dreams. At a certain point in the *sugya*, several statements are presented consecutively that open with "an x (given number) of things were said about..." From here, the discussion shifts towards other statements with a similar opening formula, which relate to other topics, including medicine. It is evident that the statement "Ten things bring a man's sickness on again..."[7] is a stand-alone textual unit that the editor of the *sugya* decided to include in this discussion on dreams based on his own considerations. It is reasonable to assume that statement was mentioned in a different context that we cannot trace back.[8]

The intention of the speaker in this statement is not halakhic, aggadic, or moral by nature. His intention is to simply teach his listeners which foods a sick person must avoid in order to become healthy. The intention here is to transmit medical information, and therefore this is a medical teaching ("direct medical content").

---

6   The last word was translated in the Soncino edition as "cucumbers," but the common understanding of קישוא is "chate melon"; see: Zohar Amar and Efraim Lev, "Watermelon, Chate Melon and Cucumber: New Light on Traditional and Innovative Field Crops of the Middle Age," *Journal Asiatique* 299, 1 (2011): 193–204. Cf. b. Avodah Zarah 29a, where the order is different and liver appears instead of milk.

7   Amar identified the existence of "medical teachings or warnings that one must act upon" and stated that some of them are known by "the number of medical properties present in a particular plant," and "in the 'known' number of medical substances," and didn't elaborate further on this matter. Cf. Zohar Amar, "Materia Medica from the Land of Israel in the Time of the Bible, the Mishnah and the Talmud according to Written Sources," in *Health and Sickness in Antiquity* (ed. Anat Rimmon; Haifa: Hecht Museum, University of Haifa, 2006), 56–57 [In Hebrew].

8   On this matter, Ben-Yehuda, in the main introduction to his dictionary, suggested that there were Jewish medical writings from the Return to Zion (*Shivat Zion*) era and onwards. These texts were compiled into scrolls and later gathered in book form, but the book was archived due to the resistance to written books. And this, in his view, is the historical kernel of the story of the "Book of Medicines" (*Sefer harefu'ot*) that Hezekiah sent to be archived. The *baraitot* (teachings not included into the Mishnah) that open with תנו רבנן (*tanu rabanan*; 'our sages taught'), that contain medical teachings are, in Ben-Yehuda's view, remnants of this medical book. He dates these *baraitot* back to sometime before the Hasmonean era. Cf. Eliezer Ben-Yehuda, *A Complete Dictionary of Ancient and Modern Hebrew* (Jerusalem: General Federation of Jewish Labour in Eretz-Israel, 1948–1959), 1:56–57.

Two genres

When observing, even briefly, the talmudic medical teachings in their entirety, one notices immediately that they are not monolithic. There are different styles and medical approaches, reflecting a variety of medical cultures. Within these, two distinct genres of literature are clearly noticeable. One genre is characterized by short, concise statements, and very simple medical teachings: "do this and not this." In this genre the medical content is mostly in Hebrew, with almost no magical elements. The medical instructions in this genre are straightforward, with only basic components. The prescriptions typically involve only a single plant. The directive is so simple, that even the method of processing (such as crushing, cutting, shaking, mixing with wine, vinegar, or water) is not mentioned. In this genre quantities are rarely mentioned, either. In contrast, the second genre of direct medical content is characterized by long, detailed, and often complicated prescriptions, which include quantities. Statements of this genre are generally in Babylonian Aramaic, and include an abundance of magic.[9]

The first genre can be demonstrated with Rabbi Yohanan's statement regarding *tsaraʿat*:[10]

> R. Yohanan stated: Why are there no lepers in Babylon? —Because they eat beet,drink beer and bathe in the waters of the Euphrates. (b. Ketuboth 77b)

---

9 Shaul Shaked begins one of his many articles on the various representations of magic thus: "Any one working within the field of magic in Judaism in Late Antiquity and the early Middle Age knows the difficulties besetting any attempt to define it. Despite these difficulties, which exist in Judaism just as they do in any religious culture, there are not very many cases of hesitation when one tries to identify magic texts in practice." Shaul Shaked, "'Peace Be upon You, Exalted Angels': On Hekhalot, Liturgy and Incantation Bowls," *Jewish Studies Quarterly* 2 (1995): 197–219; here: 197. This is also my impression from the medical magical texts in the Talmud. An explanation for this impression can be found in what Yuval Harari calls his "quasi-ostensible" definition of magic, in which he relies on Wittgenstein's principle of "family resemblance." As a focus for "what is a Jewish magical text?," Harari suggests the oath and the address to metaphysical powers, thus defining two additional, more expansive circles of texts which have some kind of "family resemblance" to the core texts (oaths). The quality of the resemblance determines whether a text is magical or not, and to what extent it is magical in relation to other texts. See Yuval Harari, *Early Jewish Magic: Research, Method, Sources* (Jerusalem: Bialik Institute and Ben-Zvi Institute, 2010), 122–134 [In Hebrew]. For a comprehensive, broad, and fascinating survey of magic and scholarly attempts to define it, see ibid., 5–121. My description of the direct medical content in the second genre is based on the initial findings of my doctoral dissertation, in which I will thoroughly examine these matters.

10 Much ink has been spilled on the identification of *tsaraʿat* (cf. Preuss, *Biblical and Talmudic Medicine*, 323–327). Amar already showed that the biblical *tsaraʿat* was translated as leprosy by Josephus, the Septuagint, and the Vulgate, and thus has been identified in Christian tradition—and continues to be so identified in the modern medical world—with Hansen's disease. However, Amar showed that the obvious symptoms of Hansen's disease mentioned in the Talmud are identified there as *sheḥin* rather than *tsaraʿat*. Zohar Amar, "What Is *sheḥin* in the Language of the Sages?" *Assia* 19 (2005): 61–69 [In Hebrew]. Therefore, talmudic *tsaraʿat* should not be identified with leprosy/Hansen's disease, and the term should remain transliterated for the time being.

אמר רבי יוחנן: מפני מה אין מצורעין בבבל? מפני שאוכלין תרדין, ושותין שכר, ורוחצין במי
פרת. (כתובות עז ע"ב)

The statement is a medical teaching. Rabbi Yohanan's intention was to present ways
by which *tsara'at* can be prevented. The guidelines are very simple and do not refer to
quantities or complicated prescriptions; the statement is articulated in Hebrew, and
is free of magic. These features point strongly to the first category of instructions. A
medical teaching of the second genre is found in tractate Gittin:

> To stop bleeding at the nose he should bring a *Kohen* whose name is Levi and
> write Levi backwards, or else bring any man and write, I Papi Shila bar Sum-
> ki, backwards, or else write thus: *Ta'am Deli Beme Kesaf, Ta'am Deli Be-Me
> Pegam.* Or else he can take root of clover and the rope of an old bed and papy-
> rus and saffron and the red part of a palm branch and burn them all together
> and then take a fleece of wool and weave two threads and steep them in vinegar
> and roll them in the ashes and put them in his nostrils. Or he can look for a wa-
> tercourse running from east to west and stand astride over it and pick up some
> clay with his right hand from under his left leg and with his left hand from
> under his right leg and twine two threads of wool and rub them in the clay and
> put them in his nostrils. Or else he can sit under a gutter pipe while they bring
> water and pour over him saying, 'As these waters stop, so may the blood of A,
> son of the woman B, stop'. (Bab. Talmud, Gittin 69a)

לדמא דאתי מנחירא—ליתי גברא כהן דשמיה לוי, וליכתוב ליה לוי למפרע.
ואי לא, ליתי איניש מעלמא, וניכתוב ליה אנא פפי שילא בר סומקי למפרע.
ואי לא, ניכתוב ליה הכי, טעם דלי במי כסף טעם דלי במי פגם.
ואי לא, ליתי עיקרא דאספסתא ואשלא דפורייא עתיקא, וקורטסא ומוריקי וסומקא דלוליבא,
ונקלינהו בהדי הדדי, וליתי גבבא דעמרא וניגדול תרתי פתילתא, ולטמיש בחלא וניגדבל
בקיטמא הדין, וניתיב בנחיריה.
ואי לא, ליחזי אמת המים דאזלת ממזרח כלפי מערב, ונפסע וניקום חד כרעא להאי גיסא וחד
כרעא להאי גיסא, ונישקול טינא בידיה דימינא מתותי כרעא דשמאליה, ובידיה דשמאלא
מתותי כרעא דימיניה, וניגדול תרתי פתילתא דעמרא וניטמיש בטינא, וניתיב בנחיריה.
ואי לא, ליתיב תותי מרזבא וניתו מיא,[11] ולישדו עליה ולימרו: כי היכי דפסקי הני מיא
ליפסוק דמיה דפלניא בר פלניתא. (גיטין סט ע"א)

Before us is a series of prescriptions for treating the flow of blood from the nostrils.
In this textual unit, written in Babylonian Aramaic, there is plenty of magic, the prescriptions are complicated and some include quantities. Both "natural" medical practice and forms of magic can be identified in the text.[12]

---

11 The variant in MS Vatican 130 reads: ליקו תותיה נורא וניתי כוזא דמיא.

12 In the first three prescriptions, the medical teaching is based on an amulet, the fourth is through
    "natural" medical practice, the fifth delineates a magic ritual, and the sixth delineates treatment
    through sympathetic magic as a remedy for the blood dripping from the nostrils. In Geller's
    discussion of the medical list from b. Gittin 68b–69a, he refers to some of these prescriptions

Focusing on genre A

Almost all appearances of the first genre, which is concise, written mainly in Hebrew, and lacks magic, in the literature of the sages is to be found in the Talmuds, in which there are some 180 directives that fit these criteria.[13] Of these, approximately 90 percent are found in the Babylonian Talmud, and approximately 10 percent in the Jerusalem Talmud. The analysis of the contents of the directives provides the following findings:

1   Prevention-diagnosis-treatment

The directives of the first genre contain content relating to three important medical categories: prevention, diagnosis, and treatment. Below is an example of a medical teaching relating to prevention:

> But thus did Shmuel say: A drop of cold water in the morning, and bathing the hands and feet in hot water in the evening, is better than all the eye-salves in the world. (Bab. Talmud, Shabbat 108b)

> אלא הכי אמר שמואל: טובה טיפת צונן שחרית, ורחיצת ידים ורגלים בחמין ערבית, מכל
> קילורין שבעולם. (שבת קח ע"ב)

Kilor is a sticky paste condensed into a capsule, made of medical herbs, which was used mainly for intestinal diseases, as well as the treatment of eye diseases, by applying the paste to the eyes when dissolved in a variety of liquids.[14] Shmuel, the Babylonian sage known even to the sages of the Israel for his useful *kilor*s, explains in this statement that it is better to be mindful regarding hand and foot hygiene in order to prevent disease, than to treat it with *kilor*s after it appears.

The treatment category among the directives involves instructions that are meant to cure a disease or to ease symptoms. For example:

> Rami b. Abba stated: A mil's walk or a little sleep removes the effects of wine. (Bab. Talmud, Eruvin 64b)

> אמר רמי בר אבא: דרך מיל, ושינה כל שהוא מפיגין את היין. (עירובין סד ע"ב)

---

and connects them to Babylonian medicine. Markham J. Geller, "An Akkadian Vademecum in the Babylonian Talmud," in *From Athens to Jerusalem* (ed. Samuel Kottek and Manfred Horstmanshoff; Rotterdam: Erasmus, 2000), 19–21. In a separate discussion, Geller describes the existence of "natural" medical practice alongside "magic medicine" in Babylonian medicine. Cf. Markham J. Geller, *Ancient Babylonian Medicine: Theory and Practice* (Chichester, UK: Wiley-Blackwell, 2010), 8–10. I will add that Jewish medicine is present in this text from Gittin.

13 Aviad Recht, *"The Regimens of Health of the Rabbinic Sages"* (MA thesis, Bar-Ilan University, 2012), 16–36 [In Hebrew]. The cataloging of Talmudic materials cannot reflect all the existing dimensions of the text. It is partial by its very nature and perhaps even inherently so. Nonetheless, such cataloging creates real contributions. This is also true with respect to the MA thesis on which this article is based. Although my decision-making process and method can be challenged on specific points, the overall findings remain firm, as they are based on large-scale findings.

14 For further details see Ravid Krener, *"Materia Medica of the Land of Israel in the Roman Period"* (Ph.D. diss., Bar-Ilan University, 2007), 260–261. [In Hebrew]

In order to ease symptoms of drunkenness, Rami Bar-Aba recommends a short walk or a quick nap. This directive does not include a medical imperative to go for a walk or to take a nap in order to prevent disease. It is a medical response to a given sickness (drunkenness). Another example:

> Rabbi said: Vinegar restores the soul. (Bab. Talmud, Yoma 81b).

דתניא, רבי אומר: חומץ משיב את הנפש. (יומא פא ע"ב)

Rabbi does not recommend that one should drink vinegar frequently Rather, he teaches that vinegar restores the soul, namely, that when exhausted, vinegar is useful. These two medical teachings can be classified within the treatment category. Directives that describe a medical condition but do not provide information regarding actual actions related to treatment or prevention fall in the category of diagnosis:[15]

> R. Hiyya taught: As the leaven is wholesome for the dough, so is blood wholesome for a woman. (b. Ketubbot 10b)

תני רבי חייא: כשם שהשאור יפה לעיסה, כך דמים יפים לאשה. (כתובות י ע"ב)

Rabbi Hiyya states that the flow of blood is good for women during menstruation. However, this directive does not contain any actual prescription on how to reach this desired state, or how to refrain from its reversal. An analysis of the teachings of the first genre demonstrates that within the fields of classical medicine (prevention, treatment, and diagnosis) the majority of directives deal with prevention.[16] The breakdown is: prevention (approximately 66 percent), treatment (approximately 18 percent), and diagnosis (approximately 16 percent).

2   The practicalities: using materials from the natural world and physical activities

The medical teachings of the first genre can be divided into two kinds: those that prescribe the use of products from the natural world (plants and animals), and prescriptions for proper physical activities.[17] In response to Rav's halakhic ruling, "one who eats dates should not teach," the Stam raises a question (metivi) from a textual unit that provides a medical teaching:

> An objection was raised. Dates are wholesome morning and evening, in the afternoon they are bad, at noon they are incomparable. And they remove three things: evil thought, stress of the bowels, and abdominal troubles. (b. Ketubbot 10b)

---

15 It would have been preferable to provide a positive characterization of the rabbis' method of diagnosis, as classical medical books (such as that of Asaf the Physician) did. However, to date I have not found in this genre a methodical theory of diagnosis upon which the rabbis' advice is based.

16 For the method I use to classify the directives, see Recht, *"Regimens,"* 38–39, and the references to the detailed appendix that classifies the directives.

17 Directives included under the diagnosis category do not appear in this section.

תמרים: שחרית וערבית—יפות, במנחה—רעות, בצהרים—אין כמותן; ומבטלות שלשה דברים:
מחשבה רעה, וחולי מעים, ותחתוניות. (כתובות י ע״ב)

In this medical teaching we see a recommendation for the use of a product from the plant kingdom—dates.[18] In contrast, the medical teachings of Raba's brothers deal with maintaining health through proper physical activity:

> His brothers sent [the following message] to Rabbah: ...If you are not coming up, however, beware [we advise you] of three things. Do not sit too long, for [long] sitting aggravates one's abdominal troubles; do not stand for a long time, because [long] standing is injurious to the heart; and do not walk too much, because [excessive] walking is harmful to the eyes. Rather [spend] one third [of your time] in sitting, one third in standing and one third in walking. Standing is better than sitting when one has nothing to lean against. (b. Ketubbot 111a)

שלחו ליה אחוהי לרבה...ואם אין אתה עולה, הזהר בשלשה דברים: אל תרבה בישיבה—
שישיבה קשה לתחתוניות, ואל תרבה בעמידה—שעמידה קשה ללב, ואל תרבה בהליכה—
שהליכה קשה לעינים, אלא שליש בישיבה, שליש בעמידה, שליש בהילוך, כל ישיבה שאין
עמה סמיכה—עמידה נוחה הימנה. (כתובות קיא ע״א)

Sitting, standing, and walking are routine, daily activities. Raba's brothers warn him that each should be done in the right proportion, in order to avoid a variety of diseases and illness. Additional routine activities appear in the medical teachings, such as intercourse, sleep, using the bathroom, and more. Examination of these materials reveals that approximately 62 percent of the directives deal with the use of products from the natural world, and approximately 38 percent relate to physical activities.[19]

3 Products from the natural world: eating versus external application

Animal and plant products can be used for medicine whether by ingestion or by external application—as ointments or poultices, through smelling the scent directly or inhaling vapor, and more, all of which were common in ancient medicine.

In the following directive, two prescriptions are provided together, one for eating and one for rubbing:

> R. Huna said: If one finds a garden-rocket he should eat it, if he can, and if not he should pass it over his eyes. (b. Yoma 18b)

אמר רב הונא: המוצא גרגיר אם יכול לאכלו—אוכלו, ואם לאו—מעבירו על גבי עיניו.
(יומא יח ע״ב)

---

18 This *sugya* teaches us about the authority of medical teachings from the perspective of the sages themselves. The editor of the *sugya* challenges Rav with a medical statement. This demonstrates that the editor views the medical statement as valid and authoritative as much as the halakhic statement (and using the word *metivi* before the statement within the *sugya* strengthens this argument).

19 Recht, "Regimens," 40–41.

When we classify directives according to methods of use, this one, which presents two medical usages for garden-rocket (eating and applying to the eyes), appears in both categories. When we examined the methods used with natural products in all the medical teachings of the first genre, the results were unequivocal. In 94.5 percent of the cases, instructions were to eat the substance, and the rest recommended other methods (rubbing and smelling only).[20]

4   No directives for using drugs

In the Talmuds we find mention of numerous drugs such as *samteri*, *anigron*, theriac, *kahal*, and more—yet medication is absent from the directives of the first genre. All references to organic substances mention foodstuffs, such as garlic, onion, radish, cabbage, turnip, wheat, date, fig, walnut, citron, and olive. Furthermore, even when referring to these foods, there are almost no pharmaceutical descriptions, and no preparation of medical compounds. The instructions for the use of these products are to eat them.

To briefly summarize the above:

1   A textual phenomenon was presented of medical teachings appearing mainly in the Babylonian Talmud that are meant to transmit medical information, as a goal in and of itself.
2   I focused on one genre of medical teachings that is characterized by short and concise statements, written similarly to baraitot, mishnayot, and memrot. The language in this genre is mainly Hebrew and the style is simple. Directives in the genre have almost no magical content.
3   The medical teachings in this genre promote mainly preventative medicine, based on nutrition and physical activity, without mentioning drugs.

I would like to argue that medical teachings of the first genre are in fact a known Greek medical genre, namely that of the "health regimen."[21]

---

20 Recht, "Regimens," 40–41.
21 The genre is known by a number of terms, beginning with Περί Διαίτης in the Hippocratic corpus, which Jones (*Hippocrates*, 224–225) translated as "regimen." Galen's book Γαληνόυ Ὑγεινῶν (*Galenos hygeinon*) was translated to Latin as *De sanitate tuenda* (Claudii Galeni, *Opera omnia*, ed. D. Carlus Gottlob Kühn [Lipsiae, n.p., 1825], vol. 6), and to English as "Hygiene" (R. M. Green, ed., *A Translation of Galen's Hygiene* [Springfield: Thomas, 1951]). Maimonides's book is called in Arabic *Fī tadbīr al-ṣiḥḥa* and in Ibn Tibbon's translation to Hebrew, *Hanhagat haberi'ut* (Moshe Ben Maimon, *Regimen sanitatis*, ed. Suessmann Muntner [Jerusalem: Mossad Harav Kook, 1957]). Recently, in discussions of the topic the terms "lifestyle" and "diet and regimen" have been used. In light of all these names, and the changes in the meanings of terms over time, I have preferred to use the medieval term and called the genre "health regimen."

A Greek genre

The genre of "health regimen" was founded, or at least developed into a coherent and systematic field of knowledge, by Greek scholars from the fifth century BCE and onwards. This is a uniquely Greek field, compared with other systems of medicine in neighboring and Near Eastern regions.

The main emphasis in ancient medicine was on reaction to sickness. Preventative actions occur naturally, of course: intuitively one would eat foods that warms the body when cold (or use a blanket for cover, etc.). A more advanced method for preserving health existed in cultures that maintained religious codes, such as refraining from impurity and ostracizing individuals who suffer from lesions and secretions. These religious codes indicate that there was an awareness of hygiene and sanitation. Similarly, warnings meant to distance people from demons in fact distanced people from sources of sickness. Yet, the accumulation of knowledge and the development of religious legal systems did not create an organized field meant to preserve health. Such a development began in classical Greece, and was first assembled in the Hippocratic corpus. This field, called "health regimen," involves the transformation of instinctive reactions into a medical field based on theory, which deals with diagnosis and prognosis, written and catalogued with great detail. Its practice meant ensuring a careful daily regimen that is standardized and productive (maximalism), involves proper nutrition and physical activity, and is intended to preserve and protect the individual's natural well-being.

In the following pages, I will compare the rabbinic literature cited above to the following classic Greek medical writings: *Regimen in Health*,[22] *Regimen II*,[23] and *Reg-*

---

22 In Galen's days, this text was part of *On the Nature of Man* and it seems that it was written by Hippocrates himself or his student Polybus. It dealt with nutrition and exercise; its first part is intended for the general public, and the second for athletes. *Hippocrates*, W. H. S. Jones et. al., ed. and trans., LCL (London: Heinemann, 1967), vol. 4, pp. xxvi–xxix. [Volume 4, pages 44–59 (*Regimen in Health*);

23 *Hippocrates* 4, 298–365. Its author is unknown, and from Galen's days onwards there are differences of opinion on this. It is dated to approximately 400 BCE. It describes foods, exercises, and the treatment of illnesses through proper regimen. See Galen, *On the Properties of Foodstuffs* (ed. Owen Powell; Cambridge: Cambridge University Press, 2003), 36–37; John Wilkins, "The Social and Intellectual Context of *Regimen II*," in *Hippocrates in Context* (ed. Philip J. van der Eijk; Leiden: Brill, 2005), 121–122, 126.

24 The editor of *Regimen I* writes that it is unclear who the author is, and to which school of thought he belongs. It seems that this is a later eclectic text, which a Hellenistic editor added as an introduction to *Regimen II* and *Regimen III*. It is a theoretical text, not necessarily related to the field of health regimen, and therefore not relevant to the discussion.

25 *Hippocrates* 4, 366–419. Written around 400 BCE. Like the previous text, the author of this text is also unknown, and it is not clear whether they were both written by the same author. The main topics discussed are treatment of illnesses caused by excess eating or exercise through proper regimen (*Hippocrates*, 4, xlvi).

26 *Galen*, D. Carlus Gottlob Kühn ed., *Opera Omnia*, Leipzig: n.p., 1825, is the full edition of Galen's compositions. An English translation was published by Green, R. M., ed. and trans. *A Translation of Galen's Hygiene*, Springfield: Thomas, 1951. This text deals with various physical exercises that one should practice from birth to old age. Typically of Galen, the discussion is full of polemics and disagreements with doctors and philosophers of the day, and with his pre-

imen III[24] from the Hippocratic corpus,[25] and from the writings of Galen: *On Hygiene*,[26] and *On the Properties of Foodstuffs*.[27]

The field of health regimen in Greek medicine has several distinct features:

1   The main concern: preserving health

The author of *Regimen III* declares that he has found the optimal medical method for preserving human health. Galen also claims that one who acts in accordance with his directives will never be ill.[28] The pretentiousness of their declarations stems from dogmatic theories that inevitably lead to absolute conclusions. *Regimen III* is based on a scheme of qualities that make up and influence the body (mainly dry, moist, cold, hot). In Galen's texts the schematic approach formed the theory of the four humors (*humoralism*),[29] which was further developed to correspond with the four elements of the earth and the four seasons, so that all of nature acts in accordance with a structured system that is fixed and predictable.

The theory of the four humors claims that health is a balance between traits and body humors, and between human beings and their natural surroundings. At the core of this approach is the claim that the state of health is an inherent condition that the individual must preserve. In order to maintain good health, human beings must act in accordance with their gender and age, and adapt and prepare for internal and environmental changes that disturb healthy balances. Balance is maintained by allopathy, namely if the balance is disturbed by change, one must correct it by adopting

---

decessors. See G. E. R. Lloyd, "Galen and His Contemporaries," in *The Cambridge Companion to Galen* (ed. R. J. Hankinson; Cambridge: Cambridge University Press, 2008), 34–48. In the discussion, he shows full loyalty to Hippocrates.

27 Powell, Owen, ed., *Galen—On the Properties of Foodstuffs* (Cambridge: Cambridge University Press, 2003). This book describes the attributes and uses of animal and plant foods, and how to identify them. The uses of plant and animal substances mentioned are only as food (and not as drugs, to which Galen devoted another work, *On Medical Substances*). The declared purpose of the book is to collect, analyze, and categorize all the foodstuffs available in the Roman Empire, and creation create of a kind of encyclopedia for anyone wishing to eat the foods appropriate to his own health regimen. Apparently, it was written late in Galen's life (see *On the Properties of Foodstuffs*, 13–14); the books reference one another. In *On Hygiene* Galen refers to his book *On the Properties of Foodstuffs* on pp. 241, 255. In *On the Properties of Foodstuffs*, Galen refers readers to *On Hygiene*, p. 150. They may have been written at the same time or updated in later versions. In any event, if we accept the claims of Wilkins and Powell regarding the dating of *On the Properties of Foodstuffs*, we should also apply them to *On Hygiene*.

28 *Regimen III*, 367; Galen, *On Hygiene*, 38 and more.

29 In *Regimen I* the author declares that the world is composed of water and fire and four characteristics—cold and hot, moist and dry—respectively. In *Regimen II* and *Regimen III* the authors do not provide theoretical background. They do use these traits together with an allopathic approach in the attempt to create a balance. Yet it seems that they do not accept the notion that water and fire are the fundamental elements of the world. In any case, *Regimen II* and *Regimen III* do not include a structured approach to the four humors as it appears in Galen. For a detailed chronological description of the four humors theory and its development, from Hippocratic medicine until the Renaissance, see Vivian Nutton, "Humoralism," in *Companion Encyclopaedia of the History of Medicine*, vol. 1 (ed. William F. Bynum and Roy Porter; London: Routledge, 1993), 281–291.

the opposite inclination (through nutritional changes and physical activities). Maintaining harmony within a person and between a person and his/her surroundings preserves health and obviates the need for treating illness. An illness is simply the result of imbalance. Preventing illness is made possible by adaptation to internal and environmental changes, in advance and during changes—adaptations of the body, weather, geographic location, and the stars.

2 Nutrition and physical exercise, no drugs

As the purpose of a health regimen is to preserve health through balance, the directives provided in the books deal with maintaining a healthy lifestyle as a daily routine. They therefore do not discuss diseases and responses to them. Furthermore, medicines are seen as an aggressive intervention in the body's natural balance, and are only acceptable in drastic deviations (i. e., in cases of serious illness). However, from a literary perspective, the field of "health regimen" is slightly more complex.

Of the books from the Hippocratic corpus mentioned above, *Regimen II* is the most comprehensive. The first part of the book includes a list of foods from animal and plant sources, along with a description of their characteristics (hot, cold, moist, and dry). It does not indicate which plant is beneficial for a particular illness. This text provides an inventory, as inclusive as possible, of foods in the Hellenic geographic region.[30] In part 2, the author details physical exercises and the treatment of illnesses by appropriate regimen.

Galen adopted this structure, but separated it into different works. In *On the Properties of Foodstuffs*, he provides a list of foods and their properties, based on the list in *Regimen II* but longer, more organized, and better edited than the first. Galen carefully categorized and identified plants based on information from the entire Roman Empire.[31] In *On Hygiene*, Galen describes the daily routine of the individual at length, with far more detail than the description in *Regimen II*. In this text, he details in fact the appropriate physical activities for every stage and every age, from birth to old age.

The medical approach of the health regimen obviates treatment using drugs, since according to its theory, if an individual eats the right foods and conducts physical activities in accordance with his bodily humors, health will be preserved without external intervention by medicines. Furthermore, even if a person is sick, up to a certain point they can still regain their balance through exercise and nutrition only. Both the authors of the Hippocratic corpus and Galen refer to the field of treatment with drugs

---

30 *Regimen II* is unique in its medical approach. In contrast to many ancient medical texts that state laconically which plant is useful for which particular illness, the description in *Regimen II* of plants and the illnesses relates to their specific traits and the theory of characteristics. In other words, the Greek approach developed the idea of mechanism. Whereas other Mediterranean medical systems made do with established facts, basing themselves on empirical findings that plant X was good for illness Y, the Greeks wished to decipher the mechanism and propose a theory that would include all individual cases. Thus, *Regimen II* presents us with a more advanced medicine that allows for combinations between the manifestations of the illness and the characteristics of the plants, while matching both to physical activities.

31 Wilkins, "Context," 123; idem, Foreword to *On the Properties of Foodstuffs*, 4–5.

as secondary, and as reactions to situations when the balances have been violated to an extent that requires external intervention with drugs. The ideals of health in their view are based on a proper health regimen.[32]

3 No magic

The unique field of health regimen could not have developed outside of Greek medicine, which views mankind and the world from conceptions that do not include divine or magical forces. The classical Greek approach to medicine does not see illnesses as caused by external forces in the form of demons or punishment by the gods for improper behavior; rather, controlling disease is internal to the human being involved, and is based on harmonic physical laws that dictate realities for humans and nature alike. Galen will sometimes mention Asclepios, the god of medicine, but it seems that these references do not serve a medical purpose, but rather ease the process of transmitting knowledge in a culturally aware manner to the masses, in order to preserve customs and heritage.[33]

Conclusion: a rabbinic health regimen

There is a strong and intrinsic correlation between the first genre of concise rabbinic medical teachings and the Greek health regimen. The three criteria that distinguish the Greek field of health regimen, namely preventative medicine, a lifestyle based on proper nutrition and physical activities (without medicine), and the lack of magic are the very criteria that distinguish the medical teachings of the first genre of rabbinic medical teachings. It is therefore appropriate to suggest the term: "rabbinic health regimen."[34]

Rabbinic health regimen: an adapted genre

Up to this point, we have detailed the characteristics attesting to an affinity between the Greek health regimen and the rabbinic health regimen. However, the field of health regimen in the two Talmuds differs from its Greek counterpart in one fundamental aspect: the intended audience.[35] Who is the audience of the health regimen in the Greek medical writings and how is this reflected in medical teachings?

---

32 See this explicitly in Galen's opening remarks in *On Hygiene* (p. 5); this is inferred from the author of *Regimen III*'s declarations (p. 381–383).

33 Galen, *On Hygiene*, 39, 41.

34 I would like the reader to return for a moment to the point above where we discussed the division of the direct medical material into two main genres (under the heading *Two Genres*). There I mainly dwelled on the stylistic difference between the two genres, while now, after having examined the content characteristic of the first genre, I would point out that the second genre is different from the first in this respect as well. The trend of medical thought in the second genre is therapy in response to disease; the main practice there is medication, with almost no use of diet and certainly not of exercise.

35 There are additional aspects in which the differences between the Greek health regimen and the rabbinic health regimen are apparent, such as the style of writing in the medical teachings, which is suited to the literary context in which they appear. Another difference is the lack of humoralism in the rabbinic health regimen—a theory that is fundamental in this field of Greek medicine. This dimension will be discussed separately in a future article.

The author of *Regimen in Health* divides his book into two parts: the first is intended for the ordinary person, and the second is aimed at the athlete (also including directives for those overweight people who wish to lose weight and vice versa). In contrast, the authors of *Regimen II* and *Regimen III*, as well as the relevant Galenic writings, attempt to describe the optimal and ideal health regimen.[36] This can be seen in the fact that the authors of *Regimen II* and Galen in his *On the Properties of Foodstuffs* try to describe foods from the most remote regions possible, doing so in great detail.[37]

A comprehensive discussion appears, for example, in Galen's descriptions of grapes: sweet ones provide warmth and are a laxative, hard ones strengthen digestion and are nutritious over time, sour ones strengthen digestion like the hard ones but also cool the body. Grapes intended for wine have balanced effects between warmth and cold and are close to the sweet in their laxative effects. With raisins, too, Galen describes variety. There are many sweet raisins and few sour ones, but most are a mixture of sweet and hard. Galen is not satisfied with simply describing the types by their properties; he also describes them according to their region of origin. He describes the raisins of Cilicia, which are yellowish and small, as well as the sweet and black ones of this region. He also describes the raisins of Pamphylia, which are black and large, and the black and sweet raisins of Libya. He mentions that there is a wide variety of raisins in Asia.

When describing physical exercise, the Greek texts refer mainly to training in the gymnasium such as walking, running, wrestling in oil, wrestling in dust, arm exercises, breathing exercises, and more. Galen mentions that ten thousand strengthening exercises exist.

As mentioned, the author of *Regimen III* boasts that he has found the optimal path to good health. At the opening of the text, the author directs his message to the majority of men. This is what he advises the ordinary person to do during winter:

> Now first of all I shall write, for the great majority of men …
> Now in winter it is beneficial to counteract the cold and congealed season by living according to the following regimen. First, a man should have one meal that case let him take a light luncheon. The articles of diet to be used are such as are of a drying nature, of a warming character, assorted[38] and undiluted; wheaten bread is to be preferred to barley cake, and roasted to boiled meats; drink should be dark, slightly diluted wine, limited in quantity; vegetables should be reduced to a minimum, except such as are warming and dry, and so should barley water and barley gruel. Exercises should be many and of all kinds; running on the double track increased gradually; wrestling after being oiled,

---

36 Galen states explicitly that this is his aim. See, e.g., Galen, *On Hygiene*, 38–39; also *Regimen III*, 381–383. Our article provides only examples that testify to this, which have been chosen for comparison to the "rabbinic health regimen."

37 These are encyclopedic lists. The great increase in items and their inaccessible (to most of the population) sources, especially in Galen, is evidence that their aim was a maximalist and ideal description of the world's *materia medica*, thus application of their indications was possible mainly for the higher strata of the population. More on this below.

38 See Jones's note on his deliberation as to translating this: *Regimen III*, 369, n. 3.

begun with light exercises and gradually made long; sharp walks after exercises, short walk in the sun after dinner; many walks in the early morning, quiet to begin with, increasing until they are violent, and then gently finishing. It is beneficial to sleep on a hard bed and to take night walks and night runs, for all these things reduce and warm; unctions should be copious. When a bath is desired, let it be cold after exercise in the palaestra; after any other exercise, a hot bath is more beneficial. Sexual intercourse should be more frequent at this season, and for older men more than for the younger. Emetics are to be used three times a month by moist constitutions, twice a month by dry constitutions, after a meal of all sorts of food; after the emetic three days should pass in slowly increasing the food to the usual amount, and exercises should be lighter and fewer during this time. Emetics are beneficial after beef, pork, or any food causing excessive surfeit; also after excess of unaccustomed foods, cheesy, sweet or fat.[39]

It is apparent, and Farrington[40] has enlightened me in this respect, that the ordinary person cannot act in accordance with this regimen, since the layman must work and make a living. These sorts of regimens are suitable for men of the higher classes, who do not work for a living. Additionally, both in the Hippocratic writings (except for *Regimen in Health*) and in those of Galen, fatigue—a sickness caused by overeating or excessive physical activities—is the dominant disease.[41]

A description of a variety of foods and their properties, the description of a massive number of exercises, and carefully structured days—all serve the author's intention to present health regimens as a rich and fascinating field, meant only for people with free time and financial resources. For the vast majority of the population, this genre is simply irrelevant.[42]

In contrast, the rabbinic health regimen is completely different in this regard. The foods mentioned in the regimen are simple ones, such as garlic, chate melon, turnip, radish, olive, figs, dates, leek, wheat, beet, grape, onions, and beans, available to the housewife at home or at the local market. In the field of physical exercises, too, the texts are different. The directives of the rabbinic health regimen relate to the individual's existing routine, and only speak of proper conduct: how to eat, how to sleep, how to use the bathroom, how to have intercourse, and how to travel. There are no gymnastic activities in the rabbinic health regimen. Needless to say, numerous diseases and aches are mentioned, but fatigue is not one of them.

---

39 *Regimen III*, 369–73.

40 Benjamin Farrington, "The Hand in Healing: A Study in Greek Medicine from Hippocrates to Ramazzin," in Idem, *Head and Hand in Ancient Greece: Four Studies in the Social Relations of Thought* (London: Folcroft Library Editions, 1947), 2854.

41 *Regimen in Health*, 57; *Regimen II*, 359–365; Galen, *On Hygiene*, 143–184. This is the fourth of the six books of *On Hygiene*, in which Galen makes an exception to the rule of treatment through regimen, and prescribes drugs.

42 For positions similar to the one I presented (yet at odds with my position in terms of *On Regimen*'s audience), see Hynek Bartoš, *Philosophy and Dietetics in the Hippocratic* On Regimen—*A Delicate Balance of Health* (Leiden: Brill, 2015), 47–53.

It seems that the sages identified the potential of medical practices relating to a health regimen, and adopted the principles of preventative medicine, using nutrition and physical activities, and no magic. Yet practically, the wording of the medical teachings reflects a process of adaptation and adjustment. The sages changed the medical teachings into simple directives that take routine lives into consideration. In this way, they made them more suitable and relevant to their audience —the entire Jewish community, which worked for a living.

A Greek genre in the Babylonian Talmud

The appearance of the Greek genre of health regimen in the Babylonian Talmud raises questions. The intuitive expectation is for such a Greek genre to appear in the Jerusalem Talmud or other rabbinic materials from the land of Israel (to fit the classic dichotomy[43] in which materials from the land of Israel are influenced by Greco-Roman culture, whereas Babylonian writings have Babylonian influences).[44] Why then does the rabbinic health regimen, a genre with clear Greek influences, appear in the Babylonian Talmud, while it is almost nonexistent in the Jerusalem Talmud? And of course, the next question is, how did such Greek materials make their way into Babylon?

The answer to the first question has to do with the characters of the two Talmuds. The Jerusalem Talmud is more limited in the areas of its concern. It contains halakhah and aggadah but shows very little interest in adjacent fields of knowledge. The redactors of the Babylonian Talmud, in contrast, evince an anthological approach.

---

43 See Daniel Boyarin, "Hellenism in Jewish Babylonia," in *The Cambridge Companion to the Talmud and Rabbinic Literature* (ed. Charlotte Elisheva Fonrobert and Martin S. Jaffee; Cambridge: Cambridge University Press, 2007), 337–338. As for medical sources in the BT, Geller maintains this dichotomy consistently. He attributes Hellenistic motives in medical Babylonian sources as coming from *Eretz Israel*. Cf. Markham J. Geller, *Akkadian Healing Therapies in the Babylonian Talmud* (Berlin: Max Planck-Institut für Wissenschaftsgeschichte. 2004), 17–18. In another case he claims that it is difficult to assume the existence of bloodletting in Babylon because it is considered as a pure Hellenistic motive. Cf. Markham J. Geller "Bloodletting in Babylonia," in *Magic and Rationality in Ancient Near Eastern and Graeco-Roman Medicine* (ed. H.F.J. Horstmanshoff and M. Stol; Leiden: Brill, 2004), 305–324.

44 Trying to extract realistic aspects from the literature shows the following results: In terms of geography, it is impossible to reach unequivocal insights: of the 100 "health regimens" in which the name of a sage is mentioned, the majority are from the land of Israel (37, as opposed to 13 Babylonian sages). At the same time there are some 80 anonymous "health regimen" sayings, which cannot be categorized as either originating from the land of Israel or Babylonia, and their categorization might tip the balance in either direction. In contrast, the chronology is decisive: most of the "health regimen" sayings are attributed to rabbis from the fifth generation of Tannaim up to the third generation of Amoraim (i.e., from the second third of the second century CE up to the turn of the third and fourth centuries CE), with its peak in the first generation of Amoraim (the "transition period" in the first half of the third century). From the fourth generation of Amoraim onwards, "health regimen" sayings decline acutely and completely disappear (see Recht, "Regimens," 51–55). The fact that the phenomenon can be delineated most clearly in terms of chronology rather than geography, as well as the fact that this largely Greek genre appears in the Babylonian Talmud, undermines the automatic dichotomy of land of Israel/Hellenistic culture vs. Babylon/Babylonian culture, and demands a different look at the phenomenon: a diachronic one.

With regard to the genre of health regimen, this difference between the two Talmuds is seen in the fact that there are more sages from the land of Israel than ones from Babylon among those cited as having uttered such directives. In other words, the redactors of the Jerusalem Talmud were aware of these materials and still deliberately decided not to include them.[45]

As for the second question, I will briefly suggest here two possible routes by which Greek materials made their way to the Babylonian Talmud. One possible route is through the Jewish community internally—by knowledge transmitted among the sages, as part of the strong connection that existed between the population centers of Babylon and the land of Israel. These sorts of connections were a necessity in halakhic fields such as *kiddush haḥodesh* (sanctification of the month) and *'ibbur hashanim* (intercalation), that were crucial for preserving tradition, halakhic innovations, and rulings. Along with such relations, secular issues closely related to matters of holiness, such as medicine, were transmitted. The *naḥute*, messenger sages, transferred information from the sages of the land of Israel to the sages of Babylon and vice versa, including medical knowledge.[46]

Another possible route for the diffusion of knowledge of a Greek genre into Babylon is the Sassanid culture surrounding the Jewish community there. The roots of the Greek cultural presence in the Iranian region dates back to ties between Greece and

---

45 Recht, "Regimens," 51–55. A good example is as follows: "Ulla said, and some say [that] it was taught in a Baraitha: Ten cups [of wine] the scholars have instituted [to be drunk] in the house of the mourner: Three before the meal in order to open the small bowels, three during the meal in order to dissolve the food in the bowels, and four after the meal: one corresponding to 'who feed', one corresponding to the blessing of 'the land', one corresponding to 'who re-build Jerusalem', and one corresponding to 'who is good and does good'. They [then] added unto them [another] four [cups]: one in honor of the officers of the town, and one in honor of the leaders of the town, and one in honor of the Temple, and one in honor of Rabban Gamaliel. [When] they began to drink [too much] and to become intoxicated, they restored the matter to its original state" (b. Ketubbot 8b). The parallel version in the Jerusalem Talmud (y. Berakhot 3a) omits the first cups and their medical value and discusses only the cups of halakic significance: "It was taught: They drink ten cups [of wine] in a house of mourning–two before the meal, and five during the meal, and three after the meal. Regarding these three **after** the meal..." Tzvee Zahavy, trans., "Berakhot." Vol.1 of *The Talmud of the Land of Israel* (Chicago: University of Chicago Press, 1989), 116. There is a critical attitude speaking about a creative attribution by the BT as it was phrased by Stern and Bregman. Cf. Sacha Stern, "Attribution and authorship in the Babylonian Talmud," *Journal of Jewish Studies* 45,1 (1994): 28–51 and more references in note 1; Marc Bregman, "Pseudepigraphy in Rabbinic Literature," in *Pseudepigraphic Perspectives; the Apocrypha and Pseudepigrapha in Light of the Dead Sea Scrolls* (ed. Esther G. Chazon and Michael Stone; Leiden: Brill, 1999), 27–41. Still, even Stern maintains a general principle of authencity of Talmudic attributions (Stern, "Attribution," 32). In this case, I do not find it persuasive anyway. There is no clue for a faked attributions and there are positive evidences for assuming the authencity of these attributions.

46 An example: "R. Jannai sent [word] to Mar 'Ukba, Send us some of Mar Samuel's eye-salves. He sent back [word], I do indeed send [them] to you, lest you accuse me of meanness; but thus did Samuel say: A drop of cold water in the morning, and bathing the hands and feet in hot water in the evening, is better than all the eye-salves in the world" (b. Shabbat 108b). R. Yannai was a sage from the land of Israel (from the first generation of Amoraim), while Mar 'Ukba was a Babylonian sage (also of the first generation, and an exilarch); they exchange messages on a purely medical matter.

Persia at the time of the Achaemenid dynasty. The presence of Hellenistic culture in Iran increases and even became dominant after Alexander the Great conquered the region, and during the Parthian Empire. During the rule of the Sassanid dynasty (the period in which the Babylonian Talmud was composed), Zoroastrian religious fervor was a present reality. Yet alongside this trend, there was an exchange of new ideas, worldviews, and knowledge—both from Greece and Rome in the west, and from India in the east. This cosmopolitanism finds expression in the world of medicine as well. Medical writings from the era and region have not been found, but an active medical scene that was part of the pro-universalistic trend among Sassanid rulers can be identified from circumstantial, historical,[47] and linguistic[48] perspectives. Those responsible for maintaining Greek medical culture in the Sassanid Empire were Eastern Christian monks, and this connection between the monastic traditions and the Babylonian Talmud has been recently offered by Michal Bar Asher Siegal.[49] This may be an additional explanation for the appearance of health regimen in the Babylonian Talmud.[50]

To sum up, we have seen that the totality of medical content in the Talmud includes the texts of medical teachings, intended to transmit medical knowledge. One genre of these directives has been isolated and named "rabbinic health regimen," a genre that bears a close affinity to the field of health regimen in Greek medical literature. I suggested that the sages adapted the genre in order to make the contents suitable for their audience. Finally, I proposed two possible paths by which Greek content may have reached the Babylonian Talmud.

This field has not received its due share of attention in the research on ancient medicine, and may have been neglected due to its lack of glamour compared to the trends and achievement of modern medicine, which to some extent dictate the interests of scholars of ancient medicine, as well. Yet, the Greeks themselves—and possibly the sages, too—considered a healthy lifestyle the pinnacle of medicine.

---

47 Such as the victory of Shāpūr I (r. 241–272) over Aurelian; his marriage to her daughter and her arrival in Iran accompanied by Hippocratic physicians; the establishment of the hospital at Gondishāpūr by Shāpūr II (r. 309–379); and the immigration of Nestorian scholars from Edessa and Athens into the Sassanian Empire during the reign of Khusraw I (r. 531–579). See Cyril Elgood, *A Medical History of Persia* (Cambridge: Cambridge University Press, 1951), 34–57; Richard Frye, *The Golden Age of Persia: The Arabs in the East* (New York: Barnes and Noble, 1975), 22.

48 In Arab medical writings with Greek and Indian contents, remnants of Syriac and Pahlavi are to be found, demonstrating the route that this knowledge took: from Greek or Sanskrit via Syriac and Pahlavi to Arabic. It seems that this transmission took place in the medical centers of the Sassanid Empire (see for example Gül Russell, "Greece x. Greek Medicine in Persia," *Encyclopædia Iranica*, XI/4, pp. 342–357, (available online at http://www.iranicaonline.org/articles/greece-x); Frye, *Golden Age of Persia*).

49 Michal Bar-Asher Siegal, *Early Christian Monastic Literature and the Babylonian Talmud* (New York: Cambridge University Press, 2013).

50 This joins to a broader view of recent Talmudic research who finds Hellenistic motives in the Babylonian Talmud, e.g. Daniel Boyarin, *Socrates and the Fat Rabbis*, (Chicago; London: The University of Chicago Press, 2009); Richard Lee Kalmin, *Jewish Babylonia between Persia and Roman Palestine*, (New York: Oxford University Press, 2006).

Bibliography

Sources

Ben Maimon, Moshe. *Regimen sanitatis–Hanhagat haberi'ut.* Edited by Suessmann Muntner. Jerusalem: Mossad Harav Kook, 1957.

Dioscorides, Pedanius. *De materia medica.* Translated by Lily Y. Beck. Hildesheim: Olms-Weidmann, 2005.

Dioscorides, Pedanius. *De materia medica.* Translated and edited by T. A. Osbaldeston and R. P. A. Wood. Johannesburg: IBIDIS, 2000.

Epstein, Isidore, ed. and trans. *The Babylonian Talmud.* 18 vols. London: Soncino, 1961.

Galen, Claudius. *Opera Omnia,* 20 volumes. Edited by Carolus Gottlob Kühn. Leipzig: Car. Cnoblochius, 1822.

Green, R. M., ed. and trans. *A Translation of Galen's Hygiene.* Springfield: Thomas, 1951.

Hippocrates, Works. English & Greek. 11 volumes. Edited and translated by W.H.S Jones. London: Heinemann/ New York: Putnam, 1923–1931; Cambridge: Harvard University Press, 1988–2018.

Pliny the Elder. *Natural History.* Translated by H. Rackham. Cambridge, MA: Harvard University Press, 1952.

Powell, Owen, ed. *Galen—On the Properties of Foodstuffs.* Cambridge: Cambridge University Press, 2003.

Zahavy, Tzvee, *Berakhot.* Vol. 1 of *The Talmud of the Land of Israel.* Translated by T. Zahavy. Chicago: University of Chicago Press, 1989.

Literature

Amar, Zohar. "Materia Medica from the Land of Israel in the Time of the Bible, the Mishnah and the Talmud according to Written Sources." In *Health and Sickness in Antiquity.* Edited by Anat Rimmon. Haifa: Hecht Museum, University of Haifa, 1996. Pages 50–57. [In Hebrew]

—. "What is *sheḥin* in the Language of the Sages?" *Assia* 19 (2005): 61–69. [In Hebrew]

Amar, Zohar, and Efraim Lev. "Watermelon, Chate Melon and Cucumber: New Light on Traditional and Innovative Field Crops of the Middle Age." *Journal Asiatique* 299,1 (2011): 193–204.

Bar-Asher Siegal, Michal. *Early Christian Monastic Literature and the Babylonian Talmud.* New York: Cambridge University Press, 2013.

Bartoš, Hynek. *Philosophy and Dietetics in the Hippocratic* On Regimen—*A Delicate Balance of Health.* Leiden: Brill, 2015.

Ben-Yehuda, Eliezer. *A Complete Dictionary of Ancient and Modern Hebrew.* Jerusalem: 1948–1959.

Boyarin, Daniel. "Hellenism in Jewish Babylonia." In *The Cambridge Companion to the Talmud and Rabbinic Literature.* Edited by Charlotte E. Fonrobert, Martin S. Jaffee. Cambridge: Cambridge University Press 2007. Pages 336–363.

—. *Socrates and the Fat Rabbis.* Chicago: The University of Chicago Press, 2009.

Bregman, Marc. "Pseudepigraphy in Rabbinic Literature." In *Pseudepigraphic Perspectives; the Apocrypha and Pseudepigrapha in Light of the Dead Sea Scrolls.* Edited by Esther G. Chazon and Michael Stone. Leiden: Brill, 1999. Pages 27–41.

Elgood, Cyril. *A Medical History of Persia.* Cambridge: Cambridge University Press, 1951.

Farrington, Benjamin. "The Hand in Healing: A Study in Greek Medicine from Hippocrates to Ramazzini." In *Head and Hand in Ancient Greece: Four Studies in the Social Relations of Thought*. London: Folcroft Library Editions, 1947. Pages 28–54.

Frye, Richard. *The Golden Age of Persia: The Arabs in the East*. New York: Barnes and Noble, 1975.

Geller, Markham J. "Akkadian Healing Therapies in the Babylonian Talmud." Preprint Series 259. Berlin: Max Planck-Institut für Wissenschaftsgeschichte, 2004.

—. "Bloodletting in Babylonia." In *Magic and Rationality in Ancient Near Eastern and Grae-co-Roman Medicine*. Edited by H.F.J. Horstmanshoff and M. Stol. Leiden-Boston: Brill 2004. Pages 305–324.

—. "An Akkadian vademecum in the Babylonian Talmud." In *From Athens to Jerusalem*. Edited by Samuel Kottek and Manfred Horstmanshoff. Rotterdam: Erasmus, 2000. Pages 13–32.

—. *Ancient Babylonian Medicine: Theory and Practice*. Chichester, UK: Wiley-Blackwell, 2010.

Harari, Yuval. *Early Jewish Magic: Research, Method, Sources*. Jerusalem: Bialik Institute and Ben-Zvi Institute, 2010. [In Hebrew]

Kalmin, Richard L. *Jewish Babylonia between Persia and Roman Palestine*. New York: Oxford University Press, 2006.

Kerner, Ravid. *"Materia Medica of the Land of Israel in the Roman Period."* Ph.D. diss., Bar-Ilan University, 2007. [In Hebrew]

Lloyd, G. E. R. "Galen and His Contemporaries." In *The Cambridge Companion to Galen*. Edited by R. J. Hankinson. Cambridge: Cambridge University Press, 2008. Pages 34–48.

Nutton, Vivian. "Humoralism." In *Companion Encyclopedia of the History of Medicine*. Volume 1. Edited by William F. Bynum and Roy Porter. London: Routledge, 1993. Pages 281–291.

Preuss, Julius. *Biblical and Talmudic Medicine*. Translated and edited by Fred Rosner. Northvale, NJ: J. Aronson, 1994.

Recht, Aviad. *"The Regimens of Health of the Rabbinic Sages."* MA thesis, Bar-Ilan University, Ramat Gan, 2012. [In Hebrew]

Russel, Gul. "Greek Medicine in Persia." In *Encyclopedia Iranica Online*, 2012. February 16th, 2016, Online: http://www.iranicaonline.org/

Shaked, Shaul. "'Peace Be upon You, Exalted Angels': On Hekhalot, Liturgy and Incantation Bowls." *Jewish Studies Quarterly* 2 (1995): 197–219.

Steinberg, Avraham. *Chapters in the Pathology of the Talmud*. Jerusalem: Hamakhon Leheqer Harefu'ah 'al pi Hatorah [= Dr. Falk Schlesinger Institute for Medical-Halachic Research], 1975.

Stern, Sacha. "Attribution and authorship in the Babylonian Talmud." *Journal of Jewish Studies* 45,1 (1994): 28–51.

Sussmann, Yaakov. "The Oral Torah Literally Speaking: The Power of Every Jot and Tittle." In *Mehqere Talmud: Talmudic Studies*, vol. 3, a. Edited by Yaakov Sussmann and David Rosenthal. Jerusalem: Magnes, 2005. Pages 209–384.

Wilkins, John. "Foreword." In *Galen—On the Properties of Foodstuffs*. Edited by O. Powell. Cambridge: Cambridge University Press, 2003. Pages ix–xxi.

—. "The Social and Intellectual Context of Regimen II." In *Hippocrates in Context*. Edited by Philip J. van der Eijk. Leiden: Brill, 2005. Pages 121–133.

Part 3:
Historicity, Authority and Legitimacy
of Medical Knowledge:
Tradition, Transfer and Cultural Negotiations

The Physician in Bible and Talmud—
Between the Lord and the Ailing

Samuel Kottek

My first, rather provocative, question will be: Is there, in fact, a Jewish medicine? The answer is indeed a question of definition. Historiography can individualize Egyptian, Mesopotamian, Greco-Roman, and Arabic medicine(s), but no Jewish medicine can be documented; no Hebrew or Aramaic medical works from the biblical and/or Talmudic period(s) have reached us. There was, in ancient times, apparently no specific Jewish way of medical practice. There were of course Jewish healers, even physicians, who were mentioned in the Bible, and a number of them were named in the Talmud. The duty to save and even to try to save endangered human life is a foremost commandment (Heb. *piquaḥ nefesh*).[1]

In other words, there is a far-reaching topic called "Jews and medicine" and another one called "Jewish medical ethics," that includes "medicine and halakhah." Moreover, more than a century ago, Julius Preuss published (in German) a book entitled *Biblical and Talmudic Medicine* (1911),[2] which remains informative to this day, although deserving revision. Being this as it may, if "Jewish medicine" is considered to mean "medicine among the Jews," then I guess that the title is acceptable. We shall now consider the ways in which physicians were regarded in Bible and Talmud.[3]

---

1 On *piquaḥ nefesh*, see Lev 18:5: "You will keep my statutes and my judgments, which a man will do, and will live in them, I am the Lord." Our Biblical quotes are taken from *The Holy Scriptures*, English text revised and edited by Harold Fisch (Jerusalem: Koren Publishers, 1986), with some slight modifications by S.K. The topic is discussed at length in the Babylonian Talmud, Yoma 85a–b. *Babylonian Talmud* [Aramaic-Hebrew] (Jerusalem: El Hameqorot, 1948–1952); *The Babylonian Talmud*, ed. I. Epstein [Hebrew-English ed.] (London: Soncino Press, 1965–1990).

2 Julius Preuss, *Biblisch-talmudische Medizin* (Berlin: S. Karger, 1911). The work of Preuss was praised by the German medical historian Karl Sudhoff. It was translated by Fred Rosner and published in 1978: Julius Preuss, *Biblical and Talmudic Medicine* (trans. and ed. Fred Rosner; New York: Sanhedrin Press, 1978).

3 Physicians represent medical knowledge as well as medical practice. They are therefore at the core of the problem that we wish to scrutinize: Were Jewish physicians different from other contemporary physicians?

DOI: 10.13173/9783447108263.179

Physicians in the Bible

At first view, in Scripture there is only one Physician—the Lord. We read (Exod 15:26): *"... I am the Lord, your healer."*[4] And another passage states: *"I will take sickness away from the midst of you"* (Exod 23:25).[5] It seems thus that health and disease are within the Lord's exclusive will and command. We read also (Deut 32:39): *"I kill and I make alive, I wound and I heal; neither is there any that can deliver out of my hand."*

Only once in the five books of Moses do we find physicians mentioned; these were *"the servants of Joseph, the physicians."* They were supposed to embalm the corpse of Jacob, who was to be buried in the land of Canaan (Gen 50:2). However, it is known that the embalmers in ancient Egypt were not physicians. It seems likely that Joseph indeed sent his private physician(s) to be present throughout the embalming process; they would see to it that the magical and cultic ceremonies were avoided. Who could sustain such a long and disgusting process but physicians? However, there is no reference here to healing.[6]

In the other biblical books, physicians and healing are mentioned repeatedly. Some prophets achieved miraculous healing. Elijah and Elisha each revived a seemingly dead child.[7] Without going into detail, in both cases the prophet first prayed to the Lord to allow the revival. The prophet Isaiah cured King Hezekiah, whose disease was deadly, but it is clearly stated that the healing was the Lord's decision (2 Kings 20:1–7).[8] Elisha "cured" the water of the spring in Jericho (Ibid. 2:21–22), just as Moses sweetened the bitter waters in Mara (Exod 15:25). In both cases, the Lord was the "healer" of the waters.

According to the early Christian writings, the Master and his apostles performed impressive, miraculous healings, which were aimed at asserting their authority, whereas in the Hebrew Bible these healing cases are no more than an epiphenomenon. In other words, the prophets are, per definition, the representatives of the Lord's word and/or of the Lord's will.

The priests (Heb. *kohanim*) have been sometimes considered medical practitioners, particularly in the context of "biblical leprosy" (Heb. *tsara'at*). Here again, we shall

---

4 Exodus 15:26 reads: *"If you hearken diligently to the voice of the Lord and will do what is right in his sight ... and will keep all his statutes, I will put none of these diseases upon you, which I have brought on Egypt."*

5 Exodus 23:25. The context is relevant. It says that if you obey the voice of the Lord, then He will bless your bread and your water and will take sickness away from you. "Bread" stands for food and "water" for beverage. Defective or excessive alimentation was (and still is) considered a foremost cause of diseases. Health is a blessing of the Lord.

6 Preuss thought that the Bible used the term *rof'im* for the embalmers, because the Hebrew language had no specific term for a practice that was not applied by the Hebrews (cf. Preuss, *Biblical and Talmudic Medicine*, 18).

7 For the prophet Elijah, see 1 Kings 17:17–24. For Elisha, see 2 Kings 4:18–37; this case is described in more detail than the first one.

8 Isaiah first announced that King Hezekiah would die. However, the king prayed and wept; the Lord not only heard the prayer and saw the tears, but He decided that Hezekiah would enjoy fifteen more years of life. Isaiah then forwarded a treatment for the king's disease and he recovered.

not go into detail. This "disease" is indeed described in depth, and the priest was the one who diagnosed, and would even isolate the "patient" for seven, or fourteen days, in unclear cases. He was qualified to decide that the "leprous" individual was cured and could return to society. But was all this medical practice? The answer is no, it was not. The priest had no role in the healing process, and the text does not even say that he prayed for the "patient's" recovery. The chapters on *tsara'at* are in fact a theological ritual within the central theme of purity/impurity in the Bible (Lev 13–14).[9]

We further read (2 Chron 16:12) that king Asa "was diseased in his feet ...yet in his disease he did not seek the Lord, but the physicians." This has been considered proof that the Bible has a negative approach to medicine, or, rather, to physicians.[10] However, King Asa was stigmatized for having not *also* sought the Lord, or for not having sought the Lord *before* seeking the physicians.[11]

Another king, Ahaziahu, who sustained a serious accident, sent his servants in order to ask *Baal-zevuv*, the god of Ekron,[12] whether he would recover or not (2 Kings 1:2). Here neither the Lord, nor physicians, but foreign deities are sought.[13]

In the Pentateuch, human healing is simply not relevant. It is made clear that the *ultimate* healer is the Lord, the Savior. Human intervention is not brought into discredit, but it must be regarded in its obvious relativity and problematic success. Its good fortune is submitted to the Lord's will. Such an approach is not specifically Jewish. Its bearing on later readers of the Bible is that a physician should endorse a sense of humility and repel what has been so often been accused of physicians: self-conceit.[14]

---

9 The topic "Purity/Impurity in the Bible" has been widely discussed. *Tsara'at* was not just leprosy (Hansen's disease); its symptoms were not specific to one disease, I therefore call it "biblical leprosy." It is described in Leviticus chapters 13 and 14. For detailed information see Jozeph Michman, S. David Sperling and Louis Isaac Rabinowitz, *"Leprosy," in Encyclopedia Judaica. Jewish Virtual Library*, n.p. [cited 10 April 2014]. *Online:* http://www.jewishvirtuallibrary.org/jsource/judaica/ejud_0002_0012_0_12153.html.

10 See, for instance, Klaus Seybold and Ulrich B. Mueller, *Sickness and Healing* (trans. D. W. Stott, Biblical Encounters; Nashville: Abingdon, 1978), 94–96.

11 King Asa's disease was, according to the Talmud, gout. Known as *podagra* in most ancient languages, it has long been considered to be a disease affecting mainly "high society." Cf. K. C. Gritzalis, M. Karamanou and G. Androutsos, "Gout in the writings of eminent ancient Greek and Byzantine physicians." *Acta medico-historica Adriatica* 9,1 (2011): 83–88; F. Rosner, "Gout in the Bible and the Talmud," *Annals of Internal Medicine* 86,6 (1977): 833.

12 *Baal-zevuv*, the deity of Ekron, means etymologically the "Master of the Fly." Some scholars opine that this could imply a medical expertise, if it was able to deter or destroy the flies, which feast on excrement. Flies could be messengers of death: see Eccl 10:1, also Isa 7:18–19. Others thought that it could be a corruption of *Baal zevul*, "the Lord of the [high] Abode."

13 The king's messengers to Baal-zevuv were intercepted by the prophet Elijah, who told them that the king would soon die, which indeed was the case.

14 See below, in the section on physicians and surgeons in the Talmud.

Physicians as seen in the Second Temple period

Shimon Yeshu'a ben Sira lived in the third century BCE. Chapter 38 of his ethical treatise sets forth the role of the physician in society. Its first sentence, "Honor the physician before you are in need of him," has often been mistranslated. The physician has been imparted his knowledge from the Lord, and the plants that heal are the Lord's creation. Both sick people and physicians will pray to the Lord to allow the cure to succeed. Therefore, "one who places himself superior to the physician is a sinner."[15] Although the book of Ben Sira was not accepted among the canonic works of the Hebrew Bible, it was cited a number of times in the Talmud.[16] This text shows us that medicine was then readily accepted in Hebrew society, on condition that prayers be addressed to the Lord from both sides involved.

Philo of Alexandria lived in the first century CE in the Hellenistic Egyptian diaspora. In his allegorical interpretation of Scripture, he often uses metaphoric medical descriptions. Philo paraphrases the biblical sentence *"And the Lord will take away from thee all sickness"* (Deut 7:15 and Exod 23:25) as follows:

> The Lord bestows health, in the simplest sense, preceded by no illness [...], by himself only; but health that comes by way of escape from illness he bestows both through medical science and through the physician's skill, letting both knowledge and practitioner enjoy the credit of healing, though it is He himself that heals alike by these means and [also] without them.[17] (Philo, *Allegorical Interpretation* 3.178)

Philo thus differentiates between health—seen as the natural state of a human being—and health, as "an escape from illness," although prevention of disease can also be considered an "escape" from becoming sick. We are therefore not very far from Ben Sira's approach. The knowledge (i.e., medicine) and practice are both the means by which the Lord allows healing to succeed.

Both the book of *Enoch* and the book of *Jubilees*, which date to the Second Temple period, describe how medical knowledge was transmitted to Noah, or to women, by the "Fallen Angels."[18] Neither Noah, nor the women (who were "chosen" by these angels) were called "physicians." The important lesson of these tales is that medical

---

15 Cf. Moshe Tsvi Segal, *Sefer Ben-Sira hashalem* (Jerusalem: Bialik Institute, 1972), 242–43 [in Hebrew]. In English, see Patrick W. Skehan and A. A. Di Lella, *The Wisdom of Ben Sira* (New York: Doubleday, 1987).

16 The conclusion of Ben Sira's chapter on physicians is worth a quote: "Whoever behaves haughtily before a physician commits a sin before the Creator." In early Jewish medical ethics, both physicians and patients were asked to show humility before the Lord's command over disease. On Talmudic quotes of Ben Sira, see Benjamin G. Wright, "B. Sanhedrin 110b and rabbinic knowledge of Ben Sira," in *Treasures of Wisdom—studies in Ben Sira and the book of Wisdom* (ed. N. Calduch-Benages and J. Vermeleyen; Leuven: University Press, 1999), 41–50.

17 See in the *Works of Philo*, translated by F. H. Colson, G. H. Whitaker and Ralph Marcus, 12 vols., LCL (Cambridge, MA: Harvard University Press, 1929–68).

18 See my paper, Samuel Kottek, "Magic and Healing in Hellenistic Jewish Writings," *Frankfurter Judaistische Beiträge* 27 (2000): 1–16.

knowledge was seen as stemming from a divine origin, the angels being the transmitters. It is not quite clear whether the transmission was allowed by the Lord or not. It is interesting to note that this tale, also known as *midrash Noah*, appears as an introduction to the first known medical treatise in Hebrew, *Sefer Asaf Harofe*', which dates to the seventh or eighth century.[19]

Physicians in the Talmud

The Talmud, a wide-ranging development of the Oral Law, was composed over some seven centuries, if we include the Mishnah, from the second century BCE until the early sixth century CE. The Talmudists included in their discussions a large amount of data on their social environment, including on medicine and physicians. Practitioners were often praised, but sometimes there were problems between them and the rabbis. Let us describe one particular case.

Benjamin and the rabbis

Benjamin (alias *Minyomi*) was a physician who lived in the third century CE, at the time of Rava. He once revealed to Rava the formula of a specific ointment that was efficient on all kinds of wounds. Rava disclosed the formula to the public. Benjamin and his sons were quite distressed to have lost their secret panacea (b. Shabbat 133b). Consequently, they became opposed to the sages.[20] We learn from this story that the rabbinic authority decided that such a widely efficient drug should not remain private property, but should be disclosed to the public. On the other hand, it is well known that many physicians and/or pharmacists had some specific formulas, which could yield an enjoyable income, even until modern times.

Physicians in their environment

We shall now consider a case that may perhaps be considered paradigmatic. A woman suffered a discharge from her private parts, described as red peelings. The question was not about the diagnosis of the discharge, but whether the woman was prohibited to her husband, as is the case when there is an issue of blood from the matrix. The caretakers went to ask Abba[21] (called a "surgeon" several times in the Talmud),

---

19 *Sefer Asaf Harofe*': The introduction to the book of Assaf was first printed separately under the title Sefer Noaḥ by Adolf Jellinek in his six-volumes work, Adolf Jellinek, *Bet hamidrash: Sammlung kleiner Midraschim und vermischter Abhandlungen aus der älteren jüdischen Literatur* (6 vols.; Leipzig: F. Nies, 1853–1877), vol. 3, p. 156. Asaf is cited as one of the main early medical authorities, between Hippocrates and Dioscorides, followed by Galen. See my brief excursus on Asaf in Samuel Kottek, "Sefer Assaph ha-Rofe (Jewish medical text)," in *The Encyclopedia of Ancient History. Wiley Online Library*, 2012, n.p. [cited 17 January 2014]. Online: https://doi.org/10.1002/9781444338386.wbeah11210. See also Ronit Yoeli-Tlalim's and Tamás Visi's contribution to this volume.

20 The children of Benjamin openly put the belief in rabbinical authorities in doubt, and were therefore considered 'epiqorsim (heretics, or sceptics). See b. Sanhedrin 99b.

21 Abba: He is known as Abba Ummna (Abba the "surgeon"). He was praised by the rabbis for his strict principles of modesty, decency, charity, and altruism. See b. Ta'anit 21b and below note 37, "Surgeons in the Talmud."

but he was unable to answer. He forwarded the question to the rabbis, and the latter forwarded it further to the physicians. They answered as follows: "This woman has a wound in her womb, from which these red peelings issue. Put them into water, if they dissolve therein, the woman is impure" (b. Niddah 22b). This test showed that the peelings were, or contained, blood from the womb. A second case is reported in the Talmud, with the same succession of referees.[22]

This shows us that the "surgeon" (actually a bloodletter) was closest to the families there and then; the next to be consulted were the rabbinic authorities, who might have previously tackled such a case. The physicians came last, but not least. The rabbis were obviously open and mindful of the physicians' opinions.

Mar Samuel (third century CE), who belonged to the first generation of Amoraim,[23] headed the Talmudic academy in Nehardea, Babylonia. He was also known as a trained astronomer and physician. In Julius Preuss's book on *Biblical and Talmudic Medicine* there are more than eighty references to Samuel, which cover a wide range of medical topics. We shall only discuss a few of them.[24]

Samuel was a scientist. He used to study the digestive tract with the following test: He asked the patient to swallow a hard egg much reduced in size through repeated boiling and gathered it at the other end of the bowels. We do not know how the results were interpreted. Such a "test" has not been documented so far anywhere else (b. Nedarim 50b).

Samuel once examined an aborted fetus and declared that it was forty-one days old, which was afterwards authenticated (b. Niddah 25b). This is important regarding abortion: We are told (b. Yevamot 69b) that the embryo is considered like water until the fortieth day of pregnancy.

Samuel's ethical standards were notable. We are told that he repeatedly examined his young female servant in order to gather precise information on the chronology of sexual development. He then gave her money "for the shame she sustained." Other rabbis retorted: "Why did you do this, she is your slave!" —"Sure, he answered, but she is here in order to work for me, not in order to be ashamed" (b. Niddah 47a). This is indeed medical ethics, going even further than the practice of the law.

Thodos (alias Theodorus) was a physician who once came "with a group of physicians" to examine a number of human bones in order to decide whether there was a problem of "impurity of the tent" (Heb. *tum'at 'ohel*).[25] He was apparently known as a specialist in human osteology (b. Nazir 52a). It is not clear whether the physicians

---

22 In this case, the woman had a discharge of something like red hairs. The verdict of the physicians was quite similar to the preceding case. On rabbis seeking advice from physicians and other medical experts, see the contribution by Tirzah Meacham to this volume.

23 Amoraim: the generations of rabbis who were the followers and exegetes of the early rabbinic sages, the *Tannaim*, who produced the Mishnah. The Amoraic rabbis lived from approximately 200 to 500 CE.

24 On Samuel, the physician, see Fred Rosner, *Medicine in the Bible and Talmud* (New York: Ktav, 1977), 156–170.

25 This impurity (Heb. *tum'at 'ohel*) means that if someone is under the same roof (or covering) as a corpse, he becomes impure. Cf. m. Ohalot 3:1. Thodos was able to acknowledge that these bones were remains of several corpses and that there was less than half the number of bones of

who came with him were colleagues who appreciated his anatomical knowledge, or students. Thodos might well have learned medicine in Alexandria, where anatomy and physiology were then taught more in depth than anywhere else.

Legal principles of medical practice

Liability of physicians

The statement that a physician who practiced with license from court would not be sanctioned in a case in which he caused some damage to his patient involuntarily appears in three different places in the Tosefta.[26] It seems that this rule was not included in the Mishnah because it only concerned a marginal part of society, physicians.

We read in the Tosefta, t. Gittin 4:6: "A certified physician [Heb. *rofe' 'umman*][27] who has practiced under court license and has caused damage, if involuntarily—he is free, if voluntarily—he will be condemned—for the ordinance of the world [Heb. *mipne tiqqun ha'olam*]."

The Tosefta in t. Bava Qamma 6:17 states again that causing involuntary damage does not entail liability, but there is an addition: "however his [the physician's] retribution is referred to Heaven (Heb. *masur lashamayim*)." The Lord will be able to judge whether there has been some degree of carelessness or inaccuracy in diagnosis or treatment, in which case the Lord will chastise him.

Moreover, t. Bava Qamma 9:11 reads: "If he has injured [or mutilated, Heb. *hibbel*] more than was opportune, he is liable." This is most probably addressed at surgeons, although it could also be applied to excessive medication. In case the physician has caused the death of his patient (again, a certified physician with a license from court), then he must retire to a city of refuge (t. Makkot 2:5).

This detailed legislation on physicians' liability is indeed impressive. A few interesting details must still be considered. First, here *rofe' 'umman* does not mean a physician-surgeon, but rather a certified physician, that is, an accomplished, well-trained practitioner. Second, *mipne tiqqun ha'olam* means that if this were not ruled so leniently, nobody would enter medical practice, and people are in need of physicians. Third, the "cities of refuge"[28] existed only as long as there was a temple in Jerusalem and a high priest. After the destruction, the rule could be that the physician who caused the death of his patient should remove his practice to another place, a common-sense solution.

The license allegedly given by the court to practice is quite surprising. In ancient times there was no medical licensing in other cultures. Even in the Middle Ages, it

---

one single individual. "Impurity of the tent" is only one aspect of the very complicated laws of purity/impurity.

26 The Tosefta (t.) is a collection of halakic and aggadic records from the time of the Mishnah, which were not included in the final editing of the Mishnah, at the beginning of the 3rd century CE. See *Tosephta*, ed. by M. S. Zuckermandel (Jerusalem: Wahrmann, 1970).

27 Here *'umman* is not the "surgeon" (or the bloodletter). It derives from the root *'emun*, meaning "reliable, trustworthy."

28 The cities of refuge were six towns where anyone who killed someone accidentally could flee and be protected from any revenge. He could not leave this shelter before the demise of the high priest. See Num 35:6–28.

was a rare and local occurrence. However, no details are given on how and by whom (judges? trained physicians?) such a license was awarded.[29]

Additionally, in several places cited above, the special case of embryotomy[30] is mentioned. If the practitioner who dismembered the fetus during childbirth in order to save the mother caused damage or even death to her, the same rules apply.

Such deontological rules are really impressive. There was thus indeed a Jewish way of practicing medicine, as documented in the Tosefta.

Wages of physicians

The Talmud does not speak directly of wages, however there is an enlightening proverb, which says "A physician who heals for nothing is worth nothing" (Heb. *'asya demagen bemagen, magen shave*).[31] The context is as follows: Someone has hurt another individual. He says: "I shall bring to you a physician who will treat you gratis." The other then answers with the said proverb, which means that he does not put his trust in such a physician who heals gratis.

Later rabbis felt that in principle a physician should heal without payment, for he performs a mitzvah, which can sometimes get close to *piquah nefesh* (saving life).[32] The rabbis, however, decided that physicians (like judges and teachers) can be compensated for their strain and for the time spent (Heb. *tirhah ubattalah*).[33]

Physicians' social status

Physicians were often praised and consulted by the sages in Talmudic times. We read that "they asked the physicians," or "they consulted the experts" (Heb. *sha'alu labeqiyim*). The latter were not necessarily physicians; there have always been experienced

---

29 It is not stated whether there were trained physicians who had to examine the candidate before the court, or whether the candidate had to show some certificate from his teacher(s). Maimonides in his "Rules for Judges" (*Hilkhot Sanhedrin* 2:1) indicates that judges should master a vast amount of expertise, among which medicine is the first field cited. Moses b. Maimon, *Mishneh Torah*, 2 vols. (New York: Binah, 1947). See Joshua Leibowitz, "The Problem of Medical Licence in Hebrew Sources," *Koroth* 7,5–6 (1977): 47–53.

30 Embryotomy means dismembering of the embryo. In case the mother in childbirth was in serious danger, it was a legal procedure to destroy the fetus in order to save her. Such a procedure was prohibited by the church fathers, who opined that both mother and (unborn) child were living beings and the Lord would decide who would live and who would die.

31 See b. Bava Qamma 85a. This applies even if the person who caused the injury is himself a trained physician: the injured individual is entitled to require another practitioner.

32 *Piquah nefesh*: See above, n. 1. If healing the sick is considered a religious duty, you should—in principle—perform it without expecting remuneration.

33 This was stated, in medieval time, by Nahmanides (Rabbi Moses ben Nahman, 1194–1270) in his *Sefer torat ha'adam, 'inyan hasakanah*, in *Kitvei Rabbenu Moshe ben Nahman*, 2 vols., ed. Hayim Dov Shavel (Jerusalem: Mosad ha-Rav Kook, 1964), 2: 22–45, and followed by Rabbi Joseph Karo, in *Shulhan 'Arukh, Yore de'ah*, chapter 336 (ed. Z. H. Presler and S. Havlin; Jerusalem: Ketuvim, 1993). More on physicians' fees in Immanuel Jakobovits, *Jewish medical ethics: a comparative and historical study of the Jewish religious attitude to medicine and its practice* (New York: Bloch, 1967), 222–228.

laypersons who were widely accepted as being knowledgeable. Moreover, trained practitioners were not easily available everywhere.[34] However, an important Talmudic adage determines:

> A scholar should only live in a township where ten things are to be found: a judicial court, a charity fund, a synagogue, a public bath, public latrines, a physician, a "surgeon," a scribe, a butcher and a teacher for the children. (b. Sanhedrin 17b)

Thus, both a physician and a surgeon (i.e., a bloodletter) were considered social desiderata for a Talmudic scholar. This does not mean, of course, that this was the case at any time and in any place. A public bath and public latrines are also relevant to public health.[35]

On the other hand, physicians were sometimes depreciated, even vilified. Already in the Mishnah, we find the following affirmation (m. Qiddushin 4:14): "The best of physicians—to Gehenna!" No context and no explanation are appended to this strange statement. Neither is it discussed in the corresponding Talmudic Gemara (but see below). Later commentators have tried to find acceptable reasons for such a severe judgment of doctors. To quote one of them: "A physician who believes he is the best of all will be condemned to Gehenna."[36] It is well known that physicians have often been considered conceited, in non-Jewish sources as well, for being in charge of life and death. We understand better now how important it is for a physician to consider himself as an intermediate between the Lord and the patient.

Surgeons in the Talmud

The surgeon is called 'umman in the Talmud.[37] As mentioned above, the "surgeon" Abba was first consulted for a case of gynecological pathology. This person is cited several times in the Talmud, one incident of which is particularly noteworthy.

Abba Ummna (Abba the surgeon)[38] performed bloodletting and his method is described in detail. Women and men were treated separately. When a woman came to him, he would cover her with a special dress, which would only lay bare the place where he would incise the vein. He did not require payment, but placed a box out-

---

34 It says in b. Bava Qamma 46b: "Whoever is in pain should consult a physician." However, since it often happened that the physician came from far off, then "the eye may well be blinded before he arrives" (b. Bava Qamma 85a). Eye diseases were then considered, with good reasons, as serious afflictions.

35 Private lavatories were in ancient times a clear mark of luxury. Therefore, there was indeed a need for public latrines. On this topic, see Preuss, *Biblical and Talmudic Medicine*, 546–550. Cf. also the contribution of Estee Dvorjetski on hygiene and public health in this volume.

36 See the commentary of Rabbi Samuel Edels (1555–1641) in his *Hiddushei Halakhot* (חידושי הלכות), ad loc, in Babylonian Talmud (1951). Salomon Ibn Verga (ca. 1460–1554) writes in *Shevet Yehudah*, chapter 41 (ed. Azriel Shohat; Jerusalem: Mosad Bialik, 1947), that the physician should always feel as if Gehenna is open before him and ready to engulf him in case he is negligent in his work.

37 See my paper entitled "The Surgeon as Depicted in Talmudic Literature," in *Proceedings of the 37th International Congress on the History of Medicine* (Galveston: Institute for the Medical Humanities, 2002), 275–279.

38 Abba Ummna: 'ummna is the Aramaic equivalent to 'umman in Hebrew.

side his shop into which the patients could insert whatever sum they wished or could afford. Young students were told they were free of any fees, and he would even offer the needy some money, so that they would be able to eat something after bloodletting. He said: "Go and refresh your soul" (b. Ta'anit 21b). Mar Samuel[39] ruled that after bloodletting one should drink at once and eat within the time one needs to walk half a mile (b. Shabbat 129a–b). Clearly, it appears that Abba Ummna was highly appreciated by the sages and served as an example of ethical and unselfish behavior. He allegedly received a daily salute from the Heavenly Academy,[40] an honor to which even high-ranking cited Talmudists were not entitled (cf. ibid.).

The following is a discussion of diverse professions that are either advocated or contra-indicated by the Talmudic authorities. Those who perform bloodletting are judged as follows:

> Our rabbis taught: "Ten things were told regarding the bloodletter [Heb. gara']:[41] He walks on his side, he is conceited, he leans back when seated; he has a grudging and evil eye; he eats much and excretes little; he is suspected of sexual abuse, of robbery and of bloodshed." (b. Qiddushin 82b)

This quote needs some explanation. The three first remarks denote conceit and mannerism, which is in tune with what was said about physicians in the Mishnah. Grudging and "evil eye" mean that he wants to earn money and wishes for people to become sick and need to be bled. He eats much, being often invited by well-to-do patients; he excretes little, for the food is healthy and well prepared there. Sexual relations with women, while being alone with them, can be a risk. Robbery has been related to the fact that some women might "steal" money from their husbands in order to go to the surgeon. Finally, he may be incriminated of bloodshed, if he draws too much blood from his patient, more than was requested.

This accumulation of negative characteristics seems rather excessive. It stands in sharp contrast to the description of Abba Ummna. It must, however, be put in its context. The Talmudists are discussing the following question: What kind of trade or profession should be chosen by a father for his son? It should be, they contend, a job that is "clean and easy." In other words, a business that is physically and morally spotless and manageable without vulnerable aspects. We are therefore presented with a list of possible pitfalls that could befall a bloodletter.

We find there a whole list of trades and professions that should be avoided, some of them considered unclean, others dangerous, or even both. The only professions that are somewhat related to medicine are barbers and bath attendants.[42]

---

39 On Samuel the physician, see above, n. 24.
40 The "Heavenly Academy" features a virtual meeting of demised Talmudic scholars in heaven. The idea is that earlier generations of scholars would still inspire the later decisions of legal authorities.
41 *Gara'*: This denomination of the bloodletter derives from a word meaning "to deduct" or "to diminish" the blood. In another context the same word means "to shave" or "to cut the hair." We could thus consider *gara'* as an equivalent to the English term "barber-surgeon."
42 Barbers may become dangerous, owing to their instruments. Bath attendants could be consid-

While examining the context of the disparaging statement on the *'umman*, we must remember that it refers to what is asserted in the connected Mishnah: "The best of physicians—to Gehenna!" It seems that later Talmudists felt they could hardly subscribe to such a negative opinion on physicians. They therefore shifted the criticism toward the lower social stratum of medical care, the surgeons. They were considered, together with tanners and brick-layers (masons), unfit to be elected as leaders of the community (Heb. *parnas*) or guardians (Aram./Gr. *epitropos*)[43] as stated in *Derekh Eretz Zuta* 10.

Here again, we recognize that the Talmudic corpus is a multifaceted mirror of Jewish society. The outstanding portrait of Abba Ummna contradicts the deprecating statements about surgeons in general. The lesson to be kept in mind could be the following: Remember that this profession can be dangerous and beware the possible pitfalls. Take Abba as an example to be followed, and you will then be welcomed and even honored.

While I have treated physicians and surgeons separately above, this should not be understood as a clear-cut segregation between them. Several surgical procedures are mentioned in the Mishnah and Talmud that are allegedly performed by a *rofe'*. Even circumcision, dental intervention, and some surgical operations were done by *rof'im*.[44] Bloodletting remained, however, in the province of the *'umman*.

Medical practice: legitimate or not?

In b. Berakhot 60a, Rabbi Aha, a Palestinian Amora of the fourth century, is quoted as saying:

> Whoever is going to endure bloodletting should first enunciate [the following prayer]: "May it be your wish, o Lord, that this procedure be a cure for me, and [the practitioner] be a healer for me, for you are a faithful healer (Heb. *rofe' ne'eman*) and your medicine is infallible [or "certain," Heb. *'emet*]. For it is not in the ways of humans to heal, they just took to it [Heb. *'ella shenahagu*]."

> When the Babylonian Amora Abaye heard this, he exclaimed: "Nobody should utter such a prayer! For it has been ruled by Rabbi Ishmael [one of the influential mishnaic authorities] that the Holy Scriptures have stated that physicians are entitled to heal" [cf. Heb. "*verapo' yerape'*," in Exod 21:19].

This passage, in particular, shows that the question of the legitimacy of medical practice was still being discussed in the fourth century. Of course, it is more than legiti-

---

ered responsible in case someone would fall into the timbers burning under the floor, or for any other accident in the bathhouse.

43 *Epitropos*: The Greek word stands for a guardian, or overseer, or tutor; in other words (in this case) someone responsible for the health and well-being of an orphan, an old person, or a woman living alone.

44 See Preuss, *Biblical and Talmudic Medicine*, 11–12. For instance, a *rofe'* treated eye diseases (b. Kethubot 105a). Another healed wounds with herbs (Gen. Rabbah 10:6). Another explained why teeth were falling out (y. Shabbat 6:5). Regarding circumcision, see b. Avodah Zarah 26b.

mate to pray to the Lord, but not to consider that people just got accustomed to go to some human healer, as if they turned their back to the Lord's healing agency.

Conclusion

In order to define "Jewish Medicine" we would have needed some medical works, if not from the biblical period, at least from the Talmudic period. However, there are no such documents available. Medical practice was not relevant in the worldview of the Pentateuch. In the other biblical books, diseases and healing are mentioned, but not particularly described. In the Talmud, the situation is quite different. We find numerous descriptions of diseases, of medications, of popular medicine, even of magical devices. We could have discussed the use of incantations and of amulets, which were rejected by the Tannaim, but accepted later by Babylonian Amoraim, although not without specific restrictions.[45] A number of physicians and rabbinic authorities who had some kind of medical knowledge are named and their practice delineated. However, there is no systematic presentation of these data.

A number of descriptions of physicians and surgeons from the Talmud have been provided, stressing particularly the legal principles applied to medical practice.

In conclusion, two elements are most important: First, ethical behavior in the Jewish tradition is quite stringent, it is the Law (Heb. *halakhah*). Second, both physicians and surgeons (rather, bloodletters) are praised on the one hand, while spurned on the other hand. This shows the plain realism of Talmudic literature. There is certainly a Jewish way of practicing medicine, if we read Talmudic descriptions positively. There is, however, I argue, no Jewish medicine.

In other words, the question of whether there is a Jewish medicine depends on the way in which the expression "Jewish medicine" is defined.

Bibliography

Sources

Babylonian Talmud. Jerusalem: El Hameqorot, 1948–1952.
The Babylonian Talmud. Edited by I. Epstein. London: Soncino Press, 1965–1990.
The Holy Scriptures. English text revised and edited by Harold Fisch. Jerusalem: Koren Publishers, 1986.
Ibn Verga, Salomon. *Shevet Yehudah*. Edited by Azriel Shohat. Jerusalem: Mosad Bialik, 1947. [In Hebrew]
Jellinek, Adolf (Aaron). *Beit hamidrash. Sammlung kleiner Midraschim und vermischter Abhandlungen aus der älteren jüdischen Literatur*. 6 vols. Leipzig: F. Nies, 1853–1877. [In Hebrew.]
Maimonides (Moses b. Maimon). *Mishneh Torah*. 2 vols. New York: Binah, 1947. [In Hebrew]

---

45 On magic healing in the Talmud, see (for instance) Markham J. Geller, *Akkadian Healing Therapies in the Babylonian Talmud* (Preprint Series 259; Berlin: Max Planck Institute for the History of Science, 2004); Online: http://www.mpiwg-berlin.mpg.de/Preprints/P259.PDF. Also Meir Bar-Ilan, "Between Magic and Religion: Sympathetic Magic in the World of the Sages of Mishnah and Talmud," *Review of Rabbinic Judaism* 5,3 (2002): 383–399.

Nahmanides (Moses b. Nahman). *Kitvei Rabbenu Moshe ben Nahman*. Edited by Hayim Dov Shavel. 2 vols. Jerusalem: Mosad ha-Rav Kook, 1964. [In Hebrew]

Philo of Alexandria. *Works of Philo*. Translated by F. H. Colson, G. H. Whitaker and Ralph Marcus. 12 vols., LCL. Cambridge, MA: Harvard University Press, 1929–1962.

Karo, Joseph. *Shulḥan ʻArukh*. Edited by Z. H. Presler and S. Havlin. Jerusalem: Ketuvim, 1993. [In Hebrew]

Segal, Moshe Tsvi. *Sefer Ben-Sira hashalem*. Jerusalem: Bialik Institute, 1972. [In Hebrew]

Skehan, Patrick W., and A. A. Di Lella. *The Wisdom of Ben Sira*. New York: Doubleday, 1987.

Tosephta. Edited by M. S. Zuckermandel. Jerusalem: Wahrmann, 1970. [In Hebrew]

Literature

Bar-Ilan, Meir. "Between Magic and Religion: Sympathetic Magic in the World of the Sages of Mishnah and Talmud." *Review of Rabbinic Judaism* 5,3 (2002): 383–399.

Geller, Markham J. *Akkadian Healing Therapies in the Babylonian Talmud*. Berlin: Max Planck Institute for the History of Science, 2004. Preprint Series 259. Cited 3 March 2015. Online: http://www.mpiwg-berlin.mpg.de/Preprints/P259.PDF.

Gritzalis, K. C., M. Karamanou and G. Androutsos. "Gout in the writings of eminent ancient Greek and Byzantine physicians." *Acta medico-historica Adriatica* 9,1 (2011): 83–88.

Jakobovits, Immanuel. *Jewish medical ethics: a comparative and historical study of the Jewish religious attitude to medicine and its practice*. New York: Bloch, 1959.

Kottek, Samuel. "Magic and Healing in Hellenistic Jewish Writings." *Frankfurter Judaistische Beiträge* 27 (2000): 1–16.

—. "The Surgeon as Depicted in Talmudic Literature." In *Proceedings of the 37th International Congress on the History of Medicine*. Edited by Chester R. Burns, Ynez Viole O'Neill, Philippe Albou, and José Gabriel Rigaú-Pérez. Galveston: Institute for the Medical Humanities, 2002. Pages 275–279.

—. "Sefer Assaph ha-Rofe (Jewish medical text)." In *The Encyclopedia of Ancient History. Wiley Online Library*, 2012. No Pages. Cited 5 February 2014. Online: https://doi.org/10.1002/9781444338386.wbeah11210

Leibowitz, Joshua. "The Problem of Medical Licence in Hebrew Sources." *Koroth* 7, 5–6 (1977): 47–53.

Michman, Jozeph, S. David Sperling and Louis Isaac Rabinowitz, "Leprosy," in Encyclopedia Judaica. *Jewish Virtual Library*. No pages. Cited 10 May 2014. Online: http://www.jewish virtuallibrary.org/jsource/judaica/ejud_0002_0012_0_12153.html.

Preuss, Julius. *Biblisch-talmudische Medizin*. Berlin: S. Karger, 1911.

—. *Biblical and Talmudic Medicine*. Translated by Fred Rosner. New York: Sanhedrin Press, 1978.

Rosner, Fred. "Gout in the Bible and the Talmud." *Annals of Internal Medicine* 86,6 (1977): 833.

—. *Medicine in the Bible and Talmud*. New York: Ktav, 1977.

Seybold, Klaus, and Ulrich B. Mueller. *Sickness and Healing*. Translated by D. W. Stott. Nashville: Abingdon, 1978.

Physicians' Expertise and Halakha:
On Whom Did the Sages Rely?

Tirzah Meacham

In this article we shall present a brief overview of healing and healers in the Bible which demonstrates both the idea that the true healer is God and the connection between sin and ill health. The indeterminate role of the human healer will be addressed. This will be followed by a short summary of the relationship of the rabbinic sages to physicians in classical rabbinic texts: Mishnah, Tosefta, Jerusalem Talmud and Babylonian Talmud.[1] We shall then examine in detail the interaction between the sages and the physicians when issues of purity, either moral or ritual, are at stake. We shall explore to what extent the medical expertise of physicians was accepted or ignored by the sages in order to maintain strict positions in reference to purity.

1

According to Jewish liturgy, the primary physician is, of course, God. This is also the view taken in the Bible.[2] In all the biblical instances below, the root רפא is used chiefly as a verb.[3] God heals Abimelekh and all his household who are stricken on ac-

---

1 Mishnah was redacted in ~200–220 CE in the Land of Israel; Tosefta was redacted about a generation later in the Land of Israel. These parallel texts were written in Middle Hebrew with primarily Greek loanwords and both have the same organization: six Orders divided into Tractates. On the relationship between these works see Harry Fox, "Introducing Tosefta: Textual, Intratextual and Intertextual Studies," in *Introducing Tosefta: Textual, Intratextual and IntertextualStudies*, (eds. Harry Fox (leBeit Yoreh) and Tirzah Meacham (leBeit Yoreh); Hoboken, New Jersey: Ktav 1999), 1–37. Jerusalem Talmud (also called Yerushalmi and Palestinian Talmud) was redacted in the Land of Israel ~375/400 CE. It is based on the Mishnah and written in a combination of Middle Hebrew and Jewish Western Aramaic with Greek and Latin loanwords. The Babylonian Talmud (also called Bavli) was composed in Babylonia and redacted ~500 CE and followed by a later redaction by *savoraim* who were post-Talmudic sages. Its language is a combination of Jewish Eastern Aramaic and Middle Hebrew II with Persian loanwords. Neither the Yerushalmi nor the Bavli covers all of the tractates in Mishnah. See Herman Strack and Günter Stemberger, *Introduction to the Talmud and Midrash* (trans. Markus Bockemuehl; Minneapolis: Fortress Press, 1996), and Shmuel Safrai, ed., *Literature of the Sages—Part One*, (Philadelphia: Fortress Press, 1987–2006). Throughout the article Mishnah =m, Tosefta =t, Yerushalmi =y and Bavli =b and in all cases followed by the name of the Tractate.

2 This is expressed in the eighth blessing of the weekday *Amidah*, a prayer recited three times each weekday while standing facing east or the Land of Israel or Jerusalem. The blessing is as follows: "Heal us Lord and we shall be healed; save us and we shall be saved for You are our praise. Please bring about a cure and complete healing for all our ailments and sufferings for You are God, King, a faithful and merciful healer. Blessed are You, O Lord, healer of the sick of His people,

---

DOI: 10.13173/9783447108263.193

count of taking Sarah into his household for concubinage after Abraham prays for him (Genesis 20:17).[3] God states "I am your healer" (Exodus 15:26), promising that the plagues in Egypt shall not be put upon the Israelites. One of the most moving prayers in the Bible is that of the anguished Moses when his sister Miriam is stricken with skin disease after she and Aaron speak against him: "Please God, heal her please" (Numbers 12:13). It should be noted that Aaron begs Moses to forgive him and Miriam for their folly before Moses beseeches God to heal her. This connection between repentance and healing indicates that disease is inflicted by God as a result of sin. Miriam is readmitted to the camp of the Israelites, presumably healed, seven days after being stricken with scale disease. God listens to Hezekiah's prayer which recounted his righteousness and heals him (II Kings 20:5; Isaiah 38:1–5). In the closing poem of Deuteronomy 32:39 God states, "See now that I myself am he! There is no god besides me. I put to death that which I bring to life; I have wounded and I will heal, and no one can be delivered out of my hand." In Psalm 6:3 we find God as the healer: "Have mercy upon me, Lord; for I am weak: Lord, heal me; for my bones are shaking." Similarly, in Psalm 30:3 we find "Lord my God I cried unto you and you healed me." God is referred to as the "healer of all your wounds" in Psalm 103:3. In Psalm 107:20 God sent word and healed. God is referred to as the "healer of the broken in heart who binds up their wounds" (Psalm 147:3). It should be noted that God first afflicts the characters mentioned above or allows them to be afflicted by others and then heals them.

There are other examples of healing in the Bible being contingent on repentance. Jeremiah's prayer (17:14) "Heal me Lord and I will be healed; save me and I will be saved for you are the one I praise," connects healing and salvation to God. God afflicts the Egyptians and heals them when they repent (Isaiah 19:22). God will heal the wounds he inflicted on the people of Zion (Isaiah 30:26). The suffering servant was afflicted by God and as a result Israel is healed (Isaiah 53:5). God heals the contrite (Isaiah 57:18–19) and God's love for Israel is represented by healing them (Hosea 11:3). Hosea exhorts Israel to repentance with God's words: "I will heal their waywardness and love them generously" (Hosea 14:5). The guilt and sin of Israel is likened to a wound without a cure (Jeremiah 30:13) but God relents and will cure forsaken Zion (Jeremiah 30:17). God promises restoration for the land of Judah and healing and cleansing for them from the sins they had committed (Jeremiah 33:6, 8). Hosea urges Israel to repent so that God can heal them (Hosea 6:1). When Israel repents and seeks

---

Israel." This acknowledgement of God as the true healer is also found in bBerakhot 60a in the prayer a person says before undergoing bloodletting.

3   The biblical text uses the same root referring to Elijah who healed/repaired the altar which had been torn down (I Kings 18:30) and to Elisha who stated that the Lord said, "I have healed this water," which was bad and making the land unproductive (II Kings 2:21).The root רפא is used in the sense of "freshening" the water of the Dead Sea so that fish can live and be harvested though the swamps and marshes will remain salty (Ezekiel 47:8–9, 11).

God, he will forgive their sins and heal their land (II Chronicles 7:14). Some wounds and ailments have no cure because the sins are too great.[4]

Although God is the true healer, human healers, physicians, and practitioners of healing arts were also attempting to heal ill and injured people. Samuel Kottek notes the tension between those who hold that the right to heal and to afflict is God's and those who hold that healing was given to human beings.[5] King Asa apparently died because he turned to physicians rather than to God for his acute foot ailment (II Chronicles 16:12–13). According to Exodus 21:19, if someone injured a person, s/he was obligated to see that the injured party was healed by medical treatment. *Mekhilta deRabbi Ishmael* (*Mishpatim, Neziqim*:6) and *Mekhilta of Rabbi Shimon ben Yohai* offer early legal exegeses of this verse from the third century CE.[6] They reiterate the obligation to heal. The latter text specifically mentions that a physician רופא direct the healing process. Certain prophets are connected with healing: both Elijah (I Kings 17: 20–23) and Elisha (II Kings 4:34–35) revive children, and Elisha aided in the cure of scale disease in Naaman (II Kings 5:10). These instances were accompanied by prayer or noted good deeds. According to Leviticus 13:18, 37; and 14:3, priests evaluated skin diseases to see whether they had spread or had healed to determine the ritual purity status of the person. For that reason, priests were often considered the physicians of the Bible, though there is no evidence that they actually practiced medicine.[7]

As we have seen above there is significant overlap between spiritual/moral realms and medicine in the Bible. Medical treatments may not be effective unless repentance occurred or righteous acts performed to stimulate divine mercy. Laura Zucconi describes a similar correspondence between medicine and religion in ancient Egypt.[8]

---

4   See, for example, the admonition texts in Deuteronomy 28:27, 35. See also Jeremiah 46:11; 51:8–9; Ezekiel 30:21; II Chronicles 21:18; 36:16; Lamentations 2:13; and Proverbs 29:1.

5   Samuel S. Kottek, "Healing in Jewish Law and Lore," in *Jews and Medicine: Religion, Culture, and Science* (ed. Natalie Berger; Tel Aviv: Beth Hatefusoth, 1995), 33–44. He notes that this tension is found not only in the Talmud but also in medieval commentaries.

6   The text in *Mekhilta deRabbi Ishmael* is used in bBerakhot 60a by Abaye to prove that the right to heal had been given to humans. In contrast, Rav Aḥa prays to God that bloodletting will be for the sake of healing because God is the true healer with authentic cures.

7   See Julius Preuss, *Medicine in the Bible and the Talmud* (trans. Fred Rosner; New York: Sanhedrin Press, 1978), 18–19; Joshua O. Leibowitz, "Biblical Medicine," in *Lexicon Mikrai*, eds. Menaḥem Solieli and Moshe Barkoz (Tel Aviv: Dvir, 1965), 807–816 [In Hebrew]. See Also Samuel S. Kottek, "Le Médecin a l'époque du Talmud: entre techne et Halakhah," *Medicina nei Secoli arte e scienza* 9/2 (1997): 313–330. Jeremiah, however, states that the prophets and the priests practiced deceit and yet claimed to heal the wounds of Israel (Jeremiah 6:14; 8:11). Ailments caused by sin cannot be cured without repentance unless it is an act of mercy on the part of God. See, for example, Jeremiah 8:22; 14:19; 15:18; Proverbs 6:15, etc. The afflictions on the people of Israel who had eaten the Passover sacrifice in ritual impurity were cured when Hezekiah purified the Temple and renewed the covenant with God (II Chronicles 30:20). Kottek, *ibid.* p. 328 n.1 refers to a lost biblical book of remedies which Hezakiah buried. See the reference to this in mPesaḥim 4:9.

8   See Laura M. Zucconi, "Medicine and Religion in Ancient Egypt," *Religion Compass* 1/1

Balance and justice (*maat*) guided not only the political order but also bodily function. Mark Geller observes the interconnection between magic and medicine, where herbal remedies were often accompanied by incantations to invoke spiritual aid or exorcism of demons.[9] James Longrigg notes that the priests in the temple of Asclepius were also physicians.[10] He qualifies this by stating that the physicians were part of a hereditary guild that had originally been connected to the temple of Asclepius.[11] Although Greek and Roman medicine developed a more rational approach from Hippocrates onwards, John Scarborough observes that the beginnings of Roman medicine attributed disease to divine displeasure.[12] Due to the strong influence of the Bible, it is possible that Jewish medical practices continued to maintain the claim for a strong connection between sin, ill health, repentance and healing.

2

We shall now turn to the relationship of the rabbinic sages to physicians. There are a number of terms used in the classical rabbinic texts to designate medical practitioners and healers. These include רופא *rofe* (from the root 'to heal' ר.פ.א.),[13] רופא מומחה *rofe mumḥeh*,[14] רופא אומן *rofe uman*[15] and בקיאין *beqi'in*[16] meaning knowledgeable and in Aramaic, אסיא *assia* (from the root 'to cure, heal' א.ס.י.). In some cases, the terms refer to a circumciser or a bloodletter but they may also refer to those who performed surgeries, such as amputation or embryotomy, or treated wounds, illnesses and fevers, and set bones. We are not informed by these texts concerning the training which they underwent, only that some were considered expert physicians who may be appointed by the religious court, *beit din*, to practice in certain situations under its auspices. Others, including women, also practised healing arts which included knowing how to compound and apply medications.[17] Among these women is the nursemaid of Abaye

---

(2007): 26–37. She holds that the *wab* priest and *sau* dealt chiefly with the divine while the healer *swnw* may have dealt with physical manifestations and symptoms.

9 See Markham Geller, *Ancient Babylonian Medicine: Theory and Practice* (Chichester, UK: Wiley-Blackwell, 2010), especially 8–10, 161–167.

10 James Longrigg, *Greek Medicine from the Heroic to the Hellenistic Age: A Sourcebook* (London: Duckworth, 1998), especially sections I.22–I.29

11 *Ibid.* section IV:13.

12 John Scarborough, *Roman Medicine* (London: Camelot Press, 1969), 15–16.

13 This word is normally translated physician or doctor but it can also refer to a circumciser according to Rashi in bBaba Batra 21a.

14 This apparently refers to a highly trained physician whose skill is recognized by many and who may be appointed by a *beit din* or a *beit din* may consult him.

15 This term generally refers to a skilled artisan; according to Rashi in bBaba Batra 21a, it refers to a bloodletter but may have a broader meaning in terms of medical practitioner.

16 Such knowledgeable people were allowed to instruct that an ill person should be fed on Yom Kippur according to mYoma 8:5, bYoma 83a.

17 See, for example, bAvodah Zarah 28a about a *matronita*, a term which is normally applied to a high-status Roman woman, here a healer whose remedy Rabbi Yoḥanan disclosed. Rashi considered the woman who treated Rabbi Yoḥanan as a *rofa mumḥah*. Tal Ilan, however, considers her to be a Jewish woman in this particular context. She bases her position on the version of

to whom he refers as *Em* (mother). This term is, however, considered by Mark Geller to come from Akkadian *ummânū* referring to a Mesopotamian scholar or medical expert belonging to a guild from whom Abaye learned medical secrets.[18] Yalta the spouse of Rav Naḥman and daughter of the Exilarch knew what foods to give to a man with a fever.[19] We find several sages mentioned in bAvodah Zarah 27a–28b who discuss medical treatments but they may have only been reporting on them rather than prescribing or performing the treatment.

Steven Oberhelman,[20] relying on Arthur Kleinman,[21] describes the coexistence of multiple modes of healthcare, each of which "explains disease and treats health-related problems; determines the healer(s) and the patient and the ways in which they interact; and fixes the course of treatment." Kleinman holds that there are three overlapping parts of a medical system, the popular, the professional, and the folk sector, any or all of which may be accessed by the patient. Those in the professional sector are acknowledged to have had training and have a reputation of experience but may not have diplomas, licenses or accreditation. Folk healers are non-professionals but they may have undergone an apprenticeship rather than professional training. They are considered to have special healing powers and may have acquired their master's knowledge. The popular sector is the first level at which medical issues are recognized and its practitioners make use of advice concerning normative treatments, diets, or health regimes. Women are particularly involved in this sector as heads of the domestic arena. All the groups may invoke supernatural aid in the healing process. It is likely that a similar division into practitioners who underwent professional and practical training, apprenticeship or simply following example were present in the Talmudic era. The only clear distinction that can be made is that some physicians were appointed by the court as experts while other practitioners may have practiced or

---

the story in yShabbat 14:4, 14d which she considers the source of the story subsequently transferred to yAvodah Zarah 2:2, 40d. In yShabbat it is among the stories concerning healing on the Sabbath by Jews. The discussion there deals first with Jewish healers and then moves on to Christian and pagan healers. This leads her to conclude that the woman healer is Jewish. Her argument is attractive but is premised on redactional activity about which we have little solid criteria to evaluate. See also her discussion in Tal Ilan, *Mine and Yours are Hers: Retrieving Women's History from Rabbinic Literature* (Leiden: Brill, 1997), 263–265 and her reference there to Seth Schwartz. I do agree that there were certainly Jewish women healers, midwives, drug compounders and other kinds of female medical practitioners.

18 See, for example, bShabbat 66b, 133b, 134a, bEruvin 29b, bGittin 67ab, etc. Geller presented this position as well as some word plays on Akkadian medical terms which are found in the Babylonian Talmud at the European Association of Biblical Studies panel on Medicine in the Bible and Talmud in Leuven, July 2016. I have some reservations about Geller's position since a female medical practitioner is a plausible explanation for these texts,

19 Thus, we find her giving orders for the care of a guest who is ill in bGittin 67b.

20 Steven Oberhelman, *Dreams, Healing, and Medicine in Greece: From Antiquity to the Present* (New York: Routledge, 2016), 2–6.

21 Arthur Kleinman, *Patients and Healers in the Context of Culture: An Exploration of the Borderline between Anthropology, Medicine, and Psychiatry* (Berkeley: University of California Press, 1980), 49–50.

made medical rulings but were not covered by the protective legislation of the courts as we shall see below. Moreover, there were both male and female practitioners who had a particular expertise in compounding drugs or bandages and female midwives held a special niche in the Talmudic world. The Talmud gives us no indication of their training because it does not mention specific treatises of Hippocrates or Galen or other authorities.[22] There are, however, specific sages and some collections of medical wisdom (e.g. bGittin 68b–70a) within the Talmud. The assumption is that there was ongoing integration of unattributed medical knowledge into the Talmud. This was different than the situation in other societies in late antiquity where medical knowledge was frequently found in collections and recompiled in later encyclopedias with or without attribution to authors.[23]

Several sages who do not have the title *rofe* or *uman* nevertheless were considered medical authorities such as Shmuel (or Mar Shmuel). There are very few named physicians in classical rabbinic literature. Among them are Thodos whom we shall discuss below (mBekhorot 4:4 and bSanhedrin 33a), Theodoros who may be the same person (tOhalot 4:2, bNazir 52a),[24] Tuvia (mRosh Hashanah 1:7, bRosh Hashanah 22a) who came to give testimony concerning the new moon, and Rabbi Ami *assia* (the physician) (yBerakhot 2:3, 4c).[25] The family of Manyumi were also physicians who tore their garments when Rava revealed publicly details about a special bandage they used which may have had impact on the physician's income (bShabbat 133b).[26] Abaye also reported a treatment in his name (bAvodah Zarah 28b).

Rabbinic literature has an ambivalent relationship to physicians. According to mQiddushin 4:14 and Tractate Sofrim[27] 15:7: "the best of the physicians [is destined]

---

22 Cf. Lennart Lehmhaus and Mark Geller, "Strategies of 'Canonising' Medical Knowledge in Talmudic Discourse," in Philip van der Eijk, Mark Geller, Lennart Lehmhaus, Matteo Martelli, Christine Salazar, "Cannons, Authorities and Medical Practice in the Greek Medical Encyclopaedias of Late Antiquity and in the Talmud," in *Wissen in Bewegung. Institution—Iteration—Transfer* (eds. A. Traninger and E. Cancik-Kirschbaum; Wiesbaden: Harrassowitz Verlag, 2015), 195–221, here: 208–217.

23 Philip van der Eijk, "Introduction: The Greek Medical Encyclopaedias of Late Antiquity," in *ibid*. 195–198. There is certainly no evidence for the later phenomenon of creating a near-monolithic system in the Byzantine period described by Vivian Nutton in *Ancient Medicine* (London: Routledge, 2004), 292.

24 In bNazir 52a the name varies: Theodoros in ms. Moscow-Guenzburg 1134, Thodros/Thordoros in ms. Vatican 110, and Thodos in the Venice first edition.

25 According to Preuss, *Medicine in the Bible and the Talmud*, p. 20, Rabbi Yoḥanan and Rabbi Abbahu were each considered a *rofe mumḥeh* but are not normally referred to by that title. It should be noted, however, that it seems that that title referred to the persons who treated them rather than the sages themselves.

26 This extreme reaction is similar to the one in yShabbat and yAvodah Zarah mentioned above in note 17 where Rabbi Yoḥanan, despite his promise not to do so, reveals the remedy compounded by the *matronita,* who upon losing her unique source of income either commits suicide or converts to Judaism.

27 This is one of the fourteen *Minor Tractates* which were not "canonized." There is some dispute about the time of their redaction but much of the material seems to be tannaitic.

to Geheinom."[28] The parallel in Avot de Rabbi Natan (version a) 36 includes physicians among those who have no portion in the world to come. As we see from this, medicine was not considered the most honorable of professions. The reasons for this attitude according to medieval commentators included the fact that physicians did not exert themselves in their labor, or lacked sufficient expertise, or were prone to error. Some commentators even mentioned that some physicians refused to treat the poor.[29] Moreover, physicians were not always considered trustworthy in the moral realm as we shall see below concerning bSanhedrin 75a.[30] It is likely that more than one form of medical practice was functioning simultaneously in Babylon and the Land of Israel.

According to yQiddushin 4:12, 66b, it was forbidden to live in a city which did not have a physician *rofe*.[31] According to Rabbi Yoḥanan in bAvodah Zarah 27a, non-Jewish physicians were even allowed to circumcise Jewish boys if they were considered experts in circumcision though others disagreed with him. Medical treatment had to be available in case of injury as mentioned above and it was one of the obligations a husband and his heirs had towards his wife (mKetubbot 4:9, bKetubbot 52b). People were expected to follow the advice of the physician and it might impact on payment for physical injury if the victim did not act in accordance with the physician's instructions (tBaba Qama 9:4, bBaba Qama 85 a). Serious injuries could be treated on the Sabbath, even if it meant calling in a physician from outside the Sabbath boundaries and performing other prohibited tasks (tShabbat 15:14, bYoma 83b). If a physician were able to heal some of the defects which could disqualify a betrothal or marriage, the betrothal or marriage might be valid (tKetubbot 7:8, bKetubbot 74b). According to some opinions if a slave's master was a physician and the slave asked him to heal his eye or heal his tooth but the master accidentally blinded him or uprooted the tooth, the slave might go free (tBaba Qama 9:25, bBaba Qama, 26b, bQiddushin 24b).[32]

There were physicians who ate in ritual purity, abiding by the strict table fellowship[33] tithing laws (yDemai 3:1, 23b). Other physicians also acted in accordance with

---

28 See Samuel Kottek, "The Best of Physicians are Destined for Purgatory," *Sefer Assia* 2 (1981): 21–26. [In Hebrew].

29 Rashi (Rabbi Shlomo Yitzḥaqi, northern France 1040–1105), one of the major commentators on Bible and Talmud considers the physician someone who does not fear illness and eats well and is not humble before God and who sometimes kills the patient and may not treat a poor person (bQiddushin 82a *s.v. tov sheberofim*).

30 We shall discuss the case of a man who developed a lustful passion for a certain woman which the physicians considered this life-threatening if he did not act on his passion/lust.

31 The parallel in bSanhedrin 17b has the same term *rofe* but Rashi understands that he is to circumcise infants. It is not clear from Rashi's commentary whether that *rofe* provided other medical services. See above note 13 where Rashi also describes the *uman* as a bloodletter.

32 This is based on Exodus 21:26–27 where blinding a slave or knocking out a tooth is grounds for manumission.

33 The table fellowship refers to a Jewish group which was especially circumspect concerning issues of ritual purity and of giving the tithes and heave offerings. In Hebrew a member of this group is called *ḥaver* (pl. *ḥaverim*). They are considered to have guarded the purity of common food (*ḥullin*) in a state of ritual purity as if it were a heave offering (*terumah*) or at even higher

purity laws in reference to removal of leprous limbs on the eve of Passover by not completely severing the limb so that the leper could attach it to a thorn bush to pull it off the rest of the way. If done in that manner neither the patient nor the physician had any contact with the disconnected limb which would have caused impurity, preventing them from offering and eating the Passover sacrifice (mKeritot 3:8, with parallels in Sifra Ḥova *pareshat* 1:9 and yNazir 7:1, 55d).

Patients were expected to listen to the advice of physicians (yShabbat 14:4, 14d). When the instructions contravened halakhic norms, the sages may have chastised the patient for following them (tBaba Qama 8:13, ySotah 9:10, 24a—raising a goat in Israel) or refused to visit such a patient. If the issue were against severe halakhic restrictions the sages would then forbid following the physician's orders. We shall see, however, that in other less severe cases, the sages relied in some measure on the medical expertise of physicians when they needed help to make a medical-legal decisions. They, however, reserved the right to set halakha according to their own standards rather than relying unflinchingly on the physician's medical advice.

3

I will examine five cases in which physicians have a medical opinion that impacts on the legal opinion of the sages. The first will deal with the case of protective legislation for a sage who erred on an issue concerning ritual fitness of food. The second case will concern the physicians' input in a case concerning ritual impurity of the skull or backbone. The third case will involve a moral issue. The fourth case deals with the reactions of the sages to a remedy which is against a rabbinic prohibition to raise goats in the land of Israel. The fifth will trace the sources where tannaitic material seems to rely on the statements of the physicians. In this case, however, the Yerushalmi and the even later Bavli considerably limit the impact of the words of the physicians on the halakhic decision-making process.

The first case in mBekhorot 4:4 discusses a veterinary issue. I have included it because Thodos is considered a physician and may be Theodoros who is mentioned in another case concerning human anatomy referred to below.[34] This may indicate the close connection and possible transfer of ideas concerning animal anatomy and human anatomy.

> One who is not an expert [concerning the blemishes of the firstborn] and saw the firstborn [to determine his fitness for the priest and altar] and it was slaughtered on his word [as blemished]—behold it shall be buried and he shall pay

---

levels such as those needed for sacrifices. The implements for food preparation were also maintained at a high level of ritual purity. The people themselves were circumspect about their own ritual purity making use of pools for ritual immersion and frequent ablutions of the hands. Some scholars consider the group to be pharisaic. For a relatively recent discussion on this topic, see Jack N. Lightstone, *Mishnah and the Social Formation of the Early Rabbinic Guild: A Socio-Rhetorical Approach* (Waterloo, Ontario: Wilfrid Laurier University Press, 2002), 13–14.

34 See above note 24. See also Meir Bar-Ilan, "Medicine in Eretz Israel during the First Centuries CE," *Cathedra* 91 (Nisan 1999): 31–78, esp. 57–63 and notes.

from his house [= property]. [One who] made a judgment acquitting the guilty [or] declaring the guilty innocent [or] declaring impure the pure or declaring pure that which is impure—what he did is done and he shall pay from his house [= property]. But if he were an expert of the court, he is exempt from paying. [There was a] case concerning a cow whose uterus was removed and Rabbi Tarfon fed [the animal] to dogs and the case came before the sages and they allowed it [i.e. it could have been eaten]. Thodos the physician said: No cow or sow leaves Alexandria until they have cut out its uterus in order that it will not give birth. Rabbi Tarfon said [referring to himself]: '[There] goes your donkey [in payment for the mistake], Tarfon.' Rabbi Aqiva said to Rabbi Tarfon: You are exempt, for you are an expert of the court and every expert of the court is exempt from paying [in the event of an error].

The firstborn, if male, of cows, sheep, and goats was to be brought to the temple unless it had a certain type of blemish which would disqualify it as a sacrifice. In the first case in the Mishnah the non-expert mistakenly believed that the blemish was permanent and allowed the firstborn to be slaughtered. It should therefore have been buried as if it had died naturally and the non-expert was obligated for a quarter of the firstborn's value for sheep and goats or half of the firstborn calf's value.[35] In the continuation the Mishnah deals with compensation for mistaken judgments of non-experts while court-appointed experts are exempt. Rabbi Tarfon apparently not only declared a cow which had undergone hysterectomy *treifa*, unfit for Jewish consumption, but had the cow fed to the dogs. The case was then brought before the sages who declared it permissible for Jewish consumption on the basis of mHullin 3:2 which specifically does not disqualify a cow as *treifa* whose uterus is missing. After the sages' ruling, the statement of Thodos the physician is introduced that no cows or sows are exported from Alexandria unless they had had their uterus removed. It is not clear whether the sages are actually relying on Thodos' statement or whether a redactor inserted his statement as justification for the sages' position. The point of Thodos' statement is that a hysterectomy is not a life-threatening defect. In mHullin 3:2 we find a list of defects in cattle which are not sufficient to have them declared unfit for Jewish consumption and this includes cows which have undergone a hysterectomy. Thodos' statement is not found in that Mishnah. It appears it may have been presented in mBekhorot 4:4 to support the sages' position.

This Mishnah in Bekhorot is brought as a refutation of Rav Hamnuna to Rav Sheshet in bSanhedrin 33a.[36]

---

35 It was not considered appropriate to raise sheep and goats in the Land of Israel because of the damage they would do to crops according to mBaba Qama 7:7. As a result the fine for the mistaken judgment was less than for cattle which were permitted to be raised.

36 There are some differences in the manuscripts: Florence II-I-9, Yad Harav Herzog 1, Munich 95 all have from Beit Menaḥem while Karlsruhe—Reuchlin 2 has Rabbi Menaḥem. Moreover, only Vilna and Barko (1498) have שאמר introducing Thodos' statement.

Rav Hamnuna refuted Rav Sheshet: [Concerning a] case of a cow of the house of Menaḥem whose uterus was removed, and Rabbi Tarfon fed it to the dogs. But the case came before the sages in Yavneh and they permitted it [to be eaten] for Thodos the physician said: No cow or sow goes out from Alexandria of Egypt unless they cut out its uterus in order that it not [be able to] give birth.

Thodos' statement seems to reflect general medical or veterinary knowledge upon which the sages could rely. The inclusion of the cow, which underwent a hysterectomy in the list in mḤullin may reflect *realia* known to the redactor of the Mishnah or may be based on the sages' position in mBekhorot which may in turn be based on the statement of Thodos the physician. Since much human anatomical knowledge was obtained through animal slaughter and dissection, it is likely that medical practice crossed between human and animal cases. It is extremely likely that despite the fact that this case dealt with a veterinary issue, a physician who normally dealt with human patients was competent in animal anatomy. It should be noted that in this period nearly all human anatomy was learned from animal dissection.[37]

Our next case does involve an issue of ritual purity and again we find Thodos/Theodoros and other physicians making a statement, which is in accordance with the sages' position. The question remains whether the sages were relying on the medical statements, or were independent of them.

Rabbi Yehuda said: Rabbi Aqiva declared six things impure but retracted [his position]. [There was] a case in which they brought baskets of bones from Kefar Tavya and placed them in the air of the synagogue [not covered by a roof so that if the bones had corpse impurity, people would not have become impure by being under the same roof] in Lod; and Theodoros the physician and all of the physicians with him entered and said: There is not a backbone from a single corpse and not a skull from a single corpse. They [the sages] said: Since there are those here who declared it impure and those who declared it pure, we shall stand for a vote. They began from Rabbi Aqiva and he declared [the case] pure. They said to him: Since it was you who declared [the case] impure [and] you have declared [it] pure—they will be pure. Rabbi Shimon said: And until the day of his death, Rabbi Aqiva would declare [it] impure but if from when he died he retracted [his position][38]—I do not know. (tOhalot 4:2)

In tOhalot we also find Theodoros and the physicians making a statement in accordance with the ruling of the sages. It seems appropriate to assume that, even though not stated, the sages requested the expertise of the physicians. Despite the wording in the Mishnah, it is likely that the physicians first determined forensically that no

---

37 Herophilus was an exception. See John Scarborough, *Roman Medicine* (London: Thames and Hudson, 1969), 34–35 and Appendix III 168–170.

38 Rabbi Shimon held that Rabbi Aqiva did not retract his original declaration that the basketful of bones would cause corpse impurity. He is uncertain, however, if Rabbi Aqiva retracted his position after his death. See also Meir Bar-Ilan, "Medicine," 65–66.

complete skull from a single person or no complete backbone from a single person was present and then the sages made the halakhic ruling on the basis of that knowledge. If a complete skull or a complete spinal column from a single corpse could be reconstructed from the bone fragments, and the bones had been in the synagogue covered by a roof, this would have caused people under the same roof, especially those who had taken a Nazirite vow, to become ritually impure due to corpse impurity according to mNazir 7:2. Rabbi Aqiva apparently had originally stated that the basketful of bones would transmit corpse impurity. It is also unclear whether this was a true vote and whether Rabbi Aqiva changed his position due to the statement of the physicians or whether he was convinced or simply pressured by the majority to change his position. Rabbi Shimon is quite certain that Rabbi Aqiva did not really change his position.

The Mishnah in bNazir 49b (mNazir 7:2) gives a list of impurities for which a Nazirite must poll (remove all his hair). Included in this particular list are the spinal column and/or the skull. We find in bNazir 52a a discussion whether the *vav* in the Mishnah between the words backbone and skull is conjunctive, meaning that both the backbone and skull must be present, or disjunctive meaning that it is sufficient for either the backbone or the skull to be present to cause impurity. Later the *sugya* deals with the necessity that the backbone or the skull must be complete, even if the pieces have become separated from each other, in order to cause impurity to the Nazir. The continuation of the *sugya* brings our *baraita*.

> Come, hear: Rabbi Yehuda says: Rabbi Aqiva declared six things impure but the sages declared them pure, and Rabbi Aqiva retracted [his position]. And [there was a] case that they brought a basketful of [human] bones to the Synagogue of the Tarsians and placed it in the air. Thodos [or Theodos] the physician and all the physicians [with him] entered and they said: There is no backbone from a single corpse. The reason [that it was declared clean] is that there was not a backbone from one [corpse]; [therefore if] there was either a backbone or a skull from one [corpse]—a nazirite would poll because of it. Understand from this: We teach in the Mishnah—either a backbone or a skull. He [Todos] said it was not needed: the backbone *and* the skull from one corpse is not needed [to be mentioned]. Rather [one needs] even *either* a [complete] backbone from one corpse *or* a [complete] skull from one corpse [but this case] did not have [either]. (bNazir 52a)

In this version we find language, which will be found in yNiddah discussed below. This language indicates a necessary condition: "The reason [that it was declared clean] is that there was not a backbone from one [corpse]; [if] there was either a backbone or a skull from one [corpse]—a nazirite would poll because of it." It is, however, still in accordance with the sages' and physicians' position.

In the introduction, we saw the connection between sin and disease. Our third source deals with a case of sexual morality, that is, moral purity. In this case, however, the illness cannot be cured according to the physicians without transgressive behaviour. We find in bSanhedrin 75a the following:

Rav Yehuda said [in the name of] Rav: [There was a] case in which a certain man set his eyes on a certain woman and he became [life-threateningly] heart-sick. They came and they asked the physicians and they said: There is no cure except that she submits to sexual intercourse with him. The sages said: He should die rather than she submit to sexual intercourse with him. [The physicians said:] She should stand naked before him. [The sages said:] He should die and she should not stand naked before him. [The physicians said:] She should converse with him from behind the fence. [The sages said:] He should die and she should not converse with him from behind the fence. Rabbi Yaaqov bar Idi and Rabbi Shmuel bar Naḥmani disputed on this [issue]. One said: She was a married woman, and one said: She was a single woman. It is understandable for the one who said she was a married woman. But for the one who said that she is single, why is there such an issue? Rav Papa said: Because [such an action might be considered] a defect in the family. Rav Aḥa barei deRav Iqa said: In order that the daughters of Israel not become sexually dissolute. But he could marry her! His mind would not be calmed/eased; [it is] like that [statement] of Rabbi Yitzḥaq who said: From the day the Temple was destroyed, the de-sire for [legitimate] intercourse was taken and given to sinners as it is stated [Proverbs 9:17]: 'Stolen waters will be sweet and bread [eaten] in secret will be pleasant.' (bSanhedrin 75a)

This text hardly needs any explanation. Whatever medical remedies the physicians recommended, they could not overcome the moral objections of the sages. Conse-quently, the physicians' opinions were simply ignored by them. According to the rabbis, it was preferable that the patient die rather than transgress rabbinic norms or suggest that a woman do so.

Our next source deals with the rabbinic prohibition to raise goats in the land of Israel because of their destructive nature. A physician prescribes fresh goat's milk as a remedy for a sage's illness. We find in tBaba Qama 8:13 the following:

> ... They said about Rabbi Yehuda ben Baba that all of his actions were for the sake of Heaven except that he raised small animals [= goats]. Thus one time he became ill and the physician came to him and said: There is no remedy except fresh milk. He purchased a nanny goat and tied her to the bed post and would suckle from her fresh milk when he was groaning [from his illness]. One time the sages sought to visit him. They said how can we enter [to visit] when ban-dits are with him in the house. But when he died the sages examined his deeds and they found no transgression except that one. He [Rabbi Yehuda ben Baba] also said in the hour of his death: I know that I have no transgression except this one that I ignored the words of my colleagues.

There are a few slight changes in the version in ySotah 9:10, 24a: more than one phy-sician recommends the remedy which is to be taken whenever he is groaning because of his illness and Rabbi Yehuda ben Baba makes his statement concerning his life's transgressions before the sages check his life's actions. Apparently, the sages felt that it would have been better that he had not taken the remedy and perhaps then would not have died as he would have been without sin.

Our final set of sources seems to demonstrate that the weight of the physician's opinion in the sages' determination of *halakhah* may have changed from Tosefta to Yerushalmi to Bavli. In order to understand the context of our texts concerning Rabbi Tzadoq, we must understand mNiddah 3:1–2a. The start of mNiddah chapter 3 deals with spontaneous abortions at various stages of gestation or discharge of pathological tissue to determine whether the woman's ritual impurity is due to birth impurity or menstrual impurity or to another cause.

> 3:1 She who aborts a piece [of tissue]—if there is blood with it, she is impure but if not, she is pure. Rabbi Yehuda says: Whether or not [there is blood with it], she is impure.
> 3:2a She who aborts a kind of rind, a kind of hair, a kind of dust, a kind of insect—[all of which are] red—she places it in water. If it dissolves, she is impure; but if not, she is pure.
> 3:2b She who aborts [something] like a fish, locusts, creeping and crawling things—if there is blood with them, she is impure; but if not, she is pure [...] (mNiddah 3:1–2)

It is likely that mNiddah 3:1 refers to a very early spontaneous abortion in which the uterine lining has overgrown the implantation site. A small piece of tissue, which is the product of conception is expelled along with the uterine overgrowth. It is improbable that any piece of tissue would have been expelled without accompanying blood, although a piece of tissue could have been retained due to its size after the rest of the uterine lining is expelled as blood and menstrual detritus. The blood would cause her to be ritually impure due to menstruation while the piece of tissue has no status in terms of birth impurity.

The following Mishnah 3:2a gives examples of red material in the shape of small rinds, hair, dust/clods of earth, and flying insects. These must be placed in water to see if they dissolve which would demonstrate that they were simply blood clots. If they do not dissolve, and no other blood accompanies their discharge, she is considered to be ritually pure because there is no menstrual blood and because the material is not considered a fetus. This is followed in 3:2b by a list including fish, locusts, reptiles and other swarming creatures and reiterates the requirement that blood accompany the discharged material in order that she become menstrually impure. The Talmud states that these two *mishnaiot* interact so that if there is some ritually impure blood in either case, she is considered impure due to menstruation, but if there is no accompanying blood the material is placed in water to see if it dissolves.

We shall now turn to another tannaitic source, tNiddah 4:3–4 which uses some of the language (rind, hair) which we saw in mNiddah 3:2. Two cases are brought before Rabbi Tzadoq. He apparently did not feel qualified to answer the questions and brought them before the sages in Yavneh. They in turn sought expert advice from physicians. We find in tNiddah 4:3–4:

> Rabbi Elazar bar Rabbi Tzadoq said: [My] father brought two cases from Tivin to Yavneh. [One was of a] case in which a certain woman would abort red, rind-like [discharges]. They came and asked Rabbi Tzadoq and Rabbi Tzadoq went and asked the sages. And the sages sent and called for the physicians. They [the physicians] said: She has an injury inside [her uterus]—for that reason she aborts some kind of red rinds.
>
> Another case [was] concerning a woman who would abort red hairs. And they came and asked Rabbi Tzadoq and Rabbi Tzadoq went and asked the sages. And the sages sent and called for the physicians. They said: She has a mole in her inner parts [= uterus]—for that reason she aborts red hairs.

As in the Mishnah, these cases concern women who are having a uterine discharge which apparently is not blood. The protocol presented in Tosefta is noteworthy: the local authority is asked first but if he does not have an answer, he takes it to a center in which there are many sages. In the event that the sages need further expert opinion, they call in physicians implying that their expertise might have impact on the sages' legal decision.

The reason the physicians give in the first case is somewhat difficult to understand from the point of view of *realia*. They are apparently making a parallel from an external wound, which would scab over, and later shed the scab or have it knocked off or scratched off, and then in turn would create a new scab which would later be shed, etc. This is the norm for an external injury which is exposed to air. The blood and plasma from the wound dry out and harden on contact with the air. This is not the case in the moist internal environment of the uterus. The wound could heal but there would not be scab formation so it would make it improbable for her to shed rind-like scabs from the wound.

The physicians' diagnosis in the second case is also problematic from the point of view of *realia*. Again, the physicians are relating to an external phenomenon—the existence of a mole from which hairs grow and can be shed—to the existence of a mole inside her uterus which they believed behaves in a similar manner. Normal moles are on the surface of the skin, or subdermal, but not internal. They are often pigmented and may have hairs growing from them. Elsewhere I suggested that these cases are most probably referring to placental breakdown after embryonic or fetal death but before the actual miscarriage.[39] As the margins of the placenta begin to disintegrate, pieces of the blood-filled capillaries may separate from the surrounding tissue and be expelled separately. They resemble red hairs. Similarly, red, rind-like discharges may

---

39 Tirzah Meacham, "Mishnah Tractate Niddah with Introduction—A Critical Edition with Notes on Variants, Commentary, Redaction and Chapters in Legal History and Realia," 2 vols. (Ph.D. diss., The Hebrew University, Jerusalem, 1989) [In Hebrew]. Volume I, 243–80. See also Meir Bar-Ilan, "Medicine," 66–67 who connects the circumstances to knowledge of Soranus in note 134.

be other parts of the disintegrating placenta. The fact of an unsuccessful pregnancy may not become known until the delayed miscarriage occurs.

If a woman were having a uterine discharge of this type, she would need a halakhic decision in reference to her current purity status. If this substance were expelled without liquid blood, the question arising in Tosefta is similar to the question arising in mNiddah 3:2: either the woman would be ritually pure or the substance would be placed in water to see if it dissolved implying that it is blood. In the latter case, she would be ritually impure due to menstruation but not childbirth. It should be noted that the Tosefta and parallel mishnah do not mention that the woman may have been pregnant.

What is significant for our discussion is that tNiddah 4:3–4 does not indicate in any manner that there is disagreement with the opinion of the physicians. It seems that the sages who called for the physicians to give their expert opinion also accepted their diagnosis. The red, rind-like material and the red, hair-like material are not considered to cause menstrual impurity and certainly do not cause birth impurity. The discussion in the Talmudim gives us a somewhat different picture. We shall continue our discussion with yNiddah 3:2, 50c:

> She who aborts dry blood: Rabbi Lazar says: She is impure. Rabbi Yose ben Ḥanina said: She is pure... The *baraita* is in dispute with Rabbi Yose ben Ḥanina: [There was] a case concerning a certain woman who would abort red, rind-like [tissue] and the case came before [the] sages and they sent and called for the physicians. And they [the physicians] said to them: She has an injury inside. Again [there was a] case concerning a certain woman who would cast off [something] like red hairs [from her uterus] and the case came before [the] sages and they sent and called for the physicians. And they [the physicians said to them: she has a mole from inside her. [She is pure only] because she has a mole and because she has an injury. Behold if she did not have a mole and did not have an injury—no [she would not be pure]. On this they dispute with him and his [Rabbi Yose ben Ḥanina's position] cannot be upheld.

The first difficulty in this *sugya* is the idea of a woman aborting dry blood. Menstrual blood, even if dry, can still transmit menstrual impurity (mNiddah 7:1). In order to become dry, the liquid elements of blood would have to be removed. This would occur outside the body by normal dehydration. This process could not be accomplished in the moist environment of the uterus. The Talmud, however, is adamant that the case is one in which the blood was dry from the start. It does not use the term for clotted blood, *dam qarush*, which is used elsewhere referring to liquid blood which clotted, but rather *dam yavesh*, dry blood.

Our *baraita* is then brought as a difficulty for Rabbi Yose ben Ḥanina's position because his statement is general, referring to aborting all types of dry blood, while our *baraita* refers only to red, rind-like and red, hair-like materials which are aborted. This is further qualified by asserting that the physicians' statement in the *baraita* that she has an internal [uterine] injury or mole is a necessary qualification for these discharges to be considered pure. As a result, this qualification is considered a rejection of Rabbi Yose ben Ḥanina's position. The *baraita* itself uses the physicians' statement as an explanation of the phenomenon, but the Yerushalmi reinterprets it as a necessary condition. It is not clarified how a uterine injury or the existence of a mole in the uterus could be ascertained.

We shall now turn to the use of this *baraita* in the Babylonian Talmud. Here, too, the context is the discussion of aborting dry blood in bNiddah 22ab:

> Rabbi Yose bar Ḥanina asked Rabbi Elazar: Dry blood—what is it[s status in terms of the woman who aborts it]? The Merciful One said [Leviticus 15:19]:'when the flow of her blood shall flow'—until it surely flows; moist—yes, dry—no. Or perhaps: this [statement] 'when the flow of her blood shall flow' is [simply] the matter [process] of the thing, and even dry blood would also [be considered to flow]? ... He [Rabbi Yose bar Ḥanina] said to him: I am not questioning moist [blood] which became dry for I am questioning [what was] dry [blood] from the start. This, too, they have taught [mNiddah 3:2]:[40]'She who aborts a kind of rind, a kind of hair, a kind of dust, a kind of insect—[all of which are] red—she places it in water. If it dissolves, she is impure; but if not, she is pure.' Rabbah said: When it does not dissolve—it is a creature in its own right. And are there [creatures] such as this? Yes, but it is taught: Rabbi Elazar bar Rabbi Tzadoq said: [My] father brought two cases from Tivin to Yavneh. [One was] case in which a certain woman would abort red rind-like [discharges]. They came and asked Rabbi Tzadoq and Rabbi Tzadoq asked the sages. And the sages asked the physicians. They said to them: This woman has an injury from inside [her uterus] from which she aborts rind-like [tissue]. You shall place them in water and if they dissolve, she is impure.
>
> Another [was a] case concerning a woman who would abort something like red hairs. And they came and asked Rabbi Tzadoq and Rabbi Tzadoq asked the sages and the sages asked the physicians. They said to them: This woman has a mole in her inner parts [= uterus] –from it she aborts red hairs. You shall place [them] in water, if they dissolve, she is impure.

The changes in the *baraita* as it is found in tNiddah 4:3–4 and as it is brought in the Babylonian Talmud are significant. An extra condition has been added to both sections: 'You shall place [them] in water, if they dissolve, she is impure.' In the Tosefta, it appears that the sages simply accept the diagnosis of the physicians and do not require the extra step of placing the material in water. That also seems to be the case in the Yerushalmi. In the Bavli there is harmonization between the *baraita* as it appears in Tosefta and mNiddah 3:2 which requires soaking in water as a test. It should be noted that in yNiddah the section concerning soaking appears on the discussion of the inter-textual readings between the first part of mNiddah 3:2 on the rind-like, hair-

---

40 The text of the biblical verses and the Mishnah are brought in single quotation marks to aid the reader in understanding the text.

like, dust-like and insect-like abortions which are to be placed in water from mNiddah 3:3 concerning fish-like, locust-like, creeping creature-like and *sheratzim*-like[41] abortions which are impure if accompanied by blood. For both cases, soaking in water and checking for blood are required. This discussion in yNiddah takes place before our question arises concerning the woman who aborts dry blood but is not applied to our question.

We now have three different levels of acceptance by the sages of the position of the physicians:

1) tNiddah ends with their diagnosis leading us to believe that the sages accepted it without condition.
2) yNiddah attempts to relate mNiddah 3:2 to our *baraita* in order to limit the application of the physicians' statement to only those two cases and not any other case in Mishnah.
3) bNiddah which harmonistically reads mNiddah 3:2 and its conditions of soaking in water and accompanying blood to our *baraita*. As a result, the medical diagnosis of the physicians is limited in the case of a purity issue.

Do we understand from this example that there was a growing hesitation on the part of the sages to accept medical diagnoses in general or only those which had impact on the status of ritual purity or impurity? Or is this simply a case of the Talmudim reflecting the increased tendency for legal stringencies in reference to menstrual impurity? Or is it some combination of rabbinic suspicion about the medical profession and the validity of the diagnoses of physicians along with intensified concern for ritual purity connected with uterine blood?

In the first case brought above, dealing with protective legislation for the sage who erred on an issue concerning ritual food, the physician's judgment concerning the fitness for consumption of animals, which had undergone a hysterectomy, was accepted. The source merely sought to avoid penalizing the sage who was unaware of the physicians' judgement and its incorporation into mHullin 3:2. Rabbi Tarfon, considered a third generation Tanna, lived after the destruction of the second Temple until the revolt of Bar Kokhba but before the redaction of the Mishnah. It is possible, therefore, that the opinions in mBekhorot 4:4 protected him because mHullin 3:2 was not widely known or perhaps had not yet been composed in final form. In the second case, the sages also accepted the position of Theodorus, the physician, and those physicians who accompanied him concerning the skeletal remains. Their examination of the bones may have been made to distinguish between human and animal bones but subsequently they attempted to distinguish between human bones from different people. This could have been possible if the differences were in the size of the vertebrae and skull.[42]

---

41 *Sheratzim* are creatures, which are ritually impure when they are dead and impart a high level of ritual impurity. The usage here may not refer to the eight creatures noted in Leviticus but to a variety of small creatures.
42 The concern was whether a complete spinal column from one individual was among the bones.

The third case refers to physicians attempting to treat a man who had developed a lust for a certain woman, which was considered to put him into a dangerous, perhaps even life-threatening, condition. This case is reported by Rav Yehuda in the name of Rav, both early Babylonian *amoraim*. The recommendations of the physicians were simply disregarded because they so clearly contradicted the normative morality of the sages. In the fourth case, Rabbi Yehuda ben Baba accepted the physicians' suggested treatment for his extremely painful stomach condition, despite the fact that it was contrary to rabbinic norms. Goats were considered to be destructive animals but their fresh milk was the prescribed treatment for his condition. Despite the fact that Rabbi Yehuda ben Baba kept the goat tied to his bedstead where it could not harm the property of others, the rabbis who had intended to visit him considered the treatment recommended by the physicians as transgressive. It seems that the rabbis would have rejected the suggested treatment apparently believing that Rabbi Yehuda ben Baba would not have died had he not accepted the treatment. He is considered to have been among the third generation Tannaim and one of the ten martyrs in Hadrian's persecution.

The final case deals with a question concerning the ritual purity status of uterine discharges. Rabbi Elazar bar Rabbi Tzadoq was another Tanna of the third generation. As noted above, in the original source in tNiddah 4:3 the sages seem to accept the judgment of the physicians, as there is no additional comment or condition put on their words. We find in yNiddah and bNiddah stipulations limiting the application of the diagnosis of the physicians to particular circumstances. It is likely that the tendency to become ever stricter in reference to purity laws concerning uterine blood is the basis for the Talmudic sages limiting the weight of the physicians' statements.

Several rabbinic statements demonstrate the progression toward greater stringency in matters of ritual impurity due to uterine blood. Ritual bathing is not required in Leviticus 15 for women with normal menstruation or an abnormal uterine discharge of blood or in Leviticus 12 concerning birth blood or blood of purification. The chiastic structure or of Leviticus 15 makes it likely that since people who had contact with the menstruous woman were required to ritually bathe, she herself was also required to ritually bathe. An anonymous statement in Sifra, a tannaitic legal exegesis of the book of Leviticus, states that the phrase 'in her flesh' in Leviticus 15:19 means that blood which has left the uterus but is still inside the vagina nevertheless establishes the woman as ritually impure due to menstruation.[43] This is the position in mNiddah 5:1 and codified as law. The preposition *bet* has the meaning of both 'in' and 'on' in Biblical Hebrew. The latter meaning could be interpreted as only when menstrual blood reached the outside of the woman's body and was found on her external genitalia would she be considered ritually impure. This is likely the way the majority of women in the world become cognizant that menstruation has begun. It is possible that the understanding of the preposition to mean inside the vagina had to

---

If pelvic bones had been examined, it is possible that the physicians also could have determined the sex of the person to whom the bones belonged as they were aware that the female pelvis was broader to accommodate the birth of a child. See bEruvin 18b.

43 Sifra, Zavim *pereq* 6:4 according to the Weiss edition in the Bar Ilan Responsa Project 24.

do with the fact that during intercourse a male has contact with the woman internally. This, then, is a protective measure to prevent transgression of the prohibition on intercourse during menstrual impurity in Leviticus 18:19 and 20:18. The fact that in other cases ritual impurity, which is found within the body or in an unexposed place like the armpit or belly folds, does not transmit impurity indicates that additional stringencies were placed upon uterine blood.[44]

Hillel the Elder in mNiddah 1:1 held that women were always in a presumptive state of ritual impurity due to the possible discharge of uterine blood. This created a situation of retroactive impurity in which only an intrusive internal examination by the woman could demonstrate that there had been no uterine discharge of blood from the current examination to the previous examination. Hillel nevertheless suspected that discharge of uterine blood could occur immediately after the examination necessitating frequent internal examinations. Although the sages accepted the concept of retroactive ritual impurity, they limited it to twenty-four hours. Nevertheless, the requirement for internal examinations with a checking cloth remained in force in the time of the Mishnah for those women dealing with ritually pure foods and currently is used to verify that uterine discharge has ceased. It is possible that the strict Zoroastrian purity laws concerning such bodily discharges influenced Hillel who came from Babylon.

Sifra adds a clarification to Leviticus 15:25 concerning the number of days of uterine bleeding beyond normal menstruation (assumed to be completed within seven days) would change the woman's status from a menstruant to a woman with abnormal uterine bleeding.[45] This was established as three consecutive days during the eleven days which the sages established as the minimum number of days between one menstrual cycle and the next.[46] This necessitated constant reckoning so that there could be a distinction between normal menstruation and abnormal uterine bleeding. It was not problematic for women who had a regular cycle because if there were no prolonged period or mid-cycle bleeding they could go from period to period because the eleven days were established as a minimum. Irregular bleeding, however, required frequent interval examinations. Rabbi Judah the Patriarch, a descendent of Hillel the Elder and considered to be the redactor of the Mishnah, decreed in Sadot that if a woman saw blood one day she sits in impurity for that day and six more. This could be a reckoning of the seven days of menstrual impurity. If she saw blood two days in a row, she sits in impurity those two days and six additional days. This added an

---

44 See the discussion in bNiddah 41b–42b. Ultimately the statement in Sifra that a woman became ritually impure if uterine blood were found in the vagina even if it had not reached the outside of her body became embedded in the law due to a "decree of the verse" in bNiddah 42b.

45 Sifra *Zavim*, *pereq* 7:10 and bNiddah 38a. If a woman's period extended one or two days beyond the seven days of menstruation, she was in the category of minor *zavah* requiring only waiting one day or two days for the discharge to cease and she could undergo ritual bathing without the obligation of waiting seven days and bringing a sacrifice.

46 The derivation of eleven days is nowhere noted but it was the accepted number in mNiddah 4:4 and 10:8, bNiddah 36b and 72a. In Sifra *Tzav pereq* 11:6, bNiddah 72b, bMenaḥot 89a and the Vilna edition of yBerakhot 5:1, it is considered to be "a law for Moses from Sinai." This refers to a law which is not found in the Bible but has a legal status nearly equal to a biblical law.

additional day to the normal seven days of menstrual impurity. If, however, she saw blood for three consecutive days she was required to remain impure until she had seven days without any uterine discharge.[47] This removed the woman from the category of normal menstruation (*niddah*) to a category of abnormal uterine bleeding (*zavah*), conflating these very distinct biblical categories. No reason was given for this stringency but some later commentaries explain that in this area, there were no sages and the people were ignorant. Other statements by later sages understand his decree as being a general decree. This is expanded further by a statement of Rabbi Zeira, "The daughters of Israel became strict with themselves so that even if they see [a drop of] blood like a mustard [seed in size], they sit [in impurity] because of it seven clean days. Rav Ḥuna in yBerakhot 5:1 (8d) has a different version which does not include the daughters of Israel: "She who sees a drop [of blood] like a mustard [seed in size] sits [in impurity] and keeps seven clean days." Rav Ḥuna gave this as an example of an undisputed law. These statements and their many parallels testify to the significance of this ruling.[48] It seems that the line of the Patriarch, established by Hillel the Elder, was particularly circumspect concerning ritual purity. The archaeological evidence shows many bathing pools for ritual purification adjacent to the House of the patriarch.

I have demonstrated elsewhere the tendency of the rabbinic sages to become ever stricter in reference to purity laws concerning uterine blood.[49] In my opinion, this is more likely to be the basis for the Talmudic sages limiting the weight of the physicians' statements. This situation, combined with the moral gap evident in the case of moral purity mentioned in our third and fourth examples of consultation with medical experts had an effect of decreasing the role physicians played in the sages' decisions in amoraic times. Ultimately, the contribution of medical experts did not override rabbinic concerns with ritual and moral purity. This seems to be in accordance with the ambivalent status of physicians in the eyes of the sages.

Bibliography

Sources

Tosephta (based on the Erfurt and Vienna Codices). Edited by M.S. Zuckermandel. Jerusalem, 1970.
Babylonian Talmud; Vilna Edition.
Jerusalem Talmud; Venice Edition (1522–1524).

---

47 His decree and the following statement by Rabbi Zeira are found in bNiddah 66a.
48 Rava and Rav Papa did not accept it as a universal decree but rather as a custom in bNiddah 66a. At some point during the geonic period, the conflation of menstruation with abnormal uterine bleeding became normative law.
49 An expanded version of the above summary can be found in my article, Tirzah Meacham, "An Abbreviated History of the Development of Jewish Menstrual Laws," in *Women and Water; Menstruation in Jewish Life and Law*, ed. Rahel Wasserfall (Hanover, Mass.: University Press New England, 1999), 23–39, and 255–261 (appendix).

Literature

Bar-Ilan, Meir. "Medicine in Eretz Israel during the First Centuries CE," *Cathedra* 91 (1999): 31–78. [In Hebrew]

Fox (leBeit Yoreh), Harry. "Introducing Tosefta: Textual, Intratextual and Intertextual Studies." In *Introducing Tosefta: Textual, Intratextual and Intertextual Studies.* Edited by Harry Fox (leBeit Yoreh) and Tirzah Meacham (leBeit Yoreh). Hoboken, New Jersey: Ktav 1999. Pages 1–37.

Geller, Markham. *Ancient Babylonian Medicine: Theory and Practice.* Chichester, UK: Wiley-Blackwell, 2010.

Geller, Markham J., Philip J. van der Eijk, Lennart Lehmhaus, Matteo Martelli, Christine F. Salazar: "Canon and Authority in Greek and Talmudic Medicine." In *Wissen in Bewegung. Institution—Iteration—Transfer* (Episteme in Bewegung. Beiträge zur einer transdisziplinären Wissensgeschichte, Bd. 1). Edited by Eva Cancik-Kirschbaum and Anita Traninger. Wiesbaden: Harrassowitz, 2016. Pages 195–221.

Ilan, Tal. *Mine and Yours are Hers: Retrieving Women's History from Rabbinic Literature.* Leiden: Brill, 1997.

Kleinman, Arthur. *Patients and Healers in the Context of Culture: An Exploration of the Borderline between Anthropology, Medicine, and Psychiatry.* Berkeley: University of California Press, 1980.

Kottek, Samuel S. "The Best of Physicians are Destined for Purgatory." *Sefer Assia* 2 (1981): 21–26. [In Hebrew]

—. "Healing in Jewish Law and Lore." In *Jews and Medicine: Religion, Culture, and Science.* Edited by Natalie Berger. Tel Aviv: Beth Hatefusoth, 1995. Pages 33–44.

—. "*Le Médecin a l'époque du Talmud: entre techne et Halakhah.*" *Medicina nei Secoli arte e scienza,* 9,2 (1997): 313–330.

Leibowitz, Joshua O. "Biblical Medicine." In *Lexicon Mikrai.* Edited by Menachem Solieli and Moshe Barkoz. Tel Aviv: Dvir, 1965. Pages 807–816. [In Hebrew]

Lightstone, Jack N. *Mishnah and the Social Formation of the Early Rabbinic Guild: A Socio-Rhetorical Approach.* Waterloo, Ontario: Wilfrid Laurier University Press, 2002.

Longrigg, James. *Greek Medicine from the Heroic to the Hellenistic Age: A Sourcebook.* London: Duckworth, 1998.

Meacham, Tirzah. "Mishnah Tractate Niddah with Introduction—A Critical Edition with Notes on Variants, Commentary, Redaction and Chapters in Legal History and Realia." 2 vols. Ph.D. diss., The Hebrew University, Jerusalem, 1989. [In Hebrew]

—. "An Abbreviated History of the Development of Jewish Menstrual Laws." In *Women and Water; Menstruation in Jewish Life and* Law. Edited by Rahel Wasserfall. Hanover, Mass.: University Press New England, 1999. Pages 23–39 and 255–261.

Nutton, Vivian. *Ancient Medicine.* London and New York: Routledge, 2004.

Oberhelman, Steven M., ed., *Dreams, Healing, and Medicine in Greece: From Antiquity to the Present.* New York: Routledge, 2016.

Preuss, Julius. *Medicine in the Bible and the Talmud.* Translated by F. Rosner. New York: Sanhedrin Press, 1978.

Safrai, Shmuel, ed., *Literature of the Sages—First Part: Oral Torah, Halakha, Mishna, Tosefta, Talmud, External Tractates.* Compendia Rerum Iudaicarum Ad Novum Testamentum II/3a. Assen: van Gorcum and Philadelphia: Fortress, 1987.

Scarborough, John. *Roman Medicine.* London: Camelot Press, 1969.

Strack, Hermann and Günter Stemberger. *Introduction to the Talmud and Midrash.* Translated by Markus Bockemuehl. Minneapolis: Fortress Press, 1996.

Zucconi, Laura M. "Medicine and Religion in Ancient Egypt," *Religion Compass* 1,1 (2007): 26–37.

The Experiments of Cleopatra:
Foreign, Gendered, and Empirical Knowledge in the Babylonian Talmud*

Shulamit Shinnar

1 Introduction

In both the Tosefta and the Babylonian Talmud tractate of Niddah, the rabbis recount a strange and horrifying tale of ancient medical experimentation on women. The story describes how, in ancient Egypt, Queen Cleopatra ordered that enslaved pregnant women be cut open in order to investigate the length of time required for a human embryo to develop fully. As a story that seems to describe ancient medical research, scholars have noted that it depicts individuals seeking empirical knowledge, that is, knowledge produced through observation.[1] Strikingly, however, the observation, in this case, is not a simple, passive act, but a graphically violent one: women's bodies are ripped apart in order to examine the embryos inside them. The story creates an intrinsic link between the pursuit of empirical knowledge about women's bodies with the brutality inflicted on women as part of the process of inquiry.[2] The story forces one to consider the people involved in empirical research—both those who observe and those who are observed—and the manner in which power differen-

* Thank you to the many people who have contributed to this paper: Thank you to Beth Berkowitz, in whose seminar on rabbinic narrative a version of this paper was first conceived. Thank you to Lennart Lehmhaus who organized the panel at the EAJS. Thank you to the anonymous reviewers and my colleague Sara Ronis whose feedback helped me refine my final version.
1 See for example: Meir Bar-Ilan, "Medicine in Eretz Israel During the First Centuries CE," *Cathedra* 91 (1989): 31–78; Madalina Vartejanu-Joubert, "The Right Type of Knowledge: Theory and Experience in Two Passages of the Babylonian Talmud," *Korot* 19 (2007): 161–180.
2 The parallels to modern examples of human experimentation have been noted by Tirzah Meacham who considered this story in relationship to contemporary examples of human experimentation, including the infamous Tuskegee experiment on African American men, as well as Nazi human experimentation. Tirzah Meacham, "Halakhic Limitations on the Use of Slaves in Physical Examinations," in *From Athens to Jerusalem: Medicine in Hellenized Jewish Lore and in Early Christian Literature* (eds. Samuel S. Kottek and Manfred Horstmanshoff; Rotterdam: Erasmus Publishing, 2000), 33–48. It might also recall the sordid roots of modern American gynecology in the experimentation on enslaved African-American women. Consider, for instance, the infamous experiments of Dr. James Marion Sims. For recent scholarship and bibliography, see: Deirdre Cooper Owens, *Medical Bondage: Race, Gender, and the Origins of American Gynecology* (Athens: The University of Georgia Press, 2017).

DOI: 10.13173/9783447108263.215

tials produced through gender, ethnicity, and class shape the production of empirical medical knowledge, an issue that remains continuingly relevant.

In rabbinic literature, the Cleopatra story becomes part of a broader discussion about rabbinic medical epistemology and the acceptable ways of producing knowledge about women's bodies, pregnancy, and fetal development. Notably, the Cleopatra story does not recount specific historical events of actual experiments, but it is a carefully crafted rabbinic narrative.[3] The story is tannaitic—produced by Sages between the first and second centuries CE in Greco-Roman Palestine—in origin, and the story draws on Greco-Roman medical traditions in order to depict these medical practices critically. The story also appears in the Babylonian Talmud, a text which is a composite of rabbinic traditions from the first through seventh centuries CE and whose anonymous redactors—known as the Stammaim or simply the Stam—lived in Babylonia between the fifth through seventh centuries CE, and edited, organized, and reshaped earlier rabbinic sources.[4] In a sugya (rabbinic textual unit) in b. Niddah 30b, the rabbis evaluate the Cleopatra story and other sources for their potential for producing knowledge about fetal development.

In this paper, I examine the production of the Cleopatra story in Greco-Roman Palestine and its later reception in the BT tractate Niddah as a case study through which to consider the conception of medical knowledge within rabbinic literature more broadly. The sugya in b. Niddah 30b is one of many passages in rabbinic literature in which the rabbis discuss topics that would be classified as "medical" in mod-

---

3   The historicity of this story has been the subject of much debate amongst scholars. Some previous studies of both rabbinic medicine and ancient medicine have treated the story as if it were a description of a historical event or have refuted its historicity. (See: Preuss, Bar-Ilan, and Meacham.) On the other hand, the historian of medicine Vivian Nutton sharply critiques these approaches and argues that there is no historic basis for Cleopatra performing experiments. Instead, he views these stories as part of the mythic description of Cleopatra as a physician. More recent works, including Rivka Ulmer's study of the story, have moved away from the debate over the historicity of the story to explore the construction of these mythic narratives. My approach follows this recent scholarship. See: Julius Preuss, *Biblical and Talmudic Medicine*, (trans. Fred Rosner; Northvale: Jason Aronson Inc., 1993), 41–45; Bar-Ilan, "Medicine in Eretz Israel During the First Centuries CE"; Shlomo Naeh, "On Two Hippocratic Concepts in Rabbinic Literature," *Tarbiz* 66, 2 (1997): 169–185; Meacham, "Halakhic Limitations on the Use of Slaves in Physical Examinations," 42–43; Vivian Nutton, "From Athens to Jerusalem: Medicine in Hellenized Jewish Lore and in Early Christian Literature (Review)," *Bulletin of the History of Medicine* 75,4 (2001): 787–788; Vartejanu-Joubert, "The Right Type of Knowledge: Theory and Experience in Two Passages of the Babylonian Talmud"; Rivka Ulmer, *Egyptian Cultural Icons in Midrash* (Berlin: Walter de Gruyter, 2009), 238–241; Vivian Nutton, *Ancient Medicine*, 2nd ed. (Milton: Routledge, 2013), 380 n. 334; Joseph Geiger, "Cleopatra the Physician," *Cathedra* 92 (1999): 193–198; Joseph Geiger, "Cleopatra the Physician," *Zutot: Perspectives on Jewish Culture* 1,1 (2001): 28–32.

4   Hereafter I may employ the following abbreviations: "Mishnah" as "m."; "Tosefta" as "t."; "Yerushalmi" as "y."; "Bavli" as "b."; "Palestinian Talmud" as "PT."; "Babylonian Talmud" as "BT." The BT includes tannaitic sources, as well sources from Palestinian and Babylonian *Amoraim*, sages who lived in the third through fifth centuries CE in Palestine and Babylonia, and Stammaitic sources.

ern contexts. In these passages, the rabbis describe anatomical features of the human body, detail physiological functions, and prescribe treatments for the maintenance of one's health. In the tractate of Niddah, through the discussions of ritual purity law, the rabbis display an interest in topics now associated with the fields of gynecology and obstetrics, namely the physiology of women, diseases particular to women, pregnancy, fetal development, and complications associated with pregnancy such as miscarriage.[5] Within the broader context of these rabbinic "medical" texts, the sugya in b. Niddah 30b stands out for the insight that it offers into the theoretical framework underlying rabbinic medical epistemology. Indeed, the sugya itself raises questions regarding the basis of the rabbis' factual assertions about the physiology of the human body.

Recent scholarship has explored the rabbis' use of multiple sources when adjudicating rabbinic law, including interpretations of scripture, received traditions, and legal reasoning.[6] Building on this scholarship, here, I examine the processes by which the rabbis make claims about the human body. For instance, on what sources of knowledge did the rabbis rely? Did they consult the Bible or rabbinic law? Or, did they look to their own physical experiences? To the scientific traditions and writings of the surrounding cultures? And, of the sources available to them, did they privilege one source of knowledge over another? These issues are of particular interest with respect to the knowledge of women's bodies in rabbinic literature because they are largely outside the embodied personal experience of rabbis as men. The sugya in b. Niddah 30b engages with these questions as the rabbis debate the appropriate sources of knowledge about fetal development. At issue is the acceptability of purity laws and

---

5   Fonrobert's work on menstrual purity opened up the examination of ritual purity law as part of the production of rabbinic medical knowledge. In this vein, work by Balberg, Kessler, and Neis have further explored the rabbinic categories relating to embryology and fetal development. Lepicard, Kiperwasser, and Kottek also study rabbinic embryology. F. Gary Cunningham et al., *Williams Obstetrics, 25e* (New York: McGraw Hill Medical Companies, 2018). Charlotte Elisheva Fonrobert, *Menstrual Purity: Rabbinic and Christian Reconstructions of Biblical Gender* (Stanford: Stanford University Press, 2000); Mira Balberg, *Purity, Body, and Self in Early Rabbinic Literature* (Berkeley: University of California Press, 2014); Gwynn Kessler, *Conceiving Israel: The Fetus in Rabbinic Narratives* (Philadelphia: University of Pennsylvania Press, 2009); Rachel Rafael Neis, "The Reproduction of Species: Humans, Animals and Species Nonconformity in Early Rabbinic Science," *Jewish Studies Quarterly* 24,4 (2017): 434–451; Etienne Lepicard, "The Embryo in Ancient Rabbinic Literature: Between Religious Law and Didactic Narratives: An Interpretive Essay," *History and Philosophy of the Life Sciences* 32,1 (2010): 21–41; Reuven Kiperwasser, "'Three Partners in a Person' The Genesis and Development of Embryological Theory in Biblical and Rabbinic Judaism," *Lectio Difficilior* (2009): 1–37; Samuel S. Kottek, "Embryology in Talmudic and Midrashic Literature," *Journal of the History of Biology* 14, (1981): 299–315.

6   Some of the recent scholarship exploring these questions in rabbinic epistemology includes: Tzvi Novick, "A Lot of Learning Is a Dangerous Thing: On the Structure of Rabbinic Expertise in the Bavli," *Hebrew Union College Annual* 78 (2007): 91–107; Chaya T. Halberstam, *Law and Truth in Biblical and Rabbinic Literature* (Bloomington: Indiana University Press, 2009); Jenny R. Labendz, *Socratic Torah: Non-Jews in Rabbinic Intellectual Culture* (New York: Oxford University Press, 2013), 67–80; Christine Hayes, *What's Divine about Divine Law?: Early Perspectives* (Princeton: Princeton University Press, 2015); Ayelet Hoffmann Libson, *Law and Self-Knowledge in the Talmud* (Cambridge: Cambridge University Press, 2018).

biblical texts—sources commonly used as the basis for the adjudication of rabbinic law—as well as the Cleopatra story as potential sources for medical knowledge.

Drawing on methodologies from the history of science and the study of gender in ancient medicine and rabbinic literature, I explore the rabbis' understanding of the production of medical knowledge and of empiricism more generally. I show that, in this sugya, the rabbis display skepticism toward the reliability of empirical knowledge, which is discussed explicitly within the rabbinic debate and heightened through various literary and rhetorical devices. At the same time, however, the text betrays an unwillingness to use traditional sources used within rabbinic texts, such as interpretations of biblical texts and rabbinic legal precedent, as a basis for medical knowledge. Ultimately, the conclusion reached in the sugya is that, despite the numerous concerns expressed in the text regarding the empirical sources, these sources remain a problematic, but viable basis for medical facts.[7]

I argue that fundamental to the rabbinic conception of and skepticism toward empiricism found within the sugya is a concern with the embodied nature of empirical knowledge. For the rabbis, the trustworthiness of the person who does the observing and of the person whose body is observed must be taken into consideration when evaluating the reliability of observations of the human body. Observations made by or about persons whom the rabbis deem as less trustworthy may be less reliable. Indeed, the rabbinic skepticism regarding the reliability of the results of the Cleopatra experiments is rooted in the rabbis' biases toward the characters involved in the story, namely non-Jews, women, and enslaved persons.

In what follows, I first introduce the theoretical frameworks from the history of science and gender studies that I employ and the halakhic (Jewish legal) framework that underlies the rabbinic discussion of fetal development. I next examine the Cleopatra story in the context of ancient Greco-Roman medical traditions. The bulk of the paper is then devoted to a diachronic analysis of the sugya in b. Niddah 30b, in which I examine the Stam's reworking of earlier sources, highlighting the later editors' particular concerns regarding gender and ethnicity in producing medical knowledge.[8]

---

7 For studies that also examine "observations" and the rabbinic attitude and skepticism toward them, see: Vartejanu-Joubert, "The Right Type of Knowledge: Theory and Experience in Two Passages of the Babylonian Talmud"; Halberstam, *Law and Truth in Biblical and Rabbinic Literature*; Richard Kalmin, "Observation in Rabbinic Literature of Late Antiquity," in *The Faces of Torah: Studies in the Texts and Contexts of Ancient Judaism in Honor of Steven Fraade* (eds. Michal Bar Asher Siegal et al.; Göttingen: Vandenhoeck & Ruprecht, 2017), 359–383.

8 The subject of stammaitic redaction has been the focus of many recent studies. Following Friedman and Rubenstein, in this article I focus on the creative hand of the stammaitic redactor. For a review of recent scholarship, see Moulie Vidas's work. Shamma Friedman, "A Critical Study of Yevamot X with a Methodological Introduction," in *Texts and Studies: Analecta Judaica I* (ed. Haim Zalman Dimitrovsky; New York: Jewish Theological Seminary of America, 1977); Jeffrey L. Rubenstein, "Criteria of Stammaitic Intervention in Aggada," in *Creation and Composition: The Contribution of the Bavli Redactors (Stammaim) to the Aggada* (ed. Jeffrey L. Rubenstein; Tübingen: Mohr Siebeck, 2005), 275–441; Moulie Vidas, *Tradition and the Formation of the Talmud* (Oxford: Princeton University Press, 2014), 1–20.

1.1 Methodology

In examining rabbinic attitudes toward empiricism, I follow the approach of historians of science who have argued that the modern processes of scientific fact-making are historically contingent phenomena. As Pamela Smith writes, "since the publication of Thomas Kuhn's *The Structure of Scientific Revolutions* [in 1962], historians of science have argued that natural knowledge and the methods of obtaining it are contingent upon and constructed within particular communities and intellectual structures." Some scholarship on the Cleopatra story has attributed its reference to empiricism to the "advanced" nature of rabbinic medical knowledge at the time, arguing either that the rabbis drew on the "leading" medical traditions of the ancient world or that the traditions on which the rabbis drew prefigured modern medical empiricism.[9] In this paper's investigation of rabbinic medical epistemology, however, I am not interested in how the rabbis may have prefigured modern medicine, but rather in the particularities of how the rabbis themselves understood medical knowledge and empiricism.[10]

Additionally, my analysis draws on existing scholarship from the study of gender in ancient medicine and rabbinic purity law. In the study of ancient medicine, scholars including Aline Rousselle, Lesley Dean-Jones, Helen King, and Rebecca Flemming have shown that ancient medical texts written by male authors often portray male doctors as authorities over female medical practitioners and female patients, even though the historical realities of these relationships may have been quite different.[11]

---

9 Bar-Ilan, "Medicine in Eretz Israel During the First Centuries CE"; Preuss, *Biblical and Talmudic Medicine*, 41–45.

10 Thomas S. Kuhn, *The Structure of Scientific Revolutions* (Chicago, IL: University of Chicago Press, 1996); Pamela Smith, "Science," in *A Concise Companion to History* (ed. Ulinka Rublack; Oxford: Oxford University Press, 2011), 268–297, here: 271–272. My discussion of the social dimension of empiricism and medical epistemology has been shaped by the scholarship of Steven Shapin. Shapin's focus on the importance of trust for understanding cultures of scientific knowledge production in the early modern period is fundamental to my understanding of how rabbinic biases towards foreigners, women, and enslaved persons frames rabbinic medical epistemological discourse. See Steven Shapin, *A Social History of Truth: Civility and Science in Seventeenth-Century England* (Chicago: University of Chicago Press, 1994), xxv–xxvi. For further exploration of the implications of Shapin's claims for the study of rabbinic medical epistemology, see Shulamit Shinnar, "'The Best of Doctors Go to Hell': Rabbinic Medical Culture in Late Antiquity (200–600 CE)" (Ph.D. Dissertation, Columbia University, 2019).

11 The body of literature on ancient gynecology is extensive. Some of the key pieces of scholarship include: Aline Rousselle, *Porneia: On Desire and the Body in Antiquity* (trans. Felicia Pheasant; Cambridge, MA: Blackwell, 1993); Lesley Dean-Jones, *Women's Bodies in Classical Greek Science* (New York: Oxford University Press, 1994); Lesley Dean-Jones, "Autopsia, Historia and What Women Know: The Authority of Women in Hippocratic Gynaecology," in *Knowledge and the Scholarly Medical Traditions* (ed. Don Bates; Cambridge: Cambridge University Press, 1995), 41–59; Helen King, *Hippocrates' Woman: Reading the Female Body in Ancient Greece* (New York: Routledge, 1998); Ann E. Hanson, "The Medical Writer's Woman," in *Before Sexuality: The Construction of Erotic Experience in the Ancient Greek World* (eds. David M. Halperin, John J. Winkler, and Froma I. Zeitlin; Princeton: Princeton University Press, 1990), 309–338; Rebecca Flemming, *Medicine and the Making of Roman Women: Gender, Nature, and Authority from Celsus to Galen* (Oxford: Oxford University Press, 2000); Fonrobert, *Menstrual Purity*.

Similarly, scholars such as Charlotte Fonrobert, Mira Balberg, Gwynn Kessler, Rachel Rafael Neis, and Chaya Halberstam have explored how rabbinic ritual law constructs the rabbis as authorities over women's bodies. From menstruation to pregnancy, the rabbis create taxonomies to describe relevant anatomy and physiology and legislate practices to govern these aspects of a woman's daily life. In my examination of rabbinic medical epistemology, I build on this scholarship to consider the ways in which rabbinic texts undermine women's expertise and knowledge of their own bodies.[12]

1.2 Halakhic background

Before I examine the rabbinic discussion of fetal development in b. Niddah 30b, it is important to clarify the specific halakhic framework that underlies this text. In particular, this sugya's discussion of fetal development takes place in the context of a technical issue pertaining to the ritual purity laws that govern menstruation and birth. Based on their interpretations of various biblical passages, the rabbis assert that certain types of vaginal secretions render women impure, including menstrual blood, vaginal discharge resulting from illness, and tissues relating to miscarriage.[13] These various types of secretions result in different fixed periods of impurity. For example, according to Leviticus 15, a menstruating woman remains impure for seven days.[14] Childbirth also renders a woman impure; Leviticus 12 states that a woman remains impure for forty days after giving birth to a male baby and eighty days after giving birth to a female baby.[15] In any case, for the rabbis, the exact nature of either

---

12 Fonrobert, *Menstrual Purity*; Mira Balberg, "Rabbinic Authority, Medical Rhetoric, and Body Hermeneutics in Mishnah Nega'im," *AJS Review* 35,2 (November 2011): 323–346; Balberg, *Purity, Body, and Self*; Kessler, *Conceiving Israel*; Halberstam, *Law and Truth in Biblical and Rabbinic Literature*; R. Neis, *The Sense of Sight in Rabbinic Culture: Jewish Ways of Seeing in Late Antiquity* (New York: Cambridge University Press, 2013); Neis, "The Reproduction of Species"; Rachel Rafael Neis, "Fetus, Flesh, Food: Generating Bodies of Knowledge in Rabbinic Science," *Journal of Ancient Judaism* 10,2 (2019): 181–210.

13 For an introduction to the laws of Niddah see: Tirzah Meacham, "An Abbreviated History of the Development of the Jewish Menstrual Laws," in *Women and Water: Menstruation in Jewish Life and Law* (ed. Rahel R. Wasserfall; Hanover: University Press of New England, 1999), 23–39; Fonrobert, *Menstrual Purity*.

14 Leviticus 15:19.

15 The numbers of days associated with the different periods in which a woman has the status of being impure are in fact more complicated, but as the various states of impurity or purity are not the focus of this paper, I have simplified it. Leviticus 12 states: "When a woman at childbirth bears a male, she shall be impure seven days; she shall be impure as at the time of her menstrual infirmity (*kidemei niddah*) …And she shall remain in a state of blood purification (*demei taharah*) for thirty-three days: she shall not touch any consecrated thing, nor enter the sanctuary until her period of purification is complete. If she bears a female, she shall be impure two weeks as during her menstruation, and she shall remain in a state of blood purification for sixty-six days." The passage distinguishes two separate states. First, immediately following giving birth a woman becomes impure as if she were in niddah. Following the first state, even though she may still be bleeding, the blood is considered pure; she is in a period of *demei taharah*. The text itself doesn't clarify the exact difference between *demei taharah* and the niddah state. And, there is

a woman's vaginal discharge or the sex of her infant must be ascertained in order to determine her ritual status.[16]

The sugya in b. Niddah 30b deals with miscarriage, a legal case that is not directly addressed in the Bible. Thus, in rabbinic law, the ritual status of a woman who miscarries is unclear. It could be argued that the ritual status of such a woman is similar to either that of a woman who has given birth or that of a menstruant. Alternatively, it might be a different legal case entirely.

According to the Mishnah, the legal status of a woman who miscarries depends on the point during pregnancy at which a miscarriage occurs. If a woman miscarries before her embryo fully develops,[17] her purity status does not change. However, if a woman miscarries after the embryo fully develops, she is treated as if she has just given birth, and she becomes impure. Since a woman's purity status after a miscarriage is contingent on the extent to which the embryo has developed at the time of the miscarriage, the Mishnah debates at what stage during pregnancy an embryo is considered fully developed.

1 A woman who miscarries[18] on the fortieth day is not suspected of having a *valad* (developed fetus.)[19] [However, if a woman miscarries] on the forty-first day, she remains [in the period of impurity] dictated by the birth of a boy, the birth of a girl, and menstruation.[20]

2 R. Ishmael says, if a woman miscarries on the forty-first day, she remains [in the period of impurity dictated by] the birth of a boy and menstruation. [If a woman

---

some debate as to what legal strictures apply to a woman in the different states. For further discussion see: Fonrobert, *Menstrual Purity*, 15–39.

16 To consider the spectrum of gender identities within rabbinic literature, see Charlotte Elisheva Fonrobert, "Regulating the Human Body: Rabbinic Legal Discourse and the Making of Jewish Gender," in *The Cambridge Companion to the Talmud and Rabbinic Literature* (eds. Charlotte Fonrobert and Martin S. Jaffee; Cambridge: Cambridge University Press, 2007), 270–294.

17 I discuss what is meant by "full developed" in my discussion of the Mishnah.

18 המפלת, literally "the one who dropped" or "the one who excreted."

19 The word used is ולד. It is unclear exactly how to translate this term. Two possibilities include the term embryo or fetus. In the fortieth day of pregnancy, from the perspective of modern embryology, it would still be considered an embryo. However, *valad* seems to imply that it is more fully formed and if one were to miscarry it is as if one gave birth to a completely formed person. Thus, I chose to translate it as "fetus," as the term carries more of that implication. See Gwynn Kessler's discussion of the challenges of using modern terminology to discuss rabbinic texts and my longer discussion below. Kessler, *Conceiving Israel*, 15–19.

20 "and menstruation" follows the Kaufman manuscript and the Vilna edition of the Bavli. Meacham's critical edition deletes this word. As the focus of this paper is the Bavli's reading of the Mishnah, I have followed the Kaufman version as the b. sugya makes the most sense with these words. "MS A50, Kaufman Manuscript of the Mishnah," in *David Kaufman and His Collection of Medieval Hebrew Manuscripts in the Oriental Collection of the Library of the Hungarian Academy of Sciences* (eds. David Kaufman, Tamás Sajó, and Kinga Dévényi; Budapest: Library of the Hungarian Academy of Sciences, 2008), 271v [cited 30 December 2018]. Online: http://kaufmann.mtak.hu/en/ms50/ms50-coll1.htm; Tirzah Meacham, "Mishnah Tractate Niddah with Introduction: A Critical Edition with Notes on Variants, Commentary, Redaction and Chapters in Legal History and Realia," vol. II (Ph.D. Dissertation, Hebrew University, 1989), 32–34.

miscarries] on the eighty-first day, she remains [in the period of impurity dictated] by the birth of a boy, the birth of a girl, and menstruation. This is because a male was finished [being developed] on the forty-first day and the female was [finished being developed] on the eighty-first.

3   And, the Sages say that the formation[21] of both a male and female are the same and occur on the forty-first day (m. Niddah 3:7).[22]

In the Mishnah, both the Sages and R. Ishmael assume that the law distinguishes two periods during pregnancy: before an embryo becomes a *valad* and afterwards. The implication is that, once the embryo reaches this stage, it is comparable, at least to some degree, to a child.[23] Precisely what characterizes the stage of being a *valad*, however, is unclear. The text here uses the term "finished," suggesting that at this stage, the *valad* is considered to be fully developed in some sense. Perhaps, as discussed elsewhere in m. Niddah, becoming a *valad* or being "fully developed" means acquiring a human appearance.[24] In any case, from the perspective of purity law, if a woman miscarries after the embryo has reached the stage of being a *valad*, the miscarriage is considered analogous to giving birth, and the woman becomes impure. However, R. Ishmael and the Sages disagree about the length of time required for an embryo to develop fully and whether male and female embryos develop at the same rate.

It is useful to note that the rabbinic conception of the stages of fetal development does not map on to that of modern western medicine.[25] The most obvious difference

---

21 "בריית". Alternatively, may be translated "creation." Another word that may also mean formation/creation used later is "יצירה."

22 All translations of rabbinic texts are my own. The text of the Mishnah follows the Kaufman manuscript with reference to the text in the Vilna edition of the Bavli and Tirzah Meacham's critical edition of the m. Niddah. Translation of the Mishnah is with reference to Herbert Danby's critical translation with my own adaptations. All numbered and lettered sections in rabbinic texts are my own and there for later reference. Texts in brackets are added for clarification. Text in parentheses further explain the terminology used in the text. Ms. A50 Kaufmann, 271v; Meacham, "Mishnah Tractate Niddah," 33; Herbert Danby, *The Mishnah* (Oxford: The Clarendon Press, 1933).

23 Within rabbinic literature, even though the parturiency of a *valad* is treated as akin to giving birth to a live child for the sake of purity law, the *valad* does not seem to have the status of a live child. As Mira Balberg argues that it is the "rabbinic view that fetuses are not fully alive creatures, and thus not full persons." Acknowledging Gwynn Kessler's analysis that within midrashic literature fetuses are considered to be part of the Israelite community, Balberg argues that the halakhic sources do not share the same view. Cf. Balberg, *Purity, Body, and Self*, 110–115, 219–221; Kessler, *Conceiving Israel*.

24 M. Niddah 3:2 "The Sages say: What does not have a human form is not accounted a *valad*." For further discussion, see Balberg, *Purity, Body, and Self*, 110–115.

25 Following Gwynn Kessler, I emphasize the difference between the rabbinic texts and modern medical models of embryology. Recognizing the ways in which this sugya and other rabbinic texts about the fetus are used in the context of modern abortion debates, it is useful to keep in mind Kessler's comment that "reading rabbinic narratives about fetuses in light of contemporary abortion debates is a kind of colonization." See Kessler, *Conceiving Israel*, 18–20, esp. 19. For an analysis of how contemporary Jewish law draws on rabbinic sources to frame issues of

between the rabbinic and modern models is R. Ishmael's position that male and female fetuses develop at radically different rates.[26] Yet, even the Sages' position that both male and female embryos become fully developed in forty-one days does not reflect modern embryological developmental milestones or models. The contemporary field of embryology divides the prenatal stages of human development into embryonic and fetal periods. The most obvious visual changes of prenatal development occur during the embryonic period, which begins with fertilization and ends on the fifty-sixth day (eighth week) of pregnancy. The transformation from embryo to fetus on the fifty-seventh day (ninth week) reflects the facts that all of the major organ systems have started to develop and that it has acquired a distinctly human appearance. Other significant stages include the first trimester, which ends on the eighty-fourth day (twelfth week) of pregnancy, and fetal viability, which is defined by the fetus' ability to survive outside the uterus. In modern first-world countries, viability may happen as early as twenty-four weeks.[27]

If we consider the stages of fetal development presented in the rabbinic text from the perspective of modern embryology, on the forty-first day, the *valad* is still in the embryonic stage of development; it is neither yet a fetus by modern definitions nor is it viable. Overall, the rabbis' claim that the *valad* is "finished" or, in some sense, "fully developed" should be understood as distinct from modern models for the stages of fetal development.[28] As other scholars have done, I translate *valad* as "fetus," to better

---

fertility, pregnancy, and abortion, see: Ronit Irshai, *Fertility and Jewish Law: Feminist Perspectives on Orthodox Responsa Literature* (Waltham: Brandeis University Press, 2012).

26 Thank you to Sasha Parets for consulting on and recommending resources for my discussion of modern embryology. See the following reference for the development stages for male, female, and intersex embryos: Keith L. Moore, T.V.N. Persaud, and Mark G. Torchia, *The Developing Human: Clinically Oriented Embryology*, 11th Edition. (Edinburgh: Elsevier, 2020), 223–262. While there are differences in the development of male and female embryos, for example in terms of fetal length, they are not major. Cf. Zoe A. Broere-Brown et al., "Sex-Specific Differences in Fetal and Infant Growth Patterns: A Prospective Population-Based Cohort Study," *Biology of Sex Differences* 7,1 (2016): 65.

27 The first trimester spans the embryonic period and the early stages of fetal development. By the end of the first trimester all major systems have developed, including the differentiation of sexual organs. The placement of fetal viability at twenty-four weeks does not speak to the low survival rates associated with live births at this early stage of pregnancy. Moore, Persaud, and Torchia, *The Developing Human*, 1–9, 65–84, 85–98; Hamisu M. Salihu et al., "Survival of Pre-Viable Preterm Infants in the United States: A Systematic Review and Meta-Analysis," *Seminars in Perinatology* 37,6, Periviable Birth: Obstetric and Neonatal Management and Counseling Issues Part 1 (2013): 389–400.

28 At day forty-one, which is during the sixth week of development, the embryo does have an increasingly human appearance. At this point, the embryo is characterized by a C-shaped curve, the early formation of upper and lower limbs and digits as well as the eyes and the beginnings of ears. As seen in m. Niddah 3:2, the rabbis view day forty-one or being a *valad* having a human appearance. However, modern embryology describes fetuses as opposed to embryos as being defined by their human appearance. See modern visualizations and descriptions of the different stages of fetal development in: Moore, Persaud, and Torchia, *The Developing Human*, 1–2, 65–84.

capture the rabbinic view that the *valad* is, in some sense, fully developed, despite the fact that it does not correspond to modern medical definitions of the term.[29]

The rabbinic conceptions of embryology are better situated in Greco-Roman medical literature, where similar issues of fetal development are debated. For example, Aristotle marked an important stage in fetal development at forty days for a male embryo and ninety days for a female embryo, figures that are similar to those in R. Ishmael's opinion. The Mishnaic dispute should be understood in the context of this broader ancient discourse on fetal development.[30]

2 Cleopatra's experiments—a detailed analysis

Looking at the Mishnah's discussion, it provides no justification for either R. Ishmael's or the Sages' views regarding the rate of fetal development. The theoretical bases for their differing positions are the subject of the Talmudic debate in b. Niddah 30b. It is in the context of exploring potential sources for knowledge about fetal development that the sugya raises the story of Cleopatra's experiments. The story appears in two slightly different versions within the sugya and in a third version within the Tosefta. The version in the Tosefta states:

> R. Ishmael said: A story is told about Cleopatra,[31] the Queen of Alexandria who brought[32] her slaves,[33] who were sentenced to death by royal decree.[34] And she cut them open,[35] and it was found that the male [fetus] was completely de-

---

29 See Kessler's discussion of the modern historiography of the terms embryo and fetus and of the challenges associated with discussing rabbinic language using modern medical terms. Kessler, *Conceiving Israel*, 15–20.

30 Aristotle, *History of Animals* 7:3 in Aristotle, *History of Animals, Volume III: Books 7–10* (trans. David M. Balme; Loeb Classical Library 439; Cambridge: Harvard University Press, 1991), 434–435. See also: Bar-Ilan, "Medicine in Eretz Israel During the First Centuries CE"; Gwynn Kessler, *"The God of Small Things: The Fetus and Its Development in Palestinian Aggadic Literature"* (Ph.D. Dissertation, The Jewish Theological Seminary, 2001), 54–55. Marten Stol, *Birth in Babylonia and the Bible: Its Mediterranean Setting* (Groningen: Styx, 2000), 17–20.

31 In the text of the Tosefta the word is גלפטרה, which is most likely another rendition of Cleopatra. The epithet "Queen of Alexandria" supports this interpretation.

32 Vienna manuscript and Venice print edition attest to the word "שהביאה" versus Zuckermandel's "שהביא." Lieberman suggests the text of this sentence is corrupted here. *MS. Vienna Codex Heb. 20, Catalogue Schwarz No. 46* (Vienna: Austrian National Library in Vienna), 304r; "Tosefta Niddah," in *Alfasi's Compendium to the Talmud, Vol II.* (Venice: Bamberger, 1521), 773b; Saul Lieberman, *Tosefet Rishonim: Perush Meyusad ʿal Kitve Yad Ha-Tosefta Ve-Sifre Rishonim u-Midrashim Be-Khitve Yad u-Defusim Yeshanim*, vol. 3 (Jerusalem: Bamberger and Wahrman, 1937), 268; Moses Samuel Zuckermandel, *Tosefta: ʿal Pi Kitvei Yad Erfurṭ u-Viyenah, ʿim Marʾeh Meḳomot ve-Ḥilufei Girsáot u-Maftehot* (Jerusalem: Sifrei Wahrman, 1970).

33 While in my own analysis I refer to "enslaved persons," in my translations I use "slave" as I think it better captures the meaning of the text. Thank you to Sara Ronis and her suggestion to incorporate theoretical critiques from the modern history of slavery into this paper.

34 "שנתחייבו מיתה למלך"—"were obligated in death for the king." In the Bavli, "הריגה למלכות."

35 Ms. Vienna—"וקרעתה." Zuckermandel and the Venice print edition "וקרעתן." Lieberman suggests the text of this sentence is corrupted. The text might also be rendered "they were cut." For

veloped after forty-one days and the female [fetus] was completely developed[36] after eighty-one [days]. They said to him: one does not bring a proof from here. And from where does one bring proof? From one who came to her husband first or from one whose husband had come back from abroad (t. Niddah 4:17).[37]

This brief and enigmatic anecdote recounts how Cleopatra initiated a research project using enslaved pregnant women to study the rate of fetal development. This story supplies very few details, and the events depicted remain opaque. The verb describing the procedures performed on these women found in the Tosefta—"*qara*"—"cut open"— only hints at the violence enacted on the enslaved women that would have been necessary to examine the embryos within their bodies. As Rivka Ulmer emphasizes, the two versions in the BT are even less clear as the text uses the euphemism "*badak*"—"inspected" to cloak the violence that surely such procedures would have entailed.[38]

Although the story is short, a close analysis reveals a carefully crafted narrative whose details would have resonated with late antique and rabbinic audiences in specific ways.[39] The Tosefta's version attests to the story's origins in Roman Palestine and its engagement with Greco-Roman medical traditions. In the transmission of the story to Sassanian Babylonia, it is unclear if details specific to Greco-Roman medicine would have resonated to the same extent in its reception in the BT. In any case, whether looking at the story in the context of Greco-Roman medicine or in the context of the broader corpus of rabbinic literature, the narrative places a striking emphasis on the foreignness and gendered nature of these experiments. The story underscores that the performers of these experiments are part of a non-rabbinic medical tradition and hints at the controversial nature of these experiments. It also highlights the rabbinic concern that the production of medical knowledge about the female body and reproduction must rely, to some extent, on the experiences of women, which are outside the personal embodied experiences of the rabbis. Ultimately, every detail of the tannaitic story serves to construct a portrait of the ancient medical traditions represented by these experiments as alien and non-rabbinic.[40]

---

references, see note 32 above. Note the difference in the language used in the Bavli version of the story.

36 The word used is נגמר which literally means "finished." Note the difference in terminology for a completely developed fetus. The Tosefta refers to an embryo being *nigmar* whereas the Babylonian Talmud refers to a *valad*.

37 My translation of the Tosefta follows the text in the Zuckermandel edition, with emendations based on Lieberman's commentary in *Tosefet Rishonim* and reference to the ms. Erfurt 773b, ms. Vienna 304r, and the Bamberger Venice 1521 print edition. For references, see note 32 above.

38 Ulmer highlights the differences between the rhetorical impact of the Tosefta as opposed to the BT's word selection. Ulmer, *Egyptian Cultural Icons in Midrash*, 238–243.

39 For further discussion of the narrativity of tannaitic sources, see: Moshe Simon-Shoshan, *Stories of the Law: Narrative Discourse and the Construction of Authority in the Mishnah* (New York: Oxford University Press, 2012).

40 Situating the story contextually is difficult because it is transmitted from Roman Palestine to the rabbinic community in Sassanian Babylonia. Tannaitic in origin, the Tosefta's version emerged within the framework of Greco-Roman medical traditions. When transmitted to Sas-

For example, the specific narrative details connect the story directly to Greco-Roman medical practices and academic centers. The figure of Queen Cleopatra is especially significant because, in antiquity, she was associated with medicine and gynecology, possibly due to the fact that there was a medical practitioner of the same name who lived sometime in the first few centuries CE. Having become associated with the study of women's medicine, by late antiquity, treatises on gynecology (as well as on cosmetics) were attributed to her. The rabbinic story thus participates in constructing the myth of Queen Cleopatra as an expert on women's health.[41]

Furthermore, the story locates the experiments in Egypt in the city of Alexandria, a location considered central to the study of medicine in the ancient world. Although dissection and vivisection of the human body were generally considered taboo in antiquity, one of the few known exceptions was Egypt in the Hellenistic era, where for a brief period in the third century BCE, dissections and possibly vivisections of humans were carried out in Alexandria by the anatomists Herophilus and Erasistratus. Like the research carried out by these historical figures, Cleopatra's experiments, as described in the narrative, are "empirical" in the sense that their aim sought to understand fetal development through anatomical dissection.[42] While the events of the experiments described in the rabbinic story are not historically accurate, the text makes it clear that the rabbis are not just discussing theoretical "foreign" medical traditions. Rather, the rabbis are sufficiently familiar with Greco-Roman medicine to locate its academic center and to associate Alexandrian medicine with the practices of dissection and vivisection.

In the transmission from Greco-Roman Palestine to Sassanian Babylonia and its reception in the BT, the story retains its stress on the foreignness of Cleopatra. The figure of Cleopatra appears only a few times in the corpus of rabbinic literature, but, in these instances, she is presented as a polemical interlocutor of the rabbis. In b. San-

---

sanian Babylonia, it is unclear if the original connotations of some of the details would have been retained or not. See my discussion later on.

41 Galen mentions Cleopatra as the name of a physician and attributes a work on cosmetics to Queen Cleopatra. And, later gynecological works were attributed to Queen Cleopatra. These included the Latin text entitled "Cleopatra's Gynecology" which was composed in or later than the fourth century CE and became popular in the later Middle Ages. Additionally, stories of Cleopatra's cruelty toward enslaved women and condemned criminals—including testing poison on them—circulated in the second century CE. Ulmer alludes to some of these traditions. Cf. Ulmer, *Egyptian Cultural Icons in Midrash*, 238–239. See also Nutton, *Ancient Medicine*, 159, 196; King, *Hippocrates' Woman: Reading the Female Body in Ancient Greece*, 185–186.; Monica Green, "The Transmission of Ancient Theories of Female Physiology and Disease through the Early Middle Ages" (Diss., Princeton University, 1985). John Scarborough, "Pharmacology and Toxicology at the Court of Cleopatra VII: Traces of Three Physicians," in *Herbs and Healers from the Ancient Mediterranean through the Medieval West* (ed. Anne Van Arsdall and Timothy Graham; Farnham: Ashgate, 2012), 7–18; Geiger, "Cleopatra the Physician."

42 There is an extensive body of literature that engages with the dissection of humans in Alexandria. For references see Heinrich Von Staden, *Herophilus: The Art of Medicine in Early Alexandria: Edition, Translation, and Essays* (Cambridge: Cambridge University Press, 1989); Nutton, *Ancient Medicine*, 130–141.

hedrin, for example, she appears alongside Romans and sectarians in a debate with the Sages over theories about the resurrection of the dead. Thus, in the BT, Cleopatra stands in the company of other polemical groups whom the rabbis see in opposition to themselves. Read in the context of the Bavli, the fact that Cleopatra directs the experiments would also have characterized the knowledge produced as foreign, polemical, and other.[43]

Another aspect of the narrative that characterizes the experiments as strange and foreign is their unethical nature. As Tirzah Meacham points out, for the modern reader, the story evokes horror at the notion of torture performed for the sake of medical inquiry.[44] This sentiment was also shared by some in antiquity, as the writings of late antique Christian authors criticize the methods employed by the aforementioned anatomists of Alexandria. For example, Tertullian, writing in the second or third century CE, described Herophilus as "the butcher who cut up innumerable persons in order to examine nature," and generally excoriated the practice of vivisection. On the other hand, other ancient authors defended the Herophilean vivisections as a necessary evil.[45] While the ethics of Cleopatra's experiments are not directly addressed in either the story or the rabbinic discussions of it, the language that the rabbis used to describe these experiments gestures toward the late antique controversy over human experimentation and, perhaps, subtly questions the morality of such practices.

The detail in the rabbinic narrative that most strikingly recalls the late-antique controversy over human dissection is that the enslaved women victims were criminals condemned to death. Various late antique authors who defended Herophilus' practice of human experimentation specifically referenced the fact that Herophilus' subjects were condemned criminals and justified their treatment on these grounds. Celsus, the first century CE author of the popular medical work *De Medicina*, defended the Herophilean vivisections as necessary in order to understand the internal workings of the human body. He argued that it is not, "as most people say, cruel that in the execution of criminals, and but a few of them, we should seek remedies for innocent people of all future ages." Similarly, pseudo-Eustathius described the dissection of criminals as necessary for the good of mankind.[46] Therefore, despite the absence of any direct

---

43 Cf. b. Sanhedrin 90b. To consider the implication for the representation of "others" in rabbinic literature and in this sugya specifically, see Christine Hayes, "Displaced Self-Perceptions: The Deployment of Minim and Romans in Bavli Sanhedrin 90b–91a," in *Religious and Ethnic Communities in Later Roman Palestine* (ed. Hayim Lapin; Potomac: University Press of Maryland, 1998), 249–289; Richard Kalmin, "Christians and Heretics in Rabbinic Literature of Late Antiquity," *The Harvard Theological Review* 87,2 (1994): 155–169; Geiger, "Cleopatra the Physician."

44 Meacham, "Halakhic Limitations on the Use of Slaves in Physical Examinations."

45 Tertullian, De Anima 10.4. Translation from: Von Staden, *Herophilus*, 187–190. See Von Staden for further discussion of this debate.

46 Celsus, *De Medicina*, Proem 23–6. Translation from: W.G. Spender, trans., *Celsus On Medicine, Volume I Books I-V (Loeb Classical Library 292)* (Cambridge: Harvard University Press, 1935). Pseudo-Eustathius, Commentarius in Hexaemeron, 788 L.53. See Lawrence J. Bliquez and Alexander Kazhdan, "'Texts and Documents': Four Testimonia to Human Dissection in Byzantine Times," *Bulletin of the History of Medicine*; Baltimore, 58,4 (1984): 554–558. Other late antique

mention of this ethical debate in the rabbinic text, the rabbis may be subtly refer-encing a broader Greco-Roman medical discourse about the Herophilean anatomy research. It is possible that, by describing the enslaved women as criminals, the text is pointing to the questionable ethics of the experiments to which they were subjected. In this way, then, the rabbis may be depicting Greco-Roman medical traditions as not simply outlandish, but immoral.

2.1 Gendered knowledge

Another distinctive element of the narrative, both in its production in Greco-Roman Palestine and in its reception in the BT, is the central role that women and their bod-ies play within the Cleopatra story. The story demonstrates the intrinsic connection between the production of knowledge about embryology and women's experiences, authority, and expertise. The knowledge produced by the story requires trusting both the claims of the women who are the characters in the story and the trustworthiness of their bodies.

In the story, knowledge of embryology is produced by experiments on the bodies of enslaved women at the command of a woman, Cleopatra. Thus, the experiments in the narrative occur within what Charlotte Fonrobert terms a "women's space," a space where women interact, exercise authority, and demonstrate expertise beyond the control of men. The representation of a "women's space," without the intrusion of male authority, the male gaze, or male expertise, is unusual in both Greco-Roman medical literature and rabbinic literature. As contemporary scholarship on gender and ancient medicine has shown, Greek and Roman medical literature, from the Hippocratic corpus to Soranus and Galen, primarily depict women receiving treat-ment from male medical practitioners. Even when female medical practitioners are represented, they are described as working under the supervision of male doctors. In this male-authored literature, it is rare to find depictions of women as the sole med-ical providers for other women, despite the fact that such situations, in reality, were most likely common in the ancient world. By presenting male doctors treating female patients and male doctors supervising midwives, Greco-Roman medical literature constructs male doctors as authorities over women's bodies. Similarly, as Fonrobert demonstrates, in the tractate of Niddah, the rabbis present themselves as hermeneutic authorities on menstrual blood and pregnancy. While Fonrobert examines examples of "women's spaces" within the framework of ritual purity law, the representation of women's authority in these examples is limited as these "women's spaces" are ulti-mately "under the indirect control of male authority."[47]

In the context of both the Greco-Roman medical traditions and the rabbinic laws relating to menstrual purity, the Cleopatra story is notable in its depiction of a woman studying other women's bodies. In this way, the story emphasizes that the knowl-

---

authors, including Iohannes Alexandrinus and Agnellus Ravennas also defend Herophilus by mentioning that his subjects were criminals. Cf. Von Staden, *Herophilus*, 187–190.

47 Fonrobert, *Menstrual Purity*, 129. The body of literature on ancient gynecology is extensive. See note 11 above.

edge produced through these experiments about fetal development is mediated solely through the observations of women. Much like the details that highlight the foreignness of these experiments, the fact that the experiments are overseen by a woman in the rabbinic narrative emphasizes their origins outside the scope of the male rabbinic gaze. Furthermore, in contrast to other "women's spaces" in rabbinic literature, these experiments are uniquely independent from the control of men; as Cleopatra is a queen, she is not under the supervision of men.[48] By attributing the direction of these brutal experiments to a woman, the rabbis imagine spaces where women hold authority over other women's bodies and where that authority is completely independent from male control as dangerous and the knowledge produced within them as potentially suspect.

In addition to depicting a "women's space," the narrative presents women's physiology as a particularly difficult object of inquiry. Indeed, the story graphically depicts how the observation of the developing embryos requires tearing open the bodies of enslaved women and ripping out the embryos from the women in which they reside. By showing that the observation of the internal workings of a woman's body requires its physical destruction, the narrative emphasizes the difficulties involved in producing knowledge about women's bodies and pregnancy.

In examining this brief anecdote, we see how the rabbis crafted a layered and complex narrative. Read within the Greco-Roman context in which it was produced, the rabbis construct a description of the study of anatomy and physiology in antiquity, centered in Alexandria, led by experts in gynecology, who performed perhaps morally questionable acts in order to gain knowledge about fetal development. Read within the broader corpus of rabbinic literature, the story presents knowledge that is empirical, as it is produced by observation of the body, but which is viewed by the rabbis as non-rabbinic, originating from foreigners and women. Understanding the nuances of this story is key to explaining the place of this story within the larger conversation about rabbinic medical epistemology in b. Niddah.

3   Bavli Niddah 30b

In b. Niddah 30b, the stammaitic editors examine the claims about the rate of fetal development in m. Niddah 3:7 and debate the appropriate sources from which to derive medical knowledge. The Cleopatra story becomes a key part of the discussion.[49]

---

48 Note that in the Tosefta, it is possible that the text assumes that a male king was involved in the experiments. The phrase for "death by royal decree" is "מיתה למלך"—"death for the king." However, as this is an unusual phrase, I think it more likely to be a variant of the Bavli's "הריגה למלכות." The Bavli's expression is more clearly referring to the monarchy in general and not a male ruling figure.

49 The division of the text into different parts reflects a simplistic presentation of the diachronic layers within the text. Sources are indicated in parantheses. The stammaitic interventions within the text are more fully accounted for in my discussion and footnotes. The text is translated according to the Vilna edition, with manuscript differences that affect the meaning noted in the footnotes. The manuscript variations are in accordance with the *Saul and Evelyn Henkind Talmud Text Database* (Jerusalem: Institute for Computerization in Jewish Life in Bar-Ilan

A (*Tannaitic Source*) It was taught in a tannaitic source: R. Ishmael[50] says: with
regard to the period of impurity and purity following the birth of a male
[child], and the period of impurity and purity following the birth of a female [child]. Just as the period of impurity and purity following the birth
of a male child corresponds to the formation of the male [fetus,] so too the
period of impurity and purity following the birth of a female [child] corresponds to the formation of the female [fetus].
They replied: one does not learn formation from the laws of impurity.

B (*Tannaitic Source*) They said to R. Ishmael, a story is told about Cleopatra
the queen of Alexandria[51] that when her female slaves were sentenced to
death by royal decree, they were inspected and it was found[52] that both [a
male and female embryo become fully developed] by the forty-first day.
He replied: I bring you proof from the Torah and you bring proof from fools!

C (*Stammaitic Source*) What was the "proof from the Torah"? If you want to
say it refers to the argument that the formation [of a fetus is] based on the
period of purity and impurity, it was said to him—we do not adjudicate
formation from the laws of impurity. Rather, the scriptural text says, "she
bears," [and thus,] the text adds an additional prenatal period in the case of
a female [fetus].[53]
But what was the "proof from fools"? It is possible that the conception of
the female [fetus] preceded that of the male [fetus] by forty days.
And the Sages?—They were made to drink a purgative drug.[54]
And R. Ishmael?—Some bodies are not affected by drugs.

D (*Tannaitic Source*) R. Ishmael said to them: A story is told of Cleopatra, the
Grecian queen[55] that when her female slaves were sentenced to death under

---

University, 2018), https://www.lieberman-institute.com/. The major textual witnesses of this
sugya discussed include: Ms. Vatican 111, Ms. Vatican 113, Ms. Munich 95, The Soncino printed edition of 1489, and the Vilna printed edition.

50 Ms. Vatican 111 and Ms. Munich 95: שמע׳ ר׳; Ms. Vatican 111 and Soncino: ר׳ ישמע

51 Ms. Vatican 113: בקלפטרא מלכה מלכת אלכסנדרס; Ms. Vatican 111: בקליאופטירה מלכא אלכסנדריא;
Ms. Munich 95: בקלפט׳ מלכ; Soncino: בקלפטר׳ מלכ׳ אלכסנדרוס; Vilna: בקליאופטרא מלכת אלסנדרוס.

52 According to Ms. Vatican 113, Ms. Munich 95: בדקו ומצאו; Soncino and Vilna: בדקן ומצאן;
Ms. Vatican 111: ובדקן.

53 Quotation from Leviticus 12:5. In this verse there is an extra usage of the word "*teled*"—"she
bears" in the case of giving birth to a female. The Stam argues that this extra verb indicates it
there is extra time added to the fetal development of a female fetus and so it takes twice as long
for a female fetus to become fully developed.

54 "נפצא," translation following Michael Sokoloff, *A Dictionary of Jewish Babylonian Aramaic of
the Talmudic and Geonic Periods* (Ramat-Gan, Israel: Bar Ilan University Press, 2002), 763. According to Ms. Vatican 113, Soncino 1489: סמא דנפצא. Ms. Munich 95: סמא דנפע׳; Ms. Vatican
111: סברא דנפצא; Vilna: סמא דנפצא.

55 Ms. Vatican 113: בקלפטרא מלכה מלכת יונים; Ms. Vatican 111: בקליאופטרה ממלכות יונים; Ms. Munich 95: בקלפטר׳ מלכ; Soncino: בקלפטר׳ מלכת יווני; Vilna: בקלפטר׳ מלכת יוונית.

a government order, they were inspected, and it was found[56] that a male [fetus] was fully fashioned on the forty-first day and a female [fetus] on the eighty-first day.

They replied: one does not bring proof from fools.

E   (*Stammaitic Source*) What is the reason?—It is possible that the female slave with the female [fetus did not conceive from her initial sexual encounter, but] waited[57] for forty days to [have sexual intercourse again], and it was only then[58] that conception occurred.[59]

And R. Ishmael?—They were handed over to a warden.

And the Sages? There is no guardian against illicit sexual behavior—and the warden himself[60] might have had sexual intercourse with them.

But is it not possible that if they had cut [open the slave pregnant with] the female [fetus] on the forty-first day, it would be found fully developed like the male [fetus]?

F   (*Amoraic Source*) Abaye said: They were equal as far as their signs were concerned.[61]

G   (*Stammaitic Source*) The Sages say: The formation of a male [fetus] and the formation of the female [fetus] are the same. The Sages [hold] the same position as the first statement made in the Mishnah! And, perhaps you want to say that this statement was to indicate that the first part of the Mishnah represents the view of the Sages, and since in an argument between an individual and a group of many, the Halakha follows the many [and thus, the Halakha is like the Sages]. However, that is obvious [and the Mishnah did not need to tell us that]. What might I have said: one might have thought that R. Ishmael's reasoning was acceptable because it is supported by scripture. However, we learn otherwise (b. Niddah 30b).

---

56 According to Ms. Vatican 113, Ms. Munich 95 Ms. Vatican 111: בדקו ומצאו; Soncino and Vilna: בדקן ומצאן.

57 There are multiple manuscript variants. It may either be "אתרח"—"it waited," perhaps referring to the act of conception or the fetus itself. Or, as Sokoloff and Jastrow suggest respectively, the word may be "איתרת" or "אתרחא"—meaning "she waited," indicating that the woman waited to engage in sexual intercourse. I have translated the text above according to Sokoloff and Jastrow as contextually it makes the most sense. Marcus Jastrow, *Dictionary of the Targumim, Talmud Bavli, Yerushalmi, and Midrashic Literature* (New York: Judaica Press, 1971), 1697; Michael Sokoloff, *A Dictionary of Jewish Babylonian Aramaic of the Talmudic and Geonic Periods* (Ramat-Gan, Israel: Bar Ilan University Press, 2002), 1232. Ms. Vatican 111: איתר; Soncino: אתר; Ms. Vatican 113: איתחר; Vilna: אייתרה.

58 The word "הדר," implies that there were two sexual encounters. Only on the second encounter does the enslaved woman become pregnant.

59 Ms. Vatican 113, Soncino, Vilna: איעבר; Ms. Vatican 111: איעבד.

60 Ms. Vatican 113, Ms. Vatican 111, Soncino, Vilna: שומר גופיה; Ms. Munich 95: שומר עצמו.

61 The interjection by the amoraic sage Abaye has him agreeing with the position of the Sages.

3.1 Structural analysis

The sugya may be divided into three major sections:

> Section I: Parts A–C consists of a tannaitic text (A–B) followed by stammaitic analysis of the tannaitic text (C). The tannaitic text provides a rationale behind the debate in the Mishnah between R. Ishmael and the Sages.
>
> Section II: In parts D–F, there is another tannaitic text (D), which is an alternate version of part B. This is followed by a stammaitic analysis of the tannaitic text (E) and a citation from an amoraic sage (F).
>
> Section III: In part G, the Stam addresses a textual issue in the Mishnah and reiterates that the legal ruling follows the opinion of the Sages.

Sections I and II parallel each other with some key differences. Each references the story of Cleopatra as a proof source for the rate of fetal development. However, in each section, the story is cited by a different rabbi in support of their views, and the supposed results that the experiments yielded are also different. Additionally, in each section, the story is subsequently rejected as a valid proof for the claims about the progress of fetal development. The doubling seen in these two sections, including the repetition of the same story with contradicting details, is a textual phenomenon seen elsewhere in the BT. This doubling may be a deliberate literary choice of the Stam, the implications of which will be considered after the sugya has been examined in its entirety.[62]

3.2 The Stam's opposing epistemological sources

When considered in conjunction with the mishnaic and toseftan sources examined previously, a feature that distinguishes b. Niddah 30b from these earlier tannaitic sources is that, in the sugya, the Stam presents Rabbi Ishmael and the Sages as representing different types of epistemological sources that stand in opposition to one another. In Parts A-B of Section I, R. Ishmael and the Sages each proffer justifications for their differing views of the duration of fetal development. The biblically-based purity laws serve as the basis for R. Ishmael's claim that male embryos develop more quickly than female embryos. According to this reasoning, since a woman remains impure for forty days after giving birth to a male child, it indicates that a male embryo takes forty days to develop fully. And, since a woman remains impure for eighty days after giving birth to a male child, R. Ishmael concludes that a female embryo takes eighty days to develop. By looking to purity law, a source that might be an acceptable

---

62 Shamma Friedman discusses examples of Bavli *sugyot* with traditions that share similar traditions with key details changed. See Shamma Friedman, "Ha-Baraitot Ba-Talmud Ha-Bavli ve-Yaḥasan Le-Maqbiloteihen Sheba-Tosefta," in *Atara L'haim: Studies in the Talmud and Medieval Rabbinic Literature in Honor of Professor Haim Zalman Dimitrovsky* (eds. Daniel Boyarin et al.; Jerusalem: Magnes, 2000), 163–201; Shamma Friedman, "A Good Story Deserves Retelling: The Unfolding of the Akiva Legend," *Jewish Studies Internet Journal* 4 (2004): 55–93; Shamma Friedman, "A Good Story Deserves Retelling: The Unfolding of the Akiva Legend," in *Creation and Composition: The Contribution of the Bavli Redactors (Stammaim) to the Aggada* (ed. Jeffrey L. Rubenstein; Tübingen: Mohr Siebeck, 2005), 71–100.

basis for adjudicating rabbinic law within rabbinic literature, R. Ishmael suggests that producing medical knowledge follows a process similar to that involved in deciding rabbinic law.[63]

However, the Sages challenge R. Ishmael's legal reasoning, stating: *"ein lomdin yetsira mitumah"*—"one does not learn *yetsira* (formation) from the laws of *tumah* (impurity)." For the Sages, the ritual laws of purity are not an acceptable precedent for *yetsira* (formation). The word *yetsira*, which might also be rendered as "creation," is used in several ways in rabbinic literature. It can refer specifically to knowledge of embryonic development, i. e., the "formation of a fetus" in the uterus, to God's original formation of man in the Genesis creation story, and to esoteric knowledge. Thus, the Sages' claim "one does not learn *yetsira* (formation) from *tumah* (impurity)," both indicates that embryonic development cannot be learned from the laws of purity and also hints more generally that these laws cannot account for the creation of the world and the divine secrets behind its functioning.[64] The Sages' critique of R. Ishmael is radical in its assertion that ritual law, law that is based on the Bible, cannot be a source of knowledge about creation.

In contrast, the justification that the Sages provide for their claims about fetal development is markedly different from R. Ishmael's; the Sages present the account of Cleopatra's experiments as their source. While R. Ishmael presents a traditional rabbinic source for his justification, the Sages present a source that, as discussed above, represents medical knowledge as emerging from observations that are the result of violent experiments performed by non-rabbis. Unsurprisingly, R. Ishmael objects to the Sages' source of medical knowledge. However, whereas the Sages objected to R. Ishmael's use of purity laws as a basis for legal reasoning, the latter criticizes the origins of the Cleopatra story stating, "I bring you proof from the Torah, and you bring proof from fools," thus, setting up "Torah" in opposition to "fools."

The view that the Cleopatra story is a "proof from fools" is reinforced in Section II part D of the sugya as well, where R. Ishmael cites the Cleopatra story to support his view that male and female embryos develop at different rates. Using the same language that R. Ishmael uses in Section I part B, once again, the Sages reject the proof because they consider it to come "from fools."[65] In rabbinic literature, the phrase

---

63 See also Vartejanu-Joubert's discussion of opposing sources of knowledge in this sugya and in rabbinic literature. Vartejanu-Joubert, "The Right Type of Knowledge."

64 For references to the formation of the fetus see: b. Yoma 75a, b. Sotah 45b, b. Sanhererin 91b, b. Hullin71a, b. Niddah 22a and 23a, y. Yebamot 4:2, 5d; y. Niddah 3:2, 50c. For references to the original creation of man in Genesis see: b. Taanit 27b, b. Ketubot 8a, b. Hullin 71a, b. Niddah 22a. There is also a reference to a *Sefer Yetsira*, through which, according to the b. Sanhedrin 65b and 67b, a rabbi is said to have created and eaten a calf. Again, associating the term "יצירה" with esoteric knowledge and the creation of beings. I have rendered it as "formation" here to differentiate it from the Mishnah's usage of בריה.

65 Looking at the version of the Cleopatra story in the Tosefta in conjunction with the sugya here, the presentation of the Cleopatra story and the biblical purity laws as different types of epistemologies seems to be the working of the stammaitic editorial hand. While Parts A-B in Section I and Parts D in Section II are presented as tannaitic, including the statement "one does not

ra'ayah min hashotim, or "proof from fools," sometimes refers to idolaters and other non-Jews when they disagree with the rabbis.[66] By describing the Cleopatra story as a "proof from fools," it highlights that the issue with the Cleopatra story is the trust-worthiness of the individuals who produced the source.[67] Because the experiments took place outside the sphere of rabbinic authority, its reliability is suspect.

3.3 Undermining gendered knowledge

Throughout the sugya, the Stam continues to heighten this perceived contrast be-tween the two opposing types of epistemological sources, strengthening the "proof from Torah" and undermining the "proof from fools." For example, it tries to find other acceptable sources that are of Torah origin that cannot be refuted. In Section I Part C, the Stam argues that the "proof from the Torah" does not refer to purity laws, as an argument was brought to undermine this derivation. Rather, it refers to a verse in Leviticus, which, when talking about the purity status of a woman who gave birth to a female, adds the word "she bears" that is unnecessary to the meaning of the verse: it is extraneous. By the rabbinic principles of legal exegesis, they may use this extra word as a basis for a legal principle, or in this case, as a basis for a claim about the rate of fetal development.[68] This biblical proof text is never challenged or refuted as a basis for knowledge about fetal development.

In contrast to the Stam's attempts to bolster the "proof from the Torah," the Stam attempts to undermine the viability of the Cleopatra story as a proof source by mo-

---

bring proof from fools," in the Tosefta, the Cleopatra story is rejected as a proof source without a specific reason given, simply "we don't bring proof from here." It is possible that the Bavli's distinction between the Cleopatra story as a "proof from fools" in opposition to the biblical argument as a "proof from the Torah" is a stammaitic innovation intended to manufacture a tension between two distinct epistemological sources.

66 The phrase "ראיה מן השוטים" appears in reference to Ben Stada, which has been interpreted as Je-sus. B. Shabbat 104b. The use of "shotim" to refer to idolaters: m. Avodah Zarah 4:7, t. Avodah Zarah 6:7, b. Avodah Zarah 54b. Often it is used in the expression "Should god destroy the world on account of fools?"—the fools referring idolaters. Peter Schäfer, *Jesus in the Talmud* (Princeton: Princeton University Press, 2007).

67 In reading the sugya's rejection of the Cleopatra story, it is interesting to note that there are no clear ethical objections raised as a critique of the Cleopatra story. Recall my earlier discussion of late antique Christian authors who explicitly polemicize against the Herophilean experiments as inhuman. Instead of a contrast between "a proof from Torah" versus a "proof from fools," one could imagine a contrast between "a proof from Torah" versus a proof derived from unethi-cal behavior. The sugya lacks a clear statement of moral indignation about these experiments. It is possible that the reference to the experiments as a "proof from fools" suggests the immorality of the people running of the experiments. However, it is also possible that the text does not address the morality of the experiments on purpose; the Stam does not see the morality of the experiments as a challenge to the trustworthiness of the knowledge produced in such circum-stances. Rather, the primary issue for the Stam is the trustworthiness of the people involved.

68 Leviticus 12:5 " But if she bears a maid-child..." The verse contains the word *teled*—"she bears." The rabbis see this word as superfluous because removing the word would not affect the mean-ing of the verse. Thus, by the rabbinic principles of textual exegesis, the word must have a legal implication.

bilizing gender biases and questioning the trustworthiness of women generally and enslaved women in particular. In both Section I Part C and Section II Part E of the sugya, the Stam is suspicious of the claims that the enslaved women make about their bodies, particularly claims involving their sexual behavior. In Section I Part C, the Stam claims:

> But what was the "proof from fools"? It might be suggested that the conception of the female [fetus] preceded that of the male [fetus] by forty days.
> And the Sages?—They were made to drink a purgative drug.
> And R. Ishmael?—Some bodies are not affected by drugs.

Here, the Stam reframes the debate between R. Ishmael and the Sages as one over the possibility of regulating the physiology of women in such a way that the rabbis would be willing to rely on the women's observations about their bodies. The Stam explains that the Cleopatra story is a "proof from fools" because the correct timing of the surgeries depends on knowing with certainty when the conception of the embryos occurred. Such knowledge, by implication, depends on trusting a woman's claims about her sexual behavior and her self-awareness about her body and whether she is pregnant. If the enslaved woman had been impregnated forty days prior to the supposed date of conception of the female embryo, the conclusion that male and female embryos develop at the same rate would have been made erroneously. Trusting the results of the Cleopatra experiments depends on trusting the enslaved pregnant woman to testify reliably regarding her sexual encounters as well as her ability to recognize the changes within her own body and to determine when she became pregnant accurately.

According to the Stam's reasoning, the Sages are willing to rely on the Cleopatra story because they believe that a method is available for determining the date of conception that does not rely on a woman's claims regarding her pregnancy; namely, by medically controlling her body. The Stam suggests that by forcing the enslaved women to consume an abortifacient drug—and, presumably, also forcing them to endure a sexual assault at a specific time—it would be possible to time the date of conception with "accuracy," that is, without relying on the word of the pregnant women. However, R. Ishmael counters that it is impossible to sufficiently regulate the bodies of women through such medications since some women may not respond to them. Ultimately, the Stam assesses the trustworthiness of the Cleopatra experiments based on whether there is a medical way to regulate the bodies of women so that their testimony is not necessary to settle the issue. The disturbing depth of the Stam's discomfort with trusting women is, thus, reflected in the extreme methods that they imagine being deployed to control women's bodies.

In Section II Part E, the Stam further develops their suspicious posture toward the enslaved women's claims about their pregnancies and the dates of conception. Here, the focus of concern is the inability to control the sexual behavior of women and particularly that of enslaved women.

> They replied: one does not bring proof from fools.
> What is the reason?—It is possible that the female slave with the female [fetus did not conceive from her initial sexual encounter, but] waited for forty days to [have sexual intercourse again], and it was only then that conception occurred.
> And R. Ishmael?—They were handed over to a warden.
> And the Sages? There is no guardian against illicit sexual behavior—and the warden himself might have had sexual intercourse with them.

The Stam is concerned that the results of the Cleopatra experiments depend on trusting the enslaved women's claims about their sexual encounters. The Stam suggests that the experiments may be untrustworthy because, after the initial sexual encounter in which it was assumed that they had conceived, these women might have had other sexual encounters forty days later. The use of the active verb "waited" indicates that the Stam views these enslaved women, despite the fact that they are being forced to have sexual intercourse as part of the experiments, to be their own sexual agents. The Stam seems to imagine the enslaved women as "licentious" whose sexual behavior is uncontrollable. The Stam's characterization of these enslaved women as "licentious" underlies their skepticism of relying on an enslaved woman's claims about her sexual encounters.[69]

In these ways, the Stam makes it clear that their primary concern is the ability to control the behavior of women. Thus R. Ishmael trusts the Cleopatra experiments because he believes it possible to control the enslaved women's sexual behavior by

---

69 My reading of the text hinges on the active verb "she waited," which implies that the enslaved woman is in control of her own sexual behavior. It would seem that the concern in this text is the supposed uncontrollable "licentious" behavior of enslaved women. This reading follows Liberman's reading of the t. Niddah 4:17 discussed previously. Saul Lieberman argues that the reason the Tosefta challenges the Cleopatra story is that it depends on the testimony of non-Jewish enslaved women, whose claims about their sexual behavior are generally viewed to be untrustworthy. As an alternate proof source, the Tosefta presents cases which specifically involve Jewish women, such as a Jewish woman who miscarries after having sex with her husband for the first time or a Jewish woman who miscarries after having sex with her husband for the first time after his prolonged travels abroad. My reading of b. Niddah sees the sugya as building on concerns already expressed in the Tosefta about the sexual behavior of enslaved women. However, the complicated manuscript tradition in b. Niddah on the word "she waited" (see note 57 above) makes it difficult to make a strong claim that the enslaved women are the subject of the verb. One could also read this text as concerned with the sexual vulnerability of the enslaved women. Indeed, scholarship on slavery in rabbinic literature has argued that the sexual vulnerability of enslaved women was something rabbis were concerned with. In this reading, the enslaved women's claims about their sexual behavior are not trustworthy because the women do not have control over their own bodies and sexual encounters. However, I think this more charitable reading of this text is less likely based on the manuscript tradition. For Lieberman's analysis of the Tosefta, see Lieberman, *Tosefet Rishonim*, 3:268. For scholarship on rabbinic views on slavery, see Judith Romney Wegner, *Chattel or Person?: The Status of Women in the Mishnah* (New York: Oxford University Press, 1988); Catherine Hezser, *Jewish Slavery in Antiquity* (New York: Oxford University Press, 2005); Labovitz, Gail, "More Slave Women, More Lewdness: Freedom and Honor in Rabbinic Constructions of Female Sexuality," *Journal of Feminist Studies in Religion* 28,2 (2012): 69–87.

placing them under the supervision of male wardens. However, the Sages believe controlling sexual behavior to be impossible, as the warden himself might sexually assault the women under his control. By suggesting that the experiments could only be trusted if a warden was guarding the enslaved women—in other words, if the experiments were regulated by a male authority figure, the Stam highlights its discomfort with the Cleopatra experiments as a "women's space."

In Sections I and II of the sugya, the Stam interprets the critique of the Cleopatra story as a "proof from fools" as a concern about whether a woman's claim about her own body may be trusted. Determining the date of conception depends on knowledge of a woman's sexual behavior or a woman's knowledge of her own body. In both Section I and II, the Stam suggests that the experiments may only be trusted if it is possible to control women, either physically regulating their bodies with medication or putting the women under the guardianship of men.[70]

The distrust of women's claims about the experience of their own bodies evident in this sugya is, of course, not unique to rabbinic literature. Scholarship on gender and ancient medicine has shown that, in Greco-Roman medical literature, male medical practitioners often treated female patient's descriptions about the experiences of their own bodies with greater suspicion than claims made by male patients. Indeed, in the modern era, gender bias continues to shape doctor-patient interactions and the experiences of women seeking medical care.[71] For the Stam, beliefs about enslaved women's bodies and their sexual behavior inform the rabbinic evaluation of the assessment of the possibility of acquiring medical knowledge through observation of their bodies.

3.4 The Sugya in context

As I have shown, the sugya repeatedly undermines the reliability of the Cleopatra story and its empirical observations. Thus, it presents the story in opposition to Torah sources and highlights its foreignness and gendered nature. When considered in its entirety, even the literary structure of the sugya can be seen as working to undermine the Cleopatra story as a reliable source for medical knowledge. A key feature of this literary structure is the repetition of the story in Sections I Part C and II Part E. In Section I, the Sages use a version of the story of Cleopatra's experiments to support their position about the rate of fetal development; in Section II, by contrast, R. Ishmael uses the same description of the experiments, but the experiments show different results. Following Shamma Friedman's argument that this textual structure of doubling the narrative with changes is an intentional literary choice on the part of the Stam, I suggest that the deployment

---

70 This is not to say that generally in rabbinic literature the rabbis are always skeptical of the claims of women. In fact, in the laws of Niddah, this trust is often fundamental to adjudicating rabbinic law. That being said, scholars such as Fonrobert, Halberstam, and Libson have explored the ways in which rabbinic ritual law adjudicates in ways that undermine the expertise claimed by women. Cf. Fonrobert, *Menstrual Purity*; Halberstam, *Law and Truth in Biblical and Rabbinic Literature*; Libson, *Law and Self-Knowledge in the Talmud*.

71 See references on gender in ancient medicine in footnote 11 and cf. especially Dean-Jones, "Autopsia, Historia and What Women Know."

of this literary technique in b. Niddah 30b serves to emphasize the doubts regarding the reliability of the Cleopatra story. If very different results are associated with the same experiments, how can traditions about such observations be trusted in the first place? The literary technique of doubling the narrative—repeating the Cleopatra story cited by different Sages but with changes to the narrative—reinforces the broader stammaitic agenda within the sugya to create an aura of doubt around the Cleopatra story.[72]

Nevertheless, despite the various critiques of the Cleopatra story adduced by the Stam, ultimately, the sugya explicitly accepts the legal position of the Sages. Within the sugya, the only actual support for the Sages' view that male and female fetuses fin-ish developing within forty days was the Cleopatra story. Within the sugya as a whole, the only proof source that has not been rejected is the biblical passage used by the Stam to support R. Ishmael's claim that male and female fetuses develop at different rates. Still, at the conclusion of the sugya, the Stam argues that, regardless of the ques-tionable sources that the Sages use to support their views about fetal development, the law still follows their position.[73]

The Stam does not always provide the legal conclusion to a sugya, and the choice to do so here serves a rhetorical purpose. The sugya has presented various potential sources of knowledge about fetal development. The Stam emphasizes different prob-lems with each source, underscoring the challenges inherent both in using the Bible or rabbinic law as a basis for medical knowledge and in trusting empirically-based claims. The conclusion of the sugya emphasizes that the various critiques of the sources of medical knowledge do not affect the adjudication of the law. Despite the fact that R. Ishmael's legal position is supported by an undisputed source based in the Torah, the law follows the Sages' position according to the legal principle of majority rules rather than the position that has the support of the best source. The concluding statement that the law follows the Sages suggests that, if the majority of the rabbis uses or trusts a problematic source—such as the Cleopatra story—as a basis for claims about medical knowledge, legal opinions based on that source remain authoritative. Despite their foreignness and their gendered nature, the Cleopatra experiments seem to be the source that determines the law. It is possible to see, in this conclusion, a wary acceptance of empirical sources of knowledge. At the same time, although the story

---

72 See note 62 above, especially: Shamma Friedman, "A Good Story Deserves Retelling."
73 In Section III of the sugya, the Stam asks a common textual question of Mishnah. They assume that the first unattributed statement in the Mishnah, "A woman who miscarries on the fortieth day is not suspect as having a fully formed fetus…," is a statement of the Sages. If so, the third state-ment in the Mishnah "and the Sages say that the creation of both a male and female are the same and occur on the forty-first day" would be redundant. Furthermore, there is no need to emphasize the Sages statement in order to demonstrate that the law follows the Sages; as a general rule, the law always follows the majority opinion over the minority. The Stam rectifies this textual problem by arguing that there is a different reason that the Mishnah repeats the Sages' claim. Namely, that one might have assumed that in this case because R. Ishmael had a better source supporting his view—his source was from the Bible, the law follows him. However, the statement is repeated to emphasize that the law follows the Sages, despite the undisputed proof text of R. Ishmael.

supports the law in this context, the skepticism expressed throughout the sugya works to limit and control the potential legal application of such sources.

Furthermore, the Stam's critical attitude towards empirical knowledge in b. Niddah 30b is not limited to the sugya itself, but rather plays an important role in framing the texts that follow it. In terms of its placement within the tractate of Niddah, this sugya precedes a long series of statements about the fetus in the uterus that extends from b. Niddah 30b through 31b. These statements range from describing the physiology of the embryo to recounting the fetus's experience within the uterus, including the famous story that a fetus is taught the entirety of the Torah in utero, but upon leaving the uterus, an angel causes the infant to forget.[74] From this perspective, the sugya in b. Niddah 30b initiates a philosophical meditation on the possibility of producing knowledge about fetal development. The juxtaposition of this sugya with the collection of rabbinic statements invites the reader to consider these sections together. Thus, the rabbis' claims about the fetus in utero are introduced by a section that foregrounds the issues of the limited sources available on the topic of fetal development and the tenuous nature of these sources.

4   Conclusions

By examining the Cleopatra story as well as the literary structure, style, and diachronic development of b. Niddah 30b, I have explored the epistemological assumptions behind the rabbis' reflections on the appropriate sources of knowledge about fetal development. The value of various epistemological sources—ritual law, biblical texts, and the Cleopatra narrative—is weighed by the Stam in their efforts to establish which sources may be used to make claims about the rate of fetal development. Even as the rabbis negotiate the potential limits of ritual law and biblical traditions when it comes to producing medical knowledge, they struggle with the concerns that empiricism raises regarding the trustworthiness of the people involved in an experimental endeavor.

Through my analysis, I have shown the ways in which the rabbis' conception of medical empiricism is intrinsically tied to the people involved in medical observations—both the observers and the observed. The sugya demonstrates how knowledge produced through such observations are shaped by the power dynamics and social tensions that govern human relationships. The Stam's treatment of the Cleopatra story captures how rabbinic biases against non-Jews, women, and enslaved persons filter into their evaluation of medical knowledge and provide the basis for their skeptical view of empiricism expressed in the sugya.

---

74 For an analysis of these texts, see Kessler, *Conceiving Israel*, 106–107.

Bibliography

Sources

Aristotle. *History of Animals, Volume III: Books 7–10.* Edited and Translated by David M. Balme. Loeb Classical Library 439. Cambridge: Harvard University Press, 1991.

Celsus. *On Medicine, Volume I Books I–V.* Translated by W.G. Spender. Loeb Classical Library 292. Cambridge: Harvard University Press, 1935.

Danby, Herbert, trans. *The Mishnah.* Oxford: The Clarendon Press, 1933.

Kaufman, David, Tamás Sajó, and Kinga Dévényi, eds. "MS A50, Kaufman Manuscript of the Mishnah." In *David Kaufman and His Collection of Medieval Hebrew Manuscripts in the Oriental Collection of the Library of the Hungarian Academy of Sciences.* Budapest: Library of the Hungarian Academy of Sciences, 2008. Online: http://kaufmann.mtak.hu/en/ms50/ms50-coll1.htm.

Meacham, Tirzah. "Mishnah Tractate Niddah with Introduction: A Critical Edition with Notes on Variants, Commentary, Redaction and Chapters in Legal History and Realia." Ph.D. Dissertation, Hebrew University, 1989.

Saul and Evelyn Henkind Talmud Text Database. Jerusalem: Institute for Computerization in Jewish Life in Bar-Ilan University. Cited 30 December 2018. Online: https://www.lieberman-institute.com/.

"Tosefta Niddah." *MS Vienna Codex Heb. 20, Catalogue Schwarz No. 46.* Vienna: Austrian National Library in Vienna. Online: https://merhav.nli.org.il/permalink/f/ldj0th/NNL_ALEPH21262636550005171.

"Tosefta Niddah." *Alfasi's Compendium to the Talmud, Vol II.* Venice: Bamberger, 1521. Cited 31 July 2019. Online: https://merhav.nli.org.il/permalink/f/ldj0th/NNL_ALEPH21238248000005171.

Zuckermandel, Moses Samuel, ed. *Tosefta: ʿal Pi Kitvei Yad Erfurṭ u-Viyenah, ʿim Marʾeh Meḳomot ve-Ḥilufei Girsàot u-Maftehot.* Jerusalem: Wahrman, 1970.

Literature

Balberg, Mira. *Purity, Body, and Self in Early Rabbinic Literature.* Berkeley: University of California Press, 2014.

—. "Rabbinic Authority, Medical Rhetoric, and Body Hermeneutics in Mishnah Negaʿim." *AJS Review* 35,2 (2011): 323–346.

Bar-Ilan, Meir. "Medicine in Eretz Israel During the First Centuries CE." *Cathedra* 91 (1989): 31–78. [In Hebrew]

Bliquez, Lawrence J., and Alexander Kazhdan. "'Texts and Documents': Four Testimonia to Human Dissection in Byzantine Times." *Bulletin of the History of Medicine* 58,4 (1984): 554–558.

Broere-Brown, Zoe A., Esme Baan, Sarah Schalekamp-Timmermans, Bero O. Verburg, Vincent W. V. Jaddoe, and Eric A. P. Steegers. "Sex-Specific Differences in Fetal and Infant Growth Patterns: A Prospective Population-Based Cohort Study." *Biology of Sex Differences* 7,1 (2016): 65.

Cooper Owens, Deirdre. *Medical Bondage: Race, Gender, and the Origins of American Gynecology.* Athens: The University of Georgia Press, 2017.

Cunningham, F. Gary, Kenneth J. Leveno, Steven L. Bloom, and Jodi S. Dashe. *Williams Obstetrics, 25e.* New York: McGraw Hill Medical Companies, 2018.

Dean-Jones, Lesley. "Autopsia, Historia and What Women Know: The Authority of Women in Hippocratic Gynaecology." In *Knowledge and the Scholarly Medical Traditions*. Edited by Don Bates. Cambridge: Cambridge University Press, 1995. Pages 41–59.

—. *Women's Bodies in Classical Greek Science*. New York: Oxford University Press, 1994.

Flemming, Rebecca. *Medicine and the Making of Roman Women: Gender, Nature, and Authority from Celsus to Galen*. Oxford: Oxford University Press, 2000.

Fonrobert, Charlotte Elisheva. *Menstrual Purity: Rabbinic and Christian Reconstructions of Biblical Gender*. Stanford: Stanford University Press, 2000.

—. "Regulating the Human Body: Rabbinic Legal Discourse and the Making of Jewish Gender." In *The Cambridge Companion to the Talmud and Rabbinic Literature*. Edited by Charlotte E. Fonrobert and Martin S. Jaffee. Cambridge: Cambridge University Press, 2007. Pages 270–294.

Friedman, Shamma. "A Critical Study of Yevamot X with a Methodological Introduction." In *Texts and Studies: Analecta Judaica* I. Edited by Haim Zalman Dimitrovsky. New York: The Jewish Theological Seminary of America, 1977. Pages 275–441. [In Hebrew]

—. "A Good Story Deserves Retelling: The Unfolding of the Akiva Legend." *Jewish Studies Internet Journal* 4 (2004): 55–93.

— "A Good Story Deserves Retelling: The Unfolding of the Akiva Legend." In *Creation and Composition: The Contribution of the Bavli Redactors (Stammaim) to the Aggada*. Edited by Jeffrey L. Rubenstein. Tübingen: Mohr Siebeck, 2005. Pages 71–100.

—. "Ha-Baraitot Ba-Talmud Ha-Bavli ve-Yaḥasan Le-Maqbiloteihen Sheba-Tosefta." In *At-ara L'haim: Studies in the Talmud and Medieval Rabbinic Literature in Honor of Professor Haim Zalman Dimitrovsky*. Edited by Daniel Boyarin et al. Jerusalem: Magnes, 2000. Pages 163–201. [In Hebrew]

Geiger, Joseph. "Cleopatra the Physician." *Cathedra* 92 (1999): 193–198. [In Hebrew]

—. "Cleopatra the Physician." *Zutot: Perspectives on Jewish Culture* 1,1 (2001): 28–32.

Green, Monica. "The Transmission of Ancient Theories of Female Physiology and Disease through the Early Middle Ages." Ph.D. Dissertation, Princeton University, 1985.

Halberstam, Chaya T. *Law and Truth in Biblical and Rabbinic Literature*. Bloomington: Indiana University Press, 2009.

Hanson, Ann E. "The Medical Writer's Woman." In *Before Sexuality: The Construction of Erotic Experience in the Ancient Greek World*. Edited by David M. Halperin, John J. Winkler, and Froma I. Zeitlin. Princeton: Princeton University Press, 1990. Pages 309–338.

Hayes, Christine. "Displaced Self-Perceptions: The Deployment of Minim and Romans in Bavli Sanhedrin 90b–91a." In *Religious and Ethnic Communities in Later Roman Palestine*. Edited by Hayim Lapin. Potomac: University Press of Maryland, 1998. Pages 249–289.

—. *What's Divine about Divine Law?: Early Perspectives*. Princeton: Princeton University Press, 2015.

Hezser, Catherine. *Jewish Slavery in Antiquity*. New York: Oxford University Press, 2005.

Irshai, Ronit. *Fertility and Jewish Law: Feminist Perspectives on Orthodox Responsa Literature*. Waltham: Brandeis University Press, 2012.

Jastrow, Marcus. *Dictionary of the Targumim, Talmud Bavli, Yerushalmi, and Midrashic Literature*. New York: Judaica Press, 1971.

Kalmin, Richard. "Christians and Heretics in Rabbinic Literature of Late Antiquity." *The Harvard Theological Review* 87,2 (1994): 155–169.

—. "Observation in Rabbinic Literature of Late Antiquity." In *The Faces of Torah: Studies in the Texts and Contexts of Ancient Judaism in Honor of Steven Fraade*. Edited by Michal Bar

Asher Siegal, Tzvi Novick, and Christine E. Hayes. Göttingen: Vandenhoeck & Ruprecht, 2017. Pages 359–383.

Kessler, Gwynn. *Conceiving Israel: The Fetus in Rabbinic Narratives*. Philadelphia: University of Pennsylvania Press, 2009.

—. "The God of Small Things: The Fetus and Its Development in Palestinian Aggadic Literature." Ph.D. Dissertation, The Jewish Theological Seminary, 2001.

King, Helen. *Hippocrates' Woman: Reading the Female Body in Ancient Greece*. New York: Routledge, 1998.

Kiperwasser, Reuven. "'Three Partners in a Person' The Genesis and Development of Embryological Theory in Biblical and Rabbinic Judaism." *Lectio Difficilior* (2009): 1–37.

Kottek, Samuel S. "Embryology in Talmudic and Midrashic Literature." *Journal of the History of Biology* 14,2 (1981): 299–315.

Kuhn, Thomas S. *The Structure of Scientific Revolutions*. Chicago, IL: University of Chicago Press, 1996.

Labendz, Jenny R. *Socratic Torah: Non-Jews in Rabbinic Intellectual Culture*. New York: Oxford University Press, 2013.

Labovitz. "More Slave Women, More Lewdness: Freedom and Honor in Rabbinic Constructions of Female Sexuality." *Journal of Feminist Studies in Religion* 28,2 (2012): 69–87.

Lepicard, Etienne. "The Embryo in Ancient Rabbinic Literature: Between Religious Law and Didactic Narratives: An Interpretive Essay." *History and Philosophy of the Life Sciences* 32,1 (2010): 21–41.

Libson, Ayelet Hoffmann. *Law and Self-Knowledge in the Talmud*. Cambridge: Cambridge University Press, 2018.

Lieberman, Saul. *Tosefet Rishonim: Perush Meyusad 'al Kitve Yad Ha-Tosefta Ve-Sifre Rishonim u-Midrashim Be-Khitve Yad u-Defusim Yeshanim*. Vol. 3. Jerusalem: Bamberger and Wahrman, 1937. [In Hebrew]

Meacham, Tirzah. "An Abbreviated History of the Development of the Jewish Menstrual Laws." In *Women and Water: Menstruation in Jewish Life and Law*. Edited by Rahel R. Wasserfall. Hanover: University Press of New England, 1999. Pages 23–39.

—. "Halakhic Limitations on the Use of Slaves in Physical Examinations." In *From Athens to Jerusalem: Medicine in Hellenized Jewish Lore and in Early Christian Literature*. Edited by Samuel S. Kottek and Manfred Horstmanshoff. Rotterdam: Erasmus Publishing, 2000. Pages 33–48.

Moore, Keith L., T.V.N. Persaud, and Mark G. Torchia. *The Developing Human: Clinically Oriented Embryology*. 11th Edition. Edinburgh: Elsevier, 2020.

Naeh, Shlomo. "On Two Hippocratic Concepts in Rabbinic Literature." *Tarbiz* 66,2 (1997): 169–185. [In Hebrew]

Neis, R. *The Sense of Sight in Rabbinic Culture: Jewish Ways of Seeing in Late Antiquity*. New York: Cambridge University Press, 2013.

Neis, Rachel Rafael. "Fetus, Flesh, Food: Generating Bodies of Knowledge in Rabbinic Science." *Journal of Ancient Judaism* 10,2 (2019): 181–210.

—. "The Reproduction of Species: Humans, Animals and Species Nonconformity in Early Rabbinic Science." *Jewish Studies Quarterly* 24,4 (2017): 434–451.

Novick, Tzvi. "A Lot of Learning Is a Dangerous Thing: On the Structure of Rabbinic Expertise in the Bavli." *Hebrew Union College Annual* 78 (2007): 91–107.

Nutton, Vivian. *Ancient Medicine*. 2nd ed. Milton: Routledge, 2013.

—. "From Athens to Jerusalem: Medicine in Hellenized Jewish Lore and in Early Christian Literature (Review)." *Bulletin of the History of Medicine* 75,4 (2001): 787–788.

Preuss, Julius. *Biblical and Talmudic Medicine*. Translated by Fred Rosner. Northvale: Jason Aronson Inc., 1993.

Rousselle, Aline. *Porneia: On Desire and the Body in Antiquity*. Translated by Felicia Pheasant. Cambridge, MA: Blackwell, 1993.

Rubenstein, Jeffrey L. "Criteria of Stammaitic Intervention in Aggada." In *Creation and Composition: The Contribution of the Bavli Redactors (Stammaim) to the Aggada*. Edited by Jeffrey L. Rubenstein. Tübingen: Mohr Siebeck, 2005. Pages 417–440.

Salihu, Hamisu M., Abraham A. Salinas-Miranda, Latoya Hill, and Kristen Chandler. "Survival of Pre-Viable Preterm Infants in the United States: A Systematic Review and Meta-Analysis." *Seminars in Perinatology* 37,6. Periviable Birth: Obstetric and Neonatal Management and Counseling Issues Part 1 (2013): 389–400.

Scarborough, John. "Pharmacology and Toxicology at the Court of Cleopatra VII: Traces of Three Physicians." In *Herbs and Healers from the Ancient Mediterranean through the Medieval West*. Edited by Anne Van Arsdall and Timothy Graham. Farnham: Ashgate, 2012. Pages 7–18.

Schäfer, Peter. *Jesus in the Talmud*. Princeton: Princeton University Press, 2007.

Shinnar, Shulamit. "'The Best of Doctors Go to Hell': Rabbinic Medical Culture in Late Antiquity (200–600 CE)." Ph.D. Dissertation, Columbia University, 2019.

Simon-Shoshan, Moshe. *Stories of the Law: Narrative Discourse and the Construction of Authority in the Mishnah*. New York: Oxford University Press, 2012.

Smith, Pamela. "Science." In *A Concise Companion to History*. Edited by Ulinka Rublack. Oxford: Oxford University Press, 2011. Pages 268–297.

Sokoloff, Michael. *A Dictionary of Jewish Babylonian Aramaic of the Talmudic and Geonic Periods*. Ramat-Gan, Israel: Bar Ilan University Press, 2002.

Stol, Marten. *Birth in Babylonia and the Bible: Its Mediterranean Setting*. Groningen: Styx, 2000.

Ulmer, Rivka. *Egyptian Cultural Icons in Midrash*. Berlin: Walter de Gruyter, 2009.

Vartejanu-Joubert, Madalina. "The Right Type of Knowledge: Theory and Experience in Two Passages of the Babylonian Talmud." *Korot* 19 (2007): 161–180.

Vidas, Moulie. *Tradition and the Formation of the Talmud*. Oxford: Princeton University Press, 2014.

Von Staden, Heinrich. *Herophilus: The Art of Medicine in Early Alexandria: Edition, Translation, and Essays*. Cambridge: Cambridge University Press, 1989.

Wegner, Judith Romney. *Chattel or Person?: The Status of Women in the Mishnah*. New York: Oxford University Press, 1988.

Public Health in Jerusalem According to the Talmudic Literature: Reality or Vision?*

Estēe Dvorjetski

The quality of the environment is one of the most fundamental factors, which have a direct influence on public health. The term 'environment' is a very broad concept. It comprises man's natural surroundings, including their ecological components, his man-made habitat, and his social environment, including its psychological components. All of these factors have a powerful direct effect on man's physical, mental and social health. The social environment—in other words, 'the public'—is of very great significance in the Jewish world-outlook. The laws, which maintain the Jewish community, are based on *halakhic* precepts and rules encompassing all areas of life and defining the links between the members of the community, the mutual relationships between individual and society, and the network of partnership and responsibility they entail. The precepts dealing with ecology constitute an inherent part of the system of laws of the Jewish world. A survey of the evidence in the Talmudic literature shows that *halakhic* rules placed great emphasis on the educational aim of strengthening consciousness of public health and developing a sense of responsibility towards the environment, as early as the Second Temple period.[1]

Concerning public health administration, the public services, which the Greek cities provided for their inhabitants, varied both in scope and in magnitude according to their size and wealth. The municipal services, which we today associate with public health, are not mentioned very frequently in antiquity. Nevertheless, there were specific officials, *astynomoi*, who were responsible for such matters as drainage and water supply. Drainage systems were in the cities and many houses had latrines, of a simple type, which were flushed by slop water. There were by-laws which pro-

---

* This paper is a part of a chapter, entitled *History of Medicine, Ecology, and Public Health in Jerusalem* derived from my forthcoming book on *Medicine, Ecology and Public Health in the Holy Land from Biblical Times to the Late Roman Period: Historical-Archaeological Perspectives*; I would like to thank the peer-reviewers and the editors for their important and useful recommendations during the reviewing and editing process of the paper.

1 For the most important studies in ecology and environment in antiquity and in ancient cultures, see Oelschlaeger 1991; Hughes 1994; Balée 1998; Hughes 2001; idem. 2005; idem. 2006; Kessel 2006; Mattern and Vött 2009; Shipley and Salmon 2011; Harris 2013, especially the introduction on pp. 1–10; Walsh 2014; Hughes 2014; For the historical approach to Jewish sources, see Kotlar 1976, 17–77; Zeligmann 1981, 7–8; Zikal 1990, 37–63; Rakover 1993, 58–93; Shinover and Goldberg 1994, 135–147; Levi 1994, 8–10; Dvorjetski 1999b, 7–8; ead. 2001.

DOI: 10.13173/9783447108263.245

vided for street cleansing and scavenging: how strictly these were enforced however is impossible to tell.[2]

'A juridical concept is central to the theme of town planning. Legislation dealt with many aspects of communal living, and the actual laws which were introduced varied greatly from city to city, reflecting the problems and difficulties of the individual town', so determines Eddie Owens while discussing the subject of town planning and the law in his landmark book *The City in the Greek and Roman World*.[3] According to him, laws operated in general in three main areas. Firstly, laws defined the relationship between the state and the individual together with the responsibility which the individual had to the community. Secondly, relations between the individual and his neighbour had to be regulated. Thirdly, the general health and well-being of the citizens and the overall maintenance of the city and its services had to be ensured. Legislation was introduced but often proved to be ineffective or inadequate. Moreover, Owens also points to a very significant problem as that it is difficult to see how such a system of private arrangement worked in practice and the fine well-made roads of the cities of the Empire could hardly have been maintained through private efforts alone. It seems likely to him that there must have been some method of commuting an individual's responsibility.

A rich collection of medical lore, ecology, and public health is found in the Talmudic literature, the authoritative collection of Jewish tradition. However, the Talmudic corpus is not a medical treatise and contains random and incidental references. Vast majority of the material deals with purity and impurity, the Temple service, and the three pilgrims' festivals. A reliable methodology for extracting history from Rabbinic sources does not exist. Jonathan Price indicates unambiguously: 'this literature presents a unique set of problems, which cannot be solved by application of techniques learned from analysis of Graeco-Roman historiography. The Rabbis were not writing history—a Greek word and concept foreign to their thinking—and in their legal and exegetical arguments they freely modified historical memories or invented them out of whole cloth'.[4] Moreover, traditions about the Second Temple were written down long after they originated and had developed orally for generations; the original 'kernel' is often encrusted with later accretions and interpretations, and may not be retrievable. Following Jonathan Price, Lee Levine argues very correctly that the Rabbinic literature material is neither ipso facto reliable nor a priori worthless. He adds that 'each reference has to be evaluated on its own merits, taking into account the date of the particular text, the nature of the evidence, its context, and what purpose (polemical, apologetic, or inspirational)' this information may have served.[5]

---

2 Owens 1991, 168–169; Crouch 1993; Liebeschuetz 2000, 51–62; Hughes 2001, 60; Cooper 2001, 12; Wilson 2008, 289.
3 Owens 1991, 166–170.
4 Price 1992, 198–199; See also Heineman 1970; Schäfer 1978, 1–16, 23–44; Visotzky 1983, 403–418; Cohen 1986, 38–39; Heinemann 1986, 41–55.
5 Levine 2002, 349; See also Schäfer 1978, 1–16, 23–44; Cohen 1986, 38–39; Heinemann 1986;

Jerusalem is a city sui generis. It was the capital, the city of David, the home of the Temple, the quintessence of holiness, the symbol of Jewish national life, and the focus of all the hopes, longings, and aspirations of Jewry. Thus, it is natural that over the generations Jerusalem's special status as the location of the Temple led to its being particularly revered as a place whose exemplary purity was meticulously preserved, and impure elements excluded. The Temple Mount complex was undoubtedly of key significance in daily life in Jerusalem. Being a constantly active shrine, on such a huge scale, it not only heightened the city's vibrancy and raised its socio-economic level, but even more it contributed to its appearance and glory. Because of its special status in the national and religious consciousness of the Jewish nation, the city figured particularly prominently in the methodological precepts connected with the quality of life and the environment, including such subjects as sewage, refuse, litter, air pollution, smoke, bad odours, noise, water pollution, and the elimination of nuisances which might endanger the health of the populace. The city of Jerusalem was highly estimated by Jews and non-Jews, and was said to serve as a model both for the citizens, the pilgrims, and for all the nations: 'God will make Jerusalem a metropolis for all the nations' (*Tanhuma, Deuteronomy*, 3, Buber ed., p. 4).[6]

Other important sources for understanding the essence of public health in Jerusalem over the period of the Second Temple are the New Testament's descriptions, Classical sources, Philo of Alexandria, Josephus, and the Cairo *Genizah* fragments.

The archaeological remnants add a very important layer, especially for the Roman era, while the written documents cannot provide a clear and complete picture.[7] The legacy of Rome on hygiene, sanitation, and organization of public health reflects their important milestone in the history of public health. The great appreciation that the Romans had for public and private hygiene is shown by innumerable aqueducts, sanitary measures, public baths and bathhouses, lavatories, and paved streets, which were widely spread in Italy and through the provinces by the Roman legions.[8]

The goals of this study are the following: firstly, to introduce the ten special regulations which were applied to Jerusalem and their presumed timing, reasons, and aims;

Price 1992, 198–199; Dvorjetski 1999a, 7; ead. [forthcoming (a)], chapter 1 on *The Source Material and Methodological Considerations*.

6   The bibliography about Jerusalem is enormous. See e.g. Büchler 1956, 24–63; Safrai 1965; Urbach 1968, 156–171; Goldman 1970, 1–5; Herr 1980, 166–177; Kasher 1980, 45–56; Amir 1980, 154–165; Gafni 1987, 5–22; Safrai and Safrai 1993, 344–371; Safrai 1998, 135–152; Gafni 1999, 35–59; Strange 2003, 97–113; Goodman 2005, 459–468; Klawans 2006; Netzer 2007, 71–91; Isaac 2010, 1–37; Balfour 2012, 6–87.

7   For the Jewish material culture in the Graeco-Roman world and Talmudic realia, see Krauss 1910–1912, I-III; idem. 1924, I-II; Sperber 1986; idem. 1993; Schäfer 1998–2002, I-III; Eliav 2002, 235–265; Miller 2003, 402–419; Fine 2005; Sperber 2006; Fonrobert and Jaffee 2007; Miller 2010, 214–243; Fine 2010; Hezser 2010; Magness 2011; Goodman and Alexander 2011; Fine 2014; Meyers 2014, 303–319; Fine and Koller 2014; Eliav 2014, 38–57; idem. 2015, 153–185; Miller 2015; Eliav 2016, 17*–27*; For the material culture in general, see Tilley, Keane, Kuechler-Fogden, Rowlands, and Spyer 2006; Hicks and Beaudry 2010; Hales and Hodos 2010.

8   See the extensive survey in Dvorjetski [forthcoming (a)], chapter 2.5 on *Hygiene, Sanitation, and Organization of Public Health: The Legacy of Rome*.

secondly, to demonstrate how the *halakha* was applied in the municipal planning of the city in the Second Temple period; and thirdly, to illuminate the quality of daily life in the Holy City of Jerusalem in which strict attention was paid to public health and hence focusing on the concern for public health—the preservation of human life, which is a supreme value in the scale of values of Jewish law.

'Ten matters were said in regard to Jerusalem': timing, reasons and aims

While most of the laws pertaining to the city are given in Tannaitic sources without explanations, or acceptable explanations, a scrutiny of the laws both in their textual and historical contexts should lead to plausible answers. The Jerusalem-laws are not uniform but belong in different categories. The more problematic of these laws are those exempting or excluding Jerusalem from the binding force of certain laws of the Torah and the prohibitions that apply to Jerusalem only.

In the Talmudic literature Jerusalem is given special consideration in several respects. However, relatively little attention has been paid to the special laws related in Tannaitic sources concerning Jerusalem. The special laws may be attributed, at first thought, to the fact that Jerusalem, the capital of the land, site of Temple and Sanhedrin and the administrative centre of the land, and the destination of the masses of pilgrims needed some special laws. An examination of the sources should reveal to what extent this holds true and whether the Rabbis had reasons of their own to suggest certain laws for Jerusalem. In order to clarify matters, the following questions have to be discussed: When did the special laws concerning Jerusalem originate? What were the Sages' motivations in suggesting the laws? Were they making mere conjectures of what they believed were, or should have been, the laws in Jerusalem of the past, and presenting these conjectures as facts? Or, did the Rabbis intend to give a blueprint for the Holy City of the future?

The *tannaitic* sources giving these laws in special lists are: *Tosefta, Nega'im*, 6:1–2, Tsukermandel ed., p. 625; *ARN I*, 35, Schechter ed., p. 104; *ARN II* 39, *ibid*., pp. 107–108; and *BT, Bava Kama* 82b.[9] They enumerate 'ten maxims with regard to Jerusalem'—special precepts relating to the city which set it apart from other places. Just to illustrate the details, hereinafter of the *baraitha* of *BT, Bava Kama* 82b:[10]

---

9 'Talmudic sources often assign structure and meaning to pre-existing practices', argues Miller [2010, 214–243, especially p. 215]. Nevertheless, he adds: 'as material finds and critical examination of the Rabbinic corpus indicate, many popular observances were not in sync with the approaches of the Rabbis, who often sought to regulate, ritualize, and define them'; As for *ARN*, it is a composition which supplements and elaborates on tractate *Avot* from the *Mishnah*. Both versions *ARN I* and *ARN II* developed from the original source. *ARN II* is considered to reflect a better tradition. All the Rabbis who are mentioned in ARN are *Tannaim*, and no *Amoraim* are cited. However, there are signs of later interference. There are also quotations of *ARN* in compositions from the 9th century. On this basis, Kister 1998, dated the final editing to the post-Talmudic period, after the 5th century CE but before the 9th century. See Lerner 1987, 360–381 and especially Ben-Eliyahu, Cohn, and Millar 2012, 57–59.

10 This Talmudic passage is presented in a completely associative manner dealing with number ten. Thus, the ten stipulations laid down by Joshua and the ten enactments which were

'Ten special regulations were applied to Jerusalem: (1) A house cannot be sold there permanently. (2) It does not bring the *eglah arufah* (heifer)[11] sacrifice. (3) It cannot be made [= adjudicated] as an Apostate City. (4) It cannot be defiled by leprosy. (5) Neither beams nor balconies are allowed in it to overhang. (6) No dunghills may be made there. (7) No furnaces are allowed there. (8) No gardens or orchards are allowed there. (9) No chickens must be raised there. (10) No dead bodies may be kept there overnight'.

עשרה דברים נאמרו בירושלים. (1 אין הבית חלוט בה. (2 ואינה מביאה עגלה ערופה.
(3 ואינה נעשית עיר הנדחת. (4 ואינה מטמאה בנגעים. (5 ואין מוציאין בה זיזין וגזוז־
טראות. (6 ואין עושין בה אשפתות. (7 ואין עושין בה כבשונות. (8 ואין עושין בה גנות
ופרדסות חוץ מגנות וורדין שהיו מימות נביאים הראשונים. (9 ואין מגדלים בה תרנגולין.
(10 ואין מלינין בה את המת.

Not all the texts list the same ten things, and in some cases, there are more than ten. In comparing these four lists we see first that the numbers of the laws vary: *BT* and *ARN II* have 10, Tosefta has 14, and *ARN I* has 16 laws listed.[12] Even more noteworthy is the fact that only four of the laws are found in all four lists, and there is a considerable discrepancy in the content of the lists. More startling still is the absence of most of these laws in the *Mishnah*. However, the *Mishnah* preserves laws, which were concerned with purity of Jerusalem, but most of them are quoted among the laws of damages and not in the tractates dealing with purity and sanctity. A few of the laws included in these lists are also found in the *Mishnah* and the *tannaitic Midrashim* or are cited in various Talmudic passages without being grouped together in special lists. In all four lists occur four laws, which pertain to uncleanness and ritual, but they are not identical in all the listings: (1) the dead may not be kept in Jerusalem overnight; (2) beams or balconies may not project over public domain; (3) no planting is permitted in Jerusalem, but the rose gardens; (4) no dunghills may be kept there.

The four *halakhot* were intended to remove from Jerusalem anything which would increase ritual impurity. Dunghills were not allowed, nor was raising chickens (which peck at dung heaps), nor burials. The purity of Jerusalem as regards certain animals, tombs, burial was stressed. None of the four laws, which are found in all four lists is included in the *Mishnah*. On the other hand, there is one law in the *Mishnah* which

---

ordained by Ezra, corresponding also to ten *batlanim*, ten persons who are released from all obligations and thus have leisure to attend to public duties. After displaying the ten special regulations applied to Jerusalem, there is a description of the Hasmoneans, Hyrcanus and Aristobulus, contending in Jerusalem.

11 A *heifer* refers to a cow that was sacrificed and whose ashes were used for the ritual purification.

12 For the manuscripts of the four lists, see Finkelstein 1950, 351–355; For the *Genizah* synopses' fragments of *ARN* of Cambridge T-S NS 226.13, 170–200, MS Parma de Rossi 327, 170–205, MS Vatican 303, 170–205, and MS München 222, 170–200, see apud Becker 2004, 244–245; See also Krauss 1924, 100–106; Finkelstein 1950, 351–369; Guttmann 1969–1970, 251–275; idem. 1972, 67–69; Urbach 1984, 23–24; Lerner 1987, 374–379; Dvorjetski 1996, 203; ead. 1999a, 7–31; ead. 1999b, 50–52; Manns 2001, 76–79; Zevin 2002, 'Jerusalem', XXV, 304–350.

is present in three of the four lists: '[Houses] in Jerusalem and outside of the Land cannot contract uncleanness from leprosy' (Mishnah *Nega'im* 12:4). This law is not included in the *ARN II* list. The prohibition of dunghills in Jerusalem is found in all four lists. However, *Tosefta, Bava Qamma,* 8, 10, clearly implies permission to have dunghills there. It allows the raising of chickens in the city provided a garden or a dunghill was at their disposal. Had there been a dunghill prohibition, raising of chickens on a dunghill could not have been permitted. The contradictory *Tannaitic* views indicate that there was no established law on this matter. It is unlikely that the prohibition of raising chickens existed at the time of the Temple. Had this been an established law, the Tosefta *Nega'im* list certainly would have included it, particularly since this list was not limited to ten items as were the lists of the *BT* and *ARN II.* However, it is possible that it existed as a custom and was later listed as a law. The incongruity of the lists becomes even more striking when we realise that even the longest list, that of *ARN I*, does not include several items found in the shorter lists. Thus *ARN I* does not have the *eglah arufah* (heifer) law found in the Talmud nor the furnace prohibition found in the Talmudic *Baraitha* nor the rulings on the Second Tithe, Lesser Holy Things, and the manure prohibition included in *ARN II.* [13]

Scholars have made various assessments of the nature of these *halakhic* laws, and the time at which they were enunciated. Adolf Büchler argues that most of these regulations are dealing with purity and impurity and their goal is to keep the Holy City purity and holiness. According to him, the laws were prescribed at the end of the Second Temple period, when the Pharisees' regime was powerful and purity spread in the Land of Israel and they could be taken to fruition.[14] Samuel Krauss says that most of them were theoretical rather than practical, since it is almost impossible to put such regulations into practice; some of them originally applied only to the Temple Mount, but later generations broadened their application to the whole of Jerusalem... the purpose of these precepts was to guarantee the cleanliness and health of Jerusalem.[15] Samuel Bialoblotzki rejects Krauss's view. He believes that, although some of the *Halakhot* of Jerusalem are ancient and may have been practised by the people rather than by its leaders, often the laws preceded their reasons; the reasons of Jerusalem laws are the result of Rabbinic thought of later generations. He claims that it is hard to imagine that in the few years preceding the destruction of the Second Temple new regulations. In his view, most of the precepts originated in traditions which became the established practice of the whole nation.[16]

Another approach was suggested by Eliezer Finkelstein. He assumes that those laws were created at the end of the Second Temple period, a short time before the destruction of the city, and were connected with the political aims of the Roman rule.[17] As against Finkelstein, Samuel Safrai emphasized that some of the precepts regarding

---

13 Guttmann 1969–1970, 252–255, 261–263; Manns 2001, 77; Zevin 2002, 'Jerusalem', XXV, 332.
14 Büchler 1911, 201–215; idem. 1912, 30–50.
15 Krauss 1924, 92; See also idem. 1907, 14–55; Cf. Guttmann 1972, 78–79.
16 Bialoblotzki 1971, 37–38.
17 Finkelstein 1950, 358–362.

Jerusalem deal with rules of purity and pollution, and ways of ensuring the purity of the city for the many pilgrims staying there.[18] This opinion is somehow similar to Frédéric Manns's concept. In his view, 'the main purpose of many *Halakhot* is to maintain the purity of the city or to give a blueprint for the Jerusalem of the future'.[19]

Alexander Guttmann demands that some of these laws or customs were in force prior to 70 CE, others after 70 CE; some have relevance even today, others are meant to be implemented upon the restoration of the Jewish State and the Temple. The predominant tendency after the fall of the Temple was to emphasize the unique and distinguished status of the city by pointing to its superiority not merely from the viewpoint of beauty, sanctity, historical past, etc. Accordingly, the *Tannaim* put in special effort in creating laws and practices that would set apart Jerusalem from all the other cities of the land. As a consequence, *halakhot* are being used in the same way as are *Aggadot*. There are the theoretical laws, which are meant to be implemented in the future upon the reestablishment of the Holy City of Jerusalem as the capital of Israel.[20]

The subject was summarized by Efraim Urbach: 'It is hard to find a common theme in these precepts, or to date them. Some of them were early, and their import was known to the *Tannaim*; others were late, and some were never put into practice'. In Urbach's view, the ten maxims about Jerusalem which are mentioned in Tosefta *Nega'im* 6,1–2, and in a parallel passage in the *BT, Bava Qamma* 82b belong to the type of antique laws, which were enacted at different times; the grounds and reasons for them are varied, and those quoted in the Rabbinic sources are not always the original ones.[21] Although the unequivocal premise of Urbach, some unreasonable proposals were suggested for the original version of Jerusalem laws, such as *ARN I* or *BT, Bava Qamma* 82b. Thus, for instance, Francis Peters is convinced that *ARN I* is an authentic reflection, somewhat idealized perhaps, of what Jerusalem should be and surely to some extent was a holy city and sharing some of the same strictures against impurity as the very House of God.[22]

Moshe Herr argues that the Jerusalem *halakhot*, whether reflecting a reality or a utopia, testify to the unique nature and holiness of the city. The status of Jerusalem and the Temple is archetypal in the *halakha*. The centrality of the city, the Temple, and ritual, both conceptually and in reality, is by nature expressed in the literary descriptions of Jews and gentiles alike. All have made pilgrimage to the Temple and sent donations to it from all over the world.[23]

---

18 Safrai 1965, 136; idem. 1996, 94–113; Knowles 2006, 77–103.

19 Manns 2001, 80.

20 Guttmann 1969–1970, 264, 274.

21 Urbach 1971, 345–346; idem. 1984, 23.

22 Peters 1985, 72; The same applies to Grossmark [2006, 263–275], who tries to prove that the *Baraitha* in *BT, Bava Qamma* 82b is the original version.

23 Herr 1980, 173–174; for the attitude of Jews and gentiles towards Jerusalem, see Urbach 1968, 156–171; Kasher 1980, 45–56; Isaac 2010, 3–5.

A new layer is added by Isaiah Gafni.[24] According to him, what is evident from these *Halakhot* is not how the city functioned in reality, but how the Sages chose to view the roles of the city and its status both during the period of the Second Temple, and after its destruction. This distinction applies also to the *Aggadic* material about Jerusalem in the writings of the Sages. Gafni clarifies that the writings of the Sages about Jerusalem were influenced by current affairs and by the special place Jerusalem had in the Judeo-Christian debate, which required a retort to the opinions of the holy city held by those who viewed themselves as the 'New Israel'.

In sum then, some of the items listed as laws in the *Baraitoth* were, in fact, merely customs or practices developed in Jerusalem as it was the site of the Temple, a seat of the Sanhedrin and the capital of the Jewish commonwealth. The precepts of the four lists are never designated as *Taqqanot* or *Gezerot* as the Eighteen Regulations issued before and during the war against the Romans in 66 CE. The *Mishnah* preserves laws, which were concerned with purity of Jerusalem, but most of them are quoted among the laws of damages and not in the tractates dealing with purity and sanctity. It is not inconceivable that various preserved *Halakhot* in Tosefta *Nega'im* prior to those in the *Mishnah*, illustrate the earliest layer of the *Baraitha* of 'Ten matters were said concerning Jerusalem'. Accordingly, it seems that some of the special rules which were crystallized in Jerusalem at an early period were applied in the course of time as municipal by-laws throughout the Land of Israel. It is not unintentionally that various reasons for applying these by-laws to other towns were found, since their fundamental concern was the systematic preservation of public health.[25]

The quality of everyday life in Jerusalem: the concern for public health

The Sages considered odours and their influence on human beings' sensations to be of cardinal importance and sensitivity. 'Three things restore a man's good spirits: sounds, sights, and smells' (*BT, Berakoth* 57b). The Talmudic literature emphasizes the necessity for and the good influence of fresh air. The story of Rabban Yohanan ben Zakkai, who taught on the Temple Mount in Jerusalem 'in the shadow of the Temple' (*JT, Avoda Zarah* 3,13 [43b]; *BT, Pesahim* 26a), is a prototype of similar behaviour by the *Tannaim* and *Amoraim*, who studied and taught in the open air throughout the Land of Israel, in the shade of buildings or beneath trees.[26] This is also the purpose of the burning of incense in the Temple twice daily, in the morning and dusk, in order to counteract the strong pungent smell caused by the killing and roasting of a great number of cattle, whose smell was 'like the smell of a slaughterhouse' (Mishnah *Tamid*, 3:4).[27] The odour of the incense reached as far as Jericho (*ibid.*, 3:8),

---

24 Gafni 1999, 36.
25 The *Baraitha* in Tosefta *Nega'im* 6,1–2, seems to be the best preserved and original text. I follow Efraim Urbach's concept: 1971, 345–346; id. 1984, 23; for the main studies on *Tosefta 'Atiḳta*, see Horowitz 1889; Albeck 1969, 150; Friedman 1993, 313–338, and especially pp. 314–315; id. 2002.
26 Büchler 1914, 485–491; Krauss 1948, 82; Margalit 1977, 152.
27 See also Maimonides, *Moreh HaNebukim*, III, 45 [trans. Pines 1963, II, 579]: 'Inasmuch as

and as a result brides in Jerusalem did not need to perfume themselves (*BT, Yoma* 39b).[28] The priestly family, the Jerusalemite spice-makers, the house of Abtinas, was in charge of mixing the incense, which was composed of eleven aromatic spices (*BT, Keritot* 6a). Only they knew the professional secret of making incense whose smoke rose straight up (Mishnah *Sheqalim* 4:5; *BT, ibid.,* 48d–49a; *ibid., Yoma* 38a; *ibid., Ketuboth* 106a). Spices were very much in demand, not only for Temple purposes but for daily personal use and for burial as well.[29] It is obvious that the daily sacrifice of more than a hundred animals would indeed be an expensive installation to erect. The ritual was also associated with hygienic precautions, for the priests and the authorities felt responsible for the health of their communities.[30]

Refuse

Talmudic sources pay special attention to the need to keep Jerusalem free of refuse. One of the ten maxims is that no dunghills be made there. The *Gemara* (*BT, Bava Qamma* 82b) gives the reason: 'on account of reptiles'.[31] The Book of *Nehemiah* mentions several times a gate called *Sha'ar Ha'Ašpōt / Sopot* (2:13; 3:13–14; 12:31). This toponym is usually translated as 'Dung Gate', based on the analogy with *II Samuel* 2:8 and *Psalms* 113:7.[32] These verses mention the city's poor people, who most probably were foraging the city dump for food. Even if we accept Benjamin Mazar to relate *špt* to *tpt*—the Tophet—which was an extramural high place in the Valley of Hinnom (*II Kings* 21:6; *II Chronicles* 33:6), we remain in an area of dirt.[33] The place Tophet involved an extensive use of fire, which produced burning waste such as ashes, soot, and charred wood. Jan Simons surmises that the location of the Gate of the pottery sherds known as the *Sha'ar HaHarsīt* in the southern side of the city (*Jeremiah* 19:2), might

many beasts were slaughtered daily in that holy place, the flesh cut into pieces, and the intestines burnt and washed, there is no doubt that if it had been left in that state its smell would have been like that of a slaughterhouse'.

28 Tucazinsky 1952, 210; Kotlar 1976, 63; Feliks 1992, 59–60; idem. 1997a, 23–32, 92–97; See also Har-El 1970, 163–165, 169; However, it seems that it is quite problematic to take the texts as historical facts.

29 Haran 1960, 113–129; Klausner 1975, 188; Ayali 1987, 22, 24, 26; Har-El 1987, 312; Preuss 1993, 437; Edersheim 1997, 111; Heger 1997, 44; Rosner 2000, 173; Ulmer 2009, 204; See also the discussion in Dvorjetski [forthcoming (a)], chapter 7.3 on *Aromatic Substances: Perfumes and Spices*.

30 The conception of personal cleanliness as both a prerequisite of holiness and an aid to physical fitness is central to Jewish tradition. Many of the Biblical commandments promote hygiene, though their stated intention was ritual purity rather than physical cleanliness. Talmudic literature is even more specific in its stress on hygiene; For the norms of purity and impurity in Second Temple Judaism and for hygienic precautions taken by the priests and authorities since ancient times, see Dvorjetski [forthcoming (a)], chapter 3.5.1 on *Hygienic Measures and Preventive Medicine*.

31 Reich and Shukron 2003, 16–17; These two archaeologists reconstructed the process of garbage removal from the city from mid-1st century BCE. There existed a steady action of refuse removal from the streets to the city-dump on the southeastern outskirts of the city. It seems to them that the location of the city-dump of the late Second Temple period in this particular part of the city had a previous long history in the late Iron Age II.

32 Simons 1952, 123; Reich and Eli Shukron 2003, 16–17; See also the discussion below.

33 Mazar 1975, 194–195.

point to a pile of garbage, as pottery vessels were the type of household item broken and discarded in antiquity more than any other type of artifact.[34]

In other cities refuse was permitted to be left outside in the street for a very short time only (Mishnah *Bava Mezia* 10:5), whereas the rule for Jerusalem was that, 'no dunghills should be made there and no dunghills should be there to the public domain' (*ARN II*, 39, Schechter ed., p. 107). It was forbidden to leave refuse in public places even when it was being collected for removal from the city. This ensured that no harm was done to pilgrims, who were strangers to Jerusalem, were unfamiliar with its approaches, and did not know how to watch out the ways and the streets.[35] In addition to the prohibition on the accumulation of refuse in public areas, the preservation of the cleanliness of the streets and public health also required continuous activity day by day: 'The markets of Jerusalem must be cleaned every day' (*BT, Bava Mezia* 26a).[36]

One of the ten maxims says: 'Gardens and orchards may not be planted there' (*ibid., Bava Qamma* 82b). The *Gemara* gives the reason: 'Because of the stench'; since they may create a bad smell. It may be that this stench arises because the gardens are manured or because of flies and reptiles, as the *Gaonim* contend.[37] From this law one may learn the degree of caution required by the legal provisions concerning the preservation of the environment; it applies not only to actions which involve direct harm to the environment, but also to the creation of conditions which may bring about a nuisance—in this case, even a bad smell. The parallel *halakha* in Tosefta (*Nega'im* 6, 1–2) to 'gardens and orchards may not be planted there' in the *BT* (*Bava Qamma* 82b) states that the city 'is neither planted nor sown nor ploughed'. *Midrash Song of Songs Rabbah* (4, 13, Greenhut ed., p. 90) says that 'Jerusalem was surrounded by 364 different types of irrigated fields. In each of them there was a camphor tree, and they were full of all sorts of perfumes, and the priests would go out there and bring whatever was required for cleansing the Temple'.[38] It seems that the ecological reason for the *halakhic* precept that Jerusalem is neither planted nor sown is the exclusion of bad odours from the city.[39] Even so, it may be that *Midrash Song of Songs Rabbah* relates to Jericho Valley—a region which was well known as one of the most fertile parts of the Land of Israel, and the only place where camphor and other types of perfume were grown.[40]

The practices of the Temple in Jerusalem provide evidence of the recycling of waste in antiquity. The underlying concept is that of public health. The surplus blood from the Temple was 'merged into the water channel in the Temple court, and flowed out to the Kidron Valley, and was sold to the gardeners as manure' (Mishnah *Yoma* 5:6).[41]

---

34 Simons 1952, 230; See also Reich and Shukron 2003, 17.

35 Finkelstein 1950, 351–352; Zeligmann 1981, 10–11; Cf. Feliks 1990, 92.

36 Margalit 1977, 149; Dvorjetski 1999b, 51; Zevin 2002, 'Jerusalem', XXV, 337.

37 Bialoblotzki 1971, 28–29; Safrai 1965, 166; Guttmann 1972, 76; Zeligmann 1981, 22; Zikal 1990, 43.

38 See also Yalkut Shimoni *Song of Songs*, 4, 34; *Tanhuma Trumah* 11; Patai 1947, 90–91.

39 Urbach 1984, 24.

40 Feliks 1997a, 46–47, 97; See also Ayali 1987, 23; Schwartz 1994.

41 It was subject to the laws of peculation, and it was forbidden to use it without payment; Rakover 1993, 60.

The plentiful waters of the 'Arrub aqueduct carried the blood and the detritus of the sacrifices and the ash-houses down to the Kidron Valley.[42] In *The Letter of Aristeas*, whose author lived at the end of the 2nd century BCE, it is conspicuous that there are slopes at fixed places to carry away the water, which washes away the blood of the sacrifices on the days of the festivals many thousands of cattle are brought thither, and the supply of water is not lessened.[43]

After being removed from the altar, the ashes of the Temple sacrifices were removed outside Jerusalem, to the north of the city (Mishnah *Zevahim* 5:2; Tosefta *Yom HaKipurim* 3, 17 [Lieberman ed., p. 247]; *BT, Zevahim* 4b).[44] It may be that they were deposited in a place where there are no strong winds, as Maimonides claims, so that they should not constitute a nuisance to the eyes when dispersed in the air.[45] In the *Gemara* opinions about the place where the ashes were located are divided: some maintain that it was to the east of the city, others to the south (*BT, Yoma* 68a-b; *ibid., Zevahim* 105b–106a). According to the tradition of the Jews of Jerusalem, the depository of the ashes was to the east of today's Meah She'arim quarter.[46]

Smoke

The Rabbis differed on the question of the proscription on the burning of olive-or vine-wood on the altar for the Temple sacrifices (Mishnah *Tamid* 2:3). Rav Aha bar Ya'akov believed that it stemmed from the precept to settle the Land of Israel, in order to prevent the destruction of olive trees and vines; Rav Papa claimed that 'any wood may be used for the sacrificial fire apart from vine and olive wood... because of the smoke' (*BT, ibid.,* 21a-b).[47] In *the Book of Jubilees* Abraham warns Isaac in his will to bring suitable sacrificial wood to the altar: 'Take caution with the wood of the offering that you do not bring wood for the offering except of such as these: cypress, bay, almond, fir, pine, cedar, juniper, fig, olive, myrtle, laurel, and asphalathos'.[48]

Smoke was liable to cause damage and harm the eyes (*Midrash Lamentations Rabbah* 2,19), but smoke from the sacrificial fire—in addition to the harm it might do to the health of those who made the sacrifices and of the public in general—was liable to make the wine for the libation unacceptable (*BT, Zevahim* 64a), or to kill the birds intended for sacrifice (*ibid. ibid.,* 63a–64a; *ibid., Menahot* 86b).

Smoke from the Menorah in the temple blackened the southern wall close to which it was situated. A discussion in the *Gemara* (*BT, Yoma* 52a) emphasizes that it constituted a nuisance for the High Priest who passed by it on *Yom Kippur* through the

42 Har-El 1987, 312; Mazar 2002, 213–217, Figs. 1, 2a–2b.
43 *The Letter of Aristeas* 88–89; On its water supply: Tacitus, *Annales*, V, 12; Cf. the citations in *Ecclesiasticus* 50,3.
44 See Henshke 1997, 25–26.
45 Maimonides, *Hilkhot Tmidin ve Musafin* 2,15; See also Freudenstein 1970, 410.
46 Istori HaParhi 1959, 77; Horowitz 1964, 131, 173; Kotlar 1976, 44.
47 Kotlar 1976, 56; Shinover and Goldberg 1994, 139–140; Dvorjetski 1999b, 46.
48 *The Book of Jubilees* XXI,12–15; See also Dvorjetski 1999a, 11; idem. 1999b, 51.

Temple on his way to the Holy of Holies: 'As to Rabbi Judah, let him enter between the candlestick and the wall. His garments would become blackened'.

It is important to note that the smoke rising from the sacrificial fire in the Temple was used for meteorological observations of the course of the winds and their influence on the year's crops (*BT, Yoma* 21b):

> 'The east wind is always good, the west wind always bad, the north wind benefits wheat when it has grown to one third [of its usual height], and is bad for olives when they are budding; the south wind is bad for wheat which has grown one third [of its normal size] and good for olives when they are budding.'

Other passages refer to the amount of water available for agriculture (*BT, Bava Bathra* 147a).[49]

Due to the unique nature and the overcrowding in the city, it seems that the prohibition on polluting the air with smoke was particularly emphasized in the municipal by-laws, in order to educate the populace and ensure their health: 'No furnace shall be made there ... because of the smoke' (*BT, Bava Qamma* 82b). Smoke, which blackens the walls and fortifications of the city, the fruit of the aesthetic creativity of every ancient city, was a disgrace to any city, and especially to the city of Jerusalem. This is depicted obviously in the description of Rome by the Palestinian *amora* Ulla, 3rd–4th century CE: 'There are...baths in it [= in Rome], and 500 windows the smoke from which goes outside the wall' (*ibid., Megillah* 6b).[50]

Three types of kilns are known from ancient times: for burning lime kiln, manufacturing glass, and for pottery. In the city of Jerusalem there was a special reason for the great number of furnaces: the Passover sacrifices were brought to the city; they were burnt in ceramic ovens (Mishnah *Ta'anit* 3:8), and each sacrifice required a separate oven (*BT, Pesahim* 76b). Most of the cooking of food at this period was done in ceramic vessels, and such a vessel had to be broken if it was declared unfit for use. It could, however, be fired anew, in which case it was considered to be new (*ibid., Zevahim* 96a). The *Baraitha* in *BT, Bava Qamma* 82b, includes this in the ten maxims concerning Jerusalem: 'No furnaces shall be made there'. The *Gemara* applies this prohibition to potters' furnaces; but it is unlikely that it was applied in practice.[51] It may be that the prohibition on the building of furnaces in Jerusalem reflects the often repeated conflict between the demand to ensure the health of the populace and the aspiration to improve its economic situation. This precept gives priority to consider-

---

49 Krauss 1924, 105; Ben-Horim 1929–1930, 23; Kotlar 1976, 56–57; Dvorjetski 1996, 202–203; idem. 1999a, 11–12; idem. 1999b, 52; Zevin 2002, 'Jerusalem', XXV, 334.

50 Stephen Newmyer 1996, 89 clarifies that Ulla likely refers to attempts by the Romans to provide an effective system for removing exhaust from the heating systems of Roman baths by assuring that the windows used in such structures stood above the walls of the city, thereby preventing pollution of the air of the city of Rome by a recirculation of stale heated air inside the city'; The Soncino translator believes that Ulla is referring to the exhaust system of the enormous Baths of Diocletian built in Rome between 298 and 306 CE.

51 *BT, Hagigah* 26a; See also Bialoblotzki 1971, 27–28; Kotlar 1976, 58; Ayali 1987, 19.

ations of health.[52] In the Tosefta (*Bava Bathra* 1,10), Rabbi Nathan maintained that the prohibition on furnaces applied to cities in general: 'Furnaces are to be kept fifty cubits distant from the city'. An architect of the 6th century CE, Julian of Ascalon, a contemporary of the Byzantine Emperor Justinian I, also mentions this prohibition. Julian's treatise on *The Laws of Palestine and Its Customs* is a compilation of construction and design rules that address the prevention of nuisances and potential damages to proximate neighbours resulting from building activities associated with change and growth in the built environment.[53] His words are reminiscent of those of Rabbi Nathan in the Tosefta, who maintains that the prohibition applied to all the cities of the Land of Israel, and not only to Jerusalem.[54]

The by-laws of Jerusalem did not only employ positive expressions such as 'excluding' or standard measurements such as fifty cubits; they used unambiguously negative expressions such as 'אין עושין' [= one should not make], 'אין מקימין' [= one should not set up], or 'אין מגדלין' [= one should not raise]. It may be that most of the residents did not need legal terminology, since they were aware to the question of public health in their city, which was supposed to serve as an example and symbol for the pilgrims frequently to be found there, and because of the density of the population, which was particularly great.[55]

Acoustic nuisances

In the Graeco-Roman world, education to the avoidance of environmental noise promoted widespread consciousness as the result of urban by-laws and the legislation of the Emperors.[56] There is unique evidence from the Classical literature of another fundamental consideration of those who compiled the ecological precepts for Jerusalem with a view to the health of its population and the quality of their lives. In the 2nd century CE, the Greek orator Athenaeus from Neocratis, Egypt, wrote that the inhabitants of the city of Sybaris in southern Italy prohibited the establishment of noisy trades such as that of blacksmiths or carpenters in their town; they also prohibited the raising of chickens, lest they disturb their rest and sleep.[57]

The Talmudic literature also shows that education for the prevention of environmental noise in Jerusalem began as early as the Second Temple period.[58] The laws

---

52 Zeligmann 1981, 17; see also Spanier and Sasson 2001.
53 For Julian's treatise, see Lieberman 1971, 409–417; Hakim 2001, 4–25; Saliou 2007, 169–178; It was preserved through the manuscript tradition, as making part of *Eparchikon Biblion* and *Hexabiblos* of Harmenopulos from Thessaloniki 1345 [Nicole 1894] and which text was reconstructed by Saliou 1996.
54 Lieberman 1971, 416; Dvorjetski 1999b, 12; Guttmann 1972, 75.
55 See Yasar (Schlichter) 1950, 59–64; Dvorjetski 1999b, 12.
56 Dvorjetski 1995b, 59; On the Emperors' regulations towards noise, see Dvorjetski 1995, 59; ead. (forthcoming [a]), chapter 2.5 on *Hygiene, Sanitation, and Organization of Public Health: The Legacy of Rome*.
57 Athenaeus, *Deipnosophistae*, XII, 518c; Lieberman 1973, VIII, 748; Kotlar 1976, 50; Cf. Qimron 1994, 473–476; Dvorjetski 1999b, 18.
58 Lieberman 1973, 748.

of the High Priest of the Hasmonean dynasty, Yohanan Hyrcanus (135–104 BCE), have been preserved in the Talmudic sources. The Mishnah gives some hints of his reforms in the fields of cult and *halakha,* which were viewed favourably later on. With regard to them, it is very likely that the smiths' workshops may have been intentionally placed outside the walls as a preventive measure against noise and smoke.[59] Mishnah *Ma'aser Sheni* 5:15, reports to have banned such work from Jerusalem:

> 'Yohanan the High Priest set aside the confession of the tithes; He also abolished the awakeners (המעוררים)[60] and the stunners (הנוקפים).[61] Until his days the hammer used to smite[62] in Jerusalem. And in his days, none needed to inquire concerning *demai*-produce'.[63]

The noise of workmens' hammers is the symbol of an environmental nuisance. The Tosefta (*Sotah* 13,10), says: 'Until his days hammers did strike in Jerusalem on *Hol Hamo'ed* [= The intermediate days of the festival]; that is to say, irksome noise was heard in Jerusalem during working days on *Hol Hamo'ed*, at a period when the performance of various tasks were forbidden because of the sanctity of the festival. The *Gemara* (*BT, Sotah* 48a) represents the original sense of this early tradition and gives a similar explanation: 'Up to his days the hammer used to strike in Jerusalem on the intermediate days of the festival'.[64] It may be that certain types of work were permitted on the festival [= *Hol Hamo'ed*], but the Hasmonean ruler Yohanan Hyrcanus applied a stricter rule for Jerusalem, and decreed that even these tasks should not be performed. Hyrcanus' prohibition of hammering on these days heightened the feast's dignity. Not unintentionally, the early Jewish and Talmudic sources present him as a highly gifted high priest, conqueror, zealot against idolatry, advocate of Jewish national interests, and a pious mystic with a view for future developments.[65] Lee Levine claims that although Tosefta *Sotah* 13,10 (Lieberman ed., p. 235) interprets this decree as referring only to the intermediate days of the festival; it may well be a later, and erroneous, interpretation.[66] According to him, Hyrcanus' decree may have been a general, civic, one. Thus, the smiths' workshops may have been intentionally placed

---

59 Mishnah *Ma'aser Sheni* 5:15; *ibid., Sotah* 9:10; *ibid., Parah* 3:5; *ibid., Yadaim* 4:6; Tosefta *Sotah* 13,10; *BT, ibid.,* 48a; *ibid., Mo'ed Qatan* 11a; See Lieberman 1950, 139–143; Thoma 1994, 133–134; Levine 2002, 336; Zevin 2002, 'Jerusalem', XXV, 343.

60 Hyrcanus further forbade the liturgical custom of the 'awakeners'. See also *BT, Sotah* 48a.

61 Those who used to strike the animal between its horns before slaughtering it for a sacrifice; Thoma 1994, 134.

62 Workmens' hammers, especially smiths, worked in the Temple precinct and caused a disturbing noise of hammering (Tosefta *Sotah* 13,10; *BT, Mo'ed Qatan* 11a) on the middle days of Passover and the Feast of Tabernacles. Hyrcanus abolished work on these semi-sacred days.

63 He ordered that all *demai* produce of an *'Am HaAretz* must be tithed by the new owners; Thoma 1994, 131–132.

64 I.e., work used to be done on those days, which were a semi-festival, and Yohanan abolished the practice.

65 Danby 1933, 82; Krauss 1924, 95; Tucazinsky 1952, 209; Kotlar 1973, 9; Tabory 1995, 76; Cf. Gil 1988, 157–164; Thoma 1994, 134.

66 Levine 2002, 33; See also Lieberman 1973, VIII, 748.

outside the walls as a preventive measure against noise. Banning such work from Jerusalem, it may have been at that point that these artisans relocated outside the city walls to the north. However, scholars' opinions about the significance of the laws of Yohanan Hyrcanus have differed. Saul Lieberman maintained that Yohanan's aim was to purify the temple rites.[67] Efraim Urbach accepted Lieberman's suggestion that the object was to abolish customs connected with idolatrous rites, but added that 'the meaning of 'עד ימיו היה פטיש מכה בירושלים' [= 'until his time hammers beat in Jerusalem'] remains unexplained'. In Urbach's view, the phrase 'hammers beat' and the context in which it appears allude to 'a particular institution and custom'. Instead of the hammer, which was in use until the time of Yohanan, the use of a *magrefah*—a musical instrument with ten holes (*BT, Arakhin* 10b–11a)—to inform the priests and Levites that it was time to begin their duties was instituted.[68]

The concept of 'striking with a hammer' appears in the Talmudic corpus in connection with the law of Yohanan Hyrcanus, and is also one of the 39 trades which it is forbidden to practise on the Sabbath (Mishnah *Shabbat* 7:2). Yitzhak Gilat maintained that the list of trades originated in ancient traditions, which reflect the nature of the sacred laws of antiquity. In his view, the list of trades originated in natural observation of the works of man and his way of life, and constituted a guideline to the Sages when they came to define archetypal trades, primary occupations in each group of categories of work.[69] Thus, to the national and religious aspirations of Yohanan the High Priest and head of the Sanhedrin, we must add the concrete realistic approach for Jerusalem—education to the avoidance of environmental noise, which is known to do severe damage to health in the context of the quality of life and the environment.

Nuisances caused by animals

The requirement to eliminate public nuisances also applied to animals, which were potentially very dangerous. The Talmudic sources discuss various animals, which threaten public health. With reference to bees, for instance (Tosefta *Bava Bathra* 1,9), Rabbi Ele'azar says: 'One who raises bees is equivalent to one who raises dogs'. It may be that in both instances he is referring to the damage they cause. From *Miqṣat Ma'aśe HaTorah Scroll* we learn that the Dead Sea sect differed from their opponents on the question of whether dogs might be brought into Jerusalem. The inclusion of the prohibition of dogs in this scroll indicates the importance attributed to this question by the sect of the Judaean desert, since this scroll describes most of the controversial issues as a result of which the cult split off from the main community of Israel. This scroll gives a reason for the prohibition: fear that the dogs would eat the flesh which remained on the bones of the Temple sacrifices. Elisha Qimron and John

---

67 Lieberman 1973, VIII, 747–748.
68 Urbach 1984, 39; Mishnah *Tamid* 5:6, gives an overstated description by saying that it drowned all the voices in the city; See also *JT, Sukkah* 5,6 [55b]; *Midrash Ecclesiastes Zuta* 9,18, Buber ed., p. 127a; See also Büchler 1956, 44–51.
69 Gilat 1967, 149–151; See also Krauss 1911, 656.

Strugnell deduce that the opponents of the sect did keep dogs in Jerusalem, and the sect considered this to be a severe transgression.[70]

Interesting issue that should be pointed out that the Book of *Nehemiah* (13:16) explicitly indicates that Tyrians traders came to Jerusalem to sell fish. Other historical sources reveal that fish were a staple which was traded in international trade routes.[71] At that time, and even earlier, the 'Fish Gate' is known in the city, probably the place next to the local fish market (*Zephaniah* 1:10; *Nehemiah* 3:16). Archaeological discoveries made in close proximity to the spring located in the Kidron Valley nearby uncovered remains apparently originating from the north of the Land of Israel and perhaps Phoenicia and the Mediterranean. The earliest are dated to the end of the 9th or early 8th century BCE. Most striking findings is a greater amount (10,600 items) of fish bones, and the vast majority (about 86%) are from the Mediterranean Sea.[72]

In the laws concerning Jerusalem pigs, geese, chickens, and small cattle are also mentioned (Mishnah *Bava Qamma* 7:7; *ARN I*, 35, Schechter ed., p. 104; *ARN II*, *ibid.*, p. 107; *BT, Bava Qamma* 82b; and more). The fact that the sacrifice of pigs and the consumption of their flesh was a central item in the decrees of Antiochus IV Epiphanes, and the martyrdom of those who laid down their lives as a result of their refusal to obey these laws,[73] is sufficient support for the hypothesis that the prohibition on the raising of pigs throughout the Land of Israel is to be dated from the early Hasmonean period. This prohibition, like other laws connected with Jerusalem, is part of the system of laws dating from the early period of the Hasmonean dynasty, the days of Simeon and his son Yohanan Hyrcanus.[74] A law quoted in the *Mishnah* states: 'They may not rear small cattle in the Land of Israel, but they may rear them in Syria or in the wildernesses that are in the Land of Israel' (*Bava Qamma* 7:7). The reason for the prohibition on raising sheep and goats was certainly the desire to protect agricultural land from being spoilt by the flocks, since the shepherds did not choose their places of pasturage with care; it was also intended to encourage the cultivation of the land, and to protect natural forest—to preserve trees in inhabited places for the public benefit—since the beauty of man's environment is also of cardinal importance.[75]

The law forbidding the raising of chickens is also given a rationale: to keep unclean elements away from Jerusalem, 'No one may raise chickens in Jerusalem because of the sacrifices' (*ibid.*).[76] The *Mishnah* preserves a law which was concerned with the

---

70 Qimron and Strugnell 1994, 162–164; Qimron 1995, 474; Cf. Henshke 1997, 27.

71 Lipinski 2004, 493–545; Edelman 2005, 207–246.

72 Reich, Shukron, and Landau 2007a, 32–40; idem. 2007b, 153–169; Reich 2014, 186.

73 *II Maccabees* II,6, 18; VI,1; Josephus, *Antiquitates Judaicae* XII, 253; XIII, 243; The earliest indication of the purity of Jerusalem is an Edict (πρόγραμμα) granted to Jerusalem by Antiochus III the Great and recorded by Josephus, which forbade bringing the flesh or the hide of unclean animals into Jerusalem and forbade the rearing of such animals in the city; See Bickerman 1980, II, 44–104; Tcherikover 1982, 86–87; Stern 1983, 42, note 39; Hayes and Mandell 1998, 39–41; Manns 2001, 78–79; Levine 2002, 69.

74 Urbach 1984, 25.

75 Baer 1952, 40–41; Cohen 1978, 99–102; Ben-Shalom 1986, 36–45.

76 Guttmann 1972, 73–74; Henshke 1997, 27; Zevin 2002, 'Jerusalem', XXV, 332.

purity of Jerusalem, but it is quoted among the laws of damages, and not in the tractates dealing with purity and sanctity. The addition of geese may be interpreted in
accordance with the linguistic practice of the Talmud, since geese and chickens are
often mentioned together. In Samuel Krauss's view, the reason for the prohibitions
was because of the dirt and stench arising from the rotting bodies of the animals.[77]

A small fragment of the *Temple Scroll* from Qumran Cave 11 published by Elisha
Qimron says: 'You shall not raise chickens'.[78] The other words which have survived
indicate that other animals which were not allowed in Jerusalem were also mentioned.
The Sages who forbade the raising of chickens during the Second Temple period, according to *Miqsat Ma'ase HaTorah* treatise, permitted the keeping of dogs. Qimron
thinks that it is strange that the Sages were lenient in the matter of dogs, which are
impure beasts, and stringent in the matter of chickens, which are pure birds. This
fragment sheds light on some early legal sources referring to the purity of Jerusalem
and the sacred food eaten there.

The *Mishnah* (*Eduyot* 6:1) quotes the words of Rabbi Judah ben Abba[79] about a
chicken which was stoned in Jerusalem 'because it destroyed a soul [= a man]'. Chickens that peck among the refuse are also liable to cause damage 'because they scratch at
the walls' (Tosefta *Bava Metzia* 8,30). Half the damage is to be paid 'for the chickens
which scrabble among the dough and the fruit or peck [...] if they scratch at the rope
holding the bucket, and it falls and is broken [...] if they get into the garden and break
off the young shoots and injure the vegetables [...] if the chicken darts from place to
place and does damage with its body' (*ibid., Bava Qamma* 2,1).

The Peristereon (περιστερεῶν) [= the dovecot] situated to the east of the Tyropoeon
close to the Kidron Valley and above the Siloam ravine, is apparently the place where
doves were bred and brought up for the Temple sacrifices. It is referred to only by Josephus,[80] and was also an area which caused ecological damage,[81] since the dovecote
is included in the precepts which deal with the avoidance of nuisances in the urban
environment. So, it is cited in Mishnah *Bava Bathra* 2:5: 'One must keep his dovecote at fifty cubits' distance from a town, and he may not build a dovecote on his own
property unless there is a space of fifty cubits in every direction'.[82]

---

77 Krauss 1924, 104–105.
78 Qimron 1995, 473–474.
79 The name Rabbi Judah ben Abba appears in the manuscripts of Kaufman, Parma, Cambridge,
    and in a *Genizah* fragment; See Katsh 1970, 95; In the *Defusim* it remains Rabbi Judah ben Bava.
80 Josephus, *Bellum Judaicum* V, 505; Avi-Yonah [1956a, 319] assumes that this is one of the rocks
    near the village of Siloam, where pigeons were bred for sacrifices; Ussishkin [1974, 70–72] sug-
    gests that Josephus referred to the description of small openings of burial caves from the Iron
    Age, which were visible to all, who stood on the south-eastern hill of City of David. Those re-
    minded him of typical niches of dovecotes [= columbaria]; Cf. Reich and Shukron [2004, 187],
    who follow Avi-Yonah's opinion and rejects Ussishkin's theory; Reich 2014, 187–188.
81 Avi-Yonah 1975, 177, 242; See the map in Bahat 1994, 19: *The Second Temple Period: 538 BCE–
    70CE.*
82 See Tosefta *Bava Bathra* 1,7; See also Zikal 1990, 88–89; Dvorjetski 1999b, 15.

Sanitary inspection, urban planning, and the beauty of the city

On the 15th of the month of Adar, after the winter rains and before the arrival of large numbers of pilgrims for the Passover pilgrimage, the Court would send out agents to repair the paths, the roads, the streets, and pools of water, the water sources and the reservoirs (Mishnah *Sheqalim* 1:1; Tosefta, *ibid*. 1:1–2). Among the tasks which were permitted on *Hol Hamo'ed* because of the needs of the populace and care for their health were repairing the damage to public property in good time: aqueducts which had been damaged or blocked up by earth, and repairing the damage to public water-pipes, clearing them, removing the accumulated refuse and blockages, and repairing the reservoirs.[83] In Mishnah *Mo'ed Qatan* 1:2, the Sages differ about the appropriate timing: 'Rabbi Ele'azar ben Azzariah says, "During mid-festival and during the Seventh year they may not dig a new water-channel." But the Sages say: "During the Seventh Year they may dig a new water-channel, and during mid-festival they may repair what has been broken down; they may repair damaged water-ways in the public domain and clean them out; and they may repair roads, open places, and pools of water, and perform all public needs and mark the graves"'.

All the city's inhabitants, including orphans and scholars, were required to pay taxes and participate in the expenses of the water project (*BT, Bava Bathra* 8a). In addition to the activities organized by the authorities and inhabitants of the city, there is evidence that some individuals contributed to the digging of wells for public use at their own initiative. Shimeon from Sachnin was a member of the *boule* and dug wells, channels and caves for the pilgrims (*Ecclesiastes Rabbah* 4,17). So did Nehonia 'the trench-digger', who was appointed by the Temple and dealt with digging wells and cisterns (Mishnah *Sheqalim* 5:1; Tosefta *Bava Qamma* 6:5; *BT, ibid*. 50a).[84]

The usage of the Temple sacrifices' treasure for building an aqueduct made uproar among the Jewish people at the time of the Roman procurator Pontius Pilate (26–36 CE);[85] but then apparently, they accepted the idea, because according to Mishnah *Sheqalim* 4:2, it is allowed to use the money kept in the Chamber of the treasure for repairing the aqueduct.

Originating at the foot of the Temple Mount and flowing into a pool, the waters of the Siloam were the symbol of pure water. The waters of the Siloam were looked after meticulously, and Josephus declares, 'for so we called that fountain of sweet and abundant water'.[86] In *Midrash Lamentations Rabbah* 19 (Buber ed., p. 15), Jeremiah is represented as saying to the people of Israel: 'Had you been worthy, you would be

---

83 Safrai 1965, 112, 158; Kotlar 1976, 76; Shinover and Goldberg 1994, 183–186; Safrai 1995, 232–234; Dvorjetski (forthcoming [a]), chapter 9.2 on *Water Supply and Systems, Drainage, Sewers, and Aqueducts*.

84 Delitzsch 1877, 40; Avi-Yonah 1956b, 418; Safrai 1995, 249–250; Zevin 2002, 'Jerusalem', XXV, 329–330.

85 Josephus, *Bellum Judaicum* II,187; Avi-Yonah 1956b, 418; Dvorjetski (forthcoming [a]), chapter 10.2, on *The History of Medicine, Sanitation, and Hygiene in Jerusalem from Biblical Times to the Late Roman Period*.

86 Josephus, *Bellum Judaicum* V,140.

dwelling in Jerusalem and drinking the waters of Siloam whose waters are clean and sweet'.[87] They were used for libations in the Temple (Mishnah *Sukkah* 4:9; *BT, ibid.* 48a). When water for guilt offerings was needed, children would ride down to the Siloam well on oxen, holding stone cups, which they filled from the well (Mishnah *Parah* 3:2). It is said that the priests 'when they ate much of the sacred flesh, used to drink the water of the Siloam, which was digested in their bowels' (*ARN I*, 35, Schechter ed., p. 105). Among those responsible for the priests, medicines and merchandise of the Temple was Ben Ahijah, who was responsible for bowel sickness (Mishnah *Sheqalim* 5:1–2). He was especially well familiar with the effect of individual types of wine on the function of the stomach and intestines (*JT, ibid.* 5,1 [48d]). However, nowhere he is addressed by the title *rophé*.[88] In the list of the Temple officials which is given in the Tosefta (*ibid.* 2,14–15), a physician is not mentioned at all. Be that as it may, the priests were subject to this illness, since 'they walked barefoot on the [stone] floor, ate meat and drank water, and became sick in their bowels' [= depending excessively on a meat diet] (*JT, ibid.* 5,2 [48d]).

When the Sages comment on the future of Jerusalem, their descriptions are the most far-reaching. Thus, for instance, *Exodus Rabbah* 15,21, which states that God will one day live water out through Jerusalem to cure any disease.[89]

As for the Temple Mount, it was forbidden to enter there in an undignified manner:

> 'A man should not enter the Temple Mount with his staff or with his shoes on or with his wallet or with his feet dust-stained; nor should he make it a short cut [= kappandria], and spitting on it [= the Mount] is forbidden, *a fortiori*' (*BT, Berakhot* 54a).[90]

The Temple Mount was paved, as was customary in the Hellenistic period in courtyards and around holy places, in order to fortify the area against strong rains and to prevent erosion of the soil, dirty, and destruction of the floor as a result of the many visitors to the Temple Mount and the Temple. It appears that not only sacred sites were paved; public areas of the city were also covered with some sort of paving: 'the markets of Jerusalem had to be cleaned every day' (*ibid., Bava Metzia* 26a). Thus, not only one central market, but all or most of them were subject to sanitary inspection (*JT, Ma'aser Sheni* 5,4 [56b]). It may be that Jerusalem was paved with marble by the 18,000 building workmen who were released from their work in the Temple at the time of King Herod Agrippa II[91] for social reasons, in order to provide employment, but it was also done in order to prevent soil erosion and dirt in the streets.[92] The pil-

---

87 Funk 1912, 191, 222; Eisenstein 1952, V, 123; Hecker 1956, 195–199; Har-El 1970, 135–147; Preuss 1993, 531; Kottek 1994, 54.

88 Preuss 1993, 14, 572; See also Safrai 1983, 214; Hoenig 1989, 61–63.

89 Urbach 1971, 348.

90 Cf. Tosefta *Berakhot* 7,19: See also Safrai 1999, 23.

91 Josephus, *Antiquitates Judaicae* XX, 222; Jeremias 1969, 12–13; Mazar 1975, 210; See also Schwartz 1987.

92 Kotlar 1976, 87.

grims who entered the Temple court from the Tyropoeon or one of the Ḥuldah gates, or who passed over the viaduct leading from the Upper City, saw a vast court paved with many-coloured stones and surrounded by porticoes with columns of white stone.[93] The floors of the Temple were also suitably treated. Philo of Alexandria, who related to Jerusalem not as the capital of a state, but primarily as 'a holy city', stated that the chief function of the Levites was to guard the Temple night and day, to sing while sacrifices were being made, and 'some of them sweep the colonnades and court-yards, remove the refuse, and attend to cleanliness'.[94]

The Rabbis looked favourably on the Romans' sanitary works for the benefit of the public: 'What does the King [= Emperor] do with this money? He builds... lavatories for the needs of the poor' (*Exodus Rabbah* 31,11).[95] There were snakes, scorpions, mice, and other vermins in the lavatories (*Genesis Rabbah* 10,7, Theodor-Albeck ed., p. 81; *BT, Berakhot* 23a; *ibid., ibid.* 62a–b).[96] There were disinfectants and means of purifying impure and malodorous air in the privy: 'One should not make a blessing over perfumes of the privy, or oil which is meant to purify the filth' (*ibid., ibid.* 53a); 'a saucer of *pleiton*, which was placed in the place of filth' (*Sanhedrin* 108a); and also 'a tub of balsam which was put in the filthy place' (*Tanhuma Noah* 58,5).[97]

The ten Jerusalem maxims also deal with the planning of building in such a way that it will not harm the majority of the populace. Both public and private building had to be executed in such a way that the welfare of the people of the capital should not be impaired or endangered. 'Neither beams nor should balconies be allowed to project... not to cause harm to the pilgrims for the festivals' (*BT, Bava Qamma* 82b). Jerusalem belongs to all the people of Israel, and the rule with regard to an entrance or a courtyard is the same as that relating to public space.[98]

No one was allowed to be buried inside the city of Jerusalem except the Kings of the House of David and the prophetess Ḥuldah. Because of the prevailing western winds, burial sites were usually on the east or south of the city. The necropolis of Jerusalem is therefore concentrated on the northern, eastern and southern sides of the city, although occasional graves have also been found on the west.[99]

---

93 Josephus, *Bellum Judaicum* V,192; See also Avi-Yonah 1975, 217.

94 Philo, *De Specialibus Legibus* I, XXXII, 156; Safrai 1956, 370–371; Daniel-Nataf 1991, II/I, 263–264. See also Kasher 1980, 49–60; Amir 1980, 154–165.

95 For other parallel sources, see the discussion in Dvorjetski 2007, 279–280; See also Schwartz 1998, 44–45.

96 Kohut 1926, 71–72; Eisenstein 1975: 'Beth HaKisse', 42; Dvorjetski 1999b, 19–20; ead. 2016, 48–100.

97 *Pleiton* is an aromatic oil made of rose leaves or other perfume; Albeck 1959: VI, 120; Jastrow 1995: 'PlLw, 1928 , vol. I, p. 303; Sokolff, 2002,p. 71; For the connection between pleiton', 1141; Lw, 1928 , vol. I, p. 303; Sokolff, 2002,p. 71; For the connection between plFeliks 1994, 31; on balsam, see Löw 1924: I, 303; Feliks 1994: s.v. 'Balsam'; idem. 1997b, 275–296; Sokoloff 2002, 71. On the connection between those two, Lw, 1928 , vol. I, p. 303; Sokolff, 2002, p. 71; For the connection between plsee *Masekhtot Derech Eretz* 1,3, ed. Higger, pp. 160–161.

98 Krauss 1924, 97–99, 102; Zeligman 1981, 25; Shinover and Goldberg 1994, 219; Zevin 2002: 'Jerusalem', XXV, 331–335, 338.

99 See, for instance, Avi-Yonah 1975, 244; Kloner and Zissu 2007; Isaac 2010, 8–10.

Facilities which were essential to the health of the majority of the populace also had to be erected in locations where they would not constitute a hindrance. 'Cavities—wells, ditches and caves—should not be dug under public space (Mishnah *Bava Bathra* 3:8). Dangerous building is forbidden in advance, lest the majority of the population suffer harm. Moreover, dangerous buildings may be destroyed: 'A tomb which harms the majority may be emptied' (*BT, Sanhedrin* 47b), with the exception of the tombs of the House of David, the tomb of Isaiah, and the tomb of Ḥuldah the prophetess, which had been in Jerusalem since the days of the First Temple 'and no man has ever touched them' (*ARN II* 39, Schechter ed., p. 54). This matter led to a dispute between Rabbi Akiva and the other Rabbis, arising from the question of the implications of impurity when the impure matter was discharged through tunnels to the Kidron Valley (*JT, Nazir* 9,3 [57d]; *Treatise Semaḥot* 14,10, Higger ed., p. 207).[100] The most important point in these versions is that Rabbi Akiva disputes an anonymous view. The view of Rabbi Akiva as given in *Semaḥot* and in Tosefta *Bava Bathra* essentially corresponds to the versions in Tosefta *Nega'im* and *ARN I* and *II*. This implies that we have here a ruling that was discussed and settled in the first half of the 2nd century CE. The *BT* ignores this ruling. It obviously considered it unrealistic and unimportant. No historical source indicates that there was a mass exhumation of graves in Jerusalem, though we know of some exhumations.[101]

As a rule, graves had to be situated fifty cubits from the city—28 metres from the outermost buildings of the city, according to the average length of a cubit (Mishnah *Bava Bathra* 2:9).[102] An examination of the location of the graves shows that the quality of the stone, topographical considerations, the natural growth and spread of the city were the most important factors in deciding their position. The *Tanna Kama* considered that there was no reason not to dig graves in any place where it was possible, as long as the required distance between the city and the cemetery was kept. Rabbi Akiva, however, believed that under all circumstances graves should not be dug to the west of the city, however difficult this was (*ibid.*). The view that one should not always aspire to the ideal, but act according to the circumstances on the ground, is exemplified in certain sites in Galilee and in Jerusalem. Few graves are to be found west of Jerusalem because the stone there is hard to dig.[103]

The fundamental precept in this matter is derived from the injunction in *Deuteronomy* 21:22–23: 'If a man has committed a sin deserving of death..., and you hang him on a tree, his body shall not remain overnight on the tree, but you shall surely

---

100 Büchler 1912, 210–211; Krauss 1924, 108–113; Guttmann 1972, 72; Dvorjetski 1999b, 15–16; Levine 2002, 322; Zevin 2002: 'Jerusalem', XXV, 334.

101 For instance, the bones of King Uzziah had been exhumed and taken elsewhere. See Sukenik 1931, 288–292; Epstein 1931, 293–294, discussing *halakhic* aspects of this exhumation. See also the discussion below.

102 Stern 1963, 846–852.

103 Kloner 1980, 267.

bury him that day, so that you do not defile the land which the Lord your God is giving you as an inheritance'.[104]

Rabban Simeon ben Gamaliel (10 BCE–66 CE) describes the great national festival on 15th Ab, when the young maidens of Jerusalem in white dresses went forth to dance in the vineyards (Mishnah *Ta'anit* 4:8; *BT, ibid.* 31a); Mishnah *Ma'aser Sheni* 3:7, discusses the case of a tree which stands inside the walls of Jerusalem with its fruit hanging outside or *vice versa*. Even before the erection of the third northern wall, built under Agrippa I (41–44 CE), there were gardens in the area which was then enclosed by this wall. This is indicated by the name of the gate which formed the starting point of the second wall: *Gennath*, Garden Gate;[105] A channel which drained away the blood of the offerings, led underground into the Kidron Valley (Mishnah *Tamid* 4:1; *ibid. Middot* 3:2; *ibid. Meilah* 3:3; *ibid. Pesahim* 5: 8). The gardeners bought the blood from the temple-treasurers for use as fertilizer, and to use it without paying for it was to incur sacrilege (*ibid. Yoma* 5:6). Abba Shaul's statement at the top of *BT, Pesahim* 14a may indicate that Mount of Olives was cultivated in the Second Temple period, but the historicity of the remark is doubtful, since Abba Saul lived after the destruction.[106] And in an anonymous passage in *Midrash Psalms,* 48, 4 (Buber ed., pp. 275–276) the renovated Jerusalem—Jerusalem of the Messianic Age—will be even more wondrous than mighty Rome and will have more gardens, towers, arches, *nymphaea*, and water channels than the world's greatest city.[107]

Moses' command and warning on the matter of public hygiene—'and you shall have a *yad* outside the camp... and you shall dig with it and turn and cover your refuse... and your camp shall be holy' (*Deuteronomy* 23:13–15)—was translated faithfully into terms of religion and hygiene in the code of the Essenes in the period of the Second Temple. The concept of the *yad*, in the sense of a special sign marking the latrines outside the camp, is encapsulated in the distance of two thousand cubits from the camp to the place of the *yad*.[108] The Essenes' Gate was connected to the arrival of the Essenes from their settlements in the Judaean Desert, and particularly in its southern region, as in 'Ein Gedi and its surroundings.[109] Yigael Yadin located the Essenes' Gate in the south-west of the Upper City, and the position of the 'house of dung' outside the city, north-west of the Upper City.[110] It appears, however, that the position of

---

104 Some commentators have claimed that this precept was intended to prevent air pollution. The 14th century CE Talmudist Rabbi Levi ben Gershon [= HaRalbag] interprets: 'You shall not pollute your land, because of the stench which will return to that place if the body is left'; See also Bialoblotzki 1971, 30–35; Bar-Noy 1985, 43–49; Rakover 1993, 65.

105 Josephus, *Bellum Judaicum* V,146.

106 Price 1992, 245.

107 In *BT, Bava Bathra* 75b it appears in a closely parallel form in the name of Resh Lakish [= Rabbi Simeon ben Lakish], and should be dated mid-3rd century CE. Daniel Sperber [1998, 134–135] indicates that 'in this chronological context it would correspond to the Palestinian Messianic trends of the 250s CE, already noted by scholars'.

108 Horowitz 1964, 185; Brayer 1965, 160–162; Kottek 1994, 166–167.

109 Dalman 1924, 247; Safrai 1965, 119; Avi-Yonah 1975, 222, and see the map on p. 209.

110 Yadin 1972, 129; Har-El 1989, 162.

the public lavatory of Jerusalem could not have been so high, and certainly not to the west of the city, from which westerly winds frequently blow towards the city. It must have been located in a low place, so that the surplus water from the springs of 'Arrub would be able to flow down to it after leaving the Temple, and wash away the dung so that it should not turn into a breeding-place for diseases and epidemics.[111] Michael Avi-Yonah's view that the Essenes' Gate was in the south-west of Jerusalem, in the lowest part of the Lower City and at the edge of the Ben Hinnom Valley[112] seems most probable. The water could have reached this place from the Temple through a conduit, washing away the blood and refuse, and flowed outside the city down the slope to the Kidron Valley and to the east, as described in *The Letter of Aristeas*.[113]

The awareness that a lavatory, or 'house of water', was essential to the existence of a proper city and to the service of the whole population, was expressed in the fact that it was considered one of the ten services required for the fitting conduct of life in an urban unit. *BT, Sanhedrin* 17b reads the following:[114]

> 'It has been taught: a scholar should not reside in a city where the following ten things are not found [...] public baths; lavatories, a physician, a bloodletter, a scribe, and a teacher. And according to others it was said in the name of Rabbi Akiva: In the city should be several kinds of fruit, as the consuming of fruit enlightens the eyes'.

From this we may learn of the honourable status of the lavatory among the health services defined as essential. The fact that the lavatory was a public building necessitated the building of several such structures in every inhabited place, at a distance from densely populated areas (*BT, Berakhot* 62a). The precepts concerning lavatories give us exact information about their construction, their location, the way they were used and the way their upkeep was ensured. Nonetheless, they are quite rarely mentioned. They contained disinfectant materials and means of purifying noxious and malodorous air (*ibid., ibid.* 53a).[115]

A fascinating explanation to the Temple facilities which highlights the toilet's privacy of the priests is given by Jodi Magness in her remarkable book, entitled *Stone and Dung, Oil and Spit* based on the passage in the description of Mishnah *Tamid* 1:1:

---

111 Har-El 1987, 311.
112 Avi-Yonah 1956a, 312–313, map 10; idem. 1968, 26.
113 *The Letter of Aristeas* 88–89; See also Har-El 1987, 312.
114 See also *Tanna de bei Elijahu, Derech Eretz*, 1, ed. M. Ish-Shalom, p. 13; *Midrash HaGadol to Exodus* 18,21; Cf. *JT, Qiddushin* 4,12 [66d]: 'It is forbidden to live in a city in which there are no physician, no bath, and no court administering floggings and imprisoning people'.
115 Zevin 1963: 'Beth HaKisse', III, 206–310; Kraus 1924, 406–410; Hirschfeld 1987: s.v. 'Bet Kise'; Safrai 1995, 169; idem. 1999b, 19–20; Rosner 2000: s.v. 'Toilets', 311–312; Baruch and Amar 2004, 27–50; Magness 2012, 51–70; Neis 2012, 328–368. For the historical-archaeological survey, see Dvorjetski 2016, 47–100 and ead. [forthcoming (a)], chapter 9.5 on *Public Latrines and Toilets: Habits and Practices*.

'[If] one of them should have a nocturnal emission of semen, he goes out, proceeding along the passage that leads below the building—and lamps flicker on this side and on that—and he reaches the immersion room, and there was a fire there, and a privy (*byt kys' šl kbwd*) in good taste. And this was its good taste: [if] he found it locked, he knows that someone is there; [if he found it] open, he knows that no one is there. He went down and immersed and came up and dried off, and warmed himself by the fire'.[116]

Jodi Magness clarifies that the room containing the toilet used by the priests serving in the Jerusalem temple had a door that could be closed or locked to ensure privacy. Similarly, a concern for toilet privacy explains the placement of the toilet at Qumran in a room at the eastern edge of the settlement and at the extreme western end of the room. Not only was this toilet located in a roofed house like the toilets mandated by the *Temple Scroll,* but it would not have been visible to passersby. The *miqveh* associated with the toilet used by the priests in the temple was located in the Chamber of Immersion. The toilet and immersion facilities were located in underground rooms beneath the northwest side of the Temple courtyard, which sheds light on why the *Temple Scroll* mandates the placement of the toilets to the northwest of Jerusalem: 'Through that [= room in the Beit HaMoked] on the northwestern side do they go down to the room for immersion' (*ibid.* 1,6). Thus, the *Temple Scroll* mandates the placement of the lavatories in the ideal city to the northwest of the city because in the second Temple the toilet facilities were located on the northwest side.[117]

Magen Broshi has suggested that Mishnah *Tamid*'s (1:1) detailed description of the lavatory in the Jerusalem Temple is a polemical response to an attempted ban of toilets from Jerusalem—as represented in the *Temple Scroll*'s legislation.[118]

Josephus describes 'the house of dung' (βηθσώ) as being west of the Temple hall, close to the wall of the old city, and between the Hippicus Tower and the Essenes' Gate. Here, apparently, was the outlet of the water, the waste and the remains of the sacrifices, and here was located the public lavatory which served the people of the capital and the pilgrims.[119] Yigael Yadin points out that the 'house of dung', or the lavatory of Jerusalem, is mentioned in the *Temple Scroll*: 'they shall create for themselves a place with a *yad* outside the city, and go out thither. And there shall be pits within it, and the dung shall flow down into the pits'.[120]

In excavations of the Second Temple period in Jerusalem private ritual baths have been discovered in almost every building. These were used for ritual immersion rather than bathing, for which pools and baths were used. A bathroom was an unmistakable

---

116 Magness 2011, 142–144.
117 Magness 2011, 142–143.
118 Broshi 1992, 595–596.
119 Josephus, *Antiquitates Judaicae* V,141; Dalman 1930, 86; Har-El 1989, 162; Baumgarten 1996, 12–14.
120 Yadin 1990, 177–178; See also Milgrom 1990, 83–100; Henshke 1997, 5–28; Shemesh 2000, 101–110; Schiffman and Florentino 2008.

sign of an opulent house and a high standard of accommodation, and it points to the Jerusalem citizens' awareness of the need for bodily cleanliness, in addition to the religious duty of ritual immersion.[121]

The Rabbis spoke in extravagant terms of the beauty of Jerusalem and the Temple; for instance: 'He who has not seen Jerusalem in her splendor, has never seen a desirable city in his life. He who has not seen the Temple in its full construction has never seen a glorious building in his life' (*BT, Sukkah* 51b), or, 'Ten *ḳabs* of beauty descended to the world: nine were taken by Jerusalem and one by the rest of the world' (*ibid., Qiddushin* 49b).[122]

Preservation of the beauty of the individual's environment plays a cardinal role in protecting his mental health. Maimonides says: 'For him who has become a prey to melancholy, the sound of melodies and various tunes, and a walk among gardens and beautiful buildings… will restore his soul'.[123] The beauty of the city is the basis of several precepts which deal with the removal of nuisances which threaten the beauty of the environment; for example, the law which enjoins that trees and tanners should not be allowed in the city (Mishnah *Bava Bathra* 20:7; *JT, ibid.* 2,9 [13c]). In all these instances, which are liable to do harm to the honour of Jerusalem and to its beauty, and include things such as gardens, orchards and trees, which enhance its beauty but create a bad odour because they require manuring—such things must not be found in the city.[124]

Craftsmen, artisans and their nuisances

The crafts were held in high esteem in Judaism at the time: 'He who does not teach his son a craft teaches him brigandage' (*BT, Qiddushin* 29a). Jerusalem had its artisans, bakers, launderers or poulterers, weavers, fullers, and smiths.[125] The artisans would greet pilgrims bringing their first fruits to the Temple (Mishnah *Bikkurim* 3:3). It is very likely that their shops and workshops were located along a main street where these people were apt to pass, and this, in turn, may well point to Tyropoeon Valley Street.[126]

Various artisans inhabited special quarters in the big cities. During the Second Temple period wool shops and copper-workers' shops were confined to a separate quarter in Jerusalem.[127] There were special markets for different craftsmen: among others, vendours of poultry (*BT, Erubin* 101b), wool [= *šūq šel ṣammārīm)* (Mishnah *ibid.* 10:9; *BT, ibid.* 101a), leather (*ibid., Mo'ed Qatan* 27a; *ibid., Nedarim* 26b), and wines (*ibid., Hagigah* 9b). In the southern part of the Lower City, near the Dung

---

121 Avigad 1980, 139–143; Reich 1980, 225–256; idem. 2013.

122 See also *BT, Bava Bathra* 3b; Avi-Yonah 1975, 219; Segal 1979, 108; Shaviv 1992, 478.

123 Maimonides, *The Eight Chapters* 5; see also Schwarz 2011, 29–30.

124 Schepansky 1992, 123–125; It is rather the connection between the beauty of the environment and the inner beauty of the self and the care for all bodily needs. See, for instance, Balberg 2014.

125 Mishnah *Bikkurim* 3:3; *ibid. Erubin* 10:9; *ibid. Eduyot* 1:3; *ibid. Sotah* 9:10; *ibid. Ma'aser Sheni* 5:15; Tosefta *Miqva'ot* 4,10, Zuckermandel ed., p. 656; *BT, Avoda Zarah* 26a; Josephus, *Antiqutates Judaicae* XV,309.

126 Levine 2002, 346.

127 Josephus, *Bellum Judaicum* V,337; See also Jeremias 1969, 4–5, 20–21; Smith 1970, 373–375.

Gate, the despised trade of weaving was located. Each craft had its shops in its own quarter, and in fact it is likely that each had its own bazaar (*šūq*). It is likely that there were shops even in the Temple court (*ibid., Rosh Hashanah* 31a; *ibid., Shabbat* 15a; *ibid., Sanhedrin* 41a; *ibid., Avoda Zarah* 8b).

In Biblical times, heathen tradespeople were situated in the northern part of the city. *Zephaniah* (1:10–11) proclaims woes to the Fish Gate, the second quarter, the hills and the *Maktesh*,[128] all situated in the north. Verse 11 reads, 'Inhabitants of *Maktesh*, for the whole nation of Canaan is no more'. The 'nation of Canaan' probably means Phoenician traders such as are referred to in Jerusalem in *Nehemiah* 13:16. Nehemiah specifically addresses the Tyrians traders who came to Jerusalem to sell their fish. Other historical sources indicate that fish were a staple, which was traded in international trade routes.[129] The Fish Gate, lying at the point of intersection of the second north wall or the Tyropoeon Valley (*Nehemiah* 3:3; 12:39; *Zephaniah* 1:10; *II Chronicles* 33:14), took its name from Tyrian fish merchants (*Nehemiah* 13:16). This, too, attests heathen traders in the north of the city. The goldsmiths and perfumers mentioned in *Nehemiah* 3:8, presumably had their bazaar in the northern suburb west of the Temple according to Josephus[130] and the Talmudic sources.[131]

It is also possible that the division of the city of Jerusalem into two parts—the Upper and Lower cities, each with its own market (Mishnah *Sheqalim* 8:1; Tosefta *Sanhedrin* 14,14; *ibid., Hulin* 3,23; *Midrash Tannaim to Deuteronomy* 26,13, Hoffmann ed., pp. 175–176; *BT, Sanhedrin* 89a; *Lamentations Rabbah* 1,49)—was a result of consideration for the ecological and hygienic requirements of the population.[132] In the course of time Upper and Lower markets were also set up in Sepphoris, Tiberias, and other places (*BT, Avoda Zarah* 16b–17a; *ibid., Yoma* 11a; *ibid., Erubin* 54b). Some craftsmen, weavers, goldsmiths, and tanneries worshipped in separate synagogues, because of their strong and fetid odour. 'It is recorded of the synagogue of the טו(ו)רסיים [= 'coppersmiths'] in Jerusalem that they sold it to Rabbi Eliezer and he used it for his own purposes' (*ibid., Megillah* 26a). Similar arrangements were later made in Lydda and Tiberias (*ibid., ibid.*).[133] A strong odour emanating from a man whose work involves a noisome smell constitutes grounds for divorce on the part of a woman, who finds it intolerable (*ibid., Ketuboth* 77a). It was said of the Dung Gate, which was the most polluted quarter of the city, there is 'no more despised place in Jerusalem than the Dung Gate' (Tosefta *Eduyot* 1:3). It was there that the most despised

---

128 Literally 'the mortar'. The meaning here is doubtful; See Jeremias 1969, 20; Smith 1970, 369.
129 Lipinski 2004, 493–545; Edelman 2005, 207–246; Reich 2014, 186.
130 Josephus, *Bellum Judaicum*, V, 313.
131 Delitzsch 1877, 32; Jeremias 1969, 18–20; Klausner 1975, 185, 188; Mazar 1975, 199–200; Reich 2014, 186; For the Talmudic references to goldsmiths and perfumers, see Dvorjetski 1993, 28–30; On the Tyrians presence there, see also the discussion below.
132 Horowitz 1964, 124–125; Jeremias 1969, 18–19; Kotlar 1973, 9; Avi-Yonah 1975, 236–240; Mazar 1978, 29–40; Dan 1990, 104–105.
133 Krauss 1966, 201; Ayali 1987, 18, 22, 25, 118; Dvorjetski 1993, 33; On the טרסיים—weavers or goldsmiths—see Dvorjetski (forthcoming [a]), chapter 5 on *The Occupational Medicine of the Employee*.

workmen, the weavers, lived: 'you have no more degraded craft than weaving' (Mishnah *ibid*. 1:3; and Tosefta *Qiddushin* 5:14). We are informed in this context that some of them worked in the area of the Dung Gate (Mishnah *Eduyot* 1:3), in the southern extremity of the city, where the Kidron, Tyropoeon, and Ben Hinnom Valleys meet. It is described in the *Tannaitic* sources that 'two weavers came from the Dung Gate in Jerusalem and gave testimony in the name of Shemaiah and Avtalion that three *logs* of drawn water invalidate the immersion pool, and Sages confirmed their report' (Tosefta *ibid*. 1:3). In other words, two learnt weavers who transmitted teachings regarding *miqva'ot*.[134]

The Bible several times mentions a 'fuller's field' ('שדה כובס') which lay outside the walls of Jerusalem, near a watercourse and on one of the main access roads (*II Kings* 18:17; *Isaiah* 7:3; 36:2). One might imagine, quite reasonably, that fulleries in Jerusalem were situated outside the walls, precisely because fulling was such an unpleasant, noisy and smell activity. The fuller had to render the cloth from the looms watertight by teasing together the fibres. The north-east corner of the northernmost wall formed the so-called 'fuller's tomb'.[135] Heathen fullers (*qaṣrārīn*) have been supposed to live in the Upper City, but wrongly. There was a rule that spittle was regarded as clean in the whole town except that found in the Upper City (Mishnah *Sheqalim* 8:1).

Josephus mentions only once the Tyropoeon (τυροποιῶν), literally means 'Valley of the Cheesemakers', which 'divides the hill of the Upper City from that of the Lower [City], extends down to Siloam', an abundant spring of sweet water. In another passage, this valley is simply called the 'central valley'.[136] It is undoubtedly the valley now called *el-Wad*, which bisects the Old City from the Damascus Gate in the north of the Dung Gate in the south. It constituted a quarter for industry and crafts, and ensured very favourable climatic conditions for the residential area.[137] The name Tyropoeon, 'Valley of the Cheesemakers' has not yet been satisfactorily interpreted.[138] Jerusalem was never a large centre for dairy produce and cattle raising, and it is hardly likely that those engaged in cheese-making should have the main valley of the town named after them, especially as this activity was not a separate craft but a part of dairy production. It has been suggested that there is a Biblical reference to a Cheese Gate in *Nehemiah* (3:13), where *Safot*, meaning 'cream' or 'cheese' (*II Samuel* 17:29), is given in place of *Ashpot*—dung, but this variant is undoubtedly a simple mistake of the copyist.[139] Quite interesting that a Greek inscription on the sarcophagus of a cheese-maker on the slopes of the Mount of Olives reads: 'Young Judah, the proselyte, a cheese-maker'.[140]

---

134 Dvorjetski 1999b, 15; Levine 2002, 346.
135 Josephus, *Bellum Judaicum* V,147. See also Robertson 1986, 22; Ayali 1987, 137–138; Bradley 2002, 36.
136 Josephus, *Bellum Judaicum* V,136, 140.
137 Har-El 1989, 158–160.
138 Kotlar 1973, 9–10; Segal 1979, 108; see the discussion below.
139 Har-El 1970, 181, 240; Avi-Yonah 1975, 239; Kotlar 1976, 44; Day 1989, 27; Robertson-Smith [1957, 377] and others connect *Tophet* with the root špt by appealing to the Hebrew word *'Ašpōt*, allegedly meaning 'ash-heap', refuse-heap, dunghill.
140 Bagatti and Milik 1958, 95.

Other proposals regarded the Tyropoeon as a corruption of some Hebrew or Aramaic name with a similar sound,[141] but none of these are really convincing. However, Joachim Jeremias assumes that the toponym of Tyropoeon derives from the city of Tyre, and the Fish Gate took its name from the Tyrian fish merchants, since Tyrians traders came to Jerusalem for selling fish, as mentioned above (*Nehemiah* 13:16).[142] Recently, Ronny Reich suggested a similar interpretation focusing on the significant Phoenician artifacts in the Tyropoeon Valley and in the City of David, which illustrate the presence of Phoenicians dating to the end of the 9th century or the beginning of the 8th century BCE.[143]

The raising of pigeons for sacrifices was clearly a desideratum and might well explain the many columbaria (small niches in caves here interpreted as dovecotes) found throughout Judaea. In the vicinity of Jerusalem itself, twenty-four columbaria were built in artificial caves hewn into bedrock and four others were in constructed structures. These columbaria were found scattered around the Old City walls in all directions. Despite the difficulty in dating such installations, the overwhelming majority can be confidently placed in the late Second Temple period.[144]

A Hebrew inscription found in the burial cave near Bethphage in the vicinity of Jerusalem and dating from the period of the Second Temple includes a list of Jewish names of men employed in a local manufactory preparing ossuaries including fathers and sons engaged in the same craft, such as potters.[145]

According to Meir Ben-Dov, it cannot be definitely established that there were facilities for light industry in the houses of the quarter below the Temple Mount. This characterized the city of Jerusalem in the Byzantine era, as distinct from the Second Temple period, during which buildings devoted to industry and handicrafts were situated outside the city. In his view, not all the archaeological evidence confirms this view.[146]

Daily life in the Holy City of Jerusalem: reality and rationalism

The Talmudic sources' descriptions of Jerusalem are coloured by its eternal sacredness in the life of the people of Israel, by its overwhelming beauty and by its wealth of *Torah* and wisdom. The texts open with standard phrases such as 'There are ten measures of beauty in the world: nine in Jerusalem, and one in the rest of the world'; 'There are ten measures of wisdom in the world: nine in Jerusalem, and one in the rest of the world' (*ARN II* 48, Schechter ed., p. 132). In addition, 'ten wonders were performed for our fathers in the Temple' like: 'a woman never miscarried from the scent

---

141   Among the suggestions were *Gei HaToref* and *Gei Tura Ẓiyyon*, neither of which makes much sense. See Avi-Yonah 1975, 240, note 149.
142   Jeremias 1969, 20.
143   Reich and Shukron 2004, 185–189; Reich 2014, 186.
144   See Kloner's survey 2000, 61*–66*; See also Shiloh 1984, 9, Pls. 16:1, 17.1 and Fig. 13; Kloner 1997, 25–31; Levine 2002, 348; Zissu 2009, 30–37.
145   Orfali 1923, 253–260; Klausner 1975, 188; For similar lists of workers found also at Bethphage and now exhibited in the Louvre Museum in Paris, see Dussaud 1923, 241–249.
146   Ben-Dov 1985, 246–247.

of the sacrificial meat. The sacrificial meat never became spoiled. No fly was ever seen in the slaughterhouse... A snake or scorpion never did harm in Jerusalem' (Mishnah *Avot* 1:1). *ARN I* (35, Schlechter ed., p. 103) adds further details throwing light on the veraciousness of the texts: 'No man was ever injured in Jerusalem; No fire ever broke out in Jerusalem; No structures ever collapsed in Jerusalem'. It would appear that number ten is typological, and that its only purpose is to praise, eulogize and glorify the city, and attribute to it every positive characteristic. This, apparently, also applies to the ten city by-laws, not all of which have identical grounds or justification; for, as has been remarked above, the reasons given by our sources are not always the original reasons for their enactment.[147]

Most of the characteristics attributed to the city of Jerusalem are good in conception, but unattained in practice.[148] Despite the prohibition on the breeding of pigs there is evidence that they were in fact bred; similarly, despite the ordinance 'No dog shall be kept unless it is secured by a lead' (Mishnah *Bava Qamma* 7:7), dogs were in fact afforded complete freedom, and in the Tosefta (*Kelim, Bava Qamma* 1:6) the High Priest's dog is mentioned. Dogs are mentioned in connection with sacred food in some other sources. The dog is here conceived of as an unclean animal that should be kept away from the sacred food, and is coupled with pigs; At times of war dogs and geese were employed: 'It would be a case in which they surrounded the town with bells, chains, irons, geese, chickens, and military apparatus' (*JT, Gittin* 3,4 [45a]). In *BT, Ketuboth* 27a, 'Rabbi Levi replied: "When they placed round the town chains, dogs, trunks of trees and geese"'. To the mishnaic prohibition of the keeping of chickens (*Bava Qamma* 7:7), the *Tosefta* adds the stipulation: 'If there is a garden or dung-heap before them it is permitted (*ibid.*, 8,10). The expression 'chicken breeder', or 'brought chickens into his house' (Tosefta *Bava Bathra* 3,5), and the evidence of Rabbi Judah ben Bava regarding a rooster which was stoned in Jerusalem because it pierced the skull of a child (*BT, Berakhot* 27a) indicates a radical change compared with the *halakha*.[149] People continued to rear small cattle unhesitatingly since the *halakha* is one thing and the realities of life another.[150] In certain sources dating from after the destruction of the Temple an inclination to restrict the application of the prohibition and lighten it can be discerned (Tosefta *Bava Qamma* 8,12, 14; *ibid., Yevamot* 3,3–4). Several scholars advanced the idea that this issue may be connected with economic changes in this period.[151]

---

147 Number ten also appears in regard of degrees of holiness (*Mishnah, Kelim,* 1:6–9); See also Büchler 1956, 35; Urbach 1971, 347; Sperber 1982, 55–56; Urbach 1984, 23; Kister 1998, 184; Becker 2004, 234, 238, 343; on the literary model which opens in numerical statement, see Shin'an 1990, 85–102.

148 See the summary in Dvorjetski 1999b, 21–23; See also Krauss 1924, 106.

149 Krauss 1924, 107; Tucazinsky 1952, 209.

150 Ish-Shalom 1899, 1–7.

151 On the prohibition of raising small cattle for reasons of maintaining the land and the trees, see Alon 1967, I, 173–176; Urbach 1984, 22–23; Rakover 1993, 42–43; Cf. Gulak 1940–1941, 181–189.

The reason for the prohibition on burying the dead or keeping a body in Jerusalem was doubtless in order to ensure the purity of the city and the health of its inhabitants. From the *baraitoth* it appears that this ordinance was put into practice: 'All graves are subject to removal except for the grave of a king and the grave of a prophet' (Tosefta *Bava Bathra* 1,11; See also *JT, Nazir* 9,2 [57d]; *Tractate Semaḥot* 14,10, Higger ed., p. 207). Thus, for instance, an inscription of Uzziah King of Judah, 'Hereto were brought Uzziah's bones the King of Judah. And not to open', telling of the removal of his bones proves that the *halakha* was in fact observed, and confirms the view of Rabbi Akiva that, 'Also the grave of a king and the grave of a prophet are subject to removal' (*Tosefta, Bava Bathra*, 1, 11). The *II Book of Chronicles* (26:23) states that Uzziah was buried in the 'field of burials belonging to the Kings', since they said 'he is a leper', rather than in the tombs of the Kings, who had an indulgence annulling the impurity.[152]

The precept in the Tosefta *(Bava Bathra* 1,11) differs from the laws dealing with a grave, which is removed because it is in the city. It is probable that the removal of the King's tomb to which Rabbi Akiva referred—apparently that described in the inscription—also took place because of the extension of the boundaries of the city; for it was necessary to ensure the purity of the area which was added to the city.[153] Levi Rahmani is convinced that the tablet's inscription of Uzziah, in the square script of late Second Temple period, most likely comes from a resting place to which his bones must have been transferred at that late period. He relies upon two Biblical indications that the extension of the city westward brought with it the evacuation of earlier Israelite tombs, such as those discovered west of the Temple Mount and as well as Uzziah's late inscription. *Ezekiel*'s words, 'Let them put away... the carcasses of their Kings, far from me ...' (43:7–9), seem to show some uneasiness at that time about burials, even of Kings, inside the city. This also may be indicated by *Jeremiah*, whose words about the evacuation of tombs in a rebuilt and enlarged Jerusalem mention 'the whole valley of the dead bodies and the ashes' (31:38–40). [154]

We also learn from Josephus that it was not customary to bury the dead inside the city: he tells of the request of the people of Jerusalem to remove their dead from the city, even when it was under siege.[155] Tannaitic sources also show that it was customary to bury the dead outside the city; for instance, in the well-known description of Rabban Yohanan ben Zakkai, who was taken out of Jerusalem with the help of his pupils during the siege. The gatekeepers asked them who is this?, They replied, 'A dead man. Do you not know that dead bodies should not be left inside Jerusalem?' So they replied: 'If he is dead, take him out. And they took him out' (*ARN I* 35, Schechter ed., p. 23).[156] In another tradition, also from the time of the siege of Jerusalem, it

---

152 Sukenik 1931, 288–292; Epstein 1931, 293–294; Guttmann 1972, 72; Dvorjetski 2011–2012, 233–234; Yardeni and Price 2010, I/I, 603–604, Fig. 602; and see there the comprehensive bibliography.
153 Safrai 1965, 137.
154 Rahmani 1981, 233.
155 Josephus, *Antiquitates Judaicae* V,518.
156 See the versions in *BT, Gittin* 56a–b; *Lamentations Rabbah* 1, Buber ed., pp. 65–66; *ARN I* 4,

is said: 'Halakha. A corpse is not kept overnight in Jerusalem. When they took the deceased out for burial, those that were burying the dead were given over into the hands of the enemy' (Sifra Behuqotai 6, Weiss ed., 112a). This tradition combines two prohibitions: that on leaving a dead body unburied, which was observed outside Jerusalem as well; and that on burying the dead in Jerusalem, which applied to the city of Jerusalem alone.

Another Halakha concerning the cleanness of Jerusalem is given by Rabbi Joshua ben Hanania, who lived in Jerusalem before the destruction of the Second Temple. The Mishnah (Ohalot 7:1) discusses the position of solid tomb memorials indicating that if one leaned a hut against it, would be unclean. Regarding this mishnah, the Tosefta (ibid. 7, 16) says that Rabbi Judah did not declare these booths that leaned on the dead, clean except for the purpose of eating the Paschal lamb: 'Rabbi Judah said in the name of Rabbi Joshua, "the booths that were leaned are pure in order to eat the Paschal lambs"'.[157] Even after they eliminated the tombs from the city, there remained monuments and they permitted those eating the Paschal lambs to lean their booths against the monuments and to eat their sacrifice in the Mishnah always means eating it in the city.

Towards the end of the Second Temple period opposition to excessive rigorousness was expressed. 'On one occasion bones were found in Jerusalem, in the woodshed' [of the Temple], on the right hand side of the Eastern Gate—the entrance to the women's section. The Rabbis considered that the whole of Jerusalem should be declared impure, for fear that these bones came from unidentified graves, which might raise doubts about the purity of the whole environment. Rabbi Joshua ben Hanania's argument—'It would be a shame and a disgrace for us to declare our [holy] house to be impure?'—convinced them not to take this step (Tosefta Eduyot 3,3). In the following generation it is reported in the BT, Zevahim 113a: 'Rabbi Yohanan refuted Resh Lakish: "On one occasion they found [human] bones in the Wooden Chamber,[158] and they desired to declare Jerusalem unclean. Whereupon Rabbi Joshua rose to his feet and exclaimed: Is it not a shame and disgrace to us that we declare the city of our fathers unclean."'![159] This indicates certain cultural tensions and the two passages from Tosefta and BT do not only mirror a historical development but also, or even more so, a cultural and religious one that was rather persistent in later Rabbinic traditions.

The religious precept forbidding planting and sowing in Jerusalem, and 'planting trees there, apart from the rose garden which had existed since the days of the early prophets' (Tosefta Nega'im 6,2) should be seen as a law for the expansion of the building area in the city. The boundaries of Jerusalem could be expanded only by order of 'a King, a prophet, or the sacred stones (urim ve-tumim/ אוּרִים וְתֻמִּים) and the Sanhedrin of seventy-one', accompanied by a special ritual (BT, Shevuot 14a).[160] An-

---

Schechter ed., pp. 22–23; ARN II 6, ibid., p. 19; Neusner 1970, 115–120; Alon 1977, 269–313; Schäfer 1979, 43–101; Tropper 2005, 133–149.

157 Manns 2001, 80.
158 The place where the wood was kept for the altar. See Patrich 2011, 222.
159 See also Lieberman 1939, 185; Zevin 2002: 'Jerusalem', XXV, 336.
160 Cf. Mishnah Sanhedrin 1:5; See also Urbach 1971, 346.

other reason for the prohibition on planting, ploughing and sowing was the need to make room for more buildings, since there was not sufficient room to accommodate the crowds of pilgrims.[161]

Various sources mention cultivation in and around Jerusalem, inside the walls and outside the walls. The soil around the city was fertile. The *Mishnah* tells us that in the 'rose-garden' of Jerusalem there were also fig trees. Rabbi Judah relates an occurrence implying that there were fig trees in Jerusalem: 'Rabbi Judah said, "It once happened in a rose garden in Jerusalem that figs were sold three or four an *issar,* and neither Heave-offering nor Tithe was ever given"' (Mishnah *Ma'aseroth* 2:5). It may be that this was an ancient fig grove,[162] in which roses were also grown in the course of time, but only for a short time; or that the place was still called 'the rose garden' even though no roses grew there at the time, as we learn from the expression 'selling a vineyard, even though there are no grapes in it'.[163] The *Tosefta* does not give any reason for the prohibition on trees (Tosefta *Nega'im* 6,2), but it may be that they were excluded from Jerusalem because of the use of trees and groves in foreign cults.[164]

The prohibition on planting, whether of trees or of gardens and orchards, did not last, and the sources tell us in 'Rabbi Judah's name: The [= fuel] logs of Jerusalem were of the cinnamon trees, and when lit their fragrance pervaded the whole of Eretz-Israel' (*BT, Shabbat* 63a). It may be that by 'cinnamon trees' are meant trees and gardens which gave off a sweet smell, but were not used to make incense.[165] This text has the feel of a myth, as do other texts which mention cinnamon, since it is a tropical tree which grows in rainy regions and does not grow in the Land of Israel or the surrounding region—and, in particular, not in Jerusalem.[166] There were acacia trees in the city, which were planted close to the wall, inside and outside it (Mishnah *Ma'aser Sheni* 3:3; *ibid. Ma'aseroth* 3:10)—but they were destroyed by the enemies. *BT, Rosh Hashana* 23b, reads: 'Rabbi Yohanan said: "Every acacia tree that was taken by the invaders from Jerusalem will be restored to it by the Holy One, blessed be He, in time to come, as it says, "I will plant in the wilderness the cedar, the acacia tree" (*Isaiah* 41:19), and 'wilderness' means Jerusalem, as it is written, Zion is become a wilderness' (*ibid.* 64:9).

The Book of *Psalms* (36:9) alludes to the cultivation of perfumes, their irrigation with the temple waters and their fertilization in Jerusalem: 'And thou shalt water them with the manure of your temple, and thou shalt irrigate them with the stream of thy delights. Ezekiel is speaking of the Kidron Valley when he says: 'Along the bank of the river, on this side and that, will grow all kinds of trees used for food; their leaves will not wither, and their fruit will not fail. They will bear fruit every month, because their water

---

161 Bialoblotzki 1971, 33–34; Guttmann 1972, 74.
162 Guttmann 1972, 74; Manns 2001, 77; for soil around the city, see Avnimelech 1966, 24–31; Price 1992, 244.
163 Feliks 1997a, 64.
164 Robinson-Smith 1957, 191–196; Urbach 1984, 23.
165 Tucazinsky 1969, III, 152; Schepansky 1992, 124; Zevin 2002, 'Jerusalem', XXV, 332.
166 Feliks 1997a, 102.

flows from the sanctuary. Their fruit will be for food, and their leaves for medicine (*Ezekiel* 47:12). It should be mentioned that while excavating the Upper City in the Jewish Quarter of Jerusalem, which has been discussed above, Nahman Avigad discovered a house in which perfumes were made, with tools from the Second Temple period.[167]

It may be that the prohibition of the cultivation of gardens only applied to the Temple Mount. The words of Hecataeus of Abdera (second half of the 4th century BCE) give support to this view: he heard from the High Priest of his time that nothing was planted on the Temple Mount.[168] This was certainly strange in the eyes of a Greek, since it is quite different from the accepted custom in Greek temples, and there is, therefore, no doubt of its authenticity.[169]

Josephus mentions with pride that Herod's palace—at the highest point in Jerusalem—was well supplied with water. Magnificent gardens were also situated there. The palace was decorated with various trees, although these were probably ornamental, never intended as a source of food. Josephus calls the trees there ποικίλαι ὗλαι, which usually means forest trees, in contrast to fruit trees, δένδρα.[170] The palace was arranged in the Persian-Hellenistic manner in a series of pavilions set in an elaborate garden.[171]

In areas north of the city, as far as down to the Kidron Valley, walls, gardens, and trees were destroyed when the Romans leveled the area outside Jerusalem in preparation for their assault. In his first failure at Jerusalem, Titus became entangled in the complex of gardening trenches, walls and fences outside the walls and was almost killed. Similarly, when troops were moved from Mount Scopus to the third wall on the north side, they cleared the intervening ground of many gardens and fruit trees.[172]

Conclusions

In summing up the whole subject, we see that particular emphasis was placed on reinforcing awareness of public health, and on the development of feelings of responsibility for the natural and social environment. The recognition of the damage caused by these nuisances, and their definition as a danger to public health which could not be justified by the rule of *ḥazaka*[173]—attracted special attention. *Halakhic*-ecological reasons were the motivation of the Sages in eliminating sanitary nuisances, increasing

---

167 Avigad 1980, 130–131; Har-El 1987, 312; Dvorjetski (forthcoming [a]), chapter 7.3 on *Aromatic Substances: Perfumes and Spices*.

168 Josephus, *Contra Apionem* XXII,199; For Hecataeus of Abdera and the founding of Jerusalem, see Stern 1976, I, 20–24; Mendels 1983, 96–110; Gafni 1987, 7–8; Bolin 2003, 190–191.

169 Krauss 1924, 98–99; For the running waters and the gardens in the city, see Timochares, the Greek biographer of Antiohus VII (late 2nd century BCE) apud Stern 1976, I, 135; Bar-Kochva 2010, 458, 461, 464.

170 Josephus, *Antiquitates Judaicae* V,180–181; See also Wilkinson 1989, 83; Price 1992, 245.

171 Avi-Yonah 1975, 233; Dvorjetski (forthcoming [a]), chapter 9.7 on *Gardens and Parks: The Concept of 'Green Lungs'*.

172 Josephus, *Antiquitates Judaicae* V,57, 107, Cf. 262 and 264; Avi-Yonah 1975, 242; Price 1992, 245.

173 The halakhic concept of *ḥazaka* refers to a situation where a person's status, or the relationship between two people, is widely known and accepted.

the welfare and preserving the health of the populace, their motivation was religious. The exclusion of the sources of bad smells from residential areas, the prohibition on creating certain industries within the city, and the proscription of air pollution by industrial waste were fundamental in the Rabbinic world.

In the urban by-laws dealing with environmental pollution, which were meant to improve the health of the public, special attention was paid to Jerusalem in general and to the Temple Mount, the place of the Temple, in particular. The city—which was known as 'the metropolis of all lands' (*Exodus Rabbah* 23,10), and was highly estimated by classical authors such as Pliny the Elder, who said 'Jerusalem is by far the most famous of the cities of the East',[174] was said to serve as a model both for the pilgrims who visited it and for all the nations.[175]

According to our survey, it seems that the Talmudic sources demonstrate how the *Halakha* was applied in Jerusalem in the Second Temple period: moderation of the odours from the animal sacrifices in the Temple; the possibility of pollution by the wind; the location of the outflow of the sacrificial ashes; the Dung Gate and its place in the ecological awareness of the people of the period; the concentration of craftsmen in special quarters; the attention paid by the authorities to upkeep, repair and cleanliness of the reservoirs; the upkeep of the sewage system; the construction of synagogues for craftsmen whose odour was intolerable; and the public lavatory, a rare phenomenon in Jewish towns.

Most of the positive qualities attributed to Jerusalem are more conceptual than real. Despite the prohibition on the breeding of pigs they were bred; the same applies to dogs, which in fact afforded complete freedom, were allowed to run quite freely, and to geese and chickens. Small cattle were also kept, and after the destruction of the Temple there was a tendency to restrict and modify the application of this prohibition, apparently as a result of changes in the economy. All this proves that the *Halakha* and real life were far from identical. The typological number ten appears frequently in our sources both in relation to this subject—the urban by-laws—and in relation to the laudatory terms used for Jerusalem, as well as in the ten journeys of the Divine Presence, and in the ten miracles which our forefathers experienced in the Temple. This number glorifies the 'Holy City' in all the qualities and virtues and also applies to the ten city by-laws.

The prohibition on burial and keeping a body in the city stemmed from concern for the purity of the city and the preservation of the quality of the environment. Talmudic literature and other sources show that the *Halakha* in this respect was observed faithfully. The prohibition on planting applied only to the Temple Mount. Another reason for the prohibition on planting, ploughing and sowing was the preservation of an area for additional buildings, since the area of the city was too small for large numbers of pilgrims. The prohibition on planting trees, gardens and orchards did not

---

174 Pliny the Elder, *Naturalis Historia*, V, 70; Stern 1976, 471; idem. 2004, 519–530.
175 Patai 1947; Bietenhard 1951, 192–204; Urbach 1968, 156–171; Sperber 1982, 107–114; Safrai and Safrai 1993, 344–371; Meyers 1997, III, 232–233; Klawans 2006, 188–189.

last, and our sources tell of trees planted next to the wall, inside and outside it: acacia trees, perfume plants, the magnificent gardens of King Herod the Great, and more.

The precepts which deal with ecology constitute an inherent part of the system of laws of the Jewish world. The Talmudic literature demonstrates how the *halakha* was applied in Jerusalem in the Second Temple period reflecting the circumstances of their own time: moderation of the odours from the animal sacrifices in the Temple;[176] the possibility of pollution by the wind; the location of the outflow of the sacrificial ashes; the Dung Gate and its place in the ecological awareness of the people of the period; the concentration of craftsmen in special quarters; the attention paid by the authorities to upkeep, repair and cleanliness of the sewage system and reservoirs; the construction of synagogues for craftsmen whose odour was intolerable; the public lavatory, which is a rare phenomenon in Jewish towns.

Over the generations Jerusalem's special status as the location of the Temple led to its being particularly revered as a place whose exemplary purity was meticulously preserved, and impure elements excluded. The ecological reasons for dealing with such matters as sewage, refuse, air pollution, smoke, noise, hazards of animals, water pollution, and sanitary inspection to which little attention is given in the 'ten maxims concerning Jerusalem' and in other municipal by-laws—are part and parcel of the Rabbinic literature. They prove that public health was a central concern of those who formulated the ancient precepts, a great many of which were crystallized at the time of the Hasmoneans and became a compulsory reality. The ordinances and laws of Jerusalem—which constitute an ecological prototype—served as a classical model for urban laws in the Land of Israel for general municipal regulations, which were aimed at preserving the quality of life and the health of its inhabitants and of those who came within its gates.

Bibliography

Sources

ARN = *Avot de Rabbi Nathan.* 1887. Versions I–II. Edited by S. Schechter. Vienna: Ch. D. Lippe. [In Hebrew]

Athenaeus, *Deipnosophistae.* 1969. Translated by C.B. Gulick. *Loeb Classical Library.* London/Cambridge-Mass.: Harvard University Press.

BT = *Babylonian Talmud.* 1935–1961. Edited by I. Epstein. I–XVIII, London: Soncino Press.

Ecclesiasticus. The Old Testament Pseudepigrapha. 2008. Edited by J.H. Charlesworth. I, Garden City, NY/London: Doubleday.

JT = *Jerusalem Talmud.* 1982–1991. Translated by J. Neusner. *The Talmud of the Land of Israel.* I–XXXIV. Chicago: Chicago University Press.

---

176 Even if the Rabbis did not specifically mention their knowledge and practical experience of air pollution caused by the sacrifices in the Temple, they discussed, for example, the smoke in other places, such as in Rome (*BT, Megillah* 6b), perhaps because of the sanctity and uniqueness of the holy city, they did not mention it in the *JT, BT,* and the *Midrasim.*

Josephus, *Antiquitates Judaicae*. 1965. Translated by L.H. Feldman. *Loeb Classical Library*. London/Cambridge-Mass.: Harvard University Press.

Josephus, *Bellum Judaicum*. 1927. Translated by H. Thackeray. *Loeb Classical Library*. London/Cambridge, Mass.: Harvard University Press.

Josephus, *Vita*. 1965. Translated by H. Thackeray. *Loeb Classical Library*. London/Cambridge, Mass.: Chicago University Press.

II Maccabees. 2008. Edited by J.H. Charlesworth. *The Old Testament Pseudepigrapha*. I, Garden City, NY/London: Doubleday.

Maimonidis Commentarius in Mishnam. 1956–1966. I–III, Edited by D. Sassoon. Copenhagen: E. Munksgaard.

Maimonides, *The Eight Chapters*. 2011. Translated by M. Schwarz. Jerusalem: Yad Ben-Zvi and The Hebrew University of Jerusalem. [In Hebrew]

Maimonides, *Moreh HaNebukim (The Guide of the Perplexed)*. 1963. Translated by S. Pines. Chicago: Chicago University Press.

Midrash Genesis Rabbah. 1965. Edited by J. Theodor and Ch. Albeck. Jerusalem: Shalem. [In Hebrew]

Midrash HaGadol, Exodus. 1975. Translated by M. Margalioth. Jerusalem: HaRav Kook Institute. [In Hebrew]

Midrash Lamentations Rabbah. 1619. Pesaro Edition. [In Hebrew]

Midrash Lamentations Rabbah. 1899. Edited by S. Buber. Vilna: [n.p.]. [In Hebrew]

Midrash Rabbah. 1939–1961. Translated by H. Freedman and M. Simon. I–X, London: Soncino Press.

Midrash Tannaim, Deuteronomy. 1909. Edited by D.Z. Hoffmann. Berlin: H. Itzkowski. [In Hebrew]

Midrash Tanhuma. 1885. Edited by S. Buber. Vilna: [n.p]. [In Hebrew]

Mishnah, The Mishnah. 1933. Translated by H. Danby. London: Oxford University Press.

Mishnah, Six Orders of the Mishnah. 1952–1958. Translated by Ch. Albeck. Jerusalem/Tel-Aviv: Bialik Institute and Dvir. [In Hebrew]

Philo of Alexandria, *De Specialibus Legibus*. 1958–1962. Translated by F.H. Colson and G.H. Whitaker. *Loeb Classical Library*. London/Cambridge-Mass.: Harvard University Press.

Pliny the Elder, *Naturalis Historia*. 1958. Translated by W.H.S. Jones. *Loeb Classical Library*. London/Cambridge, Mass.: Harvard University Press.

Semahot. 1936. Edited by M. Higger. *Minor Tractates*. New York: De bei Rabanan [In Hebrew]

Sifra. 1862. Edited by I.H. Weiss. *Sifra de Bei Rav*. Vienna: J. Schlossberg. [In Hebrew]

Tacitus, *Annales*. 1925–1937. Translated by J. Jackson. *Loeb Classical Library*. London/Cambridge, Mass.: Harvard University Press.

The Book of Jubilees. 2008. Edited by J.H. Charlesworth. *The Old Testament Pseudepigrapha*. I, Garden City, NY/London: Doubleday.

The Letter of Aristeas. 1974. Translated by M. Hadas. New York: KTAV.

Tosefta. 1955–1988. Edited by S. Lieberman. I–V, New York: The Jewish Theological Seminary in America. [In Hebrew]

Tosefta. 1975. Edited by M.S. Tsukermandel. Jerusalem: Wahrman. [In Hebrew]

Literature

Albeck, Ch. 1969. *Studies in the Baraitha and the Tosefta and Their Attitude to the Talmud.* Jerusalem: HaRav Kook Institute. [In Hebrew]

Alon, G. 1967². *Studies in Jewish History during the Second Temple, the Mishna and the Talmud.* I–II, Tel-Aviv: HaKibbutz HaMeuchad. [In Hebrew]

—. 1977. *Jews, Judaism and the Classical World.* Translated by I. Abrahams. Leiden: Brill.

Amir, J. 1980. "Philo's Version of the Pilgrimage to Jerusalem." In *Jerusalem in the Second Temple Period: Abraham Schalit Memorial Volume.* Edited by A. Oppenheimer et al. Jerusalem: Yad Ben-Zvi. Pages 154–165. [In Hebrew]

Avigad, N. 1980. *The Upper City of Jerusalem.* Jerusalem: Shiqmona and The Israel Exploration Society. [In Hebrew]

Avi-Yonah, M. 1956a. "The Archaeology and Topography of Jerusalem in the Second Temple Period." In *The Book of Jerusalem: Jerusalem, Its Natural Conditions, History and Development from the Origins to the Present Day.* Edited by idem. Jerusalem: Bialik Institute and Dvir. Pages 305–319. [In Hebrew]

—. 1956b. "The Second Temple." In *The Book of Jerusalem: Jerusalem, Its Natural Conditions, History and Development from the Origins to the Present Day.* Edited by idem. Jerusalem: Bialik Institute and Dvir. Pages 392–418. [In Hebrew]

—. 1968. "Jerusalem of the Second Temple Period." *Qadmoniot* 1, 1–2: 19–27. [In Hebrew]

—. 1975. "Jerusalem in the Hellenistic and Roman Periods." In *The World History of the Jewish People: The Herodian Period.* VII, Edited by idem. Jerusalem: Magnes. Pages 206–249. [In Hebrew]

Avnimelech, M.A. 1966. "Influence of Geological Conditions on the Development of Jerusalem." *BASOR* 181: 24–31.

Ayali, M. 1987. *Workers and Craftsmen: Their Labour and Status in the Rabbinic Literature.* Givatiim: Yad La-Talmud. [In Hebrew]

Baer, Y.F. 1952. "The Historical Foundations of the Halacha." *Zion* 17: 1–55. [In Hebrew]

Bagatti, B., and J.T. Milik. 1958; repr. 1981. *Gli scavi del 'Dominus Flevit' (Monte Oliveto-Gerusalemme).* I, *La necropoli del periodo Romano.* Jerusalem: Franciscan Printing Press.

Bahat, D. 1990. repr. 1994. *The Atlas of Biblical Jerusalem.* Translated by S. Ketko. Jerusalem: Carta.

Balberg, M. 2014. *Purity, Body, and Self in Early Rabbinic Literature.* Berkeley: University of California Press.

Balfour, A. 2012. *Solomon's Temple: Myth, Conflict, and Faith.* Chichester: Wiley.

Balée, W., ed. 1998. *Advances in Historical Ecology.* New York: Columbia University Press.

Bar-Kochva, B. 2010. *The Image of the Jews in Greek Literature.* Berkeley/Los Angeles: University of California Press.

Bar-Noy, S. 1985. "On the Prohibition of Withholding Dead in General and in Jerusalem in Particular." In *Pray for the Peace of Jerusalem: The Holy City in the Halakha Legend and Thought.* Edited by J. Burris and J. Beer. Jerusalem: Ezra. Pages 43–49. [In Hebrew]

Baruch, E., and Z. Amar. 2004. "The Latrine (Latrina) in the Land of Israel in the Roman-Byzantine Period." *Jerusalem and Eretz-Israel* 2: 27–50. [In Hebrew]

Baumgarten, A.I. 1996. "The Temple Scroll, Toilet Practices, and the Essenes." *Jewish History* 10/1: 12–14.

Becker, H.J. 2004. *Geniza-Fragmente zu Avot de-Rabbi Natan.* Tübingen: Mohr Siebeck.

Ben-Dov, M. 1985. *In the Shadow of the Temple: The Discovery of Ancient Jerusalem*. New York: Harper and Row.

Ben-Eliyahu, E., et al. 2012. *Handbook of Jewish Literature from Late Antiquity, 135–700 CE*. Oxford: Oxford University Press.

Ben-Horim, N. 1929–1930. "The Eye in the Talmud." *Harofé HaIvri* 1, 2: 121–127. [In Hebrew]

Ben-Shalom, S. 1986. "Keeping Agriculture or Woodland: The Explanation of the Halakha Concerning the Prohibition of Raising Small Cattle." *Halamish* 3: 36–45. [In Hebrew]

Bialoblotzki, S. 1971. "Jerusalem in the Halakha." *Em La-Masoret: Studies and Articles*. Ramat-Gan: Bar-Ilan University Press. Pages 19–73. [In Hebrew]

Bickerman, E. 1980. *Studies in Jewish and Christian History*. II, Leiden: Brill.

Bietenhard, H. 1951. *Die himmlische Welt im Urchristentum und Spätjudentum*. Tübingen: Mohr Siebeck.

Bolin, T. M. 2003. "The Making of the Holy City: On the Foundations of Jerusalem in the Hebrew Bible." In *Jerusalem in Ancient History and Tradition*. Edited by T.L. Thompson. London: T&T Clark. Pages 171–196.

Bradley, M. 2002. "'It All Comes Out in the Wash': Looking Harder at the Roman *fullonica*." *Journal of Roman Archaeology* 15: 20–44.

Brayer, M. M. 1965. "Medicine, Hygiene and Psychology in the Scrolls Literature from the Judaean Desert." *Harofé HaIvri* 38: 145–167. [In Hebrew]

Broshi, M. 1992. "Anti-Qumranic Polemics in the Talmud." In *The Madrid Qumran Congress: Proceedings of the International Congress on the Dead Sea Scrolls, Madrid 18–21 March, 1991*. II, Edited by J. Trebolle Barrera and L. Vegas Montaner. Leiden: Brill. Pages 589–600.

Büchler, A. 1911. "La pureté lévitique d'Jérusalem et les tombeaux des Prophètes." *Revue des Études Juives* 62: 201–215.

—. 1912. "La pureté lévitique d'Jérusalem et les tombeaux des prophètes." *Revue des Études Juives* 63: 30–50.

—. 1914. "Learning and Teaching in the Open Air." *Jewish Quarterly Review, New Series* 4: 485–491.

—. 1956. "On the History of the Temple Worship in Jerusalem." In *Studies in Jewish History: The Adolph Büchler Memorial Volume*. Edited by I. Brodie and J. Rabbinowitz. London/ New York: Oxford University Press. Pages 24–63.

Crouch, D.P. 1993. *Water Management in Ancient Greek Cities*. Oxford: Oxford University Press.

Cohen, S.J.D. 1986. "The Political and Social History of the Jews in Greco-Roman Antiquity: The State of the Question." In *Early Judaism and Its Modern Interpreters*. Edited by R.A. Kraft and G.W.E. Nickelsburg. Philadelphia/Atlanta: Fortress Press. Pages 33–56.

Cohen, Y. 1978. *Chapters in the History of the Period of the Tannaim*. Jerusalem: Education and Culture Authority. [In Hebrew]

Cooper, P. F. 2001. "Historical Aspects of Wastewater Treatment." In *Decentralised Sanitation and Reuse: Concepts, Systems and Implementation*. Edited by P. Lens et al. London: IWA. Pages 11–38.

Dalman, G. 1924; repr. 1967⁴. *Orte und Wege Jesu*. Darmstadt: Wissenschaftliche Buchgesellschaft.

—. G. 1930. *Jerusalem und sein Gelände*. Gütersloh: Bertelsmann.

Dan, Y. 1990. "Internal and Foreign Trades in the Second Temple Period." In *Commerce in Palestine through the Ages*. Edited by B.Z. Kedar et al. Jerusalem: Yad Ben-Zvi. Pages 91–107. [In Hebrew]

Daniel-Nataf, S., ed. 1991. *Philo of Alexandria, Writings*. I-V, Jerusalem: Bialik Institue. [In Hebrew]

Day, J. 1989. *Molech: A God of Human Sacrifice in the Old Testament*. Cambridge/New York: Cambridge University Press.

Delitzsch, F. 1877. *Jewish Artisan Life in the Time of Our Lord*. Translated by P. Monkhouse. London: S. Bagster.

Dussaud, R. 1923. "Comptes d'ouvriers d'une entreprise funéraire juive." *Syria* 4,3: 241–249.

Dvorjetski, E. 1993. "'Tzrifa in Ascalon': A Talmudic Reality in the Art of Fine Metal Work in Eretz-Israel in the Roman and Byzantine Periods." *Tarbiz* 63,1: 27–40. [In Hebrew]

—. 1995. "The Education towards Environmental Noise in the Classical and Rabbinic Sources." In *Israel Society of Ecology and Environmental Science, Abstracts*. Haifa: Technion, Institute of Technology, Israel. Page 59. [In Hebrew]

—. 1996. "Education for the Prevention of Air Pollution in Rabbinic Literature." In *Preservation of Our World in the Wake of Change: Proceedings of the 6th International Conference of the Israeli Society for Ecology and Environmental Quality Sciences, Jerusalem, Israel, June 30-July 4*. Edited by Y. Steinberger. Jerusalem: Israel Society for Ecology and Environmental. Pages 202–203.

—. 1999a. "Public Health in Jerusalem during the Second Temple period." In *Medicine in Jerusalem through the Ages*. Edited by Z. Amar et al. Tel-Aviv: ERETZ. Pages 7–31. [In Hebrew]

—. 1999b. "Air Pollution and Public Health during the Second Temple Period, the Mishna and the Talmud." *Michmanim* 13: 46–58. [In Hebrew]

—. 2001². *Ecology and Values: Environment in Jewish Traditional Sources. Selected Sources to the Lectures*. Department of Jewish History, University of Haifa. [In Hebrew]

—. 2007. *Leisure, Pleasure and Healing: Spa Culture and Medicine in Ancient Eastern Mediterranean*. Leiden/Boston: Brill.

—. 2011–2012. "'A Leper May as Well Be Dead' (*Babylonian Talmud, Nedarim* 64b): Diagnosis, Prognosis and Methods of Treatment of 'Leprosy' throughout the Ages." *Koroth* 21: 227–254.

—. 2016. "Public Health in Ancient Palestine: Historical and Archaeological Aspects of Lavatories." In *Viewing Ancient Jewish Art and Archaeology: VeHinnei Rachel—Essays in Honor of Rachel Hachlili*. Edited by A.E. Killebrew and G. Faßbeck. Leiden: Brill. Pages 48–100.

—. [forthcoming (a)] *Medicine, Ecology and Public Health in the Holy Land from Biblical Times to the Late Roman Period: Historical-Archaeological Analysis*.

Edelman, D. 2005. "Tyrian Trade in Yehud under Artaxerxes I: Real or Fictional? Independent or Crown-Endorsed?" In *Judah and the Judeans in the Persian Period*. Edited by O. Lipschits and I. Artaxerxes. Winona Lake, IN: Eisenbrauns. Pages 207–246.

Edersheim, A. 1874; repr. 1997. *The Temple, Its Ministry and Services as They were at the Time of Jesus Christ*. Grand Rapids, MI: Eerdmans.

Eisenstein, J.D., ed. 1907–1913; repr. 1952. *Ozar Yisrael: An Encyclopedia*. I-X, Jerusalem/New York: Or Hadash. [In Hebrew]

—. 1928; repr. 1975. *A Digest of Jewish Laws and Customs*. Tel-Aviv: Shilo. [In Hebrew]

Eliav, Y.Z. 2002. "Realia, Daily Life, and the Transmission of Local Stories During the Talmudic Period." In *What Athens Has to Do with Jerusalem: Essays on Classical, Jewish and*

Early Christian Archaeology in Honor of Gideon Foerster. Edited by L.V. Rutgers. Leuven: Peeters. Pages 235–265.

Eliav, Y.Z. 2014. "Samuel Krauss and the Early Study of the Physical World of the Rabbis in Roman Palestine." *Journal of Jewish Studies* 65,1: 38–57.

—.2015. "The Material World of Babylonia as Seen from Roman Palestine: Some Preliminary Observations." In *The Archaeology and Material Culture of the Babylonian Talmud.* Edited by M. J. Geller. Leiden: Brill. Pages 153–185.

—.2016. "From Realia to Material Culture: The Reception of Samuel Krauss' Talmudische Archaologie." In *Arise, Walk through the Land: Studies in the Archaeology and History of the Land of Israel in Memory of Yizhar Hirschfeld on the Tenth Anniversary of his Demise.* Edited by J. Patrich et al. Jerusalem: The Israel Exploration Society. Pages 17*–27*.

Epstein, I. N. 1931. "To the Epitaph of Uzziahu." *Tarbiz* 2,3: 293–294. [In Hebrew]

Feliks, Y. 1990. *Agriculture in Eretz-Israel in the Period of the Bible and Talmud.* Jerusalem: R. Mass. [In Hebrew]

—.1992. *Nature and Land in the Bible: Chapters in Biblical Ecology.* Jerusalem: R. Mass. [In Hebrew]

—.1994. *Fruit Trees in the Bible and Talmudic Literature.* Jerusalem: R. Mass. [In Hebrew]

—.1997a. *Trees: Aromatic, Ornamental and of the Forest in the Bible and Rabbinic Literature.* Jerusalem: R. Mass. [In Hebrew]

—.1997b. "The History of Balsamon Cultivation in the Land of Israel." In *The Village in Ancient Israel.* Edited by S. Dar and Z. Safrai. Tel-Aviv: Eeretz. Pages 275–296. [In Hebrew]

Fine, S. 2005; rev. ed. 2010². *Art and Judaism in the Greco-Roman World: Toward a New Jewish Archaeology.* Cambridge/New York: Cambridge University Press. .

—.2014. *Art, History and the Historiography of Judaism in Roman Antiquity.* Leiden: Brill.

Fine, S. and A. Koller, eds. 2014. *Talmuda de-Eretz Israel: Archaeology and the Rabbis in Late Antique Palestine.* Berlin/Boston: De Gruyter.

Finkelstein, E.A. 1950. "The *Halakhoth* Applied to Jerusalem." *Alexander Marx Jubilee Volume on the Occasion of His 70th Birthday.* II, New York: Jewish Theological Seminary. Pages 351–369. [In Hebrew]

Fonrobert, C.E., and M.S. Jaffee, eds. 2007. *The Cambridge Companion to the Talmud and Rabbinic Literature.* Cambridge/New York: Cambridge University Press.

Freudenstein, E.G. 1970. "Ecology and the Jewish Tradition." *Judaism* 19/4: 406–414.

Friedman, S. 1993. "The Primacy of Tosefta in Mishnah-Tosefta Parallels—*Shabbat* 16, 1." *Tarbiz* 62/3: 313–338. [In Hebrew]

—.2002. *Tosefta Atiqta, Pesah Rishon: Synoptic Parallels of Mishna and Tosefta Analyzed with A Methodological Introduction.* Ramat-Gan: Bar-Ilan University Press. [In Hebrew]

Funk, S. 1912. *Die Hygiene des Talmuds.* Wien: Historische Abteilung der Internationalen Hygiene Ausstellung.

Gafni, I.M. 1987. "'Pre-Histories' of Jerusalem in Hellenistic, Jewish and Christian Literature." *Journal for the Study of the Pseudepigrapha* 1: 5–22.

—.1999. "Jerusalem in Rabbinic Literature." In *The History of Jerusalem: The Roman and Byzantine Periods (70–638 CE).* Edited by Y. Tsafrir and S. Safrai. Jerusalem: Yad Ben-Zvi. Pages 35–59. [In Hebrew]

Gil, M. 1988. "Yoḥanan the High Priest and the Priestly Dues." *Leshonenu* 52: 157–164. [In Hebrew]

Gilat, Y.D. 1967. "Hammering as One of the Principal Labour Forbidden on the Sabbath." In *Proceedings of the 4th World Congress of Jewish Studies*. I, Jerusalem: Magnes. Pages 149–151. [In Hebrew]

Goldman, S. 1970. *Jerusalem in Jewish Life and Tradition*. London: Council for Jewish-Christian Understanding.

Goodman, M. 2005. "The Temple in First Century CE Jerusalem." In *Temple and Worship in Biblical Israel*. Edited by J. Day. London/New York: T&T Clark. Pages 459–468 [= idem., *ibid*., In M. Goodman, M. 2007. *Judaism in the Roman World*. Leiden: Brill. Pages 47–58].

Goodman, M. and P. Alexander, eds. 2011. *Rabbinic Texts and the History of Late Roman Palestine*. Oxford: Oxford University Press.

Grossmark, T. 2006. "Because Kilns are not Permitted in Jerusalem (b. Zebah. 96a)." In *New Studies on Jerusalem. Proceedings of the 11th Conference*. Edited by E. Baruch et al. Ramat-Gan: Bar Ilan University Press. Pages 263–275. [In Hebrew]

Guttmann, A. 1969–1970. "Jerusalem in Tannaitic Law." *HUCA* 40–41: 251–275.

—. 1972. "Some Aspects of Theoretical *Halakhot*." In *Proceedings of the 5th World Congress of Jewish Studies*. III, Jerusalem: Magnes. Pages 67–79. [In Hebrew]

Hakim, B.S. 2001. "Julian of Ascalon's Treatise of Construction and Design Rules from Sixth-Century Palestine." *Journal of the Society of Architectural Historians* 60,1: 4–25.

Hales, S., and T. Hodos. 2010. *Material Culture and Social Identities in the Ancient World*. Cambridge: Cambridge University Press.

Haran, M. 1960. "The Uses of Incense in the Ancient Israelite Ritual." *Vetus Testamentum* 10,2: 113–129.

Har-El, M. 1970. *This Is Jerusalem*. Tel-Aviv: Am Oved. [In Hebrew]

—. 1987. "Water for Purification, Hygiene and Cult at the Temple in Jerusalem." *Eretz-Israel* 19: 310–313. [In Hebrew]

—. 1989. "The Springs of Jerusalem and the Temple." *Merhavim* 3: 158–166. [In Hebrew]

Harris, W.V., ed. 2013. *The Ancient Mediterranean Environment between Science and History*. Leiden: Brill.

Hayes, J.H., and S.R. Mandell. 1998. *The Jewish People in Classical Antiquity from Alexander to Bar Kochba*. Louisville, KY: Westminster John Knox Press.

Hecker, M. 1956. "Water Supply to Jerusalem in Ancient Times." In *The Book of Jerusalem: Jerusalem, Its Natural Conditions, History and Development from the Origins to the Present Day*. Edited by M. Avi-Yonah. Jerusalem/Tel-Aviv: Bialik Institute. Pages 191–218. [In Hebrew]

Heger, P. 1997. *The Development of Incense Cult in Israel. Ph.D. diss.*, University of Toronto.

Heineman, I. 1970. *Paths of the Aggadah*. Jerusalem: Bialik Institute. [In Hebrew]

Heinemann, J. 1986. "The Nature of the Aggadah" In *Midrash and Literature*. Edited by G.H. Hartman and S. Budick. New Haven/London: Yale University Press. Pages 41–55.

Henshke, D. 1997. "The Sanctity of Jerusalem: The Sages and Sectarian Halakha." *Tarbiz* 67,1: 5–28. [In Hebrew]

Herr, M.D. 1980. "Jerusalem, the Temple and Its Cult-Reality and Concepts in Second Temple Times." In *Jerusalem in the Second Temple Period: Abraham Schalit Memorial Volume*. Edited by A. Oppenheimer et al. Jerusalem: Yad Ben-Zvi. Pages 166–177. [In Hebrew]

Hezser, C., ed. 2010. *The Oxford Handbook of Jewish Daily Life in Roman Palestine*. Oxford: Oxford University Press.

Hicks, D., and M.C. Beaudry. 2010. *The Oxford Handbook of Material Culture Studies*. Oxford: Oxford University Press.

Hirschfeld, Y. 1987. *Dwelling Houses in Roman and Byzantine Palestine*. Jerusalem: Yad Ben-Zvi. [In Hebrew]

Hoenig, L.J. 1989. "Ben Achiya: The First Gastroenterologist in Ancient Israel?" *The Journal of Clinical Gastroenterology* 11,1: 61–63.

Horowitz, C.M. 1889. *Tosefta Atikta*. I-V, Frankfurt am Main: Private Publication. [In Hebrew]

Horowitz, I.Z. 1964. *Jerusalem in Our Literature: Geographical, Topographical and Historical Encyclopedia of Jerusalem and Its Surroundings*. Jerusalem: R. Mass. [In Hebrew]

Hughes, J. D. 1994. *Pan's Travail: Environmental Problems of the Ancient Greeks and Romans*. Baltimore/London: Johns Hopkins University Press.

—. 2001. *An Environmental History of the World: Humankind's Changing Role in the Community of Life*. London: Routledge.

—. 2005. *The Mediterranean: An Environmental History*. Santa Barbara, California.

—. 2006. *What is Environmental History?* Cambridge: Cambridge University Press.

—. 2014². *Environmental Problems of the Greeks and Romans: Ecology in the Ancient Mediterranean*. Baltimore: Johns Hopkins University Press.

Isaac, B. 2010. "Jerusalem—An Introduction." In *Corpus Inscriptionum Iudaeae/Palaestinae*. I/I, *Jerusalem*. Edited by H.M. Cotton et al. Berlin/New York: W. De Gruyter. Pages 1–37.

Ish-Shalom, M. 1899. "Four Raisings that the Sages Forbided." *Kadima* 1: 1–7. [In Hebrew]

Istori HaParhi 1959; repr. 1989. *Sefer Kaftor va-ferah*. Jerusalem: Gvil. [In Hebrew]

Jastrow, M. 1950; repr. 1995. *A Dictionary of The Targumim, The Talmud Babli and Yerusalmi, and The Midrashic Literature*. I–II, New York: Pardes.

Jeremias, J. 1962; repr. 1969³. *Jerusalem in the Time of Jesus: An Investigation into Economic and Social Conditions during the New Testament Period*. London: SCM.

Kasher, A. 1980. "Jerusalem as a 'Metropolis' in the National Consciousness of Philo." *Cathedra* 11: 45–56. [In Hebrew]

Katsh, A.I. 1970. *Ginze Mishna*. Jerusalem: HaRav Kook Institute. [In Hebrew]

Kessel, A.S. 2006. *Air, the Environment and Public Health*. Cambridge: Cambridge University Press.

Kister, M. 1998. *Studies in Avot de-Rabbi Nathan: Text, Redaction and Interpretation*. New York/Jerusalem: The Jewish Theological Seminary. [In Hebrew]

Klawans, J. 2006. *Purity, Sacrifice, and the Temple: Symbolism and Supersessionism in the Study of Ancient Judaism*. Oxford: Oxford University Press.

Klausner, J. 1975. "The Economy of Judaea in the Period of the Second Temple." In *The World History of the Jewish People*. VII, *The Herodian Period*. Edited by M. Avi-Yonah. Jerusalem: Masada Publishing. Pages 179–205.

Kloner, A. 1980. *Tombs and Burial in Jerusalem during the Second Temple Period*. Ph.D. diss., The Hebrew University of Jerusalem. [In Hebrew]

—. 1997. "Columbaria in Jerusalem." In *The 2nd Conference on Recent Innovations in the Study of Jerusalem*. Edited by Z. Safrai and A. Faust. Ramat-Gan: Bar Ilan University, The Ingeborg Rennert Center for Jerusalem Studies. Pages 25–31. [In Hebrew]

—. 2000. "Columbaria in Jerusalem." In *Jerusalem and Eretz-Israel: Arie Kindler Volume*. Edited by J. Schwartz et al. Tel-Aviv: Ingeborg Rennert Center for Jerusalem Studies and Eretz-Israel Museum. Pages 61*–66*.

Kloner, A., and B. Zissu. 2007. *The Necropolis of Jerusalem in the Second Temple Period*. Leuven: Peeters.

Knowles, M. D. 2006. *Centrality Practiced: Jerusalem in the Religious Practice of Yehud and the Diaspora during the Persian Period*. Atlanta: Society of Biblical Literature.

Kohut, H. Y. 1926². *Aruch Completum*. I-XII, New York: HaMenorah [In Hebrew]

Kotlar, D. 1973. "Ecology in Ancient Jerusalem." *HaBiosphera* 5: 8–11. [In Hebrew]

—. 1976. *Human Ecology in the Ancient World: Eretz-Israel, Greece and Rome*. Jerusalem: M. Newman [In Hebrew]

Kottek, S. S. 1994. *Medicine and Hygiene in the Works of Flavius Josephus*. Leiden/New York: Brill.

Krauss, S. 1907. "La défence d'élever du menu bétail en Palestine et questions connexes." *Revue des Études Juives* 53: 14–55.

—. 1910–1912; repr. 1966. *Talmudische Archäologie*. I–III, Leipzig: G. Fock.

—. 1922; repr. 1966. *Synagogale Alertümer*. Berlin: B. Harz.

—. 1924; repr. 1929. *Talmudic Antiquities (Qadmoniot HaTalmud)*. I-IV, Berlin: Hertz [In Hebrew]

—. 1948. "Outdoor Teaching in Talmudic Times." *Journal of Jewish Studies* 1,2: 82–84.

Lerner, M. B. 1987. "The External Tractates." In *The Literature of the Sages*. I, Oral Tora, Halakha, Mishna, Tosefta, Talmud, External Tractates. Edited by S. Safrai. Assen: Gorcum. Pages 367–403.

Levi, J. 1994. "Israel Heritage Values of Ecology as a Means of Education." *HaBiosphera* 23, 10: 8–10. [In Hebrew]

Levine, L. I. 2002. *Jerusalem: Portrait of the City in the Second Temple Period (538 B.C.E.–70 C.E.)*, Philadelphia: The Jewish Publication Society.

Lieberman, S. 1937–1939. *Tosefeth Rishonim*. I-IV, Jerusalem: Bamberger and Wahrman. [In Hebrew]

—. 1950. *Hellenism in Jewish Palestine: Studies in the Literary Transmission Beliefs and Manners of Palestine in the I Century B.C.E.–IV Century C.E.* New York: The Jewish Theological Seminary of America.

—. 1971. "A Few Words on the Book by Julian the Architect of Ascalon *The Laws of Palestine and Its Customs*." *Tarbiz* 40,4: 409–417. [In Hebrew]

Liebeschuetz, W. 2000. "Rubbish Disposal in Greek and Roman Cities." In *Sordes Urbis. La Eliminación de Residuos en la Ciudad Romana. Actas de la Reunión de Rome*. Edited by X. D. Raventós et al. Rome: L'Erma di Bretschneider. Pages 51–62.

Lipinski, E. 2004. "'Tyrians Living in Jerusalem…': The Population of Jerusalem in Antiquity." In *Itineraria Phoenicia*. Edited by E. Lipinski. Leuven: Peeters. Pages 493–545.

Löw, I. 1924–1934. *Die Flora der Juden*. I-IV, Vienna/Leipzig: Löwit.

Magness, J. 2011. *Stone and Dung, Oil and Spit: Jewish Daily Life in the time of Jesus*. Grand Rapids, MI: Eerdmans.

—. 2012. "Toilet Practices, Purity Concerns, and Sectarianism in the Late Second Temple Period." In *Jewish Identity and Politics between the Maccabees and Bar Kokhba: Groups, Normativity, and Rituals*. Edited by B. Eckhardt. Leiden/Boston: Brill. Pages 51–70.

Manns, F. 2001. 'A Response to Professor A. Shinan's Paper, "A House of Prayer for all Peoples (*Isaiah* 56:7)."' In *Jerusalem: House of Prayer for all Peoples in the Three Monotheistic Religions*. Edited by A. Niccacci. Jerusalem: Franciscan Printing Press. Pages 73–80.

Margalit, D. 1977. "Ecology (The Study of Environmental Conditions) in Our Sources." *Koroth* 7: 145–153. [In Hebrew]

Mattern, T., and A. Vött. 2009. *Mensch und Umwelt im Spiegel der Zeit: Aspekte geoarchäologischer Forschungen im östlichen Mittelmeergebiet.* Wiesbaden: Harrassowitz.

Mazar, A. 2002. "A Survey of the Aqueducts to Jerusalem." In *The Aqueducts of Israel.* Edited by D. Amit et al. Portsmouth, RI. Pages 210–244.

Mazar, B. 1975. *The Mountain of the Lord.* Garden City, NY: Doubleday.

—. 1978. "Herodian Jerusalem in Light of the Excavations South and Southwest to the Temple Mount." *Cathedra* 8: 29–40. [In Hebrew]

Mendels, D. 1983. "Hecataeus of Abdera and a Jewish 'Patrios Politeia' of the Persian Period (Diodorus Siculus XL, 3)." *Zeitschrift für Alttestamentarische Wissenschaft* 95,1: 96–110.

Meyers, E. M. 1997. "Jerusalem." In *The Oxford Encyclopedia of Archaeology in the Near East.* I–V. Edited by idem. New York/Oxford: Oxford University Press. Pages 224–237.

—. 2014. "The Use of Archaeology in Understanding Rabbinic Materials: An Archaeological Perspective." In *Talmuda de-Eretz Israel: Archaeology and the Rabbis in Late Antique Palestine.* Edited by S. Fine and A. Koller. Boston/Berlin: De Gruyter. Pages 303–319.

Milgrom, J. 1990. "The Scriptural Foundations and Deviations in the Laws of Purity of the Temple Scroll." In *Archaeology and History in the Dead Sea Scrolls.* Edited by L.H. Schiffman. Sheffield: Sheffield University Press. Pages 83–100.

Miller, S. S. 2003. "Some Observations on Stone Vessel Finds, and Other Identity Markers of Complex Common Judaism." In *Zeichen aus Text und Stein: Studien auf dem Weg zu einer Archäologie des Neuen Testaments.* Edited by S. Alkier and J. Zangenberg. Tübingen: Mohr Siebeck. Pages 402–419.

—. 2010. "Stepped Pools, Stone Vessels, and Other Identity Markers of 'Complex Common Judaism'." *Journal for the Study of Judaism in the Persian, Hellenistic, and Roman Period* 41,2: 214–243.

—. 2015. *At the Intersection of Texts and Material Finds: Stepped Pools, Stone Vessels, and Ritual Purity among the Jews of Roman Galilee.* Tübingen: Mohr Siebeck.

Neis, R. 2012. "'Their Backs toward the Temple, and Their Faces toward the East': The Temple and Toilet Practices in Rabbinic Palestine and Babylonia." *Journal for the Study of Judaism in the Persian, Hellenistic, and Roman Period* 43,3: 328–368.

Netzer, E. 2007. "The Ideal City in the Eyes of Herod the Great." In *The World of the Herods.* I, *International Conference: The World of the Herods and the Nabataeans held at the British Museum, 17–19 April, 2001.* Edited by N. Kokkinos. Stuttgart: F. Steiner. Pages 71–91.

Neusner, J. 1970². *A Life of Rabban Yohanan ben Zakkai, ca. 1–80 CE.* Leiden: Brill.

Newmyer, S. 1996. "Public Health in the Holy Land: Classical Influence and Its Legacy." In *Health and Disease in the Holy Land: Studies in the History and Sociology of Medicine from Ancient Times to the Present.* Edited by M. Waserman and S.S. Kottek. Lewiston, NY and Lampeter, Wales: Edwin Mellen Press. Pages 67–101.

Nicole, J. 1894. *Le livre du préfet: ou, L'édit de l'empereur Léon le Sage sur les corporations de Constantinople Byzantine Empire.* Geneva: Georg.

Oelschlaeger, M. 1991. *The Idea of Wilderness from Prehistory to the Age of Ecology.* New Haven/London: Yale University Press.

Orfali, G. P. 1923. "Un hypogée juif à composé de chambres taillées dans le roc Bethphagé." *Revue Biblique* 32: 253–260.

Owens, E. 1991. *The City in the Greek and Roman World.* London/New York: Routledge.

Patrich, J. 2011. "The Location of the Second Temple and the Layout of Its Courts, Gates, and Chambers: A New Proposal." In *Unearthing Jerusalem: 150 Years of Archaeological*

Research in the Holy City. Edited by K. Galor and G. Avni. Winona Lake, IN: Eisenbrauns. Pages 205–229.

Peters, F. E. 1985. *Jerusalem: The Holy City in the Eyes of Chroniclers, Visitors, Pilgrims, and Prophets from the Days of Abraham to the Beginnings of Modern Times.* Princeton: Princeton University Press.

Preuss, J. 1978; repr. 1993. *Biblical and Talmudic Medicine.* Translated and edited by F. Rosner. Northvale, N.J./London: J. Aronson.

Price, J. J. 1992. *Jerusalem under Siege: The Collapse of the Jewish State 66–70 C.E.* Leiden: Brill.

Qimron, E. 1995. "The Cock, the Dog and the Temple Scroll (11QTc)." *Tarbiz* 64,4: 473–476, [In Hebrew]

Qimron, E. and J. Strugnell. 1994. *Discoveries in the Judaean Desert: Qumran Cave 4. Miqṣat Ma'aśe Ha-Torah.* X, Oxford: Clarendon Press.

Rahmani, L.Y. 1981. "Ancient Jerusalem's Funerary Customs and Tombs: Part II." *BA* 44, 4: 229–235.

Rakover, N. 1993. *Ecology. Conceptual and Legal Aspects of the Jewish Sources.* Jerusalem: Jewish Law Library, [In Hebrew]

Reich, R. 1980. "Mishnah, Sheqalim 8:2 and the Archaeological Evidence." In *Jerusalem in the Second Temple Period: Abraham Schalit Memorial Volume.* Edited by A. Oppenheimer et al. Jerusalem: Yad Ben-Zvi. Pages 225–256. [In Hebrew]

—. 2013. *Ritual Baths during the Second Temple, the Mishna and the Talmud.* Jerusalem: Yad Ben-Zvi and Israel Exploration Society. [In Hebrew]

—. 2014. "Toponymical Remarks: Tyropoeon, Tyros, Peristereon." *Jerusalem and Eretz-Israel* 8–9: 185–189. [In Hebrew]

Reich, R. and E. Shukron. 2003 "The Jerusalem City-Dump in the Late Second Temple Period." *Zeitschrift des Deutschen Palästina-Vereins* 119,1: 12–18.

—, and E. Shukron. 2004. "The History of the Gihon Spring in Jerusalem." *Levant* 36: 211–223.

Reich R. et al. 2007a. "New Discoveries at the City of David, Jerusalem." *Qadmoniot* 40, 132: 32–40. [In Hebrew]

Reich, R. et. al. 2007b. "Recent Discoveries in the City of David, Jerusalem." *Israel Exploration Journal* 57,2: 153–169.

Robinson-Smith, W. 1957. *Lectures on the Religion of the Semites: The Fundamental Institutions.* New York: Macmillian.

Rosner, F. 2000. *Encyclopedia of Medicine in the Bible and the Talmud.* Northvale, N.J./London: J. Aronson.

Safrai, S. 1965. *Pilgrimage at the Time of the Second Temple.* Tel-Aviv: Am HaSefer. [In Hebrew]

—. 1983. "The Temple and God's Worship." In *The World History of the Jewish People:*

—. *The Herodian Period.* Edited by M. Avi-Yonah. Jerusalem: Jewish History Publications. Pages 206–237. [In Hebrew]

—. 1996. "Jerusalem in the Halacha of the Second Temple Period." In *The Centrality of Jerusalem: Historical Perspectives.* Edited by M. Poorthuis and C. Safrai. Kampen: Peeters. Pages 94–113.

—. 1998. "Jerusalem and the Temple in the Tannaitic Literature of the First Generation after the Destruction of the Temple." In *Sanctity of Time and Space in Tradition and Modernity.* Edited by A. Houtman et al. Leiden: Brill. Pages 135–152.

— 1999. "The Jews of Jerusalem during the Roman Period." In *The History of Jerusalem: The Roman and Byzantine Periods (70–638 CE)*. Edited by Y. Tsafrir and S. Safrai. Jerusalem: Yad Ben-Zvi. Pages 15–34. [In Hebrew]

— 1995. *The Jewish Community in Eretz-Israel during the Mishnah and the Talmud Periods*. Jerusalem: Zalman Shazar Center for Jewish History. [In Hebrew]

Safrai, S. and C. Safrai. 1993. "The Sanctity of Eretz-Israel and Jerusalem." In *Jews and Judaism in the Second Temple, Mishna and Talmud Period: Studies in Honor of Shmuel Safrai*. Edited by I. Gafni et al. Jerusalem: Yad Ben-Zvi. Pages 344–371. [In Hebrew]

Saliou, C. 1996. *Le traité d'urbanisme de Julien d'Ascalon: droit et architecture en Palestine au VIe siècle*. Paris: De Boccard.

—. 2007. "De la maison à la ville: le traité de Julien d'Ascalon." In *From Antioch to Alexandria: Recent Studies in Domestic Architecture*. Edited by K. Galor et al. Warsaw: Institue of Archeology, University of Warsaw. Pages 169–178.

Schäfer, P. 1978. *Studien zur Geschichte und Theologie des rabbinischen Judentums*. Leiden: Brill.

—. 1979. "Die Flucht Johanan b. Zakkais aus Jerusalem und die Gründung des 'Lehrhauses' in Jabne." *ANRW*, II.19.2: 43–101.

Schäfer, P., ed. 1998–2002. *The Talmud Yerushalmi and Graeco-Roman Culture*. I–III, Tübingen: Mohr Siebeck.

Schepansky, I. 1992. *The Takkanot of Israel*. II: *Talmudic Ordinances*. Jerusalem: HaRav Kook Institute. [In Hebrew]

Schiffman, L. H., and G. M. Florentino. 2008. *The Courtyards of the House of the Lord: Studies on the Temple Scroll*. Leiden/Boston: Brill.

Schwartz, D. R. 1987. *Agrippa I: The Last King of Judaea*. Jerusalem: Zalman Shazar Center. [In Hebrew]

Schwartz, J. 1994. "The Priests in Jericho during the Second Temple Period." *Ariel* 105–106: 52–57. [In Hebrew]

Schwartz, S. 1998. "The Hellenization of Jerusalem and Shechem." In *Jews in a Graeco-Roman World*. Edited by M. Goodman. Oxford: Oxford University Press. Pages 37–45

Segal, B. Z. 1979. *Geography in the Mishnah: Nature and Values of Sites*. Jerusalem: Institute for the Mishnah Research. [In Hebrew]

Shaviv, J. 1992. "Ornamental and Eternity: Chapter in Jewish Ecology." *Techumin* 12: 472–479. [In Hebrew]

Shemesh, A. 2000. "The Holiness of Jerusalem and Other Places according to the Temple Scroll." In *Jerusalem and Eretz-Israel: Arie Kindler Volume*. Edited by J. Schwartz et al. Tel Aviv: Ingeborg Rennert Center for *Jerusalem* Studies and *Eretz-Israel*. Pages 101–110. [In Hebrew]

Shiloh, Y. 1984. *Excavations at the City of David, 1978–1982 (Qedem, 19)*. Jerusalem: Institute of Archaeology, The Hebrew University of Jerusalem.

Shin'an, A. 1990. "The 'Opening Model' in the Eretz-Israel Aramaic Translation to the Torah and Its Contribution to the Research of the Torah's Division to Orders of Reading." *Jerusalem Studies in Hebrew Literature* 12: 85–102. [In Hebrew]

Shinover, Z., and Y. Goldberg. 1994. *Quality of Life and Environment in Jewish Sources*. Nehalim: Mofet. [In Hebrew]

Shipley, G., and J. Salmon, eds. 2011. *Human Landscapes in Classical Antiquity: Environment and Culture*. London: Routledge.

Simons, J. J. 1952. *Jerusalem in the Old Testament: Researches and Theories*. Leiden: Brill.

Smith, G. A. 1907; repr. 1970. *The Topography, Economics, and Historical Geography of Jerusalem*. Jerusalem: Ariel.

Sokoloff, M. 2002². *Dictionary of Jewish Palestinian Aramaic of the Byzantine Period*. Ramat Gan/Baltimore: Bar-Ilan University Press and Johns Hopkins University Press.

Spanier, Y., and A. Sasson. 2001. *Lime Kilns in Eretz-Israel. Symposium in Memory of the Late Samuel Avitzur*. Jerusalem: Eretz-Israel Museum and Nature Protection Society [H].

Sperber, D. 1982. *Midrash Yerushalem: A Metaphysical History of Jerusalem*. Jerusalem: The World Zionist Organization, Department for Torah Education and Culture in the Diaspora. [In Hebrew]

—. 1986. *Nautica Talmudica*. Ramat Gan: Bar Ilan University Press.

—. 1993–2006. *Material Culture in Eretz-Israel during the Talmudic Period*. I–II, Jerusalem/Ramat Gan: Bar Ilan University Press. [In Hebrew]

—. 1998. *The City in Roman Palestine*. New York: Oxford University Press.

Stern, E. 1963. "Measures and Weights." In *Encyclopedia Biblica*. IV, Jerusalem: Bialik Institute. Pages 846–852. [In Hebrew]

Stern, M. 1983³. *The Documents on the History of the Hasmonean Revolt with Commentary and Introductions*. Tel-Aviv: HaKibbutz HaMeuchad. [In Hebrew]

—. 2004. "Jerusalem, the Most Famous of the Cities of the East (Pliny, *Natural History* V, 70)." In *Studies in Jewish History: The Second Temple Period*. Edited by M. Amit et al. Jerusalem: Yad Ben-Zvi. Pages 519–530. [In Hebrew]

Stern, M. ed. 1976–1984. *Greek and Roman Latin Authors on Jews and Judaism*. I–III, Jerusalem: Israel Academy of Sciences and Humanities.

Strange, J. 2003. "Herod and Jerusalem: The Hellenization of an Oriental City." In *Jerusalem in Ancient History and Tradition*. Edited by T.L. Thompson. London: T&T Clark. Pages 97–113.

Sukenik, E. L. 1931. "An Epitaph of Uzziahu, King of Judah." *Tarbiz* 2,3: 288–292 [In Hebrew]

Tabory, J. 1995; repr. 2000. *Jewish Festivals in the Time of the Mishnah and Talmud*. Jerusalem: Magnes. [In Hebrew]

Tcherikover, A. 1961; repr. 1982. *Hellenistic Civilization and the Jews*. Translated by S. Applebaum. Philadelphia: Jewish Publication Society of America.

Thoma, C. 1994. "John Hyrcanus As Seen by Josephus and Other Early Jewish Sources." In *Josephus and the History of the Greco-Roman Period: Essays in Memory of Morton Smith*. Edited by F. Parente. Leiden: Brill. Pages 127–140.

Tilley, C., et al., eds. 2006. *Handbook of Material Culture*. London: SAGE.

Tropper, A. D. 2005. "Yohanan ben Zakkai, Amicus Caesaris: A Jewish Hero in Rabbinic Eyes." *Jewish Studies, an Internet Journal* 4: 133–149.

Tucazinsky, J.M. 1952. "Jerusalem." In *Ozar Yisrael: An Encyclopedia*. V. Edited by J.D. Eisenstein. New York: Pardes. Pages 209–221. [In Hebrew]

Ulmer, R. 2009. *Egyptian Cultural Icons in Midrash*. Berlin/New York: De Gruyter.

Urbach, E. E. 1968. "Heavenly and Earthly Jerusalem." In *Jerusalem through the Ages: The 25ᵗʰ Archaeological Convention October 1967*. Edited by J. Aviram. Jerusalem: The Israel Exploration Society. Pages 156–171. [In Hebrew]

—. 1971. "Jerusalem: Jerusalem and the Temple Mount in Jewish Law and Legend." In *Encyclopaedia Hebraica*. Jerusalem/Tel-Aviv: Encyclopaedia Publishing. Pages 344–349. [In Hebrew]

—. 1984. *The Halakha: Its Origins and Development*. Givatayim: Yad LaTalmud. [In Hebrew]

Ussishkin, D. 1974. "The Rock Called Peristereon." *Israel Exploration Journal* 24: 70–72.

Visotzky, B.I. 1983. "Most Tender and Fairest of Women: A Study in the Transmission of Aggada." *Harvard Theological Review* 76,4: 403–418.

Walsh, K. 2014. *The Archaeology of Mediterranean Landscapes: Human-Environment Interaction from the Neolithic to the Roman Period*. Cambridge/New York: Cambridge University Press.

Wilkinson, J. 1989. "Jerusalem under Rome and Byzantium 63 BC–637 AD." In *Jerusalem in History*. Edited by K.J. Asali. Brooklyn: Olive Branch Press. Pages 75–104.

Wilson, A. 2008. "Hydraulic Engineering." In *Handbook of Engineering and Technology in the Classical World*. Edited by J.P. Oleson. Oxford: Oxford University Press. Pages 285–318.

Yardeni, A., and J. Price. 2010. "Epitaph of King Uzzaiah with Aramaic Inscription 1 c. BCE–1 c. CE." In *Corpus Inscriptionum Iudaeae/Palaestinae*. I/I, *Jerusalem*. Edited by H.M. Cotton et al. Berlin/New York: De Gruyter. Pages 603–604.

Yadin, Y. 1972. "The Gate of the Essenes." *Qadmoniot* 5,19–20: 129–130. [In Hebrew]

—. 1990. *The Temple Scroll*. Tel-Aviv: Sifriyat Ma'ariv. [In Hebrew]

Yasar (Schlichter), B. 1950. "Urban Planning according to the Laws of the Torah." *HaTorah and the State* 2: 59–64. [In Hebrew]

Zeligmann, H. 1981. *Public Health in the Jewish Sources*. Ph.D. diss., The Hebrew University of Jerusalem. [In Hebrew]

Zevin, S.J., ed. 1952–2019. *Encyclopedia Talmudica: A Digest of Halachic Literature and Jewish Law from the Tannaitic Period to the Present Time*. I–XLIII, Jerusalem: The Talmudic Encyclopedia Institute. [In Hebrew]

Zikal, M. 1990. *The Environmental Quality (Ecology) in the Jewish Sources*. Ramat-Gan: Bar Ilan University, The Shut Project. [In Hebrew]

Zissu, B. 2009. "New Testament Tower? This Place is for the Birds." *Biblical Archaeology Review* 35,3: 30–37, 66–67.

Part 4:
Jewish Medical Episteme
Around the Mediterranean in the Medieval Period

Exploring Eurasian Transmissions of Medical Knowledge: Cues from the Hebrew *Book of Asaf*

*Ronit Yoeli-Tlalim**

Dedicated to the memory of Asaf Ha'rofeh Hospital, Israel

The Hebrew text referred to as *Sefer refu'ot* ("Book of Remedies") or *Sefer Asaf* ("Book of Asaf") is a very important text not only in the history of the Hebrew medical sciences, but also in the history of medicine as a whole.[1] The text is an extensive medical compendium, containing a kind of 'medical history', sections on anatomy, embryology, pulse and urine diagnosis, seasonal regimen, a medical oath and a long *materia medica* section.

This paper examines the narrative on the origins of medical knowledge as found in the *Book of Asaf*. This narrative presents the medical knowledge which follows it as deriving from Eurasian input. Narratives on the origins of knowledge such as this one both reflect and construct views on medicine and hence are important in providing a more poly-vocal history of medicine, taking into account local cultures of historiographies. More broadly, taking such accounts seriously can help to write *histories* of medicine rather than *the history* of medicine. As Nappi has pointed out, such attempts require taking local diversities in historiography seriously, and translating local differences into a meaningful common conversation.[2]

Narratives on the origins and history of medicine–and the history of knowledge more generall—are important within this scope for a number of reasons. Firstly, an analysis of how and why they were constructed can reveal important political, religious, economic and cultural factors at play at the time of construction. Secondly, narratives of this sort raise the large and complicated question of whether and to what extent such accounts actually reflect the nature of the knowledge they describe. In other words, they raise questions like: when and why does a culture/religion/state ideology choose to present/construct itself as multicultural? Are there correspondences between *being* multi-cultural and of *declaring* a culture as such?

The preface of the *Book of Asaf* has been known to scholars for a century and a half, although in ways which have caused a fair amount of confusion.[3] The preface was first

---

* Research for this paper was funded by the Wellcome Trust (grant no. 088251). I would like to thank Tamás Visi and Lennart Lehmhaus for their comments on a previous version of this paper.
1 For two recent publications, see Visi 2016 and Yoeli-Tlalim 2018.
2 As called on by Nappi in regards to the history of science at large, see Nappi 2013.
3 The following overview of the history of the study of the Introduction is based on Nutton 2012.

DOI: 10.13173/9783447108263.295

printed by Adolph Jellinek in his *Bet Hamidrash* in 1853, from the Munich ms 231. Jellinek appended the beginning of *Sefer Raziel* and the opening of *Sefer Ha'razim* to the Asaf preface and gave them the title: ספר נח (*Book of Noah*).[4] Jellinek's text was subsequently translated to German, again with the title *Book of Noah*, by A Wünsche.[5] Both Jellinek and Wünsche did not clarify that these were three separate texts. Louis Ginzburg in his *Legends of the Jews* began the process of clarification at the beginning of the 20th century.[6]

Also helping to clarifying the confusion was the important study by the Hungarian Rabbi and scholar Ludwig [Lajos] Venetianer of the *Book of Asaf*, which appeared in 1916, *Assaf Judaeus: Der aelteste medizinische Schriftsteller in hebraeischer Sprache* (Strassburg: Karl J. Tübner 1916). In that same year, Karl Sudhoff published a Latin text which was copied in the 15th century and which Sudhoff identified as deriving from the Introduction to the *Book of Asaf*.[7] The Introduction to the *Book of Asaf* was also discussed by Muntner.[8]

Versions of the introduction to the *Book of Asaf*

The manuscripts

The introduction to the *Book of Asaf* appears in the following manuscripts:

Munich Bayerische Staatsbibliothek Cod. hebr. 231; Firenze Laurenziana Plut. 88.37; British Library add.27018; Bodleian Oxford, Ms. Laud. Or. 113; Frankfurt Ms. hebr. Oct. 185; Institute of Oriental Manuscripts, Russian Acedemy of Sciences, St Petersburg Ms. A 170; Institute of Oriental Manuscripts, Russian Acedemy of Sciences, St Petersburg Ms. B 449.

Of the *Sefer Asaf* manuscripts which do not include the Introduction, mention should be made of Bodleian Oxford Ms. opp. 687 (OL 1645) (no. 2138 in Neubauer's Catalogue), which is one of three main *Asaf* manuscripts.[9]

---

4 Jellinek 1853, vol. III, xxx–xxxiii & 155–160. *Sefer Ha'razim* is a work of magical character dated to the first millennium CE, probably towards the middle of that millennium. It has survived in fragments from the Genizah and was published with many variants by Mordechai Margaliot in 1966. An English translation was prepared by Michael Morgan and published in 1983. *Sefer Raziel* is a much later work published in Amsterdam in 1701.

5 Wünsche 1909, vol. III, 201–210.

6 Ginzburg 1913, vol. 1, 154–157, 172–174.The book itself was published in 1913, but the notes which clarified the sources appeared only in 1925 (vol. 5, 172–175, 196–197).

7 Sudhoff 1916.

8 Muntner 1965, at pp. 396–407; Muntner 1957, 65–72.

9 This manuscript has been dated by Langermann to the 12th or 13th century. See Langermann 2009. On this manuscript see also Shatzmiller 1983. The manuscript includes 188 folios. Judging by its orthographic mistakes, it seems to be a copy of an earlier manuscript.

Munich Bayerische Staatsbibliothek Cod. hebr. 231

Munich Bayerische Staatsbibliothek hebr 231 is a codex of 277 folios.[10] It has been dated by Judith Olszowy-Schlanger based on preliminary paleographical indications to the 13th or 14th century and originating from Italy.[11] Previous references and studies of the *Asaf* Introduction are based on this version.

Florence Laurenziana Plut. 88.37

Florence Laurenziana Plut. 88.37 has been dated to the 14th–15th century. The *Asaf* text in Florence Laurenziana Plut. 88.37 is the first text in this codex (Fol. 1–26r), followed by six other medical texts.[12]

Bodleian Libraries, Oxford, Ms. Laud. Or. 113 (Neubauer catalogue: 2142/20)

Provence, 16th century, paper.[13] This codex is a collection of medical texts, which are numbered. The *Book of Asaf* text is four folios long (fol. 97a–98b). It includes the introduction (97a–97b) followed by the general description of the structure of the body.

British Library add.27018

This is a medical codex, which includes four separate texts. Margoliouth has dated it to the 15th century. It is written on paper and includes 22 leaves with 27 lines to a page. Leaves are missing after fol. 6, 11, and 12. Most extant leaves are slightly damaged. The last word of each folio is repeated at the beginning of the next. Margoliouth has suggested that the text is written in a peculiar Rabbinic hand of what appears to be of oriental origin.[14]

The codex includes four texts. The first text is ספר אגור –ספר (fol. 2a–14a) based on the aphorisms of Hippocrates (See Steinschneider HU, pp. 660–1).[15] The second text

---

10 Steinschneider 1875, 82–83 (pp. 106–107 in the 1895 edition).

11 Prof. Olszowy–Schlanger kindly examined a reproduction of the manuscript at my disposal. I would like to thank Prof. Olszowy–Schlanger for sharing her profound knowledge with me.

12 1. Fol. 1v–26r: *Sefer Refu'ot*;

 2. Fol. 26r–30v: Head to toe list of illnesses (incomplete; missing quire at the end);

 3. Fol. 31r–58r: ספר הראשון של פיסיקא.

 4. Fol. 58v– 73v: הספר השני אנטיאוטריאו (*Antidotarium*).

 5. Fol. 73v–84r: הספר השלישי: צירלוגיאה היא מלאכת יד.

 6. Fol. 84v–86r: ספר היקר.

 7. Fol. 86r–110r: הספר הרביעי : ספר ביאטיקו (*Viatico*).

 For a description of the codex see: Biscioni 1757, Vol. 2.

 The second text, a head to toe list of illnesses (fol. 26r– 30v), which is clearly demarcated as a separate text in Florence Laurenziana Plut. 88.37, appears at the end of Munich 231 (fols.— 267r–287r) and has been treated as part of *Sefer Asaf*. This is but one indication that what has been alluded to as *Sefer Asaf* is a composite text, which in different codices comprises of different collections.

13 Neubauer 1886 and Beit-Arié 1994.

14 Margoliouth 1965, Part III, 348.

15 Margoliouth says on the other copy of *Sefer Agur* (Harley 5527), that is it based on Constantinus Africanus' Latin version of the aphorisms of Hippocrates.

is also ascribed to Hippocrates, is titled: מידות אבוקרט (fols. 14b–16a) and is a brief treatise on signs of approaching death. The third text specifically refers to Asaf, and is titled: אלמדך להשכיל באותות הדפק מספר אסף (fols. 16a–17b)— "I shall teach you the signs of the pulse from Sefer Asaf".

The fourth text is titled: ספר עץ החיים (fols: 18b–22a, "The Book of the Tree of Life"). The title is followed by a further title: למען תגדל תפארתם על חכמי הארץ ("So that their glory shall increase among the sages of the land"). It is here we find an abbreviated version of the *Sefer Asaf* Introduction:

ויהי בבואם אל המקום ההוא וימצאו את עצי המרפא ועץ החיים וישלחו ידיהם לקחתם

ויברק עליהם להט החרב המתהפכת ויתלהטו כלם בשביבי הברק ולא נמלט מהם איש

ותעזב הרפואה מהגוים ותשבת חכמת הרופאים שש מאות ושלשים שנה עד מלוך
ארתחשסתא המלך

בימיו קם איש נבון וחכם ומלומד דעת ספרי הרפואות ומבין כל דבר ושמו אפוקראט המקדוני
ושאר חכמי הגוים

ואסף היהודי ודיסקורדיאוס הבעלכותי וגאליאנוס הכפתורי וחכמים הרבה מאד ויחדשו
עבודת הרפואה

ותהי עד היום הזה

This abbreviated Introduction is followed by the *Sefer Asaf* account of the structure of the body (fols. 19a– 22a).

Frankfurt 185, St Petersburg A 170 and St Petersburg B 449 are all modern (19th and 20th century) copies:

Frankfurt 185—has been dated to the 19th century. It is titled: *Sefer ben Noah* and contains only the Introduction (Fols. 1–7).[16]

St Petersburg A 170 has been dated to the 19th century. It consists of 11 folios. The Introduction appears on fol.1 (with no mention of India).

St Petersburg B 449 has been dated to the 20th Century and appears to be a copy of St Petersburg A 170.

Commentary of Rabbi Elhanan ben Yakar of London to Sefer Yetsirah

Zvi Langermann has brought to our attention a quote from another version of the Introduction to *Sefer Asaf*, that of Rabbi Elhanan Ben Yakar of London, probably from the year 1200, which was discussed by Yehudah Arieh Vajda:[17]

והחכמה הזאת היא גדולה ועמוקה ובארץ הינד קמו פילוסופים גדולים ודרשו וחקרו

וניסו בזאת החכמה ובימי ארתחשסתא קמו אחרים תחתם ואלה שמותם איצפוקר ההינדי
תיאופילוס המישעי מארץ מואב וגליינוס הכפתורי מארץ כפתור ואסף הירחי. ותרב חכמת
הרפואה בימים ההם כי עד הימים ההם לא ריפא אדם את חברו. והם שלחו בארץ הינד לקח
משם עצי הרפואה ודשאי הרפואה וחיות הרפואה ותגדל חכמתם והמה עשו ספרים אין קץ

---

16 According to the dating of the Jerusalem catalogue and also Roth and Prijs [1855] 1990, 58–59.
See also: Jellinek 1855, 155.

17 Langermann 2009; Vajda 1966.

לבד מספר שם בן נח אשר היה להם לפנים כי ספר שם היה סתום והיה כתוב בו לזה החולי זה
הסם ולא היה בו פיר<ו>ש הדברים ועלילות החלאים מאיזה יסוד ובמה ירפא בכח חם וקר ולח
ויבש והמה הוסיפו ופירשו כל מסיבות ועניני היסודות והגידים כמה הם ואני לא באתי לפרש
כי אם כפי הצורך לזה הספר.[18]

And this wisdom is great and deep and in the land of Hind there were great philosophers who enquired, analysed and tried this wisdom. And in the days of Artaxšaçā (Artakhshashtah, ארתחששתא, Greek: Artaxerxes), others rose in their place, and these were their names: Itspocar the Hindu, Theophilus of Mesha in the Land of Mo'ab, and Galenos the Caphtorite, of the Land of Caphtor and Asaf Ha'yerekhi (the astrologer?). And the wisdom of medicine increased in those days, since till those days no man cured another. And they sent to the Land of Hind to take the trees of medicine from there, and the herbs of medicine and the animals of medicine, and their wisdom increased and they made endless books in addition to the Book of Shem son of Noah, which they had from before, because the Book of Shem was obscure and it said: for this illness, that drug, but it did not explain the meaning and how illnesses develop, from what element, and how to cure—in the power of heat or cold, damp or dry. And they added and explained all the reasons and issues of the elements and the *gidim*[19], how many there are, and I have come but to comment as needed for this book. [20]

The Hebrew text below is based on Munich Bayerische Staatsbibliothek Cod. hebr. 231 with variant readings from Bodleian Oxford, Ms. Laud. Or. 113, Florence Laurenziana Plut. 88.37 and British Library add.27018:

Fol. 1v

ספר רפואות נקרא אסף היהודי[21]

זה ספר רפואות
אשר העתיקו חכמים[22] הראשונים מספר שם[23]
בן נח אשר נמסר[24] לנח בלובר ההר מהררי[25]

---

18 Vajda 1966, 172, lines 316–327.
19 *Gid* can mean either sinew or blood vessel.
20 My translation.
21 Plut. 88.33 begins:
בשם יי נעשה ונצליח
ספר רפואות חשוב ובדוק מרופאי הקדמונים
ספר רפואות אשר העתיקו חכמים הראשונים
In the name of God we shall proceed and be prosperous
An important book of medicine, tested by the ancient physicians
A book of medicine copied by the early sages.
22 OX Or 113 החכמים.
23 OX Or 113 בן שם בן נח.
24 OX Or 113 שנמסר.
25 OX Or 113 מהרי.

אררט אחרי²⁶ המבול כי בימים ההמה²⁷ ובעת ההיא
החלו רוחות הממזרים להתגרות בבני נח להסטות
ולהטעות ולחבל ולהכות בחלאים²⁸ ובמכאובים
ובכל²⁹ מיני מדוה הממיתים ומשחיתים את בני
אדם³⁰ אז באו כל³¹ בני נח ובניהם³² יחדו
ויספרו את³³ נגעיהם לנח אביהם ויגידו לו על
אודות המכאובים הנראים בבניהם ויבעת נח
וידע כי מעון האדם³⁴ ומדרך פשעם יתעאנו³⁵
בכל³⁶ מיני תחלואים ומדוים אז קידש³⁷
נח את בניו³⁸ ואת בני ביתו וביתו יחדו ויגש
אל המזבח³⁹ ויעל עולות ויתפלל אל האלוקים⁴⁰ ויעתר
לו וישלח מלאך אחד⁴¹ ממלאכי הפנים מן
הקדושים⁴² ושמו רפאל לכלה⁴³ את רוחות הממזרים
מתחת השמים לבלתי השחית עוד בבני האדם
ויעש המלאך כן ויכלאם אל בית המשפט⁴⁴
אך אחד מעשרה הניח להתהלך בארץ לפני שר
המשטמה⁴⁵ לרדות בם במרשיעים⁴⁶ לנגע ולענות
בהם בכל מיני מדוה תחלואים⁴⁷ ולנגע מכאובים
ואת רפואות נגעי בני אדם וכל מיני רפואות
הגיד המלאך לנח לרפא בעצי הארץ וצימחי

---

26 OX Or 113 אחר.
27 OX Or 113 ההם.
28 OX Or 113 בחליים ומכאובות.
29 OX Or 113 ולכל.
30 OX Or 113 האדם.
31 OX Or 113 – no כל.
32 OX Or 113 – no ובניהם.
33 OX Or 113 – no את.
34 OX Or 113 וידע נח כי מעון בני האדם.
35 Plut. 88.33 יתענו.
36 OX Or 113 לל.
37 OX Or 113 קדש.
38 OX Or 113 בניו ובני ובנותיו.
39 OX Or 113 אשר בנה.
40 Plut. 88.33 האלהים.
41 OX Or 113 מן הקדושים שר הפנים.
42 Plut. 88.33 מלאך אחד מן הקדושים ממלאכי הפנים.
43 OX Or 113 לכלות.
44 OX Or 113 בבית המשפט.
45 Plut. 88.33 no המשטמה. For *mastema* see also the Genizah version of the Damascus Document.
   The Damascus Document refers to Jubilees.
46 OX Or 113 להכות המרשיעים.
47 OX Or 113 ויגד המלאך לנח לרפא / מדוה ותחלואים.

האדמה ועיקריה וישלח את שרי⁴⁸
הרוחות⁴⁹ הנותרים מהם להראות לנח⁵⁰ ולהגיד לו
את עצי הרפואות עם כל דשאיהם וירקיהם
ועשביהם ועיקריהם⁵¹ וזירועיהם למה נבראו⁵²
וללמדיהו כל דברי רפואתם עד פלט למרפא
ולחיים ויכתוב נח⁵³ את הדברים האלה על
ספר ויתנהו לשם בנו הגדול⁵⁴ ומן הספר הזה
העתיקו חכמי הראשונים⁵⁵ ויכתבו ספרים הרבה
איש ואיש כלשונו ותרבה דעת הרפואה בארץ
בכל הגוים⁵⁶ אשר בחנו את ספרי הרפואות
בחכמי הודו.⁵⁷ וחכמי מקדון וחכמי מצרים כי
חכמי הודו הם שוטטו למצוא כל⁵⁸ עצי רפואות
והבשמים וחכמי ארם מצאו⁵⁹ העשבים לכל
מיניהם וזירועיהם⁶⁰ לרפא ואת פשר דברי
הספרים⁶¹ העתיקו ארמית וחכמי מקדון החלו
ראשונה לרפא בארץ וחכמי מצרים החלו⁶²
לחבר ולנחש במזרות⁶³ ובכוכבים⁶⁴ ללמד⁶⁵ את ספר
מדרש הכשדים אשר העתיק קנגרבון⁶⁶ אור בן
כשד⁶⁷ לכל מעשה החרטומים⁶⁸ ותגדל להם חכמתם⁶⁹
עד קום אסקלפינוס אחד מחכמי מקדון וארבעים

---

48 Plut. 88.33 שר.
49 OX Or 113 וישלח שר הרוחות הנותרים מהם.
50 OX Or 113 אל נח.
51 OX Or 113 no עיקריהם.
52 OX Or 113 no למה נבראו.
53 OX Or 113 ויכתוב נח כל הדברים האלה.
54 Plut. 88.33 no הגדול.
55 OX Or 113 החכמים הראשונים.
56 OX Or 113 בארץ ובכל הגויים אין חכמים אשר.
57 OX Or 113 וחכמי מצרים וכחכמת ארם כחכמי הודו.
58 OX Or 113 no כל.
59 OX Or 113 את.
60 OX Or 113 וזרעיהם.
61 OX Or 113 את פשר הדברים.
62 OX Or 113 ראשונה.
63 OX Or 113 במזלות.
64 Plut. 88.33 וכוכבים.
65 OX Or 113 וללמד ספר.
66 Plut. 88.33 קנגר בן אור.
67 OX Or 113 קינן בן כשד.
68 OX Or 113 לכל החרטומים.
69 OX Or 113 ותגדל חכמתו.

איש עמו[70] מן החרטומים מלומדי הספרים הנעתקים
וילכו הלוך בארץ ויעברו מעבר להודו אל ארץ[71]

Fol. 2v

קדמת עדן למצוא מקצת עצי החיים[72] למען
תגדל תפארתם[73] על חכמי הארץ[74] ויהי בבואם
אל המקום ההוא וימצאו את עצי המרפא[75] ועצי
עץ החיים[76] וישלחו את ידם לקחתם ויברק ה[77]
עליהם להט החרב המהפכת[78] וילהטו[79] כולם בשביבי
הברק ולא נמלט מהם איש ותעזב הרפואה מן
הרופאים[80] ותשבת חכמת הרופאים[81] שש מאות
ושלשים שנה עד מלוך ארתחשסתא[82] המלך
בימיו קם[83] איש נבון וחכם ומלומד דעת ספרי
הרפואות[84] ומבין לכל דבר[85] ושמו איפוקרט[86] המקדוני
ושאר חכמי הגוים אסף[87] היהודי[88] ודיסקרדיוס
הבעלתי[89] וגליינוס[90] הכפתורי וחכמים הרבה מאד
ויחדשו עטרת[91] הרפואה[92] ותהי עד היום הזה

---

70 OX Or 113 no עמו.

71 OX Or 113 אל ארץ נוד קדמת עדן.

72 OX Or 113 עצי הרפואה ועץ החיים.

73 OX Or 113 רפואתם.

74 BL add. 27018 (hereafter: BL) introduction text begins here. Ox Or 113 על כל חכמי הארץ.

75 OX Or 113 ואת עץ החיים הרפואה.

76 BL ועץ החיים.

77 Plut. 88.33 omits ה'.

78 OX Or 113 & BL: ויברק עליהם להט החרב המתהפכת.

79 OX Or 113 ויתלהטו.

80 Plut 88.33 מן הגוים; BL מהגויים.

81 OX Or 113 מן הגויים ותשבות הרפואה.

82 Plut 88.33 ארתחשתא.

83 OX Or 113 עמד.

84 OX Or 113 הרפואה.

85 OX Or 113 ומבין דבר מתוך דבר.

86 OX Or 113 אפוקראט המקדומי BL אפוקרט.

87 BL ואסף.

88 OX Or 113 אסף וחכמי היהודים והרבה חכמים אחרים.

89 BL ודיסקורדיאוס הבעלכותי.

90 BL וגאליאנוס.

91 BL עבודת.

92 OX Or 113 ויחדשו את עבודת הרפואה.

(fol. 1v)

The Book of Medicine [by the so-] called Asaph the Jew
This is the Book of Medicine translated by the first sages from the Book of Shem son of Noah, which was given to Noah at the Luvar Mountain, one of the Ararat Mountains[93] after the flood.

Since in those days and in that time, the evil spirits began to torment the sons of Noah, to deviate and terrorise and blow with illnesses and pain and all sorts of destructive and deadly ailments.

Then all the sons of Noah came together with their offspring and told their father Noah about all their ailments.

And they told him about the sicknesses visible in their offspring.

And Noah was terrified and he knew that it is due to human iniquity and the path of misconduct that they would contrive all sickness and ailments.

Then Noah blessed his sons and their offspring [and his household?] together.

And he went to the altar and brought sacrifice and prayed to God.

And He granted his wish and sent him one of the Angels of Presence (אחד ממלאכי הפנים), of the holy ones, and his name—*Rafa'el*,

to extinguish the evil spirits under the heaven, so as not to harm humans any longer.

And the angel did so.

And he locked them up in the house of justice.

But one out of ten—he let go in the land before the Prince of Animosity (שר המשטמה)

to reign them, the evil ones, to cause illness and pain.

And the angel told Noah about the remedies for human ailments and all sorts of ailments—

how to heal with the trees of the land and the plants

(fol. 2r) of the earth and its roots (ועיקריה).

And he sent the remaining Princes of Spirits (שרי הרוחות) to show Noah and instruct him regarding the trees of medicine along with their grass and their herbs and their vegetables and their seeds and their roots—the reason for their creation, and to teach him every detail of their healing properties.

And Noah wrote all these things in a book, and gave it to Shem, his older son. And from this book, the early sages translated and wrote many books, each one in his own language. And the knowledge of medicine increased in the land, amongst all the peoples who studied the books of medicines—[i.e.] amongst the sages of India and the sages of Macedonia[94] and the sages of Egypt.[95] The

---

93 Luvar as one of the mountains of Ararat appears also in *Jubilees* 7:1.

94 The Eastern Christian origin of *Sefer Asaf* for which I argue in Yoeli-Tlalim 2018 also explains the use here of "Macedonians" for Greeks– a usage confined to the Septuagint, specifically to *Esther* and *Maccabees*. This point has been raised by Nutton, though he suggested this indicates a Jewish source. See Nutton 2012. I would like to thank Mark Geller for raising this question.

95 OX Or 113 adds: "and the wisdom of Aram".

sages of India took to wandering in order to find the trees of medicines and
perfumes, and the sages of Aram discovered the herbs—[i.e.] all their kinds
and their seeds—in order to cure. And they translated the meaning of the
books into Aramaic [i.e. Syriac]. And the sages of Macedonia were the first
to cure in the land, and the sages of Egypt began to calculate[96] and perform
divinations with the stars and constellations, to teach the book of Babylonian
wisdom, copied by Kangar son of Ur son of Kesed[97] as well as all the deeds of
the magicians (*khartumim*).[98] And their wisdom grew
until Asclepius came, one of the Macedonian sages and forty
men with him among the magicians (*khartumim*), learned in the translated books
and they went in the land, passing beyond India to a land
(fol. 2v) east of Eden to find some of the trees of life in order to increase their
glory among the sages. And when they came to that place, they found the healing trees and the trees of the tree of life.
And they stretched their hand to take them and God thrust upon them the
flame of the swirling sword.[99] And they all burnt in the sparks of lightning
and no one escaped.
And medicine was deserted by the doctors. And the wisdom of doctors ceased
for 630 years, until the reign of Artaxšaçā (Artakhshashtah, ארתחששתא,
Greek: Artaxerxes) the King. And in the days of Artaxšaçā the King, there
rose a clever and wise man, who studied the knowledge of the books of medicines and his name: *Ippocrat* (Hippocrates) the Macedonian and the rest of the
gentiles' sages, and Asaf the Jew and Dioscorides of Ba'al[100] and Galenos of
Caphtor[101] and many other sages and they renewed the glory of medicine, and
it is living till this day...[102]

---

96 לחבר—can also mean: compose.
97 Kesed is mentioned in *Genesis* 22:22.
98 The *khartumim* are mentioned in *Genesis* 41, when they are unable to decipher Pharaoh's
    dream; in *Exodus* 7–9—in magic competitions with Moses; and in *Daniel* 1–2 and 4– when
    Daniel and his Jewish companions' wisdom exceeds that of the local *khartumim* and as inter-
    preters of Nebuchadnezzar's dreams.
99 The expression appears in *Genesis* 3:24. The *King James Bible* translates this expression as:
    "the flaming sword which turned every way". The context in *Genesis* 3: 24 is similar to here:
    God is said to have appointed the *cherubim* and the flame of the swirling sword to guard the
    way to the tree of life. Biblical commentators have discussed whether the deterrent refers to
    the sword or the flame. Rabbi David Kimkhi explains for example that it is the sight of the
    flame that is meant to frighten, i.e.: not the physical aspect, but the sight of it.
100 Perhaps referring to the mythical association of the god Ba'al with northern Syria, or some-
    times more generally: the mythical 'Mountain of the north'.
101 Biblical island; usually associated with Crete. In the Septuaginta and in the Syriac tradition,
    Caphtor was identified with Cappadocia. See: Wainwright 1956; Le Déaut and Jacques 1971.
    On this identification in the *Peshitta* and in the Syriac geographical tradition, see: Witakowski
    1993, 637, 639, and 647.
102 Munich heb 231, fols. 2r and 2v, my translation.

Links with *Jubilees* and *Enoch*

The close similarities between the introduction of the *Book of Asaf* and *Jubilees* 10: 1–14 as well as *I Enoch*, have been noted down before.[103] In *Jubilees*, a biblical apocryphal book dated to the mid–second century BCE, we find the same notion of medical knowledge as being derived from Noah and subsequently passed on to his son Shem.[104] The *Asaf* introduction also alludes to the book of *I Enoch*, in which Enoch—recounted in *Genesis* as going to heaven and not dying—transmits his divine wisdom to Metushelakh.[105] There have been two main views on the connection between the introduction to the *Book of Asaf* and *Jubilees*. One is that the *Book of Asaf* was partly based on *Jubilees*. The other is that they both preserve an older text/s known as the *Book* (or: *Books) of Noah*.[106] The *Book/Books of Noah* do not survive intact in any language. There are also no mentions of such a text in the canon lists, which suggests that the work was not widely circulated among Christians. Michael Stone has concluded that there were such literary work(s) in existence, preserved in bits in other texts such as the *Aramaic Levi Document, Jubilees* and the *Genesis Apocryphon*.[107]

The narratives as they appear in the introduction to *Book of Asaf* and *Jubilees* are generally similar, but there are some important differences. Firstly, in the *Book of Asaf* there is a far greater emphasis on the medical aspects of the story and the afflictions described are medical in nature. This medical terminology is repeated several times in the description. By comparison, in *Jubilees* 10:10 it is only when the remedies are introduced that it becomes clear that the afflictions involve illness at all. The *Book of Asaf* describes the remedies in much greater detail than in *Jubilees*. Himmelfarb has noted the difference in the angels to which the knowledge of medicine is attributed: in *Jubilees* they are anonymous angels whereas in *Sefer Asaf*, medical knowledge is attributed to a single angel: Rafa'el the arch-healing angel ('*rafa*' derives from the root 'to cure'; '*el*' means 'God'). The topos of archangels as a source of knowledge is common in *Hekhalot* literature.[108] Overall however, the introduction to *Sefer Asaf* is a more medicalised reworking of narratives found in other early Jewish sources—primarily as it serves—unlike *Jubilees*, *Enoch* or the *Hekhalot* literature—as an introduction to a substantial medical text.

The introduction to the *Book of Asaf* is an example of an "origin narrative": it recounts the origin/s of a field of knowledge, the motivation for "inventing" or "es-

---

103 See Himmelfarb 1994, particularly pp. 127–136. See also Stone 1972. The link between *Sefer Asaf* and *Jubilees* and *Enoch* has also been pointed out by Muntner 1965.
   The book of *Jubilees*, a second century BCE retelling of *Genesis* and *Exodus*, which has come down to us in Ethiopic, preserved by Ethiopic Christians. The original language of *Jubilees* was Hebrew. There is no manuscript evidence at all for the Greek version, which was the basis for the Latin and Ethiopic, although there are numerous allusions and citations. See: Bhyaro 2005.
104 See *Sefer Hayovlot*, chap. 10, verses 12–14. Hartum 1969.
105 *Genesis* 5:24.
106 See Himmelfarb 1994, particularly 127–136.
107 Stone 2006.
108 Swartz 1996.

tablishing" that kind of knowledge and the field's subsequent development.[109] Narratives of this sort have not yet made the impact they deserve in the historiography of medicine. One main reason for this is the way they appear to intertwine what is conventionally termed "mythical" and "historical". While we cannot read hagiographies and mythical accounts as straightforward historical narratives, we can—and should—take some cues from such texts as they often serve as pointers to strata otherwise forgotten or else rewritten by later historical accounts.

Narratives of universal histories and of universal histories of knowledge exemplify different ways of managing relationships between foreign and local knowledge as well as ways of negotiating cultural differences. The organization of knowledge from and about different peoples has been a powerful tool for articulating claims of empire, uniting multiplicities of locales in harmonious singularity, mirrored by a claim for comprehensiveness.[110] The *Sefer Asaf* origin narrative situates itself vis-à-vis medical knowledge deriving from other cultures. As a Hebrew text with clear Jewish characteristics, which appears to be derived from a Persian cultural milieu, transmitted via Syriac,[111] it is interlaced within a web of cross-cultural, religious, economic and political traces.

Universality

The universality constructed in *Sefer Asaf* is created through the superimposition of the notion of a universal antediluvian knowledge on the one hand together with concrete references to the known world. The correlation between the *Book of Sefer Asaf* and *Jubilees* and *Enoch* help us to unravel the nature of this universality. These sources reflect two types of universality. The first is an antediluvian one. *Enoch, Jubilees* and *Sefer Asaf* all refer to a panhuman knowledge, predating language and culture divisions. The other notion of universality is the description of the known world as found in the *Book of Jubilees*.[112] The areas of the world as described in *Jubilees* correspond to references we find in *Sefer Asaf*.

Wisdom from before the flood has fascinated humankind for as long as flood narratives existed in ancient Babylonia. "I studied inscriptions from before the flood", wrote the king of Assyria in the seventh century BCE.[113] Claims that before the flood humankind possessed precious knowledge, lost in the flood and subsequently available only to some fortunate few, were rampant in antiquity. Alien to our own notion of progression of science and knowledge, origin narratives such as these reveal rather an emphasis on priority. In the Hellenistic period, claims of priority played a major role in the cultural battle between nations on the origins of the arts and sciences. The

---

109 On origin narratives in Islamic sources, see Abbou-Hershkovitz 2008 and Brentjes 2013.
110 For Gutas's analysis of similar Sasanian texts on the origins and transmission of knowledge, see Gutas 1998, esp. 34–40. See also: van Bladel 2012. For a discussion of the Jewish case, see Reed 2014. On Pliny's *Natural History* as Roman imperial building, see Murphy 2007. I would to thank Lennart Lehmhaus for supplying this reference.
111 See Yoeli-Tlalim 2018.
112 See Scott 2002.
113 Van der Horst 2002, 139.

Babylonian scholar Berossus, writing in Greek about Babylonian culture in the late fourth or early third century BCE, claims to have 'found' the ancient writings hidden before the flood on Cronos' order to Xisutros (the "Sumerian Noah").[114] There is also a Hermetic topos of stelae containing primordial wisdom, inscribed in a sacred language from before the flood, translated after the flood, reminiscent of what we find in the *Book of Asaf*.[115] Amongst Jews, Josephus, the first century Jewish historian, also speaks about a stele which preserves ancient knowledge, otherwise lost, located in a mysterious place in the East (perhaps China?).[116] Indeed, the inscription of tablets and stones to preserve the world's ancient wisdom and to withstand future world destructions by water or fire is a common topos in many Jewish and Christian sources of the first centuries CE.

As has been argued with respect to the origins of Jewish science as it emerges in the *Book of Enoch* and *Book of Jubilees*, in the *Book of Asaf* too, we find a cross–cultural, inter–cultural assembly of knowledge, domesticating, as Philip Alexander has put it with regard to Enoch, 'a body of alien wisdom within Jewish tradition'.[117] Like the *Book of Jubilees* and the *Book of Enoch*, the compiler of the *Book of Asaf* is constructing a direct link between a divine antediluvian knowledge and the *Book of Asaf*: the medicine in this text is presented as a *renewal* of a lost *universal* knowledge—the medical book that follows it extends Jewish writings into new domains.

Another key topos found in the introduction to the *Book of Asaf* is the notion of travel to the orient as a means of acquiring knowledge. Though this topos appears already in Greek sources on the sciences, there are a number of significant differences between the Greek accounts on one hand and the *Asaf* one on the other. Most interesting for our discussion here is that in Greek sources, Greek medicine is not presented as being a synthesis of many traditions, nor do they emphasize India as a source of medical knowledge.[118] As Karttunen has noted, while Indian physicians were known in Greek general literature, Greek classical works on medicine do not mention them.[119] Specifically on Indian medicine, Herodotus notes that certain Indians make no attempt to cure and have no medical skill at all.[120]

The social purpose of the narrative

The introduction to the *Book of Asaf* presents itself as fulfilling an ancient Jewish role of preserving and disseminating knowledge. The purpose of the introduction, as found in parallel cases of ancient science is—in the words of Charlesworth: "an

---

114 Ibid, 146. On Berossus and Greek perspectives on Babylonian sciences and culture see also: Haubold 2016; Haubold 2014; and Haubold 2013. I would like to thank Lennart Lehmhaus for supplying these references.
115 Van der Horst 2002, 144–5.
116 Ibid, 150–1.
117 For natural sciences see: Alexander 2002. For geography, see: Scott 2004.
118 See Zhmud 2006, 40–41.
119 Karttunen 1997, 232.
120 Thomas 2000, 29.

attempt to say that all the things that the Greeks revere were earlier invented by, or at least known to Jews."[121] Hence, the introduction appears to address the issue of ambivalence towards medical knowledge in early Judaism—as a defence of medicine practised by Jews.[122] This ambivalence is also found in many other early Jewish sources on healing. The *Mishnah*, for example, recounts that one of the three deeds held in favour of King Hizkiyahu was the concealment of the *Book of Medicine* (*Sefer Refu'ot*).[123] In *3 Enoch*, for example, Metatron brings down to earth secrets of healing in spite of the objection of other angels. He then passes them on to Moses, from whom the knowledge passes through Joshua, the Elders, the Prophets etc.[124] It should be noted here that a figure by the name of Asaf is mentioned as the secretary of the King Hizkiyahu (*2 Kings* 18:18 and 37; *Isiah* 36:3 and 22).[125]

A similar ambivalence reflective of an ongoing discourse between supporters of science and those who rejected it is also apparent in the Islamic sources analysed by Abbou-Hershkovitz.[126] In the Jewish case, just like in the Islamic one, we can see the construction of these narratives as reflecting attempts of the medical authors to define a place for themselves within a larger intellectual context.

Conclusion

The *Book of Asaf* is an important 'bridge of knowledge' in ancient medicine. Its compiler/s is/are in conversation with a breadth of foreign ideas, situating its knowledge as deriving from the medical systems of the Indians, the Greeks, the Syrians and the Persians. The text reveals the value of looking at the 'bridging' languages and cultures of Eurasia, in this case: Hebrew and Syriac. The Hebrew *Book of Asaf* presents us with an interesting case study on which we can attempt a contemplation on the relationship between a medical tradition and its histories. It demonstrates the importance of looking at the early histories of the history of medicine and analysing the correspondence, if any, of *being* multicultural and of *declaring* yourself as such.[127]

---

121 Charlesworth 1977, 190

122 VanderKam 1997, 20–22.

123 *Mishnah*, Pesakhim, chap. 4. Also: *Talmud Bavli*: Berakhot, chap. 1; Pesakhim, chap. 4; *Talmud Yerushalmi*: Nedarim, chap. 6; Sanhedrin, chap. 1.

124 Swartz 1996, 174–181.

125 On the figure of Asaf not necessarily being a specific historical person, but probably a legendary one associated with "knowledge of the book", see Yoeli-Tlalim 2018.

126 Abbou–Hershkovitz 2008.

127 For similar questions with regards to early Tibetan medicine see Yoeli-Tlalim 2012, and Yoeli-Tlalim 2019.

Bibliography

Sources

Manuscripts of *Sefer Asaf*:
  Munich, Bayerische Staatsbibliothek Cod. hebr. 231
  Firenze, Laurenziana Plut. 88.37
  Bodleian Oxford, Ms. Laud. Or. 113
  London, British Library add.27018

Literature

Abbou-Hershkovitz, Keren. 2008. *"The Historiography of Science between the 10th and the 14th Centuries."* PhD Thesis. BenGurion University. [In Hebrew]

Alexander, Philip. 2002. "Enoch and the Beginnings of Jewish Interest in Natural Science." In *The Wisdom Texts from Qumran and the Development of the Sapiential Thought*. Edited by Charlotte Hempel, Armin Lange and Herrmann Lichtenberger. Leuven: Leuven University Press. Pages 223–243.

Beit-Arié, Malachi. 1994. *Catalogue of the Hebrew Manuscripts in the Bodleian Library: Supplement of Addenda and Corrigenda to Vol. I (A. Neubauer's Catalogue)*. Edited by Richard A. May. Oxford: Clarendon.

Bhyaro, Siam. 2005. *The Shemihazah and Asael Narrative of 1 Enoch 6–11: Introduction, Text, Translation and Commentary with reference to Ancient Near Eastern and Biblical Antecedents*. Münster: UgaritVerlag.

Biscioni, Antonio Maria. 1757. *Bibliothecae Ebraicae Graecae Florentinae sive Bibliothecae Mediceo Laurentianae*. 2 Volumes. Florence.

Brentjes, Sonja. 2013. "Narratives of Knowledge in Islamic Societies: What do they tell us about scholars and their contexts?." *Almagest* 4:1: 74–95.

Charlesworth, James H. 1977. "Jewish Astrology in the Talmud, Pseudepigrapha, the Dead Sea Scrolls, and Early Palestinian Synagogues." *Harvard Theological Review* 70: 183–200.

Ginzburg, Louis. 1913. *The Legends of the Jews*. 7 volumes. Philadelphia: The Jewish Publication Society of America.

Gutas, Dimitri. 1998. *Greek Thought, Arabic Culture: The GraecoArabic Translation Movement in Baghdad and Early 'Abbāsid Society (2nd–4th/8th–10th centuries)*. London and New York: Routledge.

Hartum, E.S., trans. and comment. 1969. *Hasefarim Hahitsonim. Sipurei Agadah*, vol. 2. Tel-Aviv: Yavneh.

Haubold, Johannes. 2013. "Berossus." In *The Romance between Greece and the East*. Edited by Tim Whitmarsh and Stuart Thomson. Oxford: Oxford University Press. Pages 105–116.

—. 2014. "Kulturkontakt aus der Sicht des Homerlesers". In *Kulturkontakte in antiken Welten: Vom Denkmodell zum Fallbeispiel*. Edited by Robert Rollinger and Kordula Schnegg. Leuven: Peeters. Pages 325–342.

—. 2016. "Hellenism, cosmopolitanism, and the role of Babylonian elites in the Seleucid empire." In *Cosmopolitanism and empire: universal rulers, local elites, and cultural integration in the ancient Near East and Mediterranean*. Edited by Myles Lavan, Richard E. Payne and John Weisweiler. New York: Oxford University Press. Pages 89–102.

Himmelfarb, Martha. 1994. "Some Echoes of *Jubilees* in Medieval Hebrew Literature." In *Tracing the Threads: Studies in the Vitality of Jewish Pseudepigrapha*. Edited by John C. Reeves. Atlanta, Georgia: Scholars Press. Pages 115–141.

Jellinek, Adolf. 1853, *Bet ha–Midrasch. Sammlung kleiner Midraschim und vermischter Abhandlungen aus der älteren jüdischen Literatur,* Leipzig, C. W. Vollrath (6 volumes).

Karttunen, Klaus. 1997. *India and the Hellenistic World.* Studia Orientalia 83. Helsinki: Finnish Oriental Society.

Langermann, Y. Tzvi . 2009. "Was There Science in Ashkenaz?." *Simon Dubnow Institute Yearbook* 8: 1–26.

Le Déaut, Roger and Roger Jacques. 1971. *Targum des Chroniques.* Rome: Biblical Institute Press.

Margoliouth, George. 1965. *Catalogue of the Hebrew and Samaritan Manuscripts in the British Museum,* Part III. London: Trustees of the British Museum.

Muntner, Suessman, ed. 1965. "Assaf ha–rofeh, Sefer Refu'ot" [Asaf the Physician, *Book of Remedies*]. *Korot* 3: 396–422. [In Hebrew]

.— 1957. *Mavo le'Sefer Asaf Ha'rofeh: Ha'sefer ha' refu'i ha'ivri ha'kadum beyoter.* Jerusalem: Genizah. [In Hebrew]

Murphy, Trevor. 2007. *Pliny The Elder's Natural History: The Empire in the Encyclopedia.* Oxford: Oxford University Press.

Nappi, Carla. 2013. "The Global and Beyond: Adventures in the Local Historiographies of Science." *Isis* 104,1: 102–110.

Neubauer, Adolf. 1886. *Catalogue of the Hebrew Manuscripts in the Bodleian Library and in the College Libraries of Oxford.* Oxford: Clarendon.

Nutton, Vivian. 2012. "From Noah to Galen. A Medieval Latin History of Medicine." In *Ritual Healing: Magic, Ritual and Medical Therapy from Antiquity until the Early Modern Period.* Edited by Ildikó Csepregi and Charles Burnett. Firenze: SISMEL edizioni del Galluzzo. Pages 53–69.

Reed, Annette Yoshiko. 2014. "'Ancient Jewish Sciences' and the Historiography of Judaism." In *Ancient Jewish Sciences and the History of Knowledge in Second Temple Literature.* Edited by Jonathan Ben-Dov and Seth Sanders. New York: New York University Press. Pages 195–254.

Roth, Ernst and Leo Prijs. [1855] 1990. *Hebräische Handschriften, Teil 1B: Die Handschriften der Stadt und Universitätsbibliothek Frankfurt am Main.* Stuttgart: Franz Steiner.

Scott, James. 2002. *Geography in Early Judaism and Christianity: the Book of Jubilees.* Cambridge: Cambridge University Press.

—. 2004. "Review of *A Study of the Geography of 1Enoch 17–19: 'No One Has Seen What I Have Seen'* by Kelley Coblentz Bautch." *Journal of Biblical Literature* 123,4: 752–756.

Shatzmiller, Joseph. 1983. "Doctors and Medical Practices in Germany around the Year 1200: The Evidence of 'Sefer Asaph'." *Proceedings of the American Academy for Jewish Research* 50: 149–164.

Steinschneider, Moritz. 1875. *Die Hebraeischen Handschriften der K. Hof- und Staatsbibliothek in Muenchen.* Munich: Palm Hofbuchhandlung.

Stone, Michael. 1972. "Noah, Books of." In vol. 12 of *Encyclopaedia Judaica.* Edited by Cecil Roth. 16 vols. Jerusalem: Keter. Page 1198.

—. 2006. "The Book(s) Attributed to Noah." *Dead Sea Discoveries* 13,1: 4–23.

Sudhoff, Karl. 1916. "Ein neuer Text der Initia medicinae." *Mitteilungen zur Geschichte der Medizin und der Naturwissenschaften* 15: 281–288.

Swartz, Michael, D. 1996. *Scholastic Magic: Ritual and Revelation in Early Jewish Mysticism.* Princeton: Princeton University Press.

Thomas, Rosalind. 2000. *Herodotus in Context. Ethnography, Science and the Art of Persuasion.* Cambridge, Cambridge University Press.

Vajda, Yehudah Arieh. 1966. "Perush R'Elhanan Ben Yakar le'Sefer Yetsirah." *Kobez al Yad* 6,16: 147–197. [In Hebrew]

Van Bladel, Kevin. 2012. "The Arabic History of Science of Abū Sahl ibn Nawbaḫt (fl. Ca 770–809) and Its Middle Persian Sources." In *Islamic Philosophy, Science, Culture, and Religion: Studies in Honor of Dimitri Gutas.* Edited by Felicitas Opwis and David Reisman. Leiden: Brill. Pages 41–62.

Van der Horst, Pieter Willem. 2002. *Japheth in the Tents of Shem: Studies on Jewish Hellenism in Antiquity.* Leuven: Peeters.

VanderKam, James C. 1997. "The Origins and Purposes of the Book of Jubilees." In *Studies in the Book of Jubilees.* Text and Studies in Ancient Judaism 65. Edited by Matthias Albani, Jörg Frey and Armin Lange. Tübingen: Mohr Siebeck. Pages 3–24.

Visi, Tamás. 2016. "Medieval Hebrew Uroscopic Texts: The Reception of Greek Uroscopic Texts in the Hebrew 'Book of Remedies' Attributed to Asaf." In *Texts in Transit in the Medieval Mediterranean.* Edited by Y. Tzvi Langermann and Robert Morrison. University Park, PA: Pennsylvania State University Press. Pages 162–197.

Wainwright, Gerald Avery. 1956. "Caphtor–Cappadocia." *Vetus Testamentum* 6: 199–210.

Witakowski, Witold. 1993. "The Division of the Earth between Descendants of Noah in Syriac Tradition." *Aram Periodical* 5: 635–656.

Wünsche, August. 1909. *Aus Israels Lehrhallen. Kleine Midraschim zur jüdischen Eschatologie und Apokalyptik.* Leipzig: E. Pfeiffer.

Yoeli-Tlalim, Ronit. 2012. "Re-visiting 'Galen in Tibet'." *Medical History* 56,3: 355–365.

—. 2018. "Exploring Persian lore in the Hebrew *Book of Asaf.*" *Aleph. Historical Studies in Science and Judaism* 18,1: 123–145.

—. 2019. "Galen in Asia?" In *Brill's Companion to the Reception of Galen.* Edited by Petros Bouras-Vallianatos and Barbara Zipser. Leiden: Brill. Pages 594–608.

Zhmud, Leonid. 2006. *The Origin of the History of Science in Classical Antiquity.* Translated by Alexander Chernoglazov. Berlin/New York: De Gruyter.

The *Book of Asaf* and Shabatai Donolo's Hebrew Paraphrase of Hippocrates' *Aphorisms*

Tamás Visi

A major problem surrounding the *Book of Remedies* attributed to Asaf the physician (hereafter: *Book of Asaf*) is the difficulty to determine its date, provenance, and author. Moritz Steinschneider devoted a series of short articles to the Book of Remedies which provide an overview of the content of the book.[1] Steinschneider argues that the authorship of "Asaf the physician" is a fiction: according to a late midrash as well as Muslim sources Asaf ben Berekhiah was the "vizier" of the biblical King Solomon; thus, the "Book of Asaf" is a sort of pseudoepigraphical text.[2] Ludwig Venetianer, the author of the first monograph devoted to *Book of Asaf*, disagreed with Steinschneider and treated Asaf as a real person who must have lived in the Early Middle Ages.[3] Venetianer's opinion was followed by Suessmann Muntner, who argued that Asaf must have lived in the Land of Israel during the sixth century.[4] Aviv Melzer dated Asaf to as early as the third century and argued that he must have been active in Iran, in the city of Gundishapur.[5]

More recently, Elinor Lieber and Ronit Yoeli-Tlalim have returned to Steinschneider's opinion that Asaf ben Berekhiah or "Asaf the physician" was not a real person.[6] The early dating of the text has been challenged too: Lieber argues for tenth-century southern Italy, and Yoeli-Tlalim finds evidence pointing to eighth-century Iran. The difference between the results of these two scholars suggests that the text itself may be a secondary compilation of disparate parts that could have come into being in different times and places. In the present paper it shall be argued that this is indeed the case.

---

1   Moritz Steinschneider, "Asaf," *Hebraeische Bibliographie*, 12 (1872): 85–88; Moritz Steinschneider, "Zur medicinischen Literatur: 4. Asaf," *Hebraeische Bibliographie* 19 (1879): 35–38, 64–70, 84–89, 105–109, [hereafter, Steinschneider, *HB*].

2   Steinschneider, *HB* 19 (1879): 35.

3   Ludwig [Lajos] Venetianer, *Assaf Judaeus: Der aelteste medizinische Schriftsteller in hebraeischer Sprache* (Strassburg: Karl J. Tübner, 1916).

4   Suessmann Muntner, *Mavo le-Sefer Asaf ha-rofe* [Introduction to the Book of Asaf the Physician] (Jerusalem: Geniza, 1957).

5   Aviv Melzer, *Asaph the Physician* (Ph.D. thesis, The University of Wisconsin, 1972), 64–69.

6   Elinor Lieber, "Asaf's *Book of Medicines*: A Hebrew Encyclopedia of Greek and Jewish Medicine, Possibly Compiled in Byzantium on an Indian Model," *Dumbarton Oaks Papers* 38 (1984): 233–249. Ronit Yoeli-Tlalim, "Exploring Persian Lore in the Hebrew *Book of Asaf*," *Aleph* 18 (2018): 123–146, and Ronit Yoeli-Tlalim's contribution to the present volume.

DOI: 10.13173/9783447108263.313

First, it should be recalled that the *Book of Remedies* is composed of various parts that include:

A Hebrew paraphrases of three works traditionally attributed to Hippocrates, name-ly the *Aphorisms*, the *Prognostics*, and the "oath."[7] One may add a fourth section based on a recently identified Greek source: Magnus of Emessa's tract on urines.[8]

B A compilation on anatomy, physiology, embryology, regimen, and food based partly on a seventh-century Syriac text composed in western Iran.[9]

C A section about herbs and other *materia medica* containing many Syriac plant names.

D Recipes, including an *antidotarium*.

E Miscellanea, including short texts on urine, pulses, and fevers.

F An introduction relating a semi-mythic history of medicine from the days of Noah to Hippocrates, Galen, and "Asaf the physician." The beginning of the text is closely related to the apocryphal *Book of Jubilees* extant only in Classical Ethiopic (Ge'ez) today.

The idea that all these texts are *not* the work of a single writer recommends itself. In fact, certain parts of the *Book of Remedies*, belonging to layer (E), are attributed to a man called *Yohanan ben Zbd'* (John, the son of Zebedee?) who is presented as a disci-ple of Asaf. The former is probably no less a fiction than the latter; nevertheless, the passages attributed to Yohanan may indeed be later additions or of a different source than the rest of the book.

An important article by Suessman Muntner published in *Koroth* in 1969 presents evidence that sheds new light on the origin of (A)-materials.[10] The implications of this article and the importance of the information contained in it have been curious-

---

7 These Greek sources have been identified by Steinschneider, *HB* 19 (1879): 87–89 and 106–108.

8 See Tamás Visi, "Medieval Hebrew Uroscopic Texts: The Reception of Greek Uroscopic Texts in the Hebrew *Book of Remedies* Attributed to Asaf," in *Texts in Transit in the Medieval Med-iterranean* (ed. Y. Tzvi Langermann and Robert G. Morrison, University Park, Pennsylvania: The Pennsylvania State University Press, 2016), 162–196.

9 Cf. Visi, ibid., 167–171. Three important updates shall be mentioned here: (1) Thomas Benfey has identified a Greek pseudo-Hippocratic text, which is parallel to the Syriac text in question; see Thomas Benfey, "A Greek Source for the *Treatise on the Composition of Man* Attributed to Aḥūdemneh Antīpaṭrōs?" *Hugoye: Journal of Syriac Studies* 22 (2019): 3–37. (2) The idea that the human body is composed of 365 parts is paralleled in one of the versions of the *Apocryphon of John,* a Gnostic text preserved in fifth-century Coptic manuscripts but had been translated from a second-century Greek original. In two of the manuscripts 365 angels create the body of Adam, each angel creating apparently one member. See Michael Waldstein and Frederik Wisse, *The Apocryphon of John: Synopsis of Nag Hammadi Codices II,1, III,1, and IV,1 with Bg 8502,2,* Nag Hammadi and Manichean Studies 33, (Leiden: Brill, 1995), 111. The text refers to "the book of Zoroaster" (*p-čŏ'me 'n-zŏroastros*) which suggests an Iranian background (the Gayōmart myth?). (3) A medieval Latin translation of this section of *Sefer Asaf* preserved important textual variants concerning the number of the bones; see Ms Vatican, BAV, lat. 623, fol. 39vd.

10 Suessmann Muntner, "Be'iqvot ktav yad hadash [B. M. 12252] le-Sefer Asaf ha-rofe ["Following a new manuscript of Sefer Asaf ha-rofe"]," *Koroth,* 4 (1969): 731–736.

ly overlooked by researchers of the subject matter, first and foremost, by its author, Suesmann Muntner himself.[11] The article presents a British Library manuscript (Or. 12252) which contains a Hebrew translation of Hippocrates' *Aphorisms*. The prologue and the epilogue of the text in the British Library manuscript explicitly identifies the text as a translation of Hippocrates' *Aphorisms* from Greek into Hebrew by certain David ben Yosef and Shabbatai ben Abraham. Muntner convincingly argues that Shabbatai ben Abraham must be identical with the well-known Jewish scholar and medical writer Shabbatai ben Abraham Donnolo, who worked in southern Italy during the tenth century, and whose knowledge of Greek and usage of Greek medical sources is well known from other sources. Therefore, this translation or paraphrase of the *Aphorisms* was probably made in tenth-century Italy by Shabbatai Donnolo and another person (a student?), David ben Yosef, connected to him.

Moreover, Muntner observed correctly that the Hebrew paraphrase of Hippocrates' *Aphorisms* included in the Book of Remedies (cf. A above) is closely related to the Donnolo-translation of the same text preserved in the British Library manuscript. In fact, save for some minor variants the two texts are exactly the same except for a number of omissions and additions the nature of which shall be discussed below. Therefore, the possibility that materials (A) in the *Book of Remedies* originate from Shabbatai Donnolo's Hebrew translations of Greek medical texts carried out in tenth-century southern Italy, and added later to the rest of the *Book of Asaf* should be considered seriously.

However, Muntner chose a different path. He stated that Shabatai Donnolo's translation of the *Aphorisms* must have been a reworking of Asaf's earlier translation. Thus, Muntner saw no reason to revise his theory that Asaf was a real person living in sixth-century *Eretz Yisrael*. The alternative that "Asaf" was dependent on Donnolo and not vice versa was not examined at all.

In the rest of this paper, I shall argue that the relationship between the two texts is the opposite of what Muntner assumed. In other words, the paraphrase of *Aphorisms* in layer (A) of the *Book of Remedies* attributed to Asaf is derived from the Donnolo-version of the same Greek text.[12] Moreover, since the style and the terminology of the translations and paraphrases making up the (A) materials are consistent, it is likely that other components of the (A) materials are also based on Donnolo's (and/or his colleagues') translations or paraphrases of the relevant Greek texts and were not part of the *Book of Remedies* before the tenth-century. Thus, both Lieber and Yoeli-Tlalim

---

11 The only exception I am aware of is Joseph Shatzmiller, "Doctors and Medical Practices in Germany around the Year 1200: The Evidence of *Sefer Asaph*," *PAAJR* 50 (1983): 149–164; here 158, note 26: "The whole relationship of *Sefer Asaph* to Shabbatai Donolo is still to be studied. It is worthwhile mentioning that a British Museum Ms. of *Sefer Asaph* mentions Shabbatai ben Avraham as very involved in its composition. See Muntner's article in *Korot* 4 (1968): 731–736."

12 Experts of the history of the Hebrew language have already suggested that Donnolo's Hebrew belongs to an *earlier* phase of the development of Hebrew than that of the book of Asaf. Cf. Samuel Kottek, "Šabbetay Donnolo en tant que médecin: anatomie et physiologie dans le Sefer ḥakmônî," in *Sabbetay Donnolo: scienza e cultura ebraica nell'Italia del secolo X* (ed. Giancarlo Lacerenza; Naples: Università degli studi di Napoli L'Orientale, 2004), 21–44; here 38.

may be right: some parts of the *Book of Remedies*, such as the (A) materials, indeed originated in tenth-century Italy, whereas other parts, perhaps the (B) materials, may have been written, at least partly, in eighth-century Iran.

If this reconstruction is correct, we may identify a significant, Greek-to-Hebrew translation program of medical texts associated with the person of Shabbetai Donnolo. This translation project is comparable to other medieval Jewish translation projects, such as the Latin-to-Hebrew translations of Doeg the Edomite, or the Arabic-to-Hebrew translations of the Tibbonide family, but it is significantly earlier than its peers. An in-depth study of this Greek-to-Hebrew translation project is a task for future research.

Muntner's edition of the *Book of Remedies*

Before analyzing the relevant primary sources, some remarks on the chapter numbers and other characteristics of Muntner's edition are in place. Muntner edited the *Book of Remedies* in a series of articles in *Koroth* from 1965 to 1972. His edition is valuable in many respects but it fails to follow clear and consistent principles. If we extract the relevant articles from their original place of publication, and put them together as a book, or pdf-file, then this "book" will have a chaotic inner structure.

The first "chapters" will contain an edition of the *Book of Remedies* on the basis of the Oxford manuscript with some variant readings from other manuscripts selected in a rather haphazard way. In the midst of these chapters, we will find the aforementioned short article on the British Library manuscript. Then Muntner publishes additional materials contained in the Oxford manuscript, even if the nature of their relationship to the *Book of Remedies* is unclear. After that long passages attested by the Florence manuscript but absent in the Oxford manuscript are printed. Next, a number of further passages attested only in the Munich manuscripts are edited. Finally, we find a full transcription of the British Library manuscript including the Donnolo-paraphrase of the *Aphorisms*.

Muntner added chapter numbers to the text that run continuously throughout his edition of various manuscripts. Therefore, the same passages of the text transcribed and printed more than one time from different manuscript receive different chapter numbers in Muntner's edition. For example, chapters 1–3 (transcribed from the Oxford manuscript) reappear as chapter 1050 (transcribed from the British Library manuscript). The Donnolo-paraphrase of the *Aphorisms* is also divided into chapters following the same method of numbering as if they were chapters of the *Book of Remedies*. Muntner must have realized that this practice is misleading; therefore, in the later "chapters" he added cross references to earlier chapter-numbers containing parallel texts.

In sum, we do have an edition of the Donnolo-paraphrase of Hippocrates' *Aphorisms* by Muntner in the journal *Koroth* in 1971, although it is disguised as a part of the *Book of Remedies* attributed to Asaf.[13] The Donnolo-paraphrase is edited as chap-

---

13 Suesmann Muntner, "Asaf ha-rofe, Sefer ha-refu'ot," *Koroth* 5 (1971): 435–473 and 603–649.

ters 1061–1300 of the *Book of Remedies*. Muntner indicates that these chapters correspond to chapters 156–420 of the same book, published in *Koroth* 4:5–7 [1968] based on the Oxford, Munich, and other manuscripts, according to the chapter numbering of his edition.[14] Due to the obscure method of Muntner's edition it is no surprise that the Donnolo-paraphrase has attracted little scholarly interest so far; as a matter of fact, its existence was hardly noticed by researchers of either Shabbetai Donnolo or the book of Asaf at all.[15]

Independently of Muntner's edition the text of Donnolo's paraphrase of the *Aphorisms* have been transcribed from the British Library manuscript and published online by the *Ma'agarim* project.[16] Thus, Muntner's transcription can be checked against the online version.

The Hebrew paraphrase of the *Aphorisms*: a general characterization

Before presenting textual arguments, a general characterization of the Hebrew paraphrase of the *Aphorisms* is necessary. First, a remark on terminology: by "*Asaf*-version" I mean that variant of the Hebrew paraphrase of the *Aphorisms* which is integrated into the *Book of Remedies* attributed to Asaf and attested in the witnesses from Bodleian, Munich, Florence, Paris, and in other manuscripts. By "Donnolo-version" I mean the Hebrew paraphrase of the *Aphorisms* as attested by the British Library manuscript. By "Hebrew paraphrase of the *Aphorisms*" I mean the common material in both versions.

The Hebrew paraphrase of the *Aphorisms* is based on the Greek original of the Hippocratic *Aphorisms*. There is no evidence pointing into the direction of an Arabic, Syriac, or Latin *Vorlage*. This has already been pointed out by Moritz Steinschneider.[17] Recently, I have compared the uroscopic passages of the Hebrew paraphrase to the Syriac version of Hippocrates' *Aphorisms* and come to the conclusion that the two versions are unrelated.[18]

The Hebrew paraphrase of the *Aphorisms* is sometimes close to a *strictu sensu* translation of the Greek original but often it expands the scope of the discussion beyond the original by adding various explicatory materials. The clearest and exceptional example of the latter phenomenon is the very beginning of the text, where Hippocrates' first aphorism is turned into a sermon on the medical profession including passages that emphasize the importance of prayer and religious piety. Such extensions, though shorter than the aforementioned one, to the kernel of the Hippocratic aphorism are

---

14 Suesmann Muntner, "Asaf ha-rofe, Sefer ha-refu'ot," *Koroth* 4 (1968): 389–443 and 531–573; the relevant section begins on p. 421
15 I find no reference to this text in either Andrew Sharf, *The Universe of Shabbetai Donnolo* (Warminster: Aris and Phillips, 1976) or Piergabriele Mancuso, *Shabbatai Donnolo's Sefer Hakhmoni* (Leiden and Boston: Brill, 2010).
16 http://maagarim.hebrew-academy.org.il/Pages/PMain.aspx?misyzira=649001
17 Steinschneider, *HB* 19 (1879): 87–89 and 106–108.
18 Visi, "Medieval Hebrew Uroscopic Texts," 183.

relatively frequently added. However, in the majority of the cases the Hebrew text contains no additions of this type.

When the Hebrew paraphrase comes closer to a translation of the Greek original, it attempts to give a precise medical sense to the all too often enigmatic Hippocratic sentences by employing *termini technici* not present in the original. For example, in Aphorisms I,2, when the Greek text says "if the matters purged be such as should be purged, the patient profits and bears up well," the Hebrew text explains that if the patient vomits or defecate that humor which is in excess in his/her body, then he/she will be relieved since the cause of the disease, namely the excess of the humor, is removed. Thus, the Hebrew paraphrase is considerably longer than the Greek original, even when it contains no explanatory additions.

A related feature is that technical terms are often rendered by circumlocutions rather than inventing a corresponding Hebrew term, or borrowing a word from cognate Semitic languages. Thus, "chronic diseases," (χρόνια νοσήματα; cf. *Aphorisms* II, 39]) a key concept of Hippocratic medicine is usually circumscribed as "diseases that affect the body continuously for many days" (חולאים המאריכים תמיד בגוף ימים רבים) or "disease that lasts for many days" (מחלה אשר תאריך ימים רבים) or similar phrases.[19] On the other hand Greek names of diseases are often transliterated.[20] Such glosses appear more often in the *Donnolo*-version, but sometimes they appear in those parts of the *Asaf*-version which have no parallel in the former.[21] It is important to note that in addition to the numerous Greek glosees, there are few Latin glosses and one Arabic gloss preserved in the *Donnolo*-version.[22]

On the other hand, the translator sometimes ignores certain nuances of the original, or clauses that qualify the main statement in the Hippocratic text. Thus, in certain respects the Hebrew paraphrase simplifies the medical content of the Greek original. One also has to reckon with the possibility that the Greek *Vorlage* of the Hebrew text was not exactly the same as any of the witnesses available today. In a particular case that will be analyzed below, the Hebrew text agrees with a variant reading preserved in a single Greek manuscript.

In addition to these reproductions of the Hippocratic aphorisms, the Hebrew paraphrase often includes general statements, or sentences introducing a topic. Such statements may take the form of "and the physicians spoke about the topic of..." or the form of "and it is appropriate for the doctor to...". Some of the introductory sentences show the influence of the Mishnah in respect of syntax and rhetoric: a *protasis* and an *apodosis* are indicated by employing the "if... then..." or the "every x is y" patterns. In

---

19 Cf. chapters 1075 and 1142 in Suesmann Muntner, "Asaf ha-rofe, Sefer ha-refu'ot," *Koroth* 5 (1971): 465 and 609.

20 Chapters 1166–1172 (Donnolo-version, Muntner's edition, *Koroth* 5 (1971): 613–616) and 229–231 (*Asaf*-version, Muntner's edition, *Koroth* 4 (1968): 431–432) contain a great number of Greek glosses, which are quite frequent in the rest of the text too.

21 Chapters 224–225 and chapter 246 (Muntner's edition, *Koroth* 4 (1968): 430–431 and 434).

22 Latin glosses: chapter 1172, 1178, and 1179. Arabic gloss: chapter 1180 (Muntner's edition, *Koroth* 5 (1971): 616–618).

some cases, the explanatory material is posited after the Hippocratic "nucleus" of the text. Thus, in the aforementioned example (*Aphorisms* I,2), we find an explanation of the theory of the four humors in a nutshell following the "nucleus" that correspond to the Greek text.

Needless to say, these additions do not render any part of the Greek text of the *Aphorisms*, even though they treat important medical topics on occasions. They may have originated partly in *scholia* added to the Hippocratic text in some Greek manuscripts or commentaries, lost or extant, on the Hippocratic corpus. Alternatively, they may reflect the learning and personal opinions of the author(s) of the Hebrew paraphrase. Some texts seem to be additions from Greek sources other than the *Aphorisms*: most remarkable is a list of twelve diseases containing Greek glosses that are partly preserved in the *Donnolo*-version (chapter 1193).[23] More research is needed to clarify the origin of such additions to the Hippocratic materials.

Yet another important characteristic of the Hebrew paraphrase is that it does not indicate the difference between the sections paraphrasing the original Hippocratic text and the sections that contain additional explanatory materials, such as the generalized statements mentioned above. One can identify the "nucleus" that corresponds to the original aphorism by comparing the Hebrew text to the Greek, but solely on the basis of the Hebrew it is impossible to discern the difference between the two types of the material. In some cases, the explanatory material is even added into the middle of the "nucleus."

The Hebrew paraphrase and the works of Shabbetai Donnolo

For a moment, let us ignore the fact that the *Donnolo*-version is explicitly attributed to Shabbetai Donnolo and David ben Yosef in the British Library manuscript. Rather, let us investigate the question whether the inherent characteristics of the "Hebrew paraphrase," that is the common material in the *Donnolo*-version and the *Asaf*-version, are similar to that of the known writings of Donnolo.

In other words, the question is whether Shabbetai ben Abraham Donnolo could possibly be the author of the Hebrew paraphrase of the *Aphorisms*? There is considerable evidence suggesting an affirmative answer. Donnolo was certainly able to read Greek scientific texts and to paraphrase their contents in Hebrew. Moreover, the presence of Latin glosses in the *Donnolo*-version corroborates that southern Italy was the place where the text was composed. The Arabic gloss mentioned in the previous section also confirms Donnolo's authorship: as is known, Donnolo was captured by Saracens and lived among Arabs for a while, and later, he learned astronomy, and perhaps medicine from a teacher from Baghdad.[24] Examining writings safely ascribed to him, Andrew Sharf has concluded that Donnolo must have been familiar with Hippocrates' *Prognostics*, that is to say, one of the Hippocratic writings included in

---

23 Similarly, chapters 1199–1201 and 1227 (Muntner's edition, *Koroth* 5 (1971): 621–622 and 626) seem to be an addition on the basis of unknown Greek sources.
24 Piergabriele Mancuso, *Shabbatai Donnolo's Sefer Hakhmoni*, 12–15; for other Arabic glosses in Donnolo's works, consult ibid., 35.

layer (A) of the *Book of Remedies*.[25] Besides these general considerations, we can find significant similarities in style and phraseology if we compare the Hebrew paraphrase to the extant writings of Donnolo.

Shabbetai Donnolo authored a compendium on pharmacology, which survived in a fragmentary form.[26] This book begins with a double title: "This is the Precious Book. This is the Book of Mixtures and Potions and Powders and Bandages and Perfumes and Anointments that are called *pplysy'* [from Greek *epiplasma*?] of the physicians, which has been composed by Shabbetai the physician, also known as Donnolo, the son of Abraham [...]"[27]

Similarly, the Hebrew paraphrase of the *Aphorisms* begins with a double title, first a short one, the *Book of Investigation*, then a longer one, which unfolds a description of the content of the book. The first title is identified with the deictic pronoun *zeh* ("this") just as is the case in Donnolo's compendium on pharmacology: "This is the *Book of Investigation* [*sefer ha-midrash*], the *Investigation of Remedies* [*midrash ha-refu'ot*] that the sages investigated and researched in order to heal and to know and to understand the matters concerning remedies and to find out the signs of plagues and diseases and pains, and also the signs of life [i.e. recovery] and death in order to understand it and teach it with the help of God who teaches man knowledge." The *Donnolo*-version adds a prologue beginning with the following words: "These are the words of the seven famous chapters called *aphorismi* [Aphorisms], the work of the sage *ipoqrat* [Hippocrates]."

As has been mentioned above the Hebrew paraphrase often begins its thematic units with general statements. One recurrent type begins with the phrase "It is appropriate for the physician/sage to..." The Hebrew word for "appropriate" is regularly *ra'uy* [ראוי] or *na'eh* [נאה literally, "beautiful," "handsome"]. The word *na'eh* is often treated as a synonym of *ra'uy* in other contexts too.[28] The same type of sentences at the beginning of textual units and employing the Hebrew word *na'eh* appear in the extant fragments of Donnolo's pharmacological book.[29]

In the Hebrew paraphrase of the *Aphorisms*, textual units are frequently introduced by general sentences containing a *protasis* and an *apodosis*. They can be expressed by

---

25　Andrew Sharf, *The Universe of Shabbetai Donnolo*, 95.

26　This text was edited in the Hebrew part of Moritz Steinschneider, *Donnolo: Pharmakologische Fragmente aus dem zehnten Jahrhundert, nebst Beiträgen zur Literatur der Salernitaner hauptsächlich nach handschriftlichen hebräischen Quellen* (Berlin: Julius Benzian, 1868). For a new edition and study, see Lola Ferre, "Donnolo's *Sefer ha-yaqar*: New Edition with English Translation," in *Sabbetay Donnolo: scienza e cultura ebraica nell'Italia del secolo X*, (ed. Giancarlo Lacerenza; Naples: Università degli studi di Napoli L'Orientale, 2004), 1–20.

27　Steinschneider, *Donnolo*, Hebrew part, 1; cf. Steinschneider's German translation and comments: ibid., German part, 124.

28　Examples for *na'eh*: ch. 168 (Muntner's edition, *Koroth* 4 (1968): 423), ch. 180 (Muntner's edition, *Koroth* 4 (1968): 425)/ ch. 1110 (Muntner's edition, *Koroth* 5 (1971): 472); ch. 188 (Muntner's edition, *Koroth* 4 (1968): 426)/ch 1120 (Muntner's edition, *Koroth* 5 (1971):.04), ch. 1186–7 (Muntner's edition, *Koroth* 5 (1971): 619).

29　See Steinschneider, *Donnolo*, Hebrew part, 1 [section 1–2].

the "if... then..." or the "everything that is x, is y" pattern, just as in the Mishnah. The same syntactic and rhetoric patterns are clearly attested in Donnolo's work as well.[30] A further stylistic similarity is the recurrent usages of the verbs *ḥaqar* and *darash* (חקר, דרש). Both means "to search, to investigate" and they frequently appear in pairs in both the *Donnolo*-version and the pharmacological fragments.

In sum, the evidence collated above strongly suggest that the author of the Hebrew paraphrase must have been Donnolo or somebody heavily influenced by him. Nevertheless, an advocate of Muntner's opinion may object that all the aforementioned peculiarities belonged originally to Asaf's work, and Donnolo just adopted these elements from Asaf's earlier Hebrew paraphrase of the *Aphorisms*.

Furthermore, a similar point can be raised if we compare the medical terminology of the works of Donnolo to the Hebrew paraphrase of the *Aphorisms* and the rest of the *Book of Remedies* attributed to Asaf. Unfortunately, such a comparison can be done only on a limited scale since much less medical terms occur in those works of Donnolo that are safely ascribed to him than in the *Book of Remedies* or the Hebrew paraphrase of the *Aphorisms*. Nevertheless, the most basic medical terms, such as the names of the four qualities, or the four elements and the four humors are exactly the same in the works of Donnolo and the Hebrew paraphrase as well as in much of layer (B) of the *Book of Remedies*. As has been mentioned, layer (B) include texts that may have been composed as early as the eighth century. Therefore, a supporter of Muntner's opinion may argue that Donnolo was, in fact, heavily influenced by the much earlier Asaf's book in respect of terminology, and perhaps this influence extended to characteristics of style, which have been enumerated above, too.

Therefore, we must investigate the relationship between the *Asaf*-version and the *Donnolo*-version of the Hebrew paraphrase of the *Aphorisms*. If this investigation leads to the conclusion that the *Donnolo*-version is the earlier of the two, then we can safely conclude that Donnolo and his colleague, David ben Yosef were the authors of this text and not a sixth-century Jewish physician in the Land of Israel hypothesized by Muntner.

Differences between the Donnolo-version and Asaf-version

The most obvious difference between the *Donnolo*-version and the *Asaf*-version is a recurrent textual variant: in the introductory sentences of the type "And the sages/physicians talked about..." the *Asaf*-version often, though not always has "Asaf" instead of "sages/physicians." Thus, in the paraphrase of *Aphorisms* I,2 the *Donnolo*-version says "And the sages talked about diarrhea..." whereas the *Asaf*-version has "And Asaf talked about diarrhea." The *Asaf*-version attributes the *Aphorisms* to Asaf the physician. As opposed to this, the prologue of the *Donnolo*-version names Hippocrates as the author of the text. Neither the prologue nor the rest of the *Donnolo*-version ever refers to Asaf at all.

---

30 Almost all the textual units of the surviving fragments begin with either of these patterns. The exceptions (sections 13, 16, 19, and 20) contain lists and begin with the phrase *elleh* ("these are...").

A stylistic difference is the recurrent occurrence of a rare Biblical Hebrew word, *kishron*, meaning "success" (cf. *Ecclesiastes 2:11, 4:4 5:10*) in the *Asaf*-version, and its absence in the *Donnolo*-version.

The *Donnolo*-version is both shorter and longer than the *Asaf*-version. It is shorter because, regrettably, long passages of the *Aphorisms* are not extant in the only surviving manuscript.[31] Probably, the British Library manuscript was copied from a deficient manuscript in which several pages were missing, and thus considerable portions of the original texts are not accessible to us. On the other hand, wherever the British Library manuscript preserves the text, it is longer than the corresponding passages in the *Book of Remedies* attributed to Asaf. In this sense, the *Donnolo*-version is longer than the *Asaf*-version.

The two texts are closely related; most of the differences between them consist of minor variants which can be explained as secondary products of textual transmission, and a number of extra passages that are absent in the *Asaf*-version, but present in the *Donnolo*-version. In a few cases, the *Asaf*-version preserved short sentences or clauses that are missing in the *Donnolo*-version. Nevertheless, all in all the textual units of the *Donnolo*-version, whenever they are preserved, are much longer than the corresponding textual units of the *Asaf*-version.

Therefore, the main research question is as follows: whether the *Asaf*-version is an abridgement of the *Donnolo*-version, or, the other way around, the latter is an interpolated version of the former. As has been mentioned, Muntner endorsed the second alternative without proposing explicit arguments in favor of it. He believed that Asaf, who was a real person, translated and paraphrased the Greek text into Hebrew, and several centuries later Shabbetai Donnolo and David ben Yosef corrected this version based on the Greek original and furnished it with further explanatory additions. This is how Donnolo's version came to be longer than Asaf's version.

A closer comparison of the two texts clearly disproves Muntner's theory. As has been mentioned above, in a number of aphorisms the Hebrew paraphrase expands the original Greek text to a considerable degree. Besides a "nucleus" which is more-or-less a translation of the original Greek text, we find explanatory sentences, which put the Hippocratic idea in a broader or more precisely defined context. These sentences may appear both before and after the "nucleus" of the section.

Now, the differences between the *Donnolo*-version and the *Asaf*-version often concern the "nucleus" itself. The *Asaf*-version, which is generally shorter than the *Donnolo*-version, omits not only much of the explanatory materials but sometimes the "nucleus" corresponding to the Hippocratic text itself as well. Sometimes a part of the

---

31 The following lacunae can be identified in the Donnolo-version: *Aphorisms* III, 11- 19 (in chapters 1164–1165, Muntner's edition, *Koroth* 5 (1971): 613); *Aphorisms* IV, 11–22 (at chapters 1190–1194, Muntner's edition, *Koroth* 5 (1971): 620–621); *Aphorisms* IV, 69–V, 5 (in chapters 1255–1256 Muntner's edition, *Koroth* 5 (1971): 630); *Aphorisms* V, 26-VII, 87 (at chapters 1280–1281, Muntner's edition, *Koroth* 5 (1971): 635). All these passages are covered in the *Asaf*-version.

"nucleus" is absent, sometimes the entire "nucleus." The hypothesis that "Asaf" paraphrased Hippocrates' *Aphorisms* by ignoring partly or entirely some of the passages
of the Greek text itself but adding long explanations to the ignored passages seems to
be extremely unlikely. On the other hand, the hypothesis that Donnolo's text is the
earlier one, and Asaf's text is its abridgment explains conveniently these textual data.
The person responsible for the abbreviation may have not been aware of the original
Hippocratic text at all, and thus had no qualms about omitting partly or entirely the
"nucleus" of the paraphrased aphorisms.

Let me provide some examples:

Aphorisms I,4

Hippocrates' text in W. H. S. Jones' translation reads: "A restricted and rigid regimen
is treacherous in chronic diseases always, in acute, where it is not called for. Again,
a regimen carried to the extreme of restriction is perilous; and in fact repletion too,
carried to extremes is perilous"[32] In the Urbinati manuscript of the Greek original the
phrase αἰεὶ πάθεσι is absent; thus the sense of the first sentence is modified to "[...] is
treacherous in chronic as well as in acute [diseases], where it is not called for." The
Hebrew paraphrase seems to reflect this textual variant.

In the *Donnolo*-version, the unit corresponding to *Aphorisms* I,4 (chapters 1074–
1075) begins with a general statement: "It is appropriate [ra'uy] for the physician to
set his mind on and research all kinds of foods and drinks that he may give to the
patients, when they suffer from diseases for a long time, when 'storms' of diseases
overwhelm them, according to their strength." The text goes on to explain that sick
people in general can absorb less food than usual, and accordingly the physician must
prescribe them to eat and drink less. On the other hand, as the disease passes, the physician should gradually increase the amount of food a patient may consume.[33]

After this general introduction the *Donnolo*-version proceeds to paraphrase Aphorism I,4 itself:

---

32 Hippocrates, *Aphorisms*, 4; see Hippocrates, vol. 4, Loeb Classical Library (ed. and trans. W. H.
   S. Jones; London and Cambridge, Mass.: William Heinemann and Harvard University Press,
   1931), 101. The Greek original (ibid., 100):
   αἱ λεπταὶ καὶ ἀκριβέες δίαιται, καὶ ἐν τοῖσι μακροῖσιν αἰεὶ πάθεσι, καὶ ἐν τοῖσιν ὀξέσιν, οὗ μὴ
   ἐπιδέχεται, σφαλεραί. καὶ πάλιν αἱ ἐς τὸ ἔσχατον λεπτότητος ἀφιγμέναι δίαιται, χαλεπαί· καὶ γὰρ
   αἱ πληρώσιες αἱ ἐν τῷ ἐσχάτῳ ἐοῦσαι, χαλεπαί.
33 *Book of Remedies*, ch. 1074–1075, according to the edition by Muntner, "Asaf ha-rofe, Sefer
   ha-refu'ot," *Koroth* 5 (1971): 465. The introductory part reads (the continuation of the text
   ["nucleus"] will be quoted in the next footnote):
   ראוי לרופא לתת שכלו ולחקור בכל מיני מאכל ומשתה הראויים להאכיל את החולים בארוך ימי תחלואיהם בהתחזק
   עליכם [צ"ל עליהם] סערות החולי להאכילם לפי משא כוחם. כי המרבה להאכיל את החולה יותר ממשא כוחו לאכול,
   יגרה עליו רוב מכאובים כי המעדיף על השובע ירע לחולה. וכאשר יתחזק החולי לרום ולהתגדל על הגוף, ראוי למעט
   מן האוכל להאכילו. ובהתחסר החולי הלוך וחסר, להימעט להוסיף על האוכל לפי כוחו החולה, עד תום ימי קץ חוליו.

In diseases that affect the body continuously for many days and also in the "sharp" and hard diseases, if [the physician] feeds the patient with fine, suitable and good food that is appropriate for his disease, but [the patient] is unable to take anything [of it] to eat it due to the great disgust [he feels] of that food, then it is bad. And similarly, if the patient eats a lot up to his satisfaction, it is bad.[34]

The Hebrew paraphrase represents a different interpretation (and partly different Greek *Vorlage*) from Jones' English translation. The terms "chronic disease" and "acute disease" are rendered through circumlocutions ("diseases that affect the body continuously for many days" vs. "sharp and hard diseases"). Whereas the standard text of Hippocrates distinguishes chronic and acute diseases as two different cases, the Hebrew paraphrase, just as the Urbinati manuscript of the Greek, ignores the difference.[35] The phrase "where it is not called for" was understood as "when the patient does not desire it [i.e. the food]" and finally, it was paraphrased as "he is unable [...] to eat it due to the great disgust of that food." The phrase "repletion [*plerosiesi*] carried out to the extreme" is rendered as "if the patient eats a lot up to his satisfaction."

In sum, the sentences cited above indeed represent the Greek original of the *Aphorisms*; they are the "nucleus" of the textual unit. The preceding passage outlining a general theory of diet during diseases is *not* a translation or paraphrase of any Greek text but an introduction, which provides the background necessary for understanding the Hippocratic aphorism. The text then continues with a similar explanatory introduction to *Aphorisms* I,5, which do not belong to the textual unit presently discussed. Having reconstructed the structure of the paraphrase of Aphorisms I,4 in the *Donnolo*-version now we can compare it to the *Asaf*-version.

The relevant unit in the *Asaf*-version appears to be corrupted at certain points. It begins with the same sentence as in the *Donnolo*-version with minor variants.[36] After that we find a short passage which is identical with a part of the Donnolo's version "introductory explanation" to *Aphorisms* I,5, that is, the section which should follow the present section. This part of the text is clearly misplaced in the *Asaf*-version.

---

34 Ibid.:

בחולאים המאריכים תמיד בגוף ימים רבים, וגם בחולאים החדים והקשים, אם תאכיל את החולה מאכל דקיק ונאה וטוב הראוי להוליו, והוא לא יוכל לקבל מאומה לאכול מרוב תיעוב האוכל רע הוא. וכמו כן אם ירבה החולה לאכול למאד לשובע רע הוא.

35 Cf. Jones, *Hippocrates*, vol. 4, 100, n. 7. The missing words are added on the margins by a second hand.

36 *Book of Remedies*, ch. 164, ed. Muntner, "Asaf ha-rofe, Sefer ha-refu'ot," *Koroth* 4 (1968): 422–423; section corresponding to the *Donnolo*-version (quoted in previous footnotes) are underlined:

וראוי לרופא לתת שכלו לחקור בכל מיני המאכל, הראוי להאכיל החולים באורך ימי תחלואיהם בהתחזק עליהם סערות החולי, להאכילם לפי משא כוחם. כי המרבה להאכיל החולה יותר ממשא כוחו לאכול יתגרה עליו הלאים ורוב מכאובים, כי המעדיף על השובע יריע לחולה. וכל דבר לפי משאו כשרון הוא. החלאים החזקים והקשים והחדים המיאשים החולים, ראוי לחוש לרפאם בחוזק יד ולא ברפיון ידים, כי הם מקריבים למות, ורבים ימותו באין דעת, כי אם ישכיל הרופא אותות הנגעים, אז יכון לרפא. וכאשר יכון הרופא לרפא חוזק החולי אשר חזק על החולה לרום ולהתגדל על הגוף הלוך וגדול, ראוי למעט מן האוכל, ובהתחסר החולי להמעט הלוך וחסור, להוסיף על האוכל לפי כוח החולה, עד תום קץ ימי חליו. ובתחילה חליו למעט מן אוכל וכלכלות החליו להוסיף על האוכל.

Then, we find the second half of the introduction to *Aphorisms* I,4, which is probably corrupted at the beginning. At the end of the unit, the *Asaf*-version contains a short addition: "And at the beginning of the disease one has to decrease the food, but when the disease is concluded, one has to increase the food." This remark may have been copied here from chapter 1082 of the Donnolo-version. However, the most important observation to be made is that the "nucleus" of *Aphorisms* I,4 in the *Donnolo*-version is *totally absent* in the *Asaf*-version.

In sum, in the *Asaf*-version we do find the introductory passage in a shortened form, but we look in vain for the "nucleus" representing the Hippocratic aphorism itself. This state of affairs can be easily explained, if we assume that the *Donnolo*-version is older than the *Asaf*-version: the person responsible for abbreviating the text must have realized that the introductory passage provides important information about diets in general, so he kept that passage in the text. The second part, which is actually based on the Greek of the *Aphorisms* seemed to explain some minor points, and thus the editor may have decided to omit it. But, on the other hand, if we follow Muntner's hypothesis, we cannot explain convincingly how could Asaf both ignore *Aphorisms* I,4 and write a short explanatory introduction to it. The idea that Donnolo added the "nucleus" to Asaf's explanatory remarks is far-fetched.

Aphorisms I,1

As has been mentioned, the very first aphorism of the collection is turned into a sermon on the medical profession in both versions of the text. Yet there are differences: the *Donnolo*-version is a longer and more clearly structured literary composition. Again the differences concern the "nucleus" of the text as well.

The famous opening lines, "[l]ife is short, the art long"[37] is only partly present in the *Asaf*-version, but it is fully represented in the Donnolo-version. The Donnolo version reads: "[...] for short [*lit.* few] is the end of the days of the life of man, but the art [*lit.* wisdom] of medicine is very long [...]."[38] In the *Asaf*-version we find: "Short [*lit.* small] is the end of the days of man [...]"[39] Again, it is unlikely that Asaf translated only half of the first aphorism and then Donnolo augmented the missing part. In all likelihood, the original text is the one which contains the full paraphrase of the aphorism.

Aphorisms II, 2

The original Hippocratic aphorism reads as follows: "When sleep puts an end to delirium it is a good sign."[40] In the *Donnolo*-version, the paraphrases of this aphorism begins with a longer explanation of 'delirium;' the Greek word itself, παραφροσύνη,

---

37 Tr. Jones, *Hippocrates*, vol. 4, 99. In the original: ὁ βίος βραχὺς, ἡ δὲ τέχνη μακρή.
38 ‏כי מעט הוא קץ ימי חיי האדם וחכמת הרפואה ארוכה היא עד מאד‎.
39 ‏קטן קץ ימי האדם‎.
40 Tr. Jones, *Hippocrates*, vol. 4, 109. In the original: ὅκου παραφροσύνην ὕπνος παύει, ἀγαθόν.

occurring in the Hippocratic text is transcribed to Hebrew.[41] Then the main point of the aphorism is explained in Hebrew, and then, the *Donnolo*-version adds further explanation: if the patient does not sleep calmly, but awakes from time to time and suffers from pains, and his eyes are red, then it is a bad sign.[42]

In the *Asaf*-version only this last sentence, which is an addition to the original Hippocratic aphorism, is attested.[43] Again the hypothesis that Asaf decided not to include *Aphorisms* II,2 in his Hebrew compendium, but still saw it necessary to add an explanatory remark to it is far-fetched. On the other hand, the hypothesis that the *Donnolo*-version was made from the Greek original, and the *Asaf*-version is a mere abridgement of it explains the textual data conveniently.

Aphorisms II, 13

According to the Hippocratic text: "When a crisis occurs, the night before the exacerbation is generally uncomfortable, the night after more comfortable."[44] In the *Donnolo*-version the "nucleus" paraphrasing the Hippocratic aphorism is preceded by an introductory remark about crisis days in general.[45] The *Asaf*-version contains only the beginning of the introductory remark.[46] The strength of this evidence is diminished by the fact that the sentence included in the *Asaf*-version ends abruptly; perhaps, the "nucleus" is omitted due to secondary textual corruption, and not due to the editor's decision.

---

41 Muntner's transcription of this word is incorrect; the Ma'agarim-website reads it as פארא פרוסיני, which clearly corresponds to Greek παραφροσύνη. Cf. http://maagarim.hebrew-academy.org.il/Pages/PMain.aspx?misyzira=649001 [cited 14 September 2015].

42 *Book of Remedies*, ch. 1103, ed. Muntner, "Asaf ha-rofe, Sefer ha-refu'ot," *Koroth* 5 (1971): 471.
כל אדם אשר יש לו חולי חד והשתנה דעתו, ויפול בחולי הנקרא פאראפרוסיכי [צ"ל פאראפרוסיני] הוא פרכוס, וידבר בבלי דעת, אם ינום וינוח וישקוט החולה בתנומתו מן החולי אות טובה הוא. ואם יכאב בחוליו וידבר בבלי דעת ופעם ינום ופעם תידד שנתו, וכאשר ינום ישקוד בפחד מידי תעורתו ועיניו מסוקרות סביב, רע הוא.

43 *Book of Remedies*, ch. 175, ed. Muntner, "Asaf ha-rofe, Sefer ha-refu'ot," *Koroth* 4 (1968): 424
ואשר יראה לך כי יכאב במחלתו וידבר בבלי דעת וינום וישקוד בפחד מדי תעורתו ועיניו מסקרות סביב, אות רעיון הוא לחולה.

44 Tr. Jones, *Hippocrates*, vol. 4, 111. In the original: Ὁκόσοισι κρίσις γίνεται, τουτέοισιν ἡ νὺξ δύσφορος, ἡ πρὸ τοῦ παροξυσμοῦ, ἡ δὲ ἐπιοῦσα εὐφορωτέρη ὡς ἐπὶ τὸ πουλύ.

45 *Book of Remedies*, ch. 1116, ed. Muntner, "Asaf ha-rofe, Sefer ha-refu'ot," *Koroth* 5 (1971): 603; the "nucleus" is underlined, variant readings from the online transcription of the *Ma'agarim*-project are added in square brackets:
וזה לך האות בכל חולה לדעת אם תמהר רפואתו לבוא. אם הלילה, אשר יהיה טרם יזיע תכבד ותגדיל ותקשה הקדחת והמצוקה להחזיק על החולה, ועת מוחרת [מחרת] למועד תהיה קלה לרוב וארוכה [וערובה] מאד בזיעת משפט טוב או באחד אות רפואה ומשפט, זה אות רפואה ממוהרת. כי כל אדם, אשר הוא מוכן להשפט מחוליו <u>כאשר יקרב ליום המשפט הלילה ההוא, אשר הוא קרוב ליום המשפט, תגדל המצוקה והקדחת על החלה, ובלילה השני, אשר יהיה לאחר יום המשפט, וייקל ויטב עד מאד, יותר מן הלילה שעבר,</u> אם נשפט כמשפט—טוב ואות חיים.

46 *Book of Remedies*, ch. 184, ed. Muntner, "Asaf ha-rofe, Sefer ha-refu'ot," *Koroth* 4 (1968): 425:
זה לך האות בכל חולה לדעת אם תמהר רפואתו לבוא אם לאן[:] הלילה אשר תהיה טרם יזיע תכבד ותקשה להחזיק על החולה ועת מחרת למועד הזה תהא קלה ועריבה מאד בזיעה.

Aphorisms II, 24

This is a long and complicated aphorism on the critical days of fever.[47] The *Donnolo*-version begins with the "nucleus" paraphrasing the Greek original (ch. 1125).[48] Then an additional explanation follows (ch. 1126).[49] The *Asaf*-version combines the first half of the "nucleus' with a shortened version of the additional explanation (ch. 193).[50] Again, we can observe that the *Asaf*-version preserves the explanatory material but ignores part of the "nucleus" representing the original Hippocratic aphorism.

Aphorisms IV,1

"Purge pregnant women, should there be orgasm, from the fourth to the seventh month, but these last less freely; the unborn child, in the first and last stages of pregnancy, should be treated very cautiously."[51]

The *Donnolo*-version (chapter 1182) introduces this aphorism with a general rule according to which pregnant women should not receive purgatives at all, since they may cause abortion. Then the "nucleus" paraphrasing the original Hippocratic aphorism follows. The reader of the *Donnolo*-version will understand that this aphorism concerns exceptional cases when pregnant women must take purgatives despite the general prohibition. After the "nucleus" an additional remark comes that points out that certain doctors give purgative to pregnant women during the first four months of the pregnancy, too. Such doctors are responsible for abortions during that period of pregnancy.[52]

---

47 Τῶν ἑπτὰ ἡ τετάρτη ἐπίδηλος ἑτέρης ἑβδομάδος ἡ ὀγδόη ἀρχή, θεωρητὴ δὲ ἡ ἐνδεκάτη αὕτη γάρ ἐστι τετάρτη τῆς δευτέρης ἑβδομάδος θεωρητὴ δὲ πάλιν ἡ ἑπτακαιδεκάτη, αὕτη γάρ ἐστι τετάρτη μὲν ἀπὸ τῆς τεσσαπεσκαιδεκάτης, ἑβδόμη δὲ ἀπὸ τῆς ἐνδεκάτης.
"The fourth day is indicative of the seven; the eighth is the beginning of another week; the eleventh is to be watched as being the fourth day of the second week; again the seventeenth is to be watched, being the fourth from the fourteenth and the seventh from the eleventh." (Tr. Jones, *Hippocrates*, vol. 4, 115.).

48 וזה לך אות ופשר לדעת כי היום הרביעי לחולה יגיד מה יהיה ביום השביעי ויום השמיני הוא תחילת השבוע השני וראה עוד גם יום אחד עשר הוא יום רביעי לשבוע השני וראה עוד גם יום שבעה עשר כי גם זה היום נחשב יום רביעי מיום ארבעה-עשר, תחשב עוד הזה שביעי מיום אחד עשר. וראה עוד גם עשרים ואחד כי גם זה היום נחשב יום שביעי מיום שמונה עשר ונחשב עוד היום הזה היום שביעי מיום טו' וזהו סוף השבוע בשלישי.

49 והאות אשר יצדק בפשר החלאים החדים ולא ימיר עד תום ארבעה עשר יום ואם לא יכנעו וישפטו להשפל בארבעה עשר יום, יאריכו עד קץ שנים עשר עד תום עשרים ואחד יום. אם יזיע החולה זיעת משפט טוב ביום השביעי, יזיע בזיעה טובה ואות משפט טוב, דע כי לקץ השבועיים ירפא ויקום.

50 וזה לך הפשר לדבר כי היום לרביעי לחולה יגיד מה יהיה ביום השביעי והשמיני עד תחילת השבוע השני, והאות אשר יצדק בפשר ולא ימיר עד תום עשרים ואחד יום. אם יזיע ביום הרביעי גם בשביעי יזיע ואם יזיע בשביעי לקץ השבועיים ירפא ויקום.

51 Tr. Jones, *Hippocrates*, vol. 4, 135. In the original: τὰς κυούσας φαρμακεύειν, ἢν ὀργᾷ, τετράμηνα καὶ ἄχρι ἑπτὰ μηνῶν, ἧσσον δὲ ταύτας· τὰ δὲ νήπια καὶ τὰ πρεσβύτερα εὐλαβέεσθαι χρή..

52 *Book of Remedies*, ch. 1182, ed. Muntner, "Asaf ha-rofe, Sefer ha-refu'ot," *Koroth* 5 (1971): 618–619; the "nucleus" is underlined:
אשה הרה אל תשקנה כל משקה תרופה חזק, ואם תעבור על המצווה, דע כי ימות הוולד בבטנה או תפיל נפל או יהא אסון, אך אחת מהרבה תמלט. <u>והנשים ההרות הצריכות לשתות משקה לכבס, אם יהיה קרבם לח ובטנם רך</u> <u>השקם ממלאות ארבעה חדשים או עד מלאות שבעה חדשים, כי ראוי להישמר בילדים בתחילת ההריון, כשהם</u>

In the *Asaf*-version (chapter 240) only the introductory remark and the additional explanation is included.[53] The "nucleus" is ignored altogether. These data can be explained along the same lines that have been pointed out in the previous sections.

Aphorisms IV, 36

"Sweats in a fever case are beneficial if they begin on the third day, the fifth, the seventh, the ninth, the eleventh, the fourteenth, the seventeenth, the twenty-first, the twenty-seventh, the thirsty-first and the thirsty-fourth, for these sweats bring diseases to a crisis. Sweats occurring on other days indicate pain, a long disease and relapses."[54]

As usual, the *Donnolo*-version reproduces the Hippocratic aphorism with additions, for example, we learn that the twenty-fourth, thirsty-seventh, and the forty-first days are also suitable for "good" sweats that bring crisis. The Hebrew paraphrase interprets the Greek text differently from Jones' English translation. The original Greek μὴ οὕτω γινόμενοι, which literally means "[if] it won't be so," is taken by Jones to refer to the possibility that sweats appear on other days, whereas the *Donnolo*-version makes it refer to the case when sweating fails to end the fever. Thus, the "critical days" enlisted in the first half of the text show whether the diseases will disappear fast, or will be prolonged.[55]

The *Asaf*-version is shorter than the *Donnolo*-version; it omits some of the elements, which are present in the original Hippocratic text, but retains some of the additions of the *Donnolo*-version, most remarkably, the "twenty-fourth day" is added to the list of days. A more dramatic difference is that the sense of the aphorism changes due to the curious omission of the middle of the sentence: the *Asaf*-version states that sweats

---

קטנים, ובעת הקרובים להוולד, כשהם גדולים. ויש אשר ירפא ההריות מתחילת ההריון עד מלאות ארבעה חדשים. ואם תשתה האשה כל דבר משקה ותפיל בעת ההיא, דע כי המשקה הפיל את הוולד. ואם מת הוולד במעיה ולא יוצא החוצה, השקנה המשקה להפילו.

53 *Book of Remedies*, ch. 240, ed. Muntner, "Asaf ha-rofe, Sefer ha-refu'ot," *Koroth* 4 (1968): 433:
אשה הרה אל תשקה כל משתה תרופה. ואם תעבור על המצוה, דע כי ימות הילד במעיה, או אסון יהיה. אך אחת מהרבה תימלט. ויש אשר ירפאו הנשים ההריות מתחילת ההריון עד מלאת ד' חדשים. ואם תפיל האשה בשנה ההיא שתשתה כל דבר משתה, דע כי המשתה הפיל הילד. ואם מת הילד במעיה ולא יצא חוץ, השקה אותה משתה להפיל.

54 Tr. Jones, *Hippocrates*, vol. 4, 145. In the original: ἱδρῶτες πυρεταίνουσιν ἢν ἄρξωνται, ἀγαθοὶ τριταῖοι, καὶ πεμπταῖοι, καὶ ἑβδομαῖοι, καὶ ἐναταῖοι, καὶ ἑνδεκαταῖοι, καὶ τεσσαρεσκαιδεκαταῖοι, καὶ ἑπτακαιδεκαταῖοι, καὶ μιῇ καὶ εἰκοστῇ, καὶ ἑβδόμῃ καὶ εἰκοστῇ, καὶ τριηκοστῇ πρώτῃ, καὶ τριηκοστῇ τετάρτῃ· οὗτοι γὰρ οἱ ἱδρῶτες νούσους κρίνουσιν· οἱ δὲ μὴ οὕτω γινόμενοι πόνον σημαίνουσι καὶ μῆκος νούσου καὶ ὑποτροπιασμούς.

55 *Book of Remedies*, ch. 1211, ed. Muntner, "Asaf ha-rofe, Sefer ha-refu'ot," *Koroth* 5 (1971): 623–624:
כל הזיעות שנקדחים המתחילות לטובה ולהקל הקדחת טובות המה. כי אם יזיעו הנקדחים ביום השלישי לחולי או ביום חמשי או ביום ז' או ביום תשעי, או ביום י"א, או ביום י"ה, או ביום י"ז או ביום עשרים ואחד, או ביום כ"ה, או ביום עשרים ושבע, או ביום ל' וא', או ביום שלשים וארבעה, או ביום ל' וד' או ביום ארבעים ואחד, אלה הזיעות שופטות החלאים להשקיטם ולהסירם מעל החולה, ואם לא תהיינה הזיעות האלה כאשר כתוב בתחילת הדבר הזה להתחיל לטובה להקל, כי אם יזיע החולה ותשקוט ותשקוט הזיעה והקדחת והחולי עומדת בחזקתם, ולא חודלים, דע כי אלה הזיעות מעידות על אותות חולי ימים רבים ותהפוכות בגוף בחולי הפכפך ושירפון.

on the critical days indicate the prolongation of the disease, without mentioning the possibility that may indicate fast recovery too.[56]

The hypothesis that the *Asaf*-version, which ignores a crucial part of the original Hippocratic aphorism, is the original paraphrase and the *Donnolo*-version is an expanded variant of it, is far-fetched again. The alternative, namely, that the *Donnolo*-version is the original paraphrase and the *Asaf*-version is its abridgement seems much more likely

However, one may consider the objection that the text of the *Asaf*-version is simply corrupted here, and thus the evidence is irrelevant. Nevertheless, in this particular case, this objection is not convincing: the Hebrew text of the *Asaf*-version is completely meaningful as it stands, and thus, it is not likely that careless scribes failed to transmit any part of it. The difference between the sense of the Greek original and the Hebrew paraphrase in the *Asaf*-version was probably created by a careless redactor, who abridged the *Donnolo*-version, and not by a careless scribe.

Aphorisms V, 10–13

These aphorisms make up a thematic unit that deals with various diseases of the throat and lung that involve sputa and spitting. The *Donnolo*-version (chapters 1260–1263) represents all the essential content of the original Hippocratic aphorisms and adds further elements to it. The *Asaf*-version (chapter 360) gives an abridged account of these aphorisms which retains some of the additions, but eliminates some of the original elements. Again, the convenient explanation is that the *Asaf*-version is derived from the *Donnolo*-version, not vice versa.

One example will suffice to illustrate this. According to the Greek *Aphorisms* V, 13 reads: "When patients spit up frothy blood, the discharge comes from the lungs."[57] In the *Donnolo*-version (ch. 1263) we find: "If someone spits up frothy blood or vomits blood, know that it comes up from the lung without doubt [*lit*. lie]."[58] The *Asaf*-version (ch. 306 *in fine*) says: "If someone vomits blood, it is from the lung without doubt."[59]

Comparing the three texts we can observe that the *Donnolo*-version contains an additional element in the *protasis*: "or vomits blood." The *Asaf*-version attests to this additional element but it omits "spits up frothy blood" of the *Donnolo*-version, which renders the *protasis* of the original Hippocratic aphorism. Thus, the *Asaf*-version retains an element of the *Donnolo*-version but omits an element of the original Greek

---

56 *Book of Remedies*, ch. 259:4, ed. Muntner, "Asaf ha-rofe, Sefer ha-refu'ot," *Koroth* 4 (1968): 436:
אדם שתאחחזנו קדחת בו, אם יזיע ביום השלישי או בחמישי או בשביעי או בתשיעי או באחד עשר או בארבעה-עשר
או בעשרים ואחד או בשלושים, כל זה יגיד על אותות חולי מאריך ימים בחלי הפכפך ושרפון

57 Tr. Jones, *Hippocrates*, vol. 4, 161. In the original: ὁκόσοι αἷμα ἀφρῶδες ἀναπτύουσι, τουτέοισιν ἐκ τοῦ πλεύμονος ἡ τοιαύτη ἀναγωγὴ γίνεται.

58 *Book of Remedies*, ch. 1263, ed. Muntner, "Asaf ha-rofe, Sefer ha-refu'ot," *Koroth* 5 (1971): 632:
כל אדם אשר ירוק מפיהו דם בקצף, או אם יקיא דם, דע כי מן הריאה הוא עולה באין כחש

59 *Book of Remedies*, ch. 306, ed. Muntner, "Asaf ha-rofe, Sefer ha-refu'ot," *Koroth* 4 (1968): 441:
כל אדם שיקיא דם, הוא מן הריאה באין כחש

text; therefore, it is probably dependent on the *Donnolo*-version and cannot be considered an independent paraphrase of the original Greek text.

Absence of counterexamples

There are no counterexamples, that is to say, cases when the *Asaf*-version preserved the "nucleus" in its entirety together with some additional explanations, whereas the *Donnolo*-version retained the additions of the *Asaf*-version but omitted the "nucleus" partly or entirely. The relationship between the two versions is asymmetrical in this respect.

Conclusion

Any of the examples enlisted above can be explained away as a result of secondary corruptions during textual transmission. However, taken together, it is extremely unlikely that all the evidence is due to a series of contingent mistakes. The same conclusion is corroborated by the lack of counterexamples. Therefore, we have a cumulative evidence in favor of the primacy of the *Donnolo*-version: since it is extremely unlikely that "Asaf" paraphrased Hippocrates by omitting partly or entirely the Hippocratic aphorism but adding explanations to the omitted parts, Muntner's hypothesis that the *Asaf*-version represents the original form of the text is untenable.

The *Asaf*-version, thus, must be considered an abridgment of the *Donnolo*-version. An important corollary to this conclusion is that the *Book of Remedies*, in the form we know it, must postdate Shabbetai Donnolo, since the latter was a source of the former. Donnolo was active in the middle of the tenth century; the year 4706 of the Jewish calendar, corresponding to 945–946 CE, is mentioned in his main work.[60] Therefore, the Hebrew paraphrase of the Aphorisms can be tentatively dated to the middle of the tenth century.

It is outside of the scope of this paper to compare the Hebrew paraphrase of Hippocrates' *Prognostics* as preserved in the *Book of Remedies* to the *Donnolo*-version of the *Aphorisms*. However, it is not beyond the point to state that a cursory comparison of the two texts suggests that the same persons authored them. Therefore, it is possible that all the (A) materials of the *Book of Remedies* derive from the Greek-into-Hebrew translations of Shabbetai Donnolo and his colleagues. Some other parts of the *Book of Remedies*, such as collections of uroscopic rules, or texts about pulse, may also turn out to be Hebrew translations or paraphrases of Greek medical texts, as has already been argued in a particular case.[61] Whether all these translations belonged to the same project of translation is a problem to be clarified in future research.

---

60 Mancuso, *Shabbatai Donnolo's Sefer Hakhmoni*, 234.
61 Visi, "Medieval Hebrew Uroscopic Texts," 172–176.

Appendix: summary of the textual evidence

The sole purpose of this table is to present the textual evidence discussed above in a convenient way. The "nucleus" corresponding to the Greek text is underlined in both Hebrew versions, whenever it can be identified. The Greek text and English translation are copied from the Loeb edition of Hippocrates' works; the Hebrew texts are copied from Muntner's edition of the *Book of Remedies*.

Aphorism	Greek / tr. Jones	Donnolo	Asaf
I,1	ὁ βίος βραχὺς, ἡ δὲ τέχνη μακρὴ Life is short, the art long.	כי מעט הוא קץ ימי חיי האדם וחכמת הרפואה ארוכה היא עד מאד.	קטן קץ ימי האדם.
I, 4	αἱ λεπταὶ καὶ ἀκριβέες δίαιται, καὶ ἐν τοῖσι μακροῖσιν αἰεὶ πάθεσι, καὶ ἐν τοῖσιν ὀξέσιν, οὐ μὴ ἐπιδέχεται, σφαλεραί. καὶ πάλιν αἱ ἐς τὸ ἔσχατον λεπτότητος ἀφιγμέναι δίαιται, χαλεπαί· καὶ γὰρ αἱ πληρώσιες αἱ ἐν τῷ ἐσχάτῳ ἐοῦσαι, χαλεπαί. A restricted and rigid regimen is treacherous in chronic diseases always, in acute, where it is not called for. Again, a regimen carried to the extreme of restriction is perilous; and in fact repletion too, carried to extremes is perilous.	ראוי לרופא לתת שכלו ולחקור בכל מיני מאכל ומשתה הראויים להאכיל את החולים בארוך ימי תחלואיהם בהתחזק עליכם [צ״ל עליהם] סערות החולי להאכילם לפי משא כוחם. כי המרבה להאכיל את החולה יותר ממשא כוחו לאכול, יגרה עליו רוב מכאובים כי המעדיף על השובע ירע לחולה. וכאשר יתחזק החולי לרום ולהתגדל על הגוף, ראוי למעט מן האוכל להאכילו. ובהתחסר החולי הלוך וחסר, להימעט להוסיף על האוכל לפי כוחו החולה, עד תום ימי קץ חולי. <u>בחולאים המאריכים תמיד</u> <u>בגוף ימים רבים, וגם בחולאים</u> <u>החדים והקשים, אם תאכיל</u> <u>את החולה מאכל דקיק ונאה</u> <u>וטוב הראוי להוליו, והוא לא</u> <u>יוכל לקבל מאומה לאכול</u> <u>מרוב תיעוב האוכל רע הוא.</u> <u>וכמו כן אם ירבה החולה</u> <u>לאכול למאד לשובע רע הוא.</u>	וראוי לרופא לתת שכלו לחקור בכל מיני המאכל, הראוי להאכיל החולים באורך ימי תחלואיהם בהתחזק עליהם סערות החולי, להאכילם לפי משא כוחם. כי המרבה להאכיל החולה יותר ממשא כוחו לאכול יתגרה עליו הלאים ורוב מכאובים, כי המעדיף על השובע יריע לחולה. וכל דבר לפי משאו כשרון הוא. החלאים החזקים והקשים והחדים המיאשים החולים, ראוי לחוש לרפאם בחוזק יד ולא ברפיון ידים, כי הם מקריבים למות, ורבים ימותו מאין באין דעת, כי אם ישכיל הרופא אותות הנגעים, אז יכון לרפא. וכאשר יכון הרופא לרפא חוזק החולי אשר חזק על החולה לרום ולהתגדל על הגוף הלוך וגדול, ראוי למעט מן האוכל, ובהתחסר החולי להמעט הלוך וחסור, להוסיף על האוכל לפי כוח החולה, עד תום קץ ימי חליו. ובתחילה חליו למעט מן אוכל וככלות החליו להוסיף על האוכל.

Aphorism	Greek / tr. Jones	Donnolo	Asaf
II, 2	ὅκου παραφροσύνην ὕπνος παύει, ἀγαθόν. When sleep puts an end to delirium it is a good sign.	כל אדם אשר יש לו חולי חד והשתנה דעתו, _ויפול בחולי הנקרא פאראפרוסיכי [צ״ל פאראפרוסינין]_ הוא פרכוס, _וידבר בבלי דעת, אם ינום וינוח וישקוט החולה בתנומתו מן החולי אות טובה הוא._ ואם יכאב בחוליו וידבר בבלי דעת ופעם ינום ופעם תידד שנתו, וכאשר ינום ישקוד בפחד מידי תעורתו משנתו ועיניו מסוקרות סביב, רע הוא.	ואשר יראה לך כי יכאב במחלתו _וידבר בבלי דעת וינום_ וישקוד בפחד מדי תעורתו ועיניו מסקרות סביב, אות רעיון הוא לחולה.
II, 13	Ὁκόσοισι κρίσις γίνεται, τουτέοισιν ἡ νὺξ δύσφορος, ἡ πρὸ τοῦ παροξυσμοῦ, ἡ δὲ ἐπιοῦσα εὐφορωτέρη ὡς ἐπὶ τὸ πουλύ. When a crisis occurs, the night before the exacerbation is generally uncomfortable, the night after more comfortable.	וזה לך האות בכל חולה לדעת אם תמהר רפואתו לבוא. אם הלילה, אשר יהיה טרם יזיע תכבד ותגדיל ותקשה הקדחת והמצוקה להחזיק על החולה, ועת מוחרת [מחרת] למועד תהיה קלה לרוב וארוכה [וערובה] מאד בזיעת משפט טוב או באחד אות רפואה ומשפט, זה אות רפואה ממוהרת. כי כל אדם, אשר הוא מוכן להשפט מחוליו _כאשר יקרב ליום המשפט הלילה ההוא, אשר הוא קרוב ליום המשפט, תגדל המצוקה והקדחת על החלה, ובלילה השני, אשר יהיה לאחר יום המשפט, ייקל ויטב עד מאד, יותר מן הלילה שעברה,_ אם נשפט כמשפט—טוב ואות חיים.	זה לך האות בכל חולה לדעת אם תמהר רפואתו לבוא אם לא[:] הלילה אשר תהיה טרם יזיע תכבד ותקשה להחזיק על החולה ועת מחרת למועד הזה תהא קלה ועריבה מאד בזיעה.
II, 24	Τῶν ἑπτὰ ἡ τετάρτη ἐπίδηλος ἑτέρης ἑβδομάδος ἡ ὀγδόη ἀρχή, θεωρητὴ δὲ ἡ ἑνδεκάτη αὕτη γάρ ἐστι τετάρτη τῆς δευτέρης ἑβδομάδος θεωρητὴ δὲ πάλιν ἡ	_וזה לך אות פשר לדעת כי היום הרביעי לחולה יגיד מה יהיה ביום השביעי ויום השמיני הוא תחילת השבוע השני וראה עוד גם יום אחד עשר כי הוא יום רביעי לשבוע השני וראה עוד גם יום שבעה עשר_	_וזה לך הפשר לדבר כי היום לרביעי לחולה יגיד מה יהיה ביום השביעי והשמיני עד תחילת השבוע השני,_ והאות אשר יצדק בפשר ולא ימיר עד תום עשרים ואחד יום. אם יזיע ביום הרביעי גם בשביעי

Aphorism	Greek / tr. Jones	Donnolo	Asaf
	ἑπτακαιδεκάτῃ, αὕτη γάρ ἐστι τετάρτη μὲν ἀπὸ τῆς τεσσαρεσκαιδεκάτης, ἑβδόμη δὲ ἀπὸ τῆς ἑνδεκάτης.	<u>כי גם זה היום נחשב יום רביעי מיום ארבעה-עשר, תחשב עוד הזה שביעי מיום אחד עשר.</u> וראה עוד גם עשרים ואחד כי גם זה היום נחשב יום שביעי מיום שמונה עשר ונחשב עוד היום הזה יום שביעי מיום ט׳ וזהו סוף השבוע בשלישי. והאות אשר יצדק בפשר החלאים החדים ולא ימיר עד תום ארבעה עשר יום ואם לא יכנעו וישפטו להשפל בארבעה עשר יום, יאריכו עד קץ שנים עשר עד תום עשרים ואחד יום. אם יזיע החולה זיעת משפט טוב ביום השביעי, יזיע בזיעה טובה ואות משפט טוב, דע כי לקץ השבועיים ירפא ויקום.	יזיע ואם יזיע בשביעי לקץ השבועיים ירפא ויקום.
	The fourth day is indicative of the seven; the eighth is the beginning of another week; the eleventh is to be watched as being the fourth day of the second week; again the seventeenth is to be watched, being the fourth from the fourteenth and the seventh from the eleventh.		
IV, 1	τὰς κυούσας φαρμακεύειν, ἢν ὀργᾷ, τετράμηνα καὶ ἄχρι ἑπτὰ μηνῶν, ἧσσον δὲ ταύτας· τὰ δὲ νήπια καὶ τὰ πρεσβύτερα εὐλαβέεσθαι χρή.	אשה הרה אל תשקנה כל משקה תרופה חזק, ואם תעבור על המצווה, דע כי ימות הוולד בבטנה או תפיל נפל או יהא אסון, אך אחת מהרבה תמלט. <u>והנשים ההרות הצריכות לשתות משקה לכבס, אם יהיה קרבם לח ובטנם רך, השקם ממלאות ארבעה חדשים או עד מלאות שבעה חדשים, כי ראוי להישמר בילדים בתחילת ההריון, כשהם קטנים, ובעת הקרובים להוולד, כשהם גדולים.</u> ויש אשר ירפא ההריות מתחילת ההריון עד מלאות ארבעה חדשים. ואם תשתה האשה כל דבר משקה ותפיל בעת ההיא, דע כי המשקה הפיל את הוולד. ואם מת הוולד במעיה ולא יוצא החוצה, השקנה המשקה להפילו.	אשה הרה אל תשקה כל משתה תרופה. ואם תעבור על המצוה, דע כי ימות הילד במעיה, או אסון יהיה. אך אחת מהרבה תימלט. ויש אשר ירפאו הנשים ההריות מתחילת ההריון עד מלאת ד׳ חדשים. ואם תפיל האשה בשנה ההיא ששתה כל דבר משתה, דע כי המשתה הפיל הילד. ואם מת הילד במעיה ולא יצא חוץ, השקה אותה משתה להפילו.
	Purge pregnant women, should there be orgasm, from the fourth to the seventh month, but these last less freely; the unborn child, in the first and last stages of pregnancy, should be treated very cautiously.		

Aphorism	Greek / tr. Jones	Donnolo	Asaf

IV, 36

Greek / tr. Jones:

ἱδρῶτες πυρεταίνουσιν ἢν
ἄρξωνται, ἀγαθοὶ τριταῖοι,
καὶ πεμπταῖοι, καὶ
ἑβδομαῖοι, καὶ ἐναταῖοι,
καὶ ἑνδεκαταῖοι, καὶ
τεσσαρεσκαιδεκαταῖοι,
καὶ ἑπτακαιδεκαταῖοι,
καὶ μιῇ καὶ εἰκοστῇ, καὶ
ἑβδόμῃ καὶ εἰκοστῇ,
καὶ τριηκοστῇ πρώτῃ,
καὶ τριηκοστῇ τετάρτῃ·
οὗτοι γὰρ οἱ ἱδρῶτες
νούσους κρίνουσιν· οἱ
δὲ μὴ οὕτω γινόμενοι
πόνον σημαίνουσι
καὶ μῆκος νούσου καὶ
ὑποτροπιασμούς.

Sweats in a fever case are
beneficial if they begin
on the third day, the
fifth, the seventh, the
ninth, the eleventh, the
fourteenth, the seven-
teenth, the twenty-first,
the twenty-seventh,
the thirsty-first and the
thirsty-fourth, for these
sweats bring diseases to
a crisis. Sweats occurring
on other days indicate
pain, a long disease and
relapses.

Donnolo:

כל הזיעות שנקדחים
המתחילות לטובה ולהקל
הקדחת טובות המה. כי אם
יזיעו הנקדחים ביום השלישי
לחולי או ביום חמשי או ביום
ז׳ או ביום תשיעי, או ביום
י״א, או ביום י״ד, או ביום
י״ז או ביום עשרים ואחד, או
ביום כ״ד, או ביום עשרים
ושבע, או ביום ל׳ וא׳, או
ביום שלשים וארבעה, או
ביום ל׳ וז׳ או ביום ארבעים
ואחד, אלה הזיעות שופטות
החלאים להשקיטם ולהסירם
מעל החולה, ואם לא תהיינה
הזיעות האלה כאשר כתוב
בתחילת הדבר הזה להתחיל
לטובה להקל, כי אם יזיע
החולה ותשקוט הזיעה
והקדחת והחולי עומדת
בחזקתה, ולא חודלים, דע
כי אלה הזיעות מעידות על
אותות מכאוב ואורך חולי
ימים רבים ותהפוכות בגוף
בחולי הפכפך ושירפון.

Asaf:

אדם שתאחזנו קדחת בו, אם
יזיע ביום השלישי או בחמישי
או בשביעי או בתשיעי או
באחד עשר או בארבעה-
עשר או בעשרים ואחד או
בשלושים, כל זה יגיד על
אותות חולי מאריך ימים בחלי
הפכפך ושרפון.

V, 13

Greek / tr. Jones:

ὁκόσοι αἷμα ἀφρῶδες
ἀναπτύουσι, τουτέοισιν ἐκ
τοῦ πλεύμονος ἡ τοιαύτη
ἀναγωγὴ γίνεται.

When patients spit
up frothy blood, the
discharge comes from
the lungs.

Donnolo:

כל אדם אשר ירוק מפיהו דם
בקצף, או אם יקיא דם, דע כי
מן הריאה הוא עולה באין
כחש.

Asaf:

כל אדם שיקיא דם, הוא מן
הריאה באין כחש.

Bibliography

Sources

Ferre, Lola. "Donnolo's *Sefer ha-yaqar*: New Edition with English Translation." In *Sabbetay Donnolo: scienza e cultura ebraica nell'Italia del secolo X.*, Edited by Giancarlo Lacerenza. Naples: Università degli studi di Napoli L'Orientale, 2004. Pages 1–20.

Hippocrates, vol. 4. Loeb Classical Library. Edited and translated by W.H.S. Jones. London and Cambridge, Mass.: William Heinemann and Harvard University Press, 1931.

London, British Library, Or. 12252, transcribed by *Ma'agarim* project. The Academy of the Hebrew Language. Online: http://maagarim.hebrew-academy.org.il/Pages/PMain.aspx?misyzira=649001

Muntner, Suessmann. "Asaf ha-rofe, Sefer ha-refu'ot." *Koroth* 4 (1968): 389–443 and 531–573; *Koroth* 5 (1971): 435–473 and 603–649.

Steinschneider, Moritz. *Donnolo: Pharmakologische Fragmente aus dem zehnten Jahrhundert, nebst Beiträgen zur Literatur der Salernitaner hauptsächlich nach handschriftlichen hebräischen Quellen*. Berlin: Julius Benzian, 1868.

Literature

Kottek, Samuel. "Šabbetay Donnolo en tant que médecin: anatomie et physiologie dans le Sefer ḥakmônî." In *Sabbetay Donnolo: scienza e cultura ebraica nell'Italia del secolo X*. Edited by Giancarlo Lacerenza. Naples: Università degli studi di Napoli L'Orientale, 2004. Pages 21–44.

Lieber, Elinor. "Asaf's *Book of Medicines*: A Hebrew Encyclopedia of Greek and Jewish Medicine, Possibly Compiled in Byzantium on an Indian Model." *Dumbarton Oaks Papers* 38 (1984): 233–249.

Mancuso, Piergabriele. *Shabbatai Donnolo's Sefer Hakhmoni*. Leiden: Brill, 2010.

Melzer, Aviv. *"Asaph the Physician."* Ph. D. Diss. The University of Wisconsin, Madison, 1972.

Muntner, Suessmann. *Mavo le-Sefer Asaf ha-rofe* (Introduction to the Book of Asaf the Physician). Jerusalem: Geniza, 1957.

—. "Be'iqvot ktav yad hadash [B. M. 12252] le-Sefer Asaf ha-rofe" ["Following a new manuscript of *Sefer Asaf ha-rofe*"]. *Koroth* 4 (1969): 731–736.

Sharf, Andrew. *The Universe of Shabbetai Donnolo*. Warminster: Aris and Phillips, 1976.

Joseph Shatzmiller, "Doctors and Medical Practices in Germany around the Year 1200: The Evidence of *Sefer Asaph*." *PAAJR* 50 (1983): 149–164.

Steinschneider, Moritz. "Asaf." *Hebraeische Bibliographie* 12 (1872): 85–88.

—. "Zur medicinischen Literatur: 4. Asaf." *Hebraeische Bibliographie* 19 (1879): 35–38, 64–70, 84–89, 105–109.

—. *Donnolo: Pharmakologische Fragmente aus dem zehnten Jahrhundert, nebst Beiträgen zur Literatur der Salernitaner hauptsächlich nach handschriftlichen hebräischen Quellen*. Berlin: Julius Benzian, 1868.

Venetianer, Ludwig [Lajos]. *Assaf Judaeus: Der aelteste medizinische Schriftsteller in hebraeischer Sprache*. Straßburg: Karl J. Tübner, 1916.

Visi, Tamás. "Medieval Hebrew Uroscopic Texts: The Reception of Greek Uroscopic Texts in the Hebrew Book of Remedies Attributed to Asaf." In *Texts in Transit in the Medieval Mediterranean*. Edited by Y. Tzvi Langermann and Robert G. Morrison. University Park, Pennsylvania: Pennsylvania State University Press, 2016. Pages 162–196.

Nu'mān al-Isrā'īlī and his Commentary to Abū Sahl al-Masīḥī's *Kitāb al-Mi'a* ("Book of the Hundred")

Y. Tzvi Langermann

I have three objectives to achieve in this brief paper. The first and most relevant objective for the theme of this volume is to add another name to the already very distinguished roster of medieval Jewish physicians and/or medical writers. In fact, I find it prudent to distinguish between individuals who are known to have been practicing physicians and those who have left us a contribution to the medical literature, without, however, there being any information about their biographies. We tend to assume, and surely this is generally a correct assumption, that those people who wrote books on medicine were practicing physicians. However, arch-skeptic that I am, I would like to see evidence for this, for example, in case histories which are noted in the books and monographs that these people wrote. More importantly, it may be the case that the books and medical texts present a theory that was not always put into practice precisely as described in the texts. I am glad to see that Max Meyerhof, himself both a practicing physician and historian of medicine, was alert to this distinction.[1] As for Nu'mān, the subject of this paper: he certainly was well-informed, and deeply interested in, theory; but so far—and I must emphasize that I have studied only a portion of the unique manuscript—I have not come across any references to his own practice.

The other two objectives do not concern the history of Jewish participation in the medical profession in any special way, but they are of no little significance. They concern two areas where the book I wish to speak about makes an important contribution to the history of medicine; hence, one can surely say that these additional tidbits indicate how important texts written by Jews are for the history of medicine in general. One is the reception of Ibn Sīnā's *al-Qānūn fī al-Ṭibb*, perhaps the most influential medical textbook ever written. If and when its reception history is told fully and properly, the story must include people like Nu'mān, who rejected Ibn Sīnā's masterpiece. Nu'mān, as we shall see, preferred earlier medical authorities; this trait was shared by the few others who also did not care much for Ibn Sīnā's *Qānūn*. The other important feature is Nu'mān's very rich list of works cited, which includes a slew of recognizable texts that are not known to have survived and personalities whose work remains basically unknown.

---

1   Max Meyerhof, "Alī ibn Rabbān aṭ-Ṭabarī, ein persischer Arzt des 9. Jahrhunderts n. Chr.," *Zeitschrift der Deutschen Morgenländischen Gesellschaft* 85 (1931): 38–68; see esp. 60, where Meyerhof describes al-Ṭabarī's *Firdaws* as a literary composition which does not give the impression that the author was involved in the actual practice of medicine.

DOI: 10.13173/9783447108263.337

Let me begin by introducing Nu'mān al-Isrā'īlī, author of a book-length commentary to *Kitāb al-Mi'a* ("Book of the Hundred"), the comprehensive medical textbook of Abū Sahl al-Masīḥī (960–1000 C.E.).[2] His full name is Nu'mān bin Abī al-Riḍā' bin Sālim bin Isḥāq. I can find no more identifying marks on this person or his oeuvre that concern his Jewishness, other than the epithet al-Isrā'īlī; but that, of course, is enough. Moritz Steinschneider devoted a few paragraphs to Nu'mān in his book on Arabic writings by Jewish authors.[3] Steinschneider speculates that our author may be the same Nu'mān who was the teacher of an author of a book on rheumatism, written around 1388. Moreover, through a line of reasoning that I cannot follow, Steinschneider also suggests that Nu'mān was the teacher of Salāḥ al-Dīn of Ḥamā, the purported author of an important book on ophthalmology.[4] These data, if correct, would locate Nu'mān in Syria sometime during the thirteenth century.

Nu'mān's book survives in a unique copy, possibly an autograph, in MS Paris, BNF arabe 2883 (= suppl. 1024), filling 207 folia.[5] In this short report I would like to give a general assessment, as well as sharing with the reader a few more gems that I have so far dug out of his book.

Fortunately, the unique copy is complete, very legible, and accurate. The full title of his work is *al-Ḥawāshiy al-Nu'māniyya li-l-Maqāṣid al-Ṭibbiyya* ("Nu'mānian Marginalia to the Medical Objectives"). *Al-Ḥawāshiy* (singular: *ḥāshiyya*) literally means "marginalia", notes that are written in the margin; but this title is misleading. It is indeed likely that the *al-Ḥawāshiy* originated in notes that Nu'mān scrawled in the margins of his copy of *Kitāb al-Mi'a*, as, indeed, many or most commentaries began their careers. If so, however, Nu'mān later collected and edited them, so that the final product, the text preserved in the manuscript at Paris, is not a series of glosses, but really a well-organized book; and its aim is not simply to clarify, but rather to expound on the meaning(s), purport(s), and objectives—all three are valid translations of *maqāṣid*—of topics within the field of medicine. There is an introduction, in which Nu'mān informs us of his motivations in writing the commentary, and something of his method as well. A list of chapter headings is also provided.

---

2   Al-Masīḥī's book has been edited by Floréal Sanagustin, *Le livre des cent questions en médecine, d'Abū Sahl ʿĪsā ibn Yaḥyā al-Masīḥī,* vol. II (Damascus: Institut Français de Damas, 2000).

3   Moritz Steinschneider, *Die arabische Literatur der Juden* (Frankfurt am Main: J. Kauffmann, 1902), entry 189, p. 246, making use of a short entry on Nu'mān in Lucien Leclerc, *Histoire de la médecine arabe,* vol. II, (Paris: Leroux, 1876), 319.

4   Salāḥ al-Dīn was identified scholars of the nineteenth century as the author of the rich compendium entitled *Nūr al-ʿUyūn wa-jāmiʿ al-funūn*; this identification is still maintained by Manfred Ullmann in his highly authoritative *Der Medizin im Islam* (Leiden: Brill, 1970), 13. The author of that book is now thought to be Abū Zakarriyā' Yaḥyā ibn Abī al-Rajā'; see Gregor Schoeler, "Der Verfasser der Augenheilkunde *K. Nūr al-ʿUyūn,*" *Der Islam* 64 (1987): 89–97.

5   It seems to be William MacGuckin baron de Slane, *Catalogue des manuscrits arabes,* (Paris: Imprimerie nationale, 1883–1895, 518–519, who first suggested that the copy is an autograph. Though the handwriting is neater than the norm for autographs, I still think the suggestion to be plausible.

When I first came across the entry on Nuʿmān in Steinschneider's book, I was struck by the very idea that someone living (as we suppose) in the thirteenth century would bother to write a commentary on *Kitāb al-Miʾa*. True, in its day Abū Sahl's book was an important text, and Abū Sahl himself, as Nuʿmān writes, was the teacher of the great Ibn Sīnā.[6] However, like just about all of the other earlier medical compendia, *Kitāb al-Miʾa* was superseded by Ibn Sīnā's *al-Qānūn fī al-Ṭibb*, which is certainly the most important medical book written in the medieval period, and one of the most repercussive medical works of all times. Many dozens, perhaps hundreds, of copies of the *Qānūn* exist, and so also many commentaries, some filling several volumes; there are several condensations, and commentaries to the condensations, and glosses to the commentaries to the condensations; there are translations into Hebrew and Latin, and commentaries in both languages; the list goes on and on. Over thirty copies exist of the Arabic text transcribed into Hebrew letters.

All of these statistics are meant to show that Ibn Sīnā's book came to dominate the medical profession like no other. However, Ibn Sīnā's book also met with some criticism and rejection. The Andalusian physicians as a rule despised it. Abū al-ʿAlāʾ Ibn Zuhr (d. 1131) is said to have found it useful only for the scraps of paper that he tore from the margins in order to write prescriptions.[7] Ibn Rushd has some harsh criticism of Ibn Sīnā's remarks on the theriac in his monograph on that remedy and in his *Kulliyāt* as well.[8] References to the *Qānūn* are conspicuously absent from Maimonides' medical writings.

Elsewhere I have suggested that the negative attitude of the Andalusian physicians to Ibn Sīnā's *Qānūn* was part of a comprehensive movement to distance themselves from the intellectual products of the Islamic East, and to construct their own alternative.[9] This does not mean, however, that the 'easterners' unanimously welcomed the *Qānūn*. Fakhr al-Dīn al-Rāzī, author of a critical commentary to Ibn Sīnā's *al-*

---

6   See note 13 below.
7   Albert Z. Iskandar, "A catalogue of Arabic manuscripts on medicine and science," in *Wellcome Historical Medical Library, vol. 2* (London: Wellcome Historical Medical Library, 1967), 36, quoting from Ibn Jumayʿ.
8   In his monograph Ibn Rushd disputes Ibn Sīnā's claim that the theriac assists the innate heat to heal all diseases, and works to preserve the health in all of the organs; see his *Kitāb al-Tiryāq* in *Rasāʾil Ibn Rushd al-Ṭibbiyya* (ed. Georges C. Anawati and Saʿīd Zāyed; Cairo: Centre de l'édition de l'héritage culturel, 1987), 397–398. The closest passage in the *Qānūn* to the one cited by Ibn Rushd is the statement in the fifth book of the *Qānūn*, (vol. 3, p. 311 in the *Būlāq* edition): "It [the theriac] effects these actions only by means of the special property of its form, which follows upon [or: is superadded to] the mixture of its components, insofar as it strengthens the pneuma and the innate heat, and it thereby assists nature against the chilling and heating contraries." Ibn Rushd spells out his differences with Ibn Sīnā with regard to compound drugs in general in *Al-Kulliyyāt fī al-Ṭibb li-Ibn Rushd* (eds. S. Shaybān and U. al-Ṭālibī; Cairo, Centre de l'édition de l'héritage culturel, 1989), 314.
9   Y. Tzvi Langermann, "Another Andalusian Revolt? Ibn Rushd's Critique of the Pharmacological Computus of al-Kindi," in *The Enterprise of Science in Islam* (ed. A.I. Sabra and J.P. Hogendijk; Cambridge, MA: M.I.T. Press, 2003), 351–372, here: 366–367.

Ishārāt wa-l-Tanbīhāt, also penned a critical commentary to the *Qānūn*.[10] ʿAbd al-Laṭīf al-Baghdādī viewed with scorn the effect the *Qānūn* had on medical education. According to him, physicians of his age learned by rote portions of the *Qānūn*, then recited them at the top of their voices in disputations, thinking that this is sufficient preparation for healing the sick. Though he preferred the ancients, Hippocrates and Galen, ʿAbd al-Laṭīf did have a high opinion of some later works, among them *Kitāb al-Miʾa*.[11]

Nuʿmān begins his commentary with an explanation why he has chosen to focus upon *Kitāb al-Miʾa* rather than the *Qānūn*. Though he ranks Ibn Sīnā among the greatest physicians, in the same class as Galen though not as excellent as he was, Nuʿmān accuses him of writing in an imprecise manner; and he notes that his work has drawn criticism. (I suspect that he has in mind the critical glosses of Fakhr al-Dīn al-Rāzī, but at the moment I have no evidence for this.) Abū Sahl al-Masīḥī, by contrast, is highly regarded by Nuʿmān's colleagues in the medical profession, who unfortunately are not named:

> Now [it is true of] many of the ancient doctors known for their excellence (*faḍl*) and famous for their knowledge, such as the outstanding physician Galen, the *raʾīs* Ibn Sīnā, and those like him, that each one of them set out to expend his effort and devote his attention to a certain composition. He (*scilicet*, each one) was determined to write it such that he would perfect and bring to completion the art that he set his design upon. Further, people by nature love themselves. The *shaykh* and *raʾīs* (Ibn Sīnā), despite his mastery and majestic capability, used many ambivalent words. People have cast doubt upon many places, which require elucidation.

Nuʿmān also hints that Ibn Sīnā included in his *Qānūn* materials that are superfluous. He continues:

> As for the outstanding physician [Galen], his discourse is too long, even if it is like a string of pearls; covering his sixteen books there is the *Kitāb al-Shukūk* of al-Rāzī,[12] and so also on the divine Hippocrates [...] One hardly finds a positive consensus concerning his work. But I have heard my colleagues who have achieved something in the science of medicine acknowledge the philosopher Abū Sahl ʿĪsā bin Yaḥyā al-Masīḥī, who is known for a writing on medicine; it is called *Kitāb al-Miʾa*, because it comprises one hundred books. Not one of those excellent [colleagues] has found the author of that book to go astray on a single [point], because he towered above the people of his time. That is because

---

10 I discuss his critique of the *Qānūn* in Y. Tzvi Langermann, "Criticism of Authority in Moses Maimonides and Fakhr al-Din al-Razi," *Early Science and Medicine* 7 (2002): 255–275.

11 Samuel M. Stern, "A Collection of Treatises by ʿAbd al-Laṭīf al-Baghdādī," *Islamic Studies* 1 (1962): 53–70, here: 62.

12 This is the "Book of Doubts", a wide ranging critique of Galen written by Abū Bakr al-Rāzī (fl. late ninth century), not to be confused with the twelfth century theologian and philosopher Fakhr al-Dīn al-Rāzī mentioned earlier; see Shlomo Pines, "Razi, critique de Galien," in *Actes du Septième Congrès International d'Histoire des Science* (Jerusalem, 1953), 480–487.

he brought together in his book branches [of knowledge] that the physician requires as well as confirmations [proofs] that the science of medicine cannot do without, without bringing in that which is extraneous.

Also, they have reported that *al-shaykh al-raʾīs* (Ibn Sīnā) was a student of his.[13] I desired to benefit from his [al-Masīḥī's] knowledge, and quickly acquired this book and studied it. I found it to be superior to most of the books on medicine. It comprises the cream of medical concepts as well as their clarification, leaving out that which is of no use.[14]

Here ends Nuʿmān's encomium to *Kitāb al-Miʾa*. What follows is an introduction to his own work which, despite its modest title, is really a well-organized *vademecum* designed to provide the physician with the basic knowledge which he must always be able to access, as swiftly and easily as possible. Nuʿmān begins by noting the vast amount of information that the physician must possess, a point emphasized by others as well, including Maimonides:

> Indeed, the ultimate purpose of medical science is to attain the improvement of every human soul in general, as well as to procure knowledge of individuals in particular; and the knowledge of the temperament of each and every one of the organs, in all of the diversity of their rankings and differences; and the relationship of one to the other [2b]. But this cannot be attained without knowledge of principles that are intimately bound to the mind; but the mind may be incapable of attaining some of these concepts, which must be present [to the mind] when he [the physician] looks for them, let alone all of them...[15]

The necessary information fills books which the doctor simply cannot carry with him everywhere he goes. To bolster this point, Nuʿmān cites Galen twice. The first citation is actually a citation of Aristotle, adduced by Galen in book ten of *On the Agreement of Hippocrates and Plato*, a book whose Arabic translation is not extant in its entirety; I discuss it in the final section of this paper. The second comes from Galen's commentary to Hippocrates' *On the Acute Diseases*. With all of this mind, Nuʿmān has decided to

> collect from the *diwān* [i.e. *Kitāb al-Miʾa*] and other books, the excellence of whose authors is not in dispute, concerning a number of issues, to the extent that I have had access to them [those books], so that it may accompany me as a sort of memoir for that which I require; it can be depended upon for the commendable principles of medicine.[16]

---

13 Though Ibn Sīnā generally boasts of being self-taught, there are reports that he studied with two physicians, one of them being al-Masīḥī; see Dimitri Gutas, *Avicenna and the Aristotelian tradition: introduction to reading Avicenna's philosophical works, second, revised and enlarged edition* (Leiden: Brill, 2014), note 20 on p. 16.

14 MS Paris ar. 2883, ff. 1b–2a.

15 Ibid, 2a–2b.

16 Ibid., 2b–3a.

In brief, then, his book is not really a commentary to *Kitāb al-Mi'a*, let alone a collection of marginalia. Nor should it be surprising that a *vademecum* gives so much space to theory, including the physics and physiology that underlie medical practice. Especially when in the service of potentates, there would often be more than one physician charged with the care of the patient, and there would be disagreement as to the proper course of action. The physician would find it helpful to be able to back up his diagnosis with some basic theory, including source references.[17]

Nu'mān's *al-Ḥawāshiy*, then, is a concise compendium of medical knowledge, arranged according to the chapters of *Kitāb al-Mi'a* and drawing primarily from that book, but supplemented with citations from a wide variety of other texts. Indeed, not a few chapters (for example, chapter eight, on the natural faculties) skip over *Kitāb al-Mi'a* completely, presenting instead Nu'mān's own synopsis of the topic, followed by an array of sources. Nu'mān states clearly that he will name his sources, and he carries through on this promise. Moreover, the additional sources do not always support or elucidate al-Masīḥī; some are critical towards him. The practical chapters of the "great *diwān*" (Nu'mān's epithet for *Kitāb al-Mi'a*) are supplemented with tried and tested remedies, those which are readily obtainable even by the poor. Nu'mān ends his introduction with a wish and a prayer (4a): "We hope to achieve for ourselves useful knowledge and productive practice, in this world and the next, from He Who possesses power and might, God Most High willing."

Historians of medicine will certainly appreciate the importance of Nu'mān's *al-Ḥawāshiy* as a repertoire of ancient and medieval sources which, in the original or in Arabic translation, are as yet unattested. I will now display three passages which serve to illustrate this feature. I have not been able to give each of these passages the thorough treatment they warrant; but even the preliminary account offered here should, I think, be a non-trivial addition to the history of medicine.

1 (MS Paris ar. 2883, f. 2b, ll. 7–11) Galen, *On the Agreement of Hippocrates and Plato*, book ten

Ḥunayn ibn Isḥāq describes in some detail his translation of this Galenic tract.[18] In his essay on his own writings, Galen tells us that this work is divided into nine books, and, indeed, there are only nine books in the Greek manuscript tradition. According to Ḥunayn, however, the book contains ten sections. A relatively long citation from book ten is cited in al-Fārābī's treatise on rhetoric, an appropriate venue, since the passage concerns the art of argumentation.[19] The passage copied by Nu'mān is actually a

---

17 In his letter to his disciple Yosef ben Yehudah, Maimonides gives this as the reason he studied books on medicine every evening: "For you know long and difficult this art is for someone who is conscientious and fastidious, and who does not wish to say anything without first knowing its proof, its source and the type of reasoning involved"; the translation is cited from my "Maimonides' Repudiation of Astrology," *Maimonidean Studies* 2 (1991): 123–158, esp. 137–138.

18 Concerning the Arabic translation of this work, which is not extant, see Manfred Ullmann, *Die Medizin im Islam* (Leiden: Brill, 1970), 40, 12.

19 For a full discussion of the Arabic translation and citation of relevant passages in Galen see

citation of Aristotle that is brought by way of Galen. I have not been able to trace the saying ascribed to Aristotle. The import of the saying is this: even though not every problem can be solved by reason, an answer may yet be found in sensory data. This notion fits the approach of the Stagirite, as elaborated, *inter alia*, at the very end of the *Posterior Analytics*.

نقل جالينوس عن ارسطوطاليس من المقالة العاشرة من اراء ابقراط وافلاطن قال ليس كل
ما يطالب به الانسان يحتاج الى جواب بل من الأشياء أشياء كثيرة تحتاج في الإجابة عنها
الى الحس

Galen transmitted in the name of Aristotle, in the tenth book of *On the Doctrines* of Hippocrates and Plato. He said: 'Not everything that a person seeks must have an answer; rather, there are many things the answer to which must [be sought by appeal] to sensation'...

2 (MS Paris ar. 2883, f. 3a, ll. 17–21) Arkhelaos, Commentary to Galen's *Therapeutics for Glaucon*

This passage was noticed already by Leclerc, who, however, has nothing more to say than this: "Ajoutons que l'on trouve cité un commentaire d'Archelaüs sur le Livre à Glaucon."[20] The name of the commentator appears in our manuscript as Arselaos (with a sign over the *sīn* indicating that it is to read as *sīn*, not *shīn*, as Leclerc would have it; but, as we shall see, it probably was transmitted elsewhere with the letter *shīn*);[21] but I think that Leclerc is correct in his identification. We possess a few fragments of medical writings by a certain Arkhelaos; though those studied thus far are not related to Galen's *Therapeutics*, Arkhelaos appears to have been steeped in the Galenic tradition. In one manuscript his name appears between those of Palladios and Stephanos of Alexandria, which, as Touaide suggests, may indicate that he belonged to the same group of "ancient physicians" from Alexandria.[22] I would like to carry this further, and propose to identify Arkhelaos with the mysterious Anqilāʾus, one of the medical authorities singled out by Ibn Abī Usaybiʾa in connection with the preparation of the so-called "Alexandrian summaries" of the core curriculum of Galenic texts.[23] Irvine and Temkin take up, and then rightly reject, the identification of Anqilāʾus with another of the five writers of the summaries, Akilaos, because the error in transcription is difficult to explain.[24] Not so, however, for Anqilāʾus: in my analysis, the *rāʾ* was

---

Phillip de Lacy, ed. and trans., *Galen on the Doctrines of Hippocrates and Plato* (Berlin: Akademie-Verlag, 1978), 42–46.

20 Leclerc, vol. II, 319.

21 On the *Ihmāl* and its implication see J.J. Witkam, "The Neglect Neglected. To Point or not to Point, that Is the question," *Journal of Islamic Manuscripts* 6 (2015): 376–408.

22 Alain Touwaide, "Arkhelaos," in *The Encyclopedia of Ancient Natural Scientists* (eds. Paul Keyser and Georgia L. Irby-Massive; London and New York: Routledge, 2008), 157–158.

23 The passage is translated from the edition of August Müller, Königsberg, vol. 1, 1884, p. 103 , by Judith T. Irvine and Owsei Temkin, "Who was Akilaos? A problem in medical historiography," *Bulletin of the History of Medicine* 77 (2003): 12–24, here: 12.

24 Irvine and Temkin, "Who was Akilaos?," especially 19.

joined, or looked to be joined, to the *shīn* which follows, and the three dots on top of the (usually) three *kursī*'s of the *shīn* were read separately, one providing the *nūn* and the other two, the *qāf*.

قال ارسلاوس في تفسيره لاغلوقن ان ابقراط وان كان قد تقادم زمانه جدا فان قوله ثابتا ولو
كنا نحن القائلين لذلك لم نكن لنصدق لان حسد اهل زماننا هذا يمنعهم ان يقيلون قولنا
فلذلك احتجنا الى شهادة القدماء

Arkhelaos said in his commentary to Glaucon that Hippocrates, even if his epoch is very ancient, what he says is yet enduring. But were we to be the ones saying it, we would not hold it to be true, because the jealousy of the people of our times does not allow them to accept what we say. For this reason, we need the testimony of times past.[25]

3   A passage from Plato, *Timaeus* (MS Paris ar. 2883, ff. 19b, l. 21–20, l. 3), on colours

قال افلاطن في طماوس واذا خلط الاشقر باللون الاسود حدث اللون العرابي هو اللون
الاخضر الذي هو صنف يتكون من الكراثي والمرة الحمراء اذا احترقت واحتدت جدا وصارت
على لون الزنجار وطبيعته

Plato said in *Timaeus* that when the colour blond (*al-ashqar*)[26] is mixed with the colour black, there is produced the colour *ʿarābī*. It is the color green (*akhḍar*), which is a type that comes about from the leek-like (*al-kurrāthī*) [colour]. When red bile is inflamed and very agitated, it takes on the colour of verdigris (*zinjār*) and its nature.

This passage is part of a long discussion on the colors of the humors, which certainly deserves to be studied in its entirety. I can here offer only a few remarks about the colors in the citation exhibited above; my analysis of even this segment is far from exhaustive, but it should contribute something towards the subject.

Plato discusses the mixing of colors in his *Timaeus* 68C. Nuʿmān uses three different words in an attempt to capture the particular shade of green that results from the mixture of blond and black. There appears to be good reason for this. The mixture of blond—or tawny, as Cornford renders πυρρός; Archer-Hind prefers "chestnut"—and black looks to be, on the basis of Cornford's translation and notes, the most problematical—and perhaps for this reason, the most interesting. The first color named by Nuʿmān is *aʿrābī*. I think it safe to assume that this is the translation of πράσιος that has reached Nuʿmān; the other two words are meant to clarify its meaning. According

---

25 I have copied out the Arabic exactly as it is in the manuscript; there are not a few obvious spelling errors which need not deter us.

26 On *al-ashqar* as blond, see A. I. Sabra, *The Optics of Ibn al-Haytham. Books I–III, On Direct Vision*, vol. II; (London: Warburg Institute, 1989), 42; cf. Ibid., 41, concerning some Arabic words for different shades of green—but the two mentioned in our passage are not mentioned there.

to Dozy, *aʿrābī* refers to "l'une des deux espèces du (Nymphae Lotus)". Bashnīn or Nymphae Lotus name the Egyptian white water-lily.

Conford renders this mixture, "tawny and black, in green (?)". In his note *ad locum*, Conford observes, "πράσιος is commonly taken to mean green like the leek (πράσον) ... If green in meant, the statement is not much more surprising than that the addition of black to red should produce a 'bilious' color (83B) ...".[27]

It is remarkable that Cornford cites here the passage from *Timaeus* 83 B which, in Nuʿmān's citation, runs together with 68 C. The passage reads, in Cornford's translation: "Or again, a yellow colour may be combined with the bitterness when the flesh decomposed by the fire of the inflammation is of recent formation. To all of these, the common name 'bile' has been given ..."[28]

Nuʿmān arrives ultimately at the shade of green associated with the leek, but unlike Plato (in Cornford's interpretation), it is not used to name directly the product of the mixture. It is, as noted, preceded by two other words, *aʿrābī*, discussed above, and *akhḍar*, the most usual Arabic word for green. Indeed, in Galen's epitome of the *Timaeus*, which survives only in Arabic, *akhḍar* is the only color named: "When the color blond (*ashqar*) is mixed with the color black, the color green (*akhḍar*) is produced from the two of them".[29]

There were practical applications for color theory in medicine, though these do not interest Nuʿmān.

Galen tells us in his *On the doctrines of Hippocrates and Plato*, Book VIII 5, 9–12, that Hippocrates would diagnose "the states of the body from the colors of the tongue"; and Diogenes of Apollonia used the color of the patient as a diagnostic tool, asserting that it reveals the dominant humor.[30] Plato's theory of color played an important role in medieval uroscopy, especially in establishing the spectrum of colors that the urine may display.[31]

Each of the four humors was associated with a colour. This theoretical issue does attract Nuʿmān's attention, and he discusses it at length. In addition to the short snippet from the *Timaeus* which we have just looked at, he cites the monograph of Qusṭā bin Lūqā on humors, and Hippocrates' *On Acute Diseases*. As stated above, a full discussion of the entire section on color must wait for another occasion.

---

27 Francis MacDonald Cornford, *Plato's cosmology: the Timaeus of Plato* (London: Kegan Paul, 1937), and frequently reprinted; I consulted the Hackett paperback, Indianapolis-Cambridge, 1997, 278. Note that this same color also appears in Aristotle who, however, considers it to be a basic color, rather than a compound one. (*On Sensation* 442 a25; *Meteorology* 372 a8).

28 Cornford, *Plato's cosmology*, 338.

29 *Galeni Compendium Timaei Platonis, aliorumgue dialogorum synopsis quae extant fragmenta*: vol. I: Plato Arabus (ed. P. Kraus and R. Walzer; London, Warburg Institute, 1951), Arabic section, 22:12–13.

30 Katerina Ierodiakonou, "Empedocles on colour and colour vision," *Oxford Studies in Ancient Philosophy* 29 (2005): 1–37, here: 11.

31 Luigi Lorio and Mario Lamagna, "Byzantine doctrines on uroscopy in the *Liber Orinalibus* of Hermogenes (codex 69 Montecassino)," *Journal of Nephrology* 24 (2011): 103–107.

Bibliography

Sources

Rushd, Ibn. "Kitāb al-Tiryāq" in *Rasā'il Ibn Rushd al-Ṭibbiyya*. Edited by Georges C. Anawa-ti and Saʿīd Zāyed; Cairo: Centre de l'édition de l'héritage culturel, 1987. Pages 397–398.

Ibn Abī Usaybi'ah, *'Uyūn al-Anbā' fī Ṭabaqāt al-Aṭibbā'*, ed. August Müller, Konigsberg, 1884.

Ibn Rushd spells out his differences with Ibn Sīnā with regard to compound drugs in gener-al in *Al-Kulliyyāt fī al-Ṭibb li-Ibn Rushd,* S. Shaybān and U. al-Ṭālibī, eds. (Cairo, 1989), p. 314.

Kraus, Paul and Richard Walzer. *Plato Arabus*. Volume I. London: Warburg Institute, 1951.

Sabra, Abdelhamid I. *The Optics of Ibn al-Haytham. Books I–III, On Direct Vision*. Vol-ume. II. London: Warburg Institute, 1989.

Literature

Gutas, Dimitri. *Avicenna and the Aristotelian tradition: introduction to reading Avicenna's phil-osophical works, second, revised and enlarged edition*. Leiden: Brill, 2014.

Ierodiakonou, Katerina. "Empedocles on colour and colour vision." *Oxford Studies in Ancient Philosophy* 29 (2005): 1–37.

Irvine, Judith T. and Owsei Temkin. "Who was Akilaos? A problem in medical historiogra-phy." *Bulletin of the History of Medicine* 77 (2003): 12–24.

Iskandar, Albert Z. "A catalogue of Arabic manuscripts on medicine and science." In *Wellcome Historical Medical Library.Vol. 2*. London: Wellcome Historical Medical Library, 1967.

Langermann, Y. Tzvi. "Maimonides' Repudiation of Astrology." *Maimonidean Studies* 2 (1991): 123–158, and 137–138.

—."Criticism of Authority in Moses Maimonides and Fakhr al-Din al-Razi." *Early Science and Medicine* 7 (2002): 255–275.

—."Another Andalusian Revolt? Ibn Rushd's Critique of the Pharmacological Computus of al-Kindi." In *The Enterprise of Science in Islam*. Edited by A. I. Sabra and J. P. Hogendijk. Cambridge, MA: M.I.T. Press, 2003. Pages 351–372 and 366–367.

Leclerc, Lucien. *Histoire de la médecine arabe: exposé complet des trad. du grec; les sciences en Orient, leur transmission à l'Occident par les traductions latines*. vol. II. Paris: Leroux, 1876.

Lorio, Luigi and Mario Lamagna. "Byzantine doctrines on uroscopy in the *Liber Orinalibus* of Hermogenes (codex 69)." *Journal of Nephrology* 24 (2011): 103–107.

MacDonald Cornford, Francis. *Plato's cosmology: the Timaeus of Plato*. Indianapolis-Cam-bridge: Hackett, 1997.

Meyerhof, Max. "Alī ibn Rabbān aṭ-Ṭabarī, ein persischer Arzt des 9. Jahrhunderts n. Chr." *Zeitschrift der Deutschen Morgenländischen Gesellschaft* 85 (1931): 38–68.

Pines, Schlomo. "Razi, critique de Galien." In *Actes du Septième Congrès International d'His-toire des Science*. Jéreusalem : 4–12 août 1953. Paris : Académie internationale d'histoire des sciences and Paris : Hermann. Pages 480–487.

Sanagustin, Floréal. *Le livre des cent questions en médecine, d'Abū Sahl 'Īsā ibn Yaḥyā al-Masīḥī*, 2 vol., Damascus: Institut Français de Damas, 2000.

Schoeler, Gregor. "Der Verfasser der Augenheilkunde K. Nūr al-'Uyūn." *Der Islam* 64 (1987): 89–97.

Slane, William MacGuckin baron de. *Catalogue des manuscrits arabes.* Paris: Imprimerie nationale, 1883–1895.

Steinschneider, Moritz. *Die arabische Literatur der Juden.* Frankfurt am Main: J. Kauffmann, 1902.

Stern, Samuel M. "A Collection of Treatises by ʿAbd al-Laṭīf al-Baghdādī." *Islamic Studies* 1 (1962): 53–70.

Touwaide, Alain. "Arkhelaos." In *The Encyclopedia of Ancient Natural Scientists.* Edited by Paul Keyser and Georgia L. Irby-Massive. London: Routledge, 2008. Pages 157–158.

Ullmann, Manfred. *Die Medizin im Islam.* Leiden: Brill, 1970.

Witkam, Jan J. "The Neglect Neglected. To Point or not to Point, that Is the question." *Journal of Islamic Manuscripts* 6 (2015): 376–408.

The Genesis of Medieval Hebrew Gynaecology:
A Preliminary Assessment[*]

Carmen Caballero Navas

This paper is a preliminary account of the progress of my work on the early stages of the reception and accommodation in Hebrew of literature and theories on female anatomy, physiology, and disease by medieval Jewish authors and translators. While the first steps of my research on the medieval Hebrew corpus of literature devoted to the care of women's health led me to specifically address the textual production and transmission of the later Middle Ages, in the course of my enquiry I have become progressively, and inevitably, interested in the beginning of these processes, and in the factors that prompted the production and dissemination of this type of literature.

The genesis of Hebrew gynaecology is intimately connected to the emergence of the Hebrew medical corpus. In the main, this is because the first Hebrew treatises on women's conditions purportedly ever produced were part of a major enterprise of translation of medical texts from Latin into Hebrew, undertaken by a translator known as 'Do'eg the Edomite,' who inaugurated the Hebrew medical corpus in the closing years of the twelfth century.[1] Furthermore, the inventory of translated texts, as well as the justification offered by the prolific translator in the prologue to his translation project, suggest that the gynaecological texts are to be understood (or were understood by him) as a 'medical specialty' encompassed in his (or his milieu's) understanding of medicine. It also suggests that the translation of the entire collection of texts was prompted by a similar concern: to make the medical corpus circulating in the West available to Jewish practitioners in order to help them keep up with contemporary trends in medicine.[2]

Albeit probably the first, *Do'eg*'s translations were not the only gynaecological texts to be made available in Hebrew in this initial phase. Around the same time, or slightly later, two other treatises were produced, associated with the Iberian Peninsula and strongly connected to the Arab medical tradition.[3]

---

[*] The research for this essay was carried out under the auspices of the research project *Language and Literature of Rabbinic and Medieval Judaism* (FFI2013–43813-P and FFI2016–78171-P), funded by the Spanish Ministry of Economy and Competitiveness. I am grateful to the anonymous referee of this essay who contributed valuable suggestions for corrections. My deepest gratitude to Monica Green for her generous advice and insightful comments on the draft version of this paper.

1 Cf. Barkai 1998; Freudenthal 2013.
2 Caballero Navas 2011a, 329–335; Freudenthal 2011a, 100–103.
3 Barkai 1998, 109–144 and 192–211, respectively. See also Caballero Navas 2019a.

DOI: 10.13173/9783447108263.349

After this remarkable beginning, and following a gap of some years, the second half of the thirteenth century bore witness to a second phase of fruitful production of gynaecological literature, based for the most part on translations from Arabic. In summary, while we know when and where the first Hebrew gynaecological treatises where produced, the factors that prompted their writing call for more investigation.

Certainly, gynaecology was one of the new trends in Latin medicine. During the so-called long twelfth century, processes of creation, diffusion, appropriation, and accommodation of literature on women's healthcare generated the Latin canon of gynaecological literature that circulated in the West until the end of the Middle Ages.[4] But it intrigues me that, if the interest of Jews in contemporary medical trends was mainly motivated by their aspiration to integrate Jewish medical practitioners into the legitimate medical system,[5] gynaecological texts—unlikely intended for male medical practice, at least at this early stage[6]—were incorporated into the incipient Hebrew medical corpus. Surely, there must have been other factors that prompted Jewish scholars from Christian milieus, who were unaware of the bulk of Greek gynaecology disseminated during late antiquity and the early Middle Ages both in Latin and Arabic,[7] to develop an interest in this sphere of medical knowledge.

The time frame between the closing years of the twelfth and the end of the thirteenth century is a key period for understanding the social and intellectual processes that determined the Jewish acquisition of medical knowledge and the integration of Jewish medical practitioners into the legitimate medical system.[8] Remarkably, nearly two-thirds of the known Hebrew texts on women's conditions were translated or written during this period.[9] Therefore, the analysis of the production and transmission of texts during this first stage may prove crucial to understanding what prompted the genesis of the textual corpus, and how it was formed and shaped.

The first focus of my study is the texts themselves. Hence, I have endeavoured to compile and describe a preliminary inventory, in which I have included treatises that circulated independently, as well as some sections on women's conditions within medical encyclopaedias that had a strong bearing on the formation of the Latin tradition of gynaecological literature and were instrumental in the formation of the Hebrew gynaecological corpus. I have paid attention to textual choices, as well as to contexts of production and dissemination and to models of appropriation. I have

---

4 Green 2000.
5 See Caballero Navas 2011a, 337–340 and Freudenthal 2011a, 100–103, and the bibliography provided by both scholars.
6 See discussion below.
7 Jewish communities established in Provence and other western Christian territories were immersed in traditional Jewish learning and in the main were unaware of the philosophical and scientific production of their host societies until approximately the mid-twelfth century. Freudenthal 1995 and 2011b.
8 See above note 2 and 5.
9 The study of Jewish medieval gynaecology was inaugurated by Ron Barkai's pioneering work in the 1990s (see bibliography). Since then, the number of identified texts and sections of texts dedicated to the care of women's health has nearly doubled, to approximately thirty.

also briefly explored the circulation of the earliest texts up to the end of the period, in order to catch a glimpse, albeit small, of the gynaecological literature available to learned Jews at the time. To that end, I have relied on the sources and quotations in the section on women's ailments in *Sēfer hayōšer*, a medical encyclopaedia written in Provence around the fourth quarter of the thirteenth century. I hope to pursue the analysis of the sources and citations in other treatises and books, as well as the manuscript distribution of the inventory of texts presented here, in future work. Finally, I have enquired into the rationale(s) behind the foundation of the gynaecological Hebrew corpus.

The end of this chapter contains an appendix with a preliminary list of the gynaecological Hebrew texts produced during the period studied.

1 In the beginning: between the closing years of the twelfth and the turn of the thirteenth century

With a few exceptions, it was not until the mid-twelfth century that scientific texts were written in Hebrew in the Christian lands of the western Mediterranean.[10] The last decade of the twelfth century witnessed the inauguration of a Hebrew medical corpus—built predominantly on translations—which, growing over the following two centuries, seems to have adequately responded to the needs of both Jewish students of medicine and practicing physicians.[11] The Hebrew corpus on gynaecology flourished under the influence of the Latin medical tradition, mainly in Provence, and followed contemporary trends favoured by Christian authors and natural philosophers. Distinctively, gynaecology became a textual specialty, and treatises on women's conditions began to circulate independently.[12]

Just as the Hebrew scientific and medical corpus relied heavily on translations (from Arabic, Latin, and some vernaculars),[13] most gynaecological texts were translated from other languages, although some had previously undergone one or more translation processes from their original language. These translation processes are enormously relevant for understanding the formation of Jewish gynaecology, as they testify to the diverse routes and modes of acquisition and accommodation of theories on female physiology and disease by Jewish medical writers, through the synthesis and adaptation of ideas and concepts from different ancient and early medieval traditions.

1.1 The Latin foundation of Hebrew gynaecology

The first known translations of gynaecological treatises into Hebrew were undertaken between 1197 and 1199 in Provence by a repentant convert, who referred to himself by the pseudonym '*Do'eg* the Edomite.' He initiated the Hebrew medical corpus by translating twenty-four medical books from Latin into Hebrew, most of them

---

10 Sela 2003.
11 Caballero Navas 2011a, 329–337.
12 Barkai 1998; Caballero Navas 2004, 80–90.
13 A recent listing of medieval Hebrew texts and their translations in Zonta 2011.

taken from the *Articella*.[14] His contribution to Hebrew gynaecology was paramount, as his impressive enterprise did not only consist of making the Latin medical texts circulating at the time available to Jewish readers by rendering them into Hebrew. Most importantly, by including among his translations three gynaecological texts as well as several medical encyclopaedias and general works that comprised important sections on women's conditions, he conveyed to a Jewish audience the synthesis of the main gynaecological traditions of antiquity as well as contemporary Latin trends.[15]

Of the three gynaecological texts, two belonged to the most widely acknowledged Latin gynaecological tradition of the time, which was made up of the translations and adaptations of Soranus of Ephesus's works. One of the routes by which ancient Greek medical texts reached the medieval Latin West was by way of Latin adaptations and translations disseminated from pre-Salernitan Italy.[16]

The longest of the two treatises, *Sēfer hatôledet* (The book on generation), derives from Muscio's fifth-sixth century Latin adaptation of Soranus's *Gynaikeia*.[17] The shorter text, *Sēfer hā'ēm 'el galinus hû' haniqrā' gyne'as* (The book on the womb by Galen, which is called *Gynaecia*), was not a Galenic work but a Hebrew translation of the Latin gynaecological treatise *De passionibus mulierum B*, an eleventh-century pre-Salernitan treatise composed of a previous version (A), the late ancient gynaecological treatises of Pseudo-Cleopatra, and some selections from Muscio.[18]

Apart from been considerably lengthier than *Sēfer hā'ēm*, *Sēfer hatôledet* presents substantive changes and additions to the Latin version, which altered the final product significantly. *Do'eg* the Edomite provided an introduction to the translation, which did not exist in the original, as well as a wide variety of Jewish elements, which consistently 'Judaized' the text. In addition to attributing the dialogue to two biblical characters—Dinah and her father Jacob—he resorted liberally to biblical and talmudic quotations and expressions, and modified, and even eliminated from the text, ideas that clash with Jewish customs and beliefs.[19]

---

14 Although Do'eg the Edomite's endeavour and the rationale behind it have received significant attention in the last few years, his cardinal contribution to the Hebrew medical corpus went unnoticed from the time of his discovery by Moritz Steinschneider until Ron Barkai 'rediscovered' him more than a century later. Lately, Gad Freudenthal has contributed essential insights into the work of this pioneering translator and the context in which he operated. See Steinschneider 1893, 711–714; Steinschneider 1888; Barkai 1998, 20–34; Freudenthal 2013.

15 For the list of Hebrew translations see, in Hebrew: Steinschneider 1888; in English translation: Barkai 1998, 20–34; and Freudenthal 2013, 118–120.

16 Hanson and Green, 1994; Green 2019.

17 Barkai 1991. Barkai suggested that *Sēfer hatôledet* might have been translated in the first half of thirteenth century by a physician who was a refugee from Granada. He later revised both the dating and authorship. Barkai 1998, 30–31.

18 For the edition and English translation of *Sēfer hā'ēm 'el galinus*, see Barkai 1998, 145–180. On *De passionibus mulierum B*, see Green 2000, 25 and 2019, 51.

19 Barkai 1991, 129–132. Barkai pondered the possibility that the 'Jewish features' were added to the treatise by a later author; see Barkai 1998, 31. Recently, Gad Freudenthal has asserted that the frame story is indeed due to a later editor, as he intends to demonstrate in a forthcoming publication authored by him, Michael McVaugh and Katelyn Mesler. See Freudenthal 2018, 46.

The third treatise, *Sēfer hasēter* (Book of the secret),[20] belongs to a new trend in gynaecological literature, stemming from Salerno, that was disseminated in Latin and numerous medieval languages beginning the twelfth century.[21] *Sēfer hasēter* is the first-ever translation from Latin into a different language of *Liber de sinthomatibus mulierum* (Book on the conditions of women) and *De ornatu mulierum* (On women's cosmetics), which are two of the three separate treatises that made up the medieval compendium that circulated under the name of *Trotula*.[22] *Do'eg* the Edomite mentioned in the prologue to his translation project that *Sēfer hasēter* 'treats some of the secrets of women and their cosmetics.'[23] However, fragments from *De ornatu mulierum* had not been identified in Hebrew until an apparently new treatise was discovered some years ago, entitled *Šě'ār yāšûb*. In fact, this was a thirteenth-century (partial?) edition of *Sēfer hasēter*, which preserved portions of the original translation that the only manuscript copy known to that date had not.[24]

In addition to these three independent gynaecological works, *Do'eg* also translated some medical books from Latin that had been previously translated from Arabic, mainly by Constantine the African at the end of the eleventh century. The translations of Greek works into Arabic (whatever the path) was a second route by which Greek medical traditions were handed down to the West. Galen's coherent explicative model of health and disease, based on the humoral theory, which he had developed from Hippocratic concepts, gained him the acknowledgement of Byzantine and Arab medical authors, who promptly endorsed the theoretical framework of his understanding of medicine. Actually, his commentaries on Hippocratic works, as he systematized and interpreted them, enabled their transmission to the Islamic world. Galen is also largely responsible for the nosology, aetiology, and therapeutics of women's diseases that would form the foundation of Arab gynaecology.[25] In his translations,

---

During the last few years I have also conducted research on this treatise, preliminary results of which have been presented at two international conferences, and will be published in a forthcoming essay entitled "Graeco-Latin Gynaecology in Jewish Robes. The Hebrew translation of Muscio's Gynaecia."

20 In this context, the figurative meaning of the Hebrew *sēter* is 'hidden [parts],' that is, 'genitalia.' However, I have deliberately rendered the term literally in order to retain the manifold meanings with which authors and translators of medieval Hebrew texts on women's healthcare invested the word. See the discussion on 'secrets of women' in Caballero Navas 2006b.

21 Barkai 1998, 61–64 (study) and 181–191 (edition and translation).

22 Green 2001.

23 Steinschneider 1888, 7; Freudenthal 2013, 119. On the literal translation of the Hebrew *sēter* (secret) and *sitrê nāšîm* (secrets of women) in this context, see note 20 above. Furthermore, '"Secrets of women," used in Hebrew medical texts as a generic term, seems to represent a way of understanding sexual difference relating to health care that takes women's health's needs as specific and connected to their sex.' Caballero Navas 2006b, 51.

24 Caballero Navas 2006a.

25 Green 1985, 85–101; and Pormann and Savage-Smith 2007, 43–45 and 51–55.

Constantine bequeathed to the Latin West the total synthesis of the ancient gynaecological traditions established by the Byzantine and Arabic writers.[26]

Do'eg also rendered Hippocrates's *Aphorisms* from Latin.[27] Although the *Aphorisms* was not a gynaecological work, most of particula V (aphorisms 28–62) was devoted to women's conditions, which made it a classic among treatises of this kind of medical literature. In addition to *Do'eg*'s translation,[28] the work had been translated into Hebrew several times by the end of the thirteenth century, for the most part with Galen's commentary. Around 1260 Hillel b. Samuel translated it from the Latin version by Constantine the African,[29] while Natan ha-Me'ati translated it from Arabic in 1283.[30] Often the *Aphorisms* was translated together with commentaries by other authors, such as Palladius, rendered from Arabic into Hebrew by Shem Ṭov ben Isaac of Tortosa in the second half of the thirteenth century in Provence,[31] or Maimonides, whose contribution to the corpus will be discussed below.

Do'eg also chose to translate into Hebrew two medical encyclopaedias that, written originally in Arabic, were among the works that Constantine handed down to the Latin West through his translations. These works included sections devoted to women's conditions that had a strong bearing on medieval Jewish gynaecology, both directly and indirectly: al-Majūsī's *Kitāb kāmil aṣ-ṣināʿā aṭ-ṭibbīya* (The complete book of the medical art), known in the West as *Pantegni*, and in Hebrew as *Sēfer mālēʾ maḥzîq* (The full [vessel] that contains);[32] and Ibn al-Jazzār's *Zād al-musāfir wa-qūt al-ḥādir* (Provisions for the traveller and nourishment for the sedentary), known in Latin throughout the Middle Ages as *Viaticum peregrinantis*, and entitled by *Do'eg* as *Sēfer yāʾîr nātîb* (The book of the illuminated road).[33]

In general, the study of (Hebrew) gynaecology has focused on treatises that circulated independently. As a consequence, the role played by general medical works (in Hebrew and in Arabic) that included sections devoted to women's ailments and their sanitary needs has passed somewhat unnoticed. However, these sections were

---

26 On the reception of Arabic medical learning in the Hebrew textual corpus, whatever the route, see Caballero Navas 2003, 2009, 43–44.
27 Steinschneider 1888, 6–8; Barkai 1998, 23; Freudenthal 2013, 118; Bos 2016, 3–6.
28 Prior to Do'eg's translation, *Sefer Asaph* or *Sefer refuot*, the first Hebrew book of medicine, which predated the launching of the Hebrew medical corpus in at least two centuries, included parts of the *Aphorisms*, together with aggadic tradition and other materials, in a consistent and deliberate attempt to link Greek medicine to Talmudic tradition. See Caballero Navas 2011a, 321–322; Bos 2016, 1–3.
29 Steinschneider 1893, 734; Bos 2016, 6–8.
30 Steinschneider 1893, 662.
31 Bos 2010, 61.
32 Steinschneider 1888, 7; Barkai 1998, 24; Freudenthal 2013, 119. It is worth noting that al-Majūsī's chapters on gynaecology (*Practica*, Book VIII) were lost and did not circulate in Latin until the thirteenth century. Prior to that date, Constantine the African's version of al-Majūsī's *Kāmil* included the description of female anatomy (*Theorica*, Book III, chapters 33–36), and a list of topical headings with basic female diseases, covering all the diseases of the reproductive organs (*Theorica*, Book IX, chapters 40–43). See Green, 1994 and 2019, 52.
33 Steinschneider 1888, 7; Barkai 1998, 25; Freudenthal 2013, 119.

widely acknowledged and exerted a significant influence on both contemporary and later works. For instance, al-Majūsī's assumptions regarding the anatomy of female genitalia, menstrual disorders, and the aetiology of uterine suffocation, together with the richness of the *materia medica* proposed in therapy, became instrumental in the development of concepts about women's healthcare until the end of the Middle Ages.[34] Thus, in addition to *Do'eg*'s early translation from Constantine's Latin rendition, all this knowledge reached Hebrew writings through Latin texts that endorsed al-Majūsī's theories. The impact of the Hebrew *Pantegni* on later medieval Hebrew medical literature on women has yet to be examined.

The sixth book of *Zād al-musāfir* or *Viaticum peregrinantis* is devoted to diseases affecting the sexual organs and contains numerous chapters (9 to 18) on women's ailments.[35] Around the thirteenth century a new Hebrew version was produced by Abraham ben Isaac—also from Constantine's eleventh-century Latin version—entitled *Sêdâ lā'ôreḥîm*.[36] The relevance of this handbook for Hebrew medicine can be measured by the fact that it was translated once more in 1259, this time from Arabic, by Moses Ibn Tibbon, who entitled it *Sêdat haderākîm*.[37] Moreover, recent research has revealed that portions of the *Zād al-musāfir/Viaticum peregrinantis*, mostly from *Do'eg*'s *Sêfer yā'îr nātîb*, can be traced in several Hebrew treatises on women's healthcare, where they had been often quoted without explicit reference to the source, namely the thirteenth-century *Sēfer 'aḥăbat nāšîm* (The book of women's love) and *Sēfer hayōšer*, and the fifteenth-century *Ša'ar hanāšîm*.[38]

Apart from *Do'eg*'s early translation from Constantine's Latin rendition, the influence of *Zād al-musāfir/Viaticum peregrinantis* reached Hebrew writings by an indirect route: the translation into Hebrew of the *Liber de sinthomatibus mulierum—Do'eg*'s *Sēfer hasēter*—on whose aetiology and therapeutics the impact of Ibn al-Jazzār's gynaecology was patent.[39] The gynaecological ideas developed by Ibn al-Jazzār were as decisive in the formation of the Hebrew gynaecological corpus as they had been for the Latin.

In summary, *Do'eg* the Edomite transmitted to medieval Jews: (a) the synthesis of Soranus's work that reached the West by way of Latin adaptations and translations, re-edited in the eleventh century in southern Italy; (b) the new trend in Latin gynaecology from Salerno; and (c) Constantine the African's synthesis of Byzantine and Arabic writers' re-elaboration of ancient Greco-Roman medical texts and 'Galenized' gynaecology, both through the rendition of Arabic versions of Greek works and through books originally written in Arabic.

---

34 Green 1985, 109–117. See also King 1998, 238–244.
35 Bos 1997.
36 Steinschneider 1893, 705.
37 Ibid., 703–704. See also Zonta 2011, 23, 32 and 99, respectively.
38 Caballero Navas 2003 and 2004, 27–30 and 87–88.
39 Green 1996, 128–131; and Caballero Navas 2006a.

1.2 A different model of appropriation of gynaecological knowledge

Around the same time that *Do'eg* embarked upon his translation project, or slightly later, two Hebrew treatises on women's conditions were circulating around the Iberian Peninsula. One of them is a short treatise that includes actual practice and (female) local customs, as well as abundant magical material. Known as *Těrûfôt lahērāyôn ha-niqrā' māgēn harô'š* (Medicaments for pregnancy, called 'the head's shield'), the text was apparently written in the late twelfth or early thirteenth century by Sheshet ben Benveniste, the head of the Jewish community of Barcelona and physician to the kings of Aragon Alfons II (1162–1196) and Pere II (1196–1213).[40] The only preserved manuscript mentions that the text was copied several times by Yehudah al-Ḥarizi, a well-known Andalusian scholar and translator who immigrated to Provence.[41] Should this testimony be accurate, it would substantiate its circulation in Provence before 1225, the year of al-Ḥarizi's death.

Meanwhile, an unknown contemporary author, apparently based in Castile, wrote a Hebrew treatise on diseases of the reproductive organs, *Zikārôn heḥŏlāyîm hahôwîm beklê hahērāyôn* (An account of the diseases of the organs of pregnancy). Ron Barkai, who edited and translated the work into English, underscored the evident impact of Arabic terminology, syntax, and style on the text. He also highlighted the profuse use of Castilian terms and the fact that the Hebrew medical and scientific terminology seems to predate the creation of a Hebrew scientific lexicon by thirteenth- and four-teenth-century translators.[42] Indeed, the treatise also has other distinctive features that connect it to the Arab medical tradition. For instance, it is divided into two parts, devoted to the diseases of male and female genitalia, respectively. This very arrangement was often employed in medical encyclopaedias by Arab authors.[43]

Further analysis has revealed striking parallels between the Hebrew treatise and Ibn Sīnā's major medical work, *Kitāb al-Qānūn fī al-ṭibb*. Book 3, which is divided into twenty-two *funūn* or treatises, systematically expounds the function and disease of each organ from head to toe. *Funūn* 20 and 21 are devoted to diseases in male and female reproductive organs, respectively. According to my ongoing investigation, the first section of the *Zikārôn* follows *fen* 20 very closely, while the second section seems to represent a further effort by the author to condense the contents of *fen* 21, which he manages to do by omitting some chapters and topics and by abbreviating some others.[44] Although further research on this treatise is still needed, it may represent the earliest adaptation of part of Ibn Sīnā's *Canon* in Hebrew.[45]

---

40 Barkai 1998, 83–86 (analysis) and 192–211 (edition and English translation). According to the online catalogue of the Institute of Microfilmed Hebrew Manuscripts at the Jewish National and University Library (Jerusalem), the title of the treatise is *Těrûfôt ûmerqāḥôt lemaḥălôt nāšîm* (Medicaments and concoctions for women's ailments).

41 Barkai 1998, 192 (Hebrew) and 198 (English).

42 Ibid. 69–76 (analysis) and 109–144 (edition and translation). Barkai rendered the title of the treatise into English as 'A Record of the Diseases Occurring in the Genital Members.'

43 For instance, *Zād al-musāfir*. See Bos 1997.

44 Caballero Navas, 2019a.

45 The *Canon* was translated for the first time into Hebrew by Natan ha-Me'ati in 1279; at roughly

These two treatises bear witness to an epistemological shift in the way in which Iberian Jews understood women's conditions and their treatment, and present—particularly the *Zikārôn*—a novel model of the appropriation of gynaecological knowledge.

The Jews of Castile and, to a lesser degree, the eastern Iberian Peninsula continued to read, copy, and even write about medicine in Arabic up to the fifteenth century. Arabic medical texts provided Castilian Jewish physicians with theoretical and practical medical knowledge and contributed to their social cohesion.[46] The Arabic medical tradition did not favour the production of independent texts on women's conditions, but preferred to include female ailments in medical encyclopaedias in the form of chapters or sections.[47] Jewish medical authors belonging to the Arabic medical tradition generally followed the same pattern, as was the case with Moses Maimonides, who included a chapter (16) dedicated to women's medical problems in his *Medical Aphorisms*.[48] In contrast, the author of the *Zikārôn*, writing in a social and scientific context in which the Arabic cultural model prevailed among Jews, deliberately created a Hebrew treatise on disorders of the reproductive organs, which, based on a major Arabic source,[49] circulated independently.

2 The thirteenth century and the shaping of the Hebrew gynaecological corpus

After an interval whose duration is difficult to determine, beginning in the second half of the thirteenth century several treatises that circulated independently were produced: (1) an abridged version of one of the Latin gynaecological treatises translated by *Do'eg*, *Sēfer hasēter*, under the title *Šě'ār yāšûb*, which has been already discussed;[50] (2) a compilation written originally in Hebrew, entitled *Sēfer 'aḥăbat nāšîm* or *Sēfer hanhāgat nāšîm* (The book of women's love or book on the regimen of women);[51] and (3) four treatises translated from Arabic, two of which were originally written in Lat-

---

the same time, Zeraḥyah Ḥen translated books 1 and 2. One century later, Joseph b. Joshua Ibn Vives ha-Lorki translated the first book and two *funūn* of the second. Counting the anonymous partial translations that have been preserved, some scholars estimate that the Canon was translated into Hebrew on at least seven occasions. See Richler 1986; Ferre 2002; Freudental and Zonta 2012, 270–271. My preliminary comparison between the *Zikārôn* and the extant Hebrew translations from book 3 reveals that the Castilian treatise is not based on them, but seems to be an earlier Hebrew synopsis of *funūn* 21 and 22 made directly from Arabic. Caballero Navas 2019a, 100–111.

46 Caballero Navas 2011a, 326–327; and García-Ballester 1994, and 2001, 454–472.

47 Cf. Green 1985, 71–128.

48 Bos 2015.

49 The *Canon* was translated into Latin under the direction of Gerard of Cremona in Toledo in 1187. His translation, most likely a collaborative project, thus bears witness to the circulation of the *Canon* in Arabic in the same milieu in which the *Zikārôn* seems to have been written. Caballero Navas 2019a, 111–116.

50 See note 24.

51 This is an anonymous Hebrew compendium of knowledge about magic, sexuality, cosmetics, gynaecology, and obstetrics, organized into three sections. Preserved in only one fifteenth-century copy, it was probably written at the end of the thirteenth century in the area of Catalonia or Provence. Cf. Caballero Navas 2004.

in and in Greek, respectively. Moreover, some general medical books that included sections on women's healthcare were produced in a like manner: four translated from Arabic, and two originally written in Hebrew.

Of the four treatises translated from Arabic, *Sēfer dînâ lĕkōl 'inyān hārehem wĕhālĕyehāh* (Dinah's book on all that concerns the womb and its diseases) is so far the only Judeo-Arabic gynaecological text contained in the whole known corpus and, according to Barkai, it has only been preserved in one fragmentary copy, apparently from the thirteenth century. The treatise is a translation of Muscio's *Pessaria*, although the source from which it was rendered is still unknown.[52] The text from the Greek tradition is *Sēfer hahērāyôn wĕhārehem lĕ'abuqraṭ* (Hippocrates's book on pregnancy and the womb). This Arabic version of *De superfoetatione*, the only translation of a Hippocratic gynaecological text that has come down to us in Hebrew, was rendered by Zerahyah ben Isaac ben Shealtiel Hen in Rome between 1277–1290.[53]

Sēfer yĕṣîrat hā'ubār wĕhanhāgat hehārôt wĕhanôlādîm (Book on the generation of the foetus and the treatment of pregnant women and newborns) is the only Hebrew translation of an Arabic gynaecological and obstetrical text by an Arabic Islamic author: *Kitāb khalq al-janīn wa-tadbīr al-ḥabālā wa-al-mawlūdīn*, written by the Andalusian physician Arib Ibn Sa'id in the tenth century.[54] Curiously, it seems to have enjoyed a wider dissemination in Jewish communities in the West than in Islamic lands, as according to Barkai, it might have been translated twice into Hebrew.[55]

Interestingly, the next treatise, *Liqûṭê rabēnû mōšeh bĕ'inyānê weset wĕhērāyôn* (Maimonides's compilation on menstruation and pregnancy), had been part of a general medical work, Maimonides's *Medical Aphorisms*, originally written in Arabic around 1185.[56] Sometime after its translation into Hebrew by Zerahyah Hen in Rome in 1277, its chapter 16, entirely dedicated to women's medical problems, became detached from the rest of the book and circulated independently.[57] It has been preserved in two manuscripts. It also enjoyed very wide circulation as a section of the general work, both in Zerahyah Hen's translation and in the version translated by Natan ha-Me'ati between 1279–1283, also in Rome.[58]

This was not the only Maimonidean contribution to the gynaecological corpus, as his *Commentary on Hippocrates's Aphorisms* with Galen's commentary was translated from Arabic by Moses Ibn Tibbon in 1257 (or 1267) in Provence, while Zerahyah Hen contributed a new translation in Rome around 1277–1290.[59] One might rightly think that Maimonides's gynaecological output was slight (chapter 16 of his *Medi-*

---

52 See Barkai 1998, 50–53 (analysis) and 97–108 (edition and English translation). On Muscio's *Pessaria*, see Green 2000, 21; Bolton 2015, 419–441 (Latin edition and English translation).
53 Zonta 2003.
54 Arib Ibn Sa'id 1956.
55 Steinschneider 1893, 671; Barkai 1998, 43 and 64.
56 Bos 2015.
57 Caballero Navas 2009, 41.
58 In the fourteenth century, an anonymous translator produced a new version. Cf. Zonta 2011, 32, 35, and 46.
59 Steinschneider 1893, 769; Zonta 2011, 32 and 35. See also Caballero Navas 2009, 35–37.

cal Aphorisms and part of particula V of the *Hippocratic Aphorisms*).[60] However, the ample diffusion enjoyed by his work guaranteed that his profoundly Galenized views on sexual difference and women's physiology reached a very wide audience of learned Jews in the Iberian Peninsula, Provence, and Italy.[61]

During the thirteenth century, some other general medical works circulated in Hebrew, originally written in Hebrew or translated from Arabic, whose content on women's ailments played an instrumental role in the formation of the Hebrew corpus. I have already briefly discussed Ibn al-Jazzār's *Zād al-musāfir*, which apart from the two translations from Latin referred to above, was translated from Arabic in 1259 by Moses Ibn Tibbon under the title *Sēdat haderākîm*.[62] Other works also translated into Hebrew were—or at least their authors were—profusely quoted in later literature (both medical and nonmedical). However, it is difficult to determine their importance in Hebrew gynaecology until further studies are undertaken. This is the case with *Kitab al-taṣrīf li-man 'agiza 'an al-ta'līf* (The recourse of him who cannot compose [a medical work of his own]), a compendium on health comprising thirty books, by the great Arab surgeon al-Zahrāwī (d.c. 1013), whose extensive section dedicated to surgery (book 30) discusses childbirth and the use of several obstetrical instruments devised by the author.[63] The *Taṣrif* was translated into Hebrew by Shem Ṭov ben Isaac of Tortosa under the title *Sēfer hašimmûš* between 1254 and 1261 in Marseilles. Moreover, it seems that some fragments of the *Taṣrif* were also rendered into Hebrew by anonymous translators.[64] Shem Ṭov ben Isaac of Tortosa also translated al-Rāzī's *Kitāb al-Manṣūrī* (Book for Almansur) from Arabic in 1264.[65]

As already mentioned, Ibn Sīnā's famous medical encyclopaedia was translated twice in the last quarter of the thirteenth century and once again in the following century, although only the first of the translations, by Natan ha-Me'ati, contained book 3, which includes a section (*fen* 21) on diseases of female reproductive organs.[66] Although both Ibn Sīnā and his *Canon* are often generically mentioned in Hebrew gynaecological texts, their bearing on them has yet to be analysed.

In the sphere of Hebrew encyclopaedias, *Ṣōrî hagûf* (Balm of the body) is a detailed and systematic work written by Natan ben Yo'el Falaquera at the end of the thirteenth century.[67] The work is divided into four parts: theory, the practice and regimen of health, a description and treatment of diseases, and a treatise on medicaments, their properties, and curative effects. In addition to a brief discussion of the function of the

---

60 In fact, I have argued elsewhere that the rest of his medical production neglects women and presents a strong male-centred stance on healthcare and sexuality. Cf. Caballero Navas 2013, 63.
61 On this diffusion, see Ferre 2009.
62 See above, notes 33, 35–38.
63 Spink and Lewis 1973. On the circulation of Gerard of Cremona's twelfth-century Latin translation of al-Zahrāwī's *Surgery* and the interest aroused by its gynaecological and obstetrical material from thirteenth century onwards, see Green 2011.
64 Feliu and Arrizabalaga 2000–2001; Bos 2010.
65 Steinscheider 1893, 725–726.
66 See notes 44 and 45.
67 Bos and Fontaine 1999. The fourth part was edited by Amar and Buchman 2004.

male and female testes and their reproductive function in the first theoretical part, the book also includes a section devoted to women's conditions, which is labelled in some manuscripts as *Sēder nāšîm misēfer Ṣōrî hagûf* (Section on women of the book 'balm of the body').[68] The author explicitly quotes Hippocrates, Galen, Ibn Sīnā, and al-Rāzī, though many of the ideas discussed are reminiscent of al-Jazzār. The chapter deals with gynaecological problems: pain, abscesses and tumours in the womb, menstrual retention, uterine suffocation (due to the retention of menstrual blood or semen, whose corrupted vapours ascend to the brain), and sterility.

Sēfer hayōšer (Book of rectitude) is a comprehensive encyclopaedia of contemporary medical knowledge, written in Provence in the last decades of the thirteenth century by a very learned medical author and practitioner. I am inclined to think that it might have been written by the translator and physician Jacob ha-Qaṭan, although further investigation is needed to reach a conclusion.[69] The book is one of the first few medical works originally written in Hebrew and reflects the perceptions of a Jewish physician during the early stages of the professionalization of medicine. Thus, it is a key witness to the strategies developed by Jewish physicians to accommodate their knowledge and practice to the new way of understanding health, disease, and healthcare in a multicultural context.[70] The work features a well-organized and very comprehensive section devoted to women's diseases—*Taḥalû'ê nāšîm min sēfer hayōšer* (Women's diseases from the 'Book of rectitude')—which contains diagnoses, aetiologies, and treatments for numerous conditions. Throughout this chapter, the author quotes ancient and contemporary medical authors and works extensively, be they Greek, Arabic, Latin, or Hebrew, although all of them seem to have been quoted from Hebrew versions. This feature makes the work an extraordinary source of information about the circulation of Hebrew medical texts in general, and of gynaecological literature in particular, among Western Jewish communities in the late thirteenth century.

3 The fortunes of the inaugural texts to the end of the first stage

Not all texts produced during the first stage of the foundation of Hebrew gynaecology had the same fate, as the popularity they enjoyed varied greatly. Some useful instruments to assess the circulation and reception of textually transmitted knowledge are: the analysis of the materiality of the manuscripts (number of extant copies, dating, geographical distribution, owners, patterns of annotation, etc.),[71] and the study of quotations included in later works. Obviously, the bulk of the texts—some of which

---

68 As, for instance, in the MS Paris, Bibliotheque Nationale, heb. 1122/6, ff. 42r–46v.
69 Some evidence points in this direction, such as the continuous self-references to two books translated by Jacob ha-Qaṭan: *Antidotarium Nicholai*, and [Roger's] *Book of [Oil and] Water*. Cf. Muntner 1947. However, the author also refers often to his 'brother' Jacob, whom he calls 'the great physician,' and to whom he attributes several treatises, such as the *Šě'ār yāšûb* (Caballero Navas 2006a). We cannot infer from those quotations whether both authors had an actual family relationship or the appellation is part of the rhetoric of the discourse.
70 Caballero Navas 2011a, 24.
71 Beit-Arié 2011.

have not been edited, or whose editions need to be revised—and the diversity of the contexts of transmission and dissemination render this a very ambitious project for which much research is still needed. Yet, in the future, the gradually growing volume of data contributed by successive studies from different quarters will enable better understanding of the afterlives of these texts.

With this goal in mind, I have analysed the quotations from gynaecological texts (or parts of texts) included in the section on women's conditions in *Sēfer hayōšer*. Through these findings, one may gain a sense of the literature of this type in Hebrew that was available to an educated physician in Provence at the end of the thirteenth century, as well as the preferences of this particular author.[72] Remarkably, this author was rather familiar with most of the works rendered by *Do'eg* the Edomite—to whom he refers thrice by his eponymous '*Do'eg*'—nearly a century earlier. However, he also drew from other books translated later both from Latin and from Arabic.

Not altogether surprisingly, two works stand out as the most profusely quoted in this section, *Šě'ār yāśûb* and *Sēfer yā'îr nātîb*. The former, attributed by the author to his 'brother' Jacob, is an abridged and edited version of *Sēfer hasēter*, discussed above. In fact, the profusion of quotations led me to identify this unknown version, which comprises previously unknown fragments from the Salernitan *De ornatu mulierum*.[73] The second work, Ibn al-Jazzār's *Zād al-musāfir* in Hebrew translation, was abundantly, though not always explicitly, cited from *Do'eg*'s version translated from Latin as *Sēfer yā'îr nātîb* but also from the 1259 translation from Arabic by Moses Ibn Tibbon, *Sêdat haderākîm*, although without attribution.[74] The fact that the author engaged with both versions (by *Do'eg* and by Ibn Tibbon) testifies to the circulation and appreciation that both seem to have enjoyed at the time in Provence. Interestingly, when referring to the early translation by *Do'eg*, the author of *Sēfer hayōšer* indistinctly used the title of the book in Latin, *Viaticum*, and in Hebrew, *Sēfer yā'îr nātîb*. However, he attributed it to various authors: *Do'eg* (the Edomite) (ff. 42r, 44r); Isaac (Israeli) (ff. 51r and 51v); and Constantine (the African) (f. 44v), to whom the author also referred once as *hakōmer* (the priest) (f. 43v).

Hippocrates's *Aphorisms* was also very popular with the author of *Sēfer hayōšer*, who had numerous versions at hand, for the work had been translated into Hebrew several times from Latin and from Arabic by the end of thirteenth century.[75] As an additional Hippocratic work, the book refers once to *Sēfer hanôlādîm* (f. 46r), which is no other than *De superfoetatione*, translated into Hebrew from an Arabic version.[76]

---

72 This book, which remains unedited, has been preserved in six manuscripts, three of which are fragmentary. For my analysis, I have relied on two of the three complete copies: Vienna, Oesterreischische Nationalbibliothek Cod hebr. 64/1, ff. 63r–83r; and Oxford, Bodleian, MS Oppenheim 180 (Cat. 2134), ff. 39v–51v (chaps. 81–99). The references have been quoted from the latter.

73 Caballero Navas 2006a.

74 Ibid., and Caballero Navas 2003.

75 See notes 27–31.

76 Zonta 2003.

The author also mentions a *Sēfer galîînus* (f. 40r), about which he does not provide enough information to ascertain whether he is referring to *Sēfer ha'ēm*,[77] whether he is indirectly quoting it, or merely making a generic reference to Galen's authority. The Islamic author al-Rāzī is also mentioned a number of times (ff. 40v, 42r, 43v, 44v, 45v, 46v, 48r, 49r–v), his name generally attached to the name of *Almaṣuri*, which is the title of his well-known medical compendium, *Book for Almansur*, which had been already translated into Hebrew from Arabic.[78] Certainly, the library available to the author of *Sēfer hayōšer* was rich and included everything from the very first books that formed the Hebrew corpus to the most up-to-date incorporations.[79] In fact, the dating of the latest translations mentioned in the book is a useful indication to assign it a tentative *terminus post quem*.

Among all these numerous works and authors, there are several intriguing absences. Some of them, such as *Zikārôn* or *Dinah's Book*, may be due to different regional trends in dissemination. It is remarkable, however, that the author, who relied on many works rendered by *Do'eg*, did not mention *Sēfer hatôledet*, a gynaecological treatise that he did not only translate but also took the time and effort to 'Judaize.'[80] However, by the thirteenth century, Muscio's *Gynaecia* had declined in popularity and the two Soranian texts translated by *Do'eg* had been completely superseded by the *Trotula* texts and the (Arabic) Galenization of gynaecology.[81] By that time, other Hebrew texts on women's healthcare scarcely quoted or mentioned them, as was the case with *Sēfer hayōšer*.

4 The rationale(s) behind the foundation of Hebrew gynaecology

As noted at the beginning of this study, the foundations of both the Hebrew medical corpus and the Hebrew textual body of literature on women's conditions are intimately connected. Jews who lived in Christian milieus shared the healthcare system with their contemporaries, both as patients and as providers. Consequently, translators, medical authors, and practitioners favoured the acquisition and accommodation of a genre of literature that was part of the corpus of knowledge sanctioned by the legitimate medical system and whose learning granted access to legitimate medical practice.[82] That is, the incorporation of gynaecology into the first group of medical texts made available in Hebrew is partly related to its role as part of the new trends in medicine. As with other aspects of medicine, medieval Jewish writers followed the trends endorsed by contemporary Christian authors.

---

77 See note 18.
78 See note 65.
79 The author quotes many other Hebrew medical works, which have not been included in this overview since they are beyond the scope of this study.
80 See above note 19.
81 Hanson and Green 1994.
82 By healthcare system, I refer both to sanctioned theoretical medical knowledge as well as to the social and legal circumstances that would regulate medical practice from the thirteenth century on. On Jewish medical training and practice in a Christian milieu, see Caballero Navas 2011a, 329–340, and the bibliography provided there.

However, this does not fully explain why early translators and authors were interested in incorporating gynaecological texts that were most likely not intended for male medical practice, at least at this early stage, into the Jewish medical corpus. Indeed, the approach of early and later medieval Hebrew texts to women's medical problems was essentially theoretical. Significantly, all the Hebrew texts were authored by and mostly addressed to men. Furthermore, many of them illustrate the interest of male physicians in differentiating their role from that of women, and endeavour to demonstrate that they (learned male physicians) hold the monopoly on theoretical knowledge, while women—such as midwives and other women mentioned in medical texts—are 'only' responsible for manipulating the female body.[83] In fact, and despite the gradual rise of male authority in gynaecology throughout the Middle Ages, the observation and manipulation of women's bodies and genitalia seem to have been the province of women until the end of the period. This was partly a result of the rhetoric of shame and concealment that aimed at restricting male access to women's bodies, but also because medical interventions involving female reproductive organs were 'differentially gendered depending on prevailing notions of expertise and competence.'[84]

Beyond the differentiation of roles, some Jewish authors also endeavoured to strip female practitioners of authority and autonomy in the practice of gynaecology, thus participating in the deliberate attempt to exclude women from legitimate practice that the professionalization of medicine entailed.[85] The author of *Sēfer hayōšer*, for example, warned women against looking for aid for their gynaecological ailments among female healers, whom he accused of administering cures that could do much harm, due to their lack of theoretical medical knowledge.[86]

One century earlier, the translator of *Sēfer hatōledet* devised a strategy to link the medical knowledge in the book to the patriarchs, whereby a fictitious Jacob staged the male appropriation of female agency in healthcare. In the book, Jacob was presented as an expert on women's conditions who answered questions about ailments associated with the female lifecycle, posed by his distressed daughter Dinah.[87] However striking the role of Jacob may seem, male authority over female physiology was not unfamiliar to a Jewish audience. Rabbinic literature had invested rabbis with authority regarding the theoretical knowledge of the bodies of women, particularly with respect to menstruation and physical examinations for menarche and other signs of puberty,

---

83 Caballero Navas 2014, 384–385. See also Caballero Navas 2019b on female medical practice in medieval Hebrew medical literature.

84 See Caballero Navas 2006b, 50–52; and Green 2013, especially on 345–346.

85 Cf. Green 2008.

86 Caballero Navas 2008, 150–151.

87 See notes 17 and 19. The possibility that the Jacob–Dinah frame story might be due to a later editor does not invalidate my contention that it was used as a strategy to legitimize Jewish (male) involvement in Graeco-Latin gynaecology in several ways, which involve rabbinic discourse (see discussion below) but also an apologetic approach that attempted to connect the origin of medicine to the Jews. For similar intents, see note 28 on *Sefer Asaph*'s deliberate attempt to link Greek medicine to Talmudic tradition.

such as the appearance of pubic hair or the growth of breasts.[88] With regard to the interpretation of impurity laws—defined in the Bible in Leviticus 11–15—the rabbis presented themselves as experts in the taxonomy of uterine blood, even if they did not themselves perform the inspection of blood and bloodstains.[89] The pioneers of Hebrew medical writing, who were all educated in traditional Talmudic-Jewish learning, might have been well acquainted with this ancient rabbinic gynaecological 'expertise'. In consequence, faced with the 'alien' body of Graeco-Arabic medicine, such knowledge of women's bodies and physiology would have appeared less 'alien' to them.

Sēfer hatôledet was translated at a time and place in which Jewish communities were still unaware of the body of Greco-Arabic knowledge with which their coreligionists from the Islamicate world had been familiar for centuries.[90] Its author, *Do'eg* the Edomite, clearly strove to eliminate religious, cultural, and social tensions from the text by altering, or even removing, certain paragraphs from the Hebrew version that were problematic from the standpoint of Jewish tradition.[91] But most importantly, he endeavoured to appropriate and transform the treatise into a distinct Jewish product, and to legitimize Jewish involvement in gynaecology by resorting to rabbinic discourse. Significantly, he adopted talmudic terminology and its categorization of female anatomy, by means of which he attempted to incorporate the rabbinic understanding of the female body into a secular body of literature and, consequently, to assert rabbinic (male) authority over gynaecological issues.[92]

Despite the uniqueness of this treatise in its deliberate 'Judaization,' other Jewish writers also relied on rabbinic and talmudic concepts of women's bodies and their functioning, which informed their attitudes and approaches to the acquisition and accommodation of theoretical medical knowledge about women.[93] One interesting example of the impact of rabbinic discourse on the shaping of medical ideas on women is the long medieval debate on the existence of female semen and women's contribution to generation, which permeated Jewish philosophical, scientific, and theological works. Judaism acknowledged the existence of female semen (b. Nid. 31a); hence, despite the ambiguity brought about by the influence of Aristotle in Jewish philosophy, the idea that women emitted semen was generally endorsed in Hebrew gynaecological texts because it fitted rabbinic discourse.[94] To all appearances, rab-

---

88 Cf. Fonrobert 2000, 103–159; and 2007. See also Balberg 2011. Both scholars call attention to the fact that traces of Hellenistic medicine can be found in the rabbinic textual corpus.

89 Balberg 2011, 331. See also Fonrobert 2000, 103–127; and Ruiz Morell 2012.

90 Cf. Freudenthal 1995 and 2011b.

91 Cf. Barkai 1991. The fact that he was a convert to Christianity did not lessen his commitment to Judaism. See Freudenthal 2013, 108.

92 Barkai 1991, 35–57. On rabbinic conceptions about women's bodies, see Fonrobert 2000, 40–67.

93 On the medieval use of rabbinic metaphors of female genitalia, see Fonrobert 2000 48–63; and Caballero Navas 2006b, 41–43.

94 The Hippocratic idea that both men and women emit seed had also been endorsed by Galen, whose authority was undisputed in medieval medicine, although he considered female sperm to be less perfect than male sperm. The notion, however, encountered with the ambiguity of 'Galenized,' Aristotelian Maimonides and the open opposition of traditionalist Naḥmanides,

binic discourse served both to sanction theories on the female body and to legitimize medical male authority over women.

When we consider that many rabbis and Jewish religious authorities—like many Christian theologians—were physicians, we can anticipate that the encounter of traditional rabbinic interest in conceptualizing female corporeality with a new interest in understanding the functioning of women's bodies on the part of medieval physicians and natural philosophers[95] facilitated Jewish acceptance of gynaecological texts. In a bidirectional process, rabbinic expertise on the female body bestowed on them authority over gynaecology, whereas their knowledge was supplemented by the concepts and theories contained in the translated texts. Consequently, halakhists and biblical commentators were provided with contemporary medical knowledge of women's physiology, which many of them chose to draw on in their legal and theological works.[96]

While I do not fully endorse Gad Freudenthal's claim that the 'immediate motivation for the [Do'eg's] translation enterprise was religious,'[97] I do believe that religion, or more accurately rabbinic culture, played an important role in the Jewish endorsement of medieval gynaecology. The reason alleged by Do'eg in his prologue—to prevent the Jewish population from consulting gentile physicians (who may recommend impure remedies)—is a topos repeated by later translators, such as Shem Ṭov ben Isaac of Tortosa, who evoked the rabbinic dictum 'we must not allow them to heal' (b. 'Abod. Zar. 27b) in the prologue to his *Sēfer haširmûš.*[98] This motivation, in my view, reflects anxiety about acculturation more than a religious concern.

Rabbinic interest in the female body justified the need to appropriate and accommodate gynaecological knowledge, whereas rabbinic expertise legitimized male authority over women's physiology and healthcare; in return, gynaecological notions acquired from written texts contributed to the expertise and authority of the rabbis over the female body and its meanings. Nonetheless, this does not necessarily mean that rabbis themselves observed and manipulated women's bodies and genitalia, or that women accepted rabbinic authority without resistance.

---

two paramount rabbinic authorities of medieval Jewish culture. See Caballero Navas 2014, 387–388; and Mosheh ben Naḥman, *Commentary on Lev. 12, 2* (Chavel 1996, 64–65).

95 On the transformation of gynaecological literature in the later Middle Ages and the interest of male physicians in women's bodies, see Green 2008.

96 Sharon Faye Koren (2004) has highlighted the use that Naḥmanides and Isaac the Blind made of contemporary medical theory to support their ideas about the evil nature of *niddah*. See also Caballero Navas 2011b.

97 Freudenthal 2013, 110.

98 Feliu and Arrizabalaga 2000–2001, 80.

Appendix. Preliminary list of the gynaecological Hebrew texts produced from the end of the twelfth to the end of the thirteenth centuries. The right-hand column shows the texts known to, and consumed by, the author of *Sēfer hayōšer*, according to its section on women's diseases.

	Date	Hebrew Translator/ Author & Place	Hebrew Title	Source Text	Language(s) of Translated Text	Section on Women of *Sēfer hayōšer*
1	1197–99	Do'eg the Edomite Provence	ספר האם אל גלינוס הוא הנקרא גינאס *Sēfer bā'ēm 'el galinus hū' haniqrā' gynē'as* Galen's book on the womb, which is called *gynaecia*	11th-century *De passionibus mulierum*, version B	Latin	ספר בגליון?
2	1197–99	Do'eg the Edomite Provence	ספר התולדת *Sēfer batōledet* The book on generation	Muscio's 5th–6th century Latin adaptation of Soranus of Ephesus's *Gynecology*	Latin adaptation from Greek	N
3	1197–99	Do'eg the Edomite Provence	ספר הסתר *Sēfer haseter* The book of the secret	[*Trotula*] *Liber de sinthomatibus mulierum; De ornatu mulierum*	Latin	מקום מליח אשר שים
4	1197–99	Do'eg the Edomite Provence	ספר אגר (אפרישמוש) *Sēfer 'aqār (aphorisms)* Book of accumulation	11th-century adaptation of Hippocrates' Aphorisms	Latin adaptation from Greek	ספר אפרישמוש
5	1197–99	Do'eg the Edomite Provence	שלם במלאכה הרפואית *Šālem bamelā'kā hārēfū'īt* The complete art of medicine	*Liber Pantegni*, 11th-century translation by Constantine the African of Al-Majūsī's *Kitāb kāmil*	Latin Original: Arabic	N
6	1197–99	Do'eg the Edomite Provence	ספר יאיר נתיב *Sēfer yā'ir nātīb* Book of the illuminating road	*Viaticum peregrinantis*, 11th-century translation by Constantine the African of Ibn al-Jazzār's *Zād al-musāfir waqut al-ḥāḍir*	Latin Original: Arabic	יאיר מקום מליח אשר שים

	Date	Hebrew Translator/ Author & Place	Hebrew Title	Source Text	Language(s) of Translated Text	Section on Women of *Sēfer hayōšer*
				Late 12th to Early 13th Century		
7	12th–13th cent.	Anonymous Castile?	זכרון בכל חולי חולים בבוטם בקלי הברייון *Zikārōn bĕḥŏlayīm baḥōwtm beklê habĕrāyōn* An account of the diseases in the organs of the pregnancy	Hebrew	The text bears significant similarities to *funūn* 20 and 21of book 3 of Ibn Sīnā's *Kitāb al-Qānūn fī al-ṭibb*	N
8	12th–13th cent.	Sheshet ben Ben-veniste ? Barcelona ?	טרפות לברייון ירוה מקרא מגן ראש *Tĕrūfōt labĕrāyōn ba-niqrā' māgēn harōʾš* Medicaments for pregnancy, called 'the head's shield'	Hebrew		N
				13th Century		
9	ca. 13th cent.?	Anonymous Iberian Peninsula?	ספר דינה לכל ענין הריון ותחלייהם *Sēfer dīnā lĕkōl 'inyān hāre-ḥem wĕḥŏlĕyĕhāb* Dinah's book on all that concerns the womb and its diseases	Translation into Judeo-Arabic of Muscio's *Pessaria*	Judeo-Arabic Arabic? Original: Greek	N
10	Second half of 13th cent.	Jacob? Provence	שאר ישוב *Šĕʾar yāšūb* A remnant shall return	Edited version of *Sēfer hašēter*, which preserves excerpts from *De ornatu mulierum*	Latin	מקרה כלום שוב ושאר
11	1257 (or 1267)	Moses Ibn Tibbon Provence	(פרוש לפרקי אבוקרט) *(Pērūš lĕpirqê ʾabuqrat)*	Moses Maimonides, *Commentary on Hippocrates's Aphorisms* (1)	Arabic	ספר אבוקראט?

	Date	Hebrew Translator/ Author & Place	Hebrew Title	Source Text	Language(s) of Translated Text	Section on Women of *Sēfer hayōšer*
12	1259	Moses Ibn Tibbon, Provence	צדת הדרכים *Ṣēdat haderākîm*	Ibn al-Jazzār's *Zād al-musā- fir waqūt al-ḥāḍir*	Arabic	צדת הדרכים
13	ca. 1260?	Hillel ben Samuel of Verona, Italy	(אפוריזמי?) Aphorisms	Hippocrates, *Aphorisms with Galen's Commentaries*	Latin translation by Constantine the African from Arabic Original: Greek	ספר אפוריזמי?
14	ca. 1270	Anonymous	ספר יצירת העובר והנהגת בהרות והנולדים *Sēfer yĕṣīrat bā'ubār wĕhan- hāgat behārōt wĕhanōlādîm* Book on the creation of the foetus and the treatment of pregnant women and newborns	10th-century Arib Ibn Sa'id's *Kitāb khalq al-janīn wa-tadbīr al-ḥabālā wa-al- mawlūdīn*	Arabic	N
15	1264	Shem Ṭov ben Isaac of Tortosa, Provence	ספר אלמנצורי *Sēfer 'almanṣūrî* Book of Almansur	al-Rāzī's *Kitāb al-Manṣūrī*	Arabic	אלמנצורי ואיר חסר בכ"י
16	1277	Zeraḥyah Ḥen, Rome	לקוטי רבנו משה בעניני וסת והריון *Liqūṭē rabēnū mōšeh bĕ'inyānê weset wĕhērāyôn* Maimonides's compilation on menstruation and pregnancy	Chapter 16 of Maimonides's *Medical Aphorisms*, detached from the rest of the book some time after its translation into Hebrew	Arabic	N. A copy has been preserved in the margins of the section on women of one of its manuscripts (Oxford, Opp. 180, Nebauer 1234)

	Date	Hebrew Translator/ Author & Place	Hebrew Title	Source Text	Language(s) of Translated Text	Section on Women of *Sēfer hayōšer*
17	ca. 1277–90	Zerahyah Ḥen Italy (Rome)	(פירוש לפירקי אבוקרט) *Pērāš lēpirqē ʾabuqraṭ* Commentary on Hippocrates's Aphorisms	Maimonides, *Commentary on Hippocrates's Aphorisms* (2)	Arabic Original: Greek	N
18	ca. 1277–90	Zerahyah Ḥen Italy (Rome)	ספר ההריון והרחם לאבוקרט *Sēfer habērāyôn wĕ hāreḥem lĕʾabuqraṭ* Hippocrates's book on pregnancy and the womb	Hippocratic *On superfetation*	Arabic Original: Greek	ספר תולדת הילדים לאבוקרט
19	1283	Natan ha-Meʾati Italy (Rome)	ספר הפרקים לאבוקרט בגאלינוס *Sēfer hapērāqîm lĕʾabuqraṭ bēpērūš gaʾlīnūs* Hippocrates's Aphorisms with Galen's Commentary	*Commentary on Hippocrates's Aphorisms*	Arabic translation by Ḥunayn Ibn Isḥāq Original: Greek	ספר אקסטרישן?
20	ca. end of the 13th cent.	Anonymous Catalonia-Provence	ספר אהבת נשים *Sēfer ʾahăbat nāšîm* The book of women's love	Shares part of contents with two French and Catalan treatises.[99]	Hebrew	N
21	ca. end of the 13th cent.	Jacob ha-Qaṭan? Provence	ספר הישר *Sēfer hayōšer* The book of rectitude		Hebrew	

99 See Caballero Navas 2004, 14, 27–30, and 95–96.

Bibliography

Sources

Amar, Zohar, and Yael Buchman, eds., 2004. *Natan Joel Falaquera, Ṣŏrî hagûf.* Ramat Gan: Bar-Ilan University. [In Hebrew]

Barkai, Ron, ed. 1991. *Les infortunes de Dinah, ou la gynécologie juive au Moyen Âge.* Paris: Cerf.

— ed. and trans. 1998. *A History of Jewish Gynaecological Texts in the Middle Ages.* Leiden: Brill.

Bolton, Lesley, ed. and trans. 2015. "An Edition, Translation and Commentary of Mustio's Gynaecia." Ph.D. diss., University of Calgary.

Bos, Gerrit, ed. and trans. 1997. *Ibn Al-Jazzār on Sexual Diseases and Their Treatment: A Critical Edition of Zād al-musāfir wa-qūt al-ḥāḍir (Provisions for the Traveller and Nourishment for the Sedentary).* London: Kegan Paul.

—,ed. and trans. 2015. *Moses Maimonides' Medical Aphorisms. Treatises 16–21. A parallel Arabic-English edition.* Provo, UT: Brigham Young University Press.

Caballero Navas, Carmen, ed. and trans. 2003. "Un capítulo de mujeres. Transmisión y recepción de nociones sobre salud femenina en la producción textual hebrea durante la Edad Medieval." *Miscelánea de Estudios Árabes y Hebraicos, Sección Hebreo* 52: 135–162.

—, ed. and trans. 2004. *The Book of Women's Love and Jewish Medieval Medical Literature on Women. Sefer ahavat nashim.* London: Kegan Paul.

—, ed. and trans. 2006a. "Algunos 'secretos de mujeres' revelados. El *Šeʾar yašub* y la recepción y transmisión del *Trotula* en hebreo." *Miscelánea de Estudios Árabes y Hebraicos. Sección Hebreo* 55: 381–425.

Chavel, Charles, ed. 1996. *Mosheh ben Nahman. Commentary on the Torah, vol. 2. Leviticus.* Jerusalem: Mossad Harav Kook. [In Hebrew]

Feliu, Eduard, and Jon Arrizabalaga, trans. 2000–2001. "El próleg de Semtov ben Issac, 'el Tortosí,' a la seva traducció hebrea del 'Tasrif ' d'Abu-l- Qasim al-Zahrawi." *Tamid* 3: 65–95.

Green, Monica H., ed. and trans. 2001. *The Trotula. A Medieval Compendium of Women's Medicine.* Philadelphia: University of Pennsylvania Press.

Spink, M. S. and G. L. Lewis, eds. and trans. 1973. *Albucasis: On Surgery and Instrument.* London: The Wellcome Institute of the History of Medicine.

Steinschneider, Moritz, ed. 1888. "Haqdāmat hamaʿātîq biktab yād paris 1190 (The preface of the copyist in the manuscript Paris 1190)." *Magazin für die Wissenschaft des Judenthums* 15: 197, 6–14 (Hebrew section).

Zonta, Mauro, ed. and trans. 2003. "A Hebrew Translation of Hippocrates' *De superfoetatione*: Historical Introduction and Critical Edition." *Aleph* 3: 97–143.

Literature

Balberg, Mira. 2011. "Rabbinic Authority, Medical Rhetoric, and Body Hermeneutics in Mishnah Negaʿim." *AJS Review* 35,2: 323–346.

Beit-Arié, Malachi. 2001. "The Production of Hebrew Scientific Books According to Dated Medieval Manuscripts." In *Science in Medieval Jewish Cultures.* Edited by Gad Freudenthal. Cambridge: Cambridge University Press. Pages 106–110.

Bos, Gerrit, and Resianne Fontaine. 1999. "Medico-Philosophical Controversies in Natan b. Yo'el Falaquera's *Sefer Sori ha-Guf.*" *Jewish Quarterly Review* 90: 27–60.

Bos, Gerrit. 2010. "Medical Terminology in the Hebrew Tradition: Shem Tov Ben Isaac, *Sefer ha-Shimmush*, book 30." *Journal of Semitic Studies* 55,1: 53–101.

—. 2016. *Novel Medical and General Hebrew Terminology. Hippocrates' Aphorisms in the Hebrew Tradition*. Journal of Semitic Studies Supplement 37. Oxford: Oxford University Press.

Caballero Navas, Carmen. 2006b. "Secrets of Women. Naming Sexual Difference in Medieval Hebrew Medical Literature." *NASHIM, A Journal of Jewish Women's Studies and Gender Issues* 12: 39–56.

—. 2008. "The Care of Women's Health: An Experience Shared by Medieval Jewish and Christian Women." *Journal of Medieval History* 34,2: 146–163.

—. 2009. "Maimonides' Contribution to Women's Health Care and His Influence on the Hebrew Gynaecological Corpus." In *Traditions of Maimonideanism*. Edited by Carlos Fraenkel. Leiden: Brill. Pages 33–50.

—. 2011a. "Medicine among Medieval Jews: The Science, the Art, and the Practice." In *Science in Medieval Jewish Cultures*. Edited by Gad Freudenthal. Cambridge: Cambridge University Press. Pages 320–342.

—. 2011b. "Palabras de rabinos, saberes de mujeres. Discursos normativos y prácticas sanitarias en torno a la menstruación." In *Temps i espais de la Girona jueva*. Edited by Silvia Planas Marcé. Girona: Patronat Call de Girona. Pages 303–310.

—. 2013. "Maimonides and his Practice of Gynaecology." In *Moses Maimonides and His Practice of Medicine*. Edited by K. Collins, S. Kottek, and F. Rosner. Haifa: Maimonides Research Institute. Pages 61–84.

—. 2014. "She Will Give Birth Immediately. Pregnancy and Childbirth in Medieval Hebrew Medical Texts Produced in the Mediterranean West." *Dynamis* 34,2: 377–401.

—. 2019a. "Del árabe al hebreo. El nacimiento de la ginecología hebrea medieval y el *Canon de medicina* de Ibn Sīnā." *Sefarad* 79,1: 89–122.

—. 2019b. "Virtuous and Wise: Apprehending Female Medical Practice from Hebrew Texts on Women's Health Care." *Social History of Medicine* 32, 4: 691–711 (Special Cluster *Learning Practice from Texts: Jews and Medicine in the Later Middle Ages*, edited by Naama Cohen-Hanegbi).

—. 2021 (forthcoming). "Graeco-Latin Gynaecology in Jewish Robes. The Hebrew translation of Muscio's Gynaecia." In *Female Bodies and Female Practitioners in the Medical Traditions of the Ancient Mediterranean World*. Edited by Lennart Lehmhaus. Tübingen: Mohr Siebeck.

Ferre, Lola. 2002. "Tras las huellas del Canon hebraico." In *Avicena, Canon medicinae: estudio y edición facsímil del ms. 2197 de la Biblioteca Universitaria de Bolonia*. Libro de estudios. Madrid: AyN Ediciones. Pages 244–287.

—. 2009. "Dissemination of Maimonides' Medical Writings in the Middle Ages." In *Traditions of Maimonideanism*. Edited by Carlos Fraenkel. Leiden: Brill. Pages 17–31.

Fonrobert, Charlotte E. 2000. *Menstrual Purity: Rabbinic and Christian Reconstructions of Biblical Gender*. Stanford, CA: Stanford University Press.

—. 2007. "The Human Body in Rabbinic Legal Discourse." In *The Cambridge Companion to the Talmud and Rabbinic Literature*. Edited by Charlotte E. Fonrobert and Martin S. Jaffee. New York: Cambridge University Press. Pages 270–294.

Freudenthal, Gad. 1995. "Science in the Medieval Jewish Culture of Southern France." *History of Science* 33: 23–58. Repr. in Gad Freudenthal. *Science in the Medieval Hebrew and Arabic Traditions*. Aldershot: Ashgate Variorum. 2005.

—. 2011a. "Arabic and Latin Cultures as Resources for the Hebrew Translation Movement." In *Science in Medieval Jewish Cultures*. Edited by Gad Freudenthal. Cambridge: Cambridge University Press. Pages 74–105.

—. 2011b. "Arabic into Hebrew. The Emergence of the Translation Movement in Twelfth-Century Provence and Jewish-Christian Polemic." In *Border Crossings: Interreligious Interaction and the Exchange of Ideas in the Islamic Middle Ages*. Edited by David Freidenreich and Miriam Goldstein. Philadelphia: University of Pennsylvania Press. Pages 124–143.

—. 2013. "The Father of the Latin-into-Hebrew Translations: 'Do'eg the Edomite', the Twelfth Century Repentant Convert." In *Latin-into-Hebrew: Texts and Studies, vol. 1*. Edited by Ressiane Fontaine and Gad Freudenthal. Leiden: Brill. Pages 105–120.

—. 2018. "The Father of the Latin-into-Hebrew Translators of the Middle Ages: Doeg the Edomite and His 24 Translations (1197–1199)." In *A Tribute to Hannah: Jubilee Book in Honor of Hannah Kasher*. Edited by Avi Elqayam and Ariel Malachi. Tel-Aviv: Idra Publishing, 23–53. [In Hebrew]

Freudenthal, Gad and Mauro Zonta. 2012. "Avicenna among Medieval Jews. The Reception of Avicenna's Philosophical, Scientific and Medical Writings in Jewish Cultures, East and West." *Arabic Sciences and Philosophy* 22,2: 217–287.

García-Ballester, Luis. 1994. "A Marginal Learned Medical World: Jewish, Muslim and Christian Medical Practitioners, and the Use of Arabic Medical Sources in Late Medieval Spain." In *Practical Medicine from Salerno to the Black Death*. Edited by Luis García-Ballester et al. Cambridge: Cambridge University Press. Pages 353–394.

—. 2001. *La búsqueda de la salud. Sanadores y enfermos en la España medieval*. Barcelona: Península.

Green, Monica H. 1985. "The Transmission of Ancient Theories of Female Physiology and Disease through the Early Middle Ages." Ph.D. diss., Princeton University.

—. 1994. "The Re-Creation of *Pantegni, Practica*, Book VIII." In *Constantine the African and 'Ali ibn al-'Abbas al-Magusi: The 'Pantegni' and Related Texts*. Edited by Charles Burnett and Danielle Jacquart. Leiden: E. J. Brill. Pages 121–160.

—. 1996. "The 'Development' of the *Trotula*." *Revue d'Historie des Textes* 26: 119–203.

—. 2000. "Medieval Gynecological Texts: A Handlist." In Eadem. *Women's Healthcare in the Medieval West: Texts and Contexts*. Aldershot: Ashgate. Appendix, Pages 1–36.

—. 2008. *Making Women's Medicine Masculine. The Rise of Male Authority in Pre-Modern Gynaecology*. Oxford: Oxford University Press.

—. 2011. "Moving from Philology to Social History: The Circulation and Uses of Albucasis's Latin *Surgery* in the Middle Ages." In *Between Text and Patient: The Medical Enterprise in Medieval & Early Modern Europe*. Edited by Florence Eliza Glaze and Brian Nance. Florence: SISMEL/Edizioni del Galuzzo. Pages 331–372.

—. 2013. "Caring for Gendered Bodies." In *Oxford Handbook of Medieval Women and Gender*. Edited by Judith Bennett and Ruth Mazo Karras. Oxford: Oxford University Press. Pages 345–361.

—. 2019, "The Recovery of 'Ancient' Gynaecology. The Humanist Rediscovery of the Eleventh-Century Gynaecological Corpus." In *Transmission of Knowledge n the Late Middle Ages and the Renaissance*. Edited by Outi Merisalo, Miika Kuha and Susanna Niiranen. Turnhout: Brepols. Pages 45–54.

Hanson, Ann Ellis, and Monica H. Green. 1994. "Soranus of Ephesus: *Methodicorum princeps*." In *Aufstieg und Niedergang der römischen Welt. Teilband II, Band 37.2*. Edited by

Wolfgang Haase and Hildegard Temporini. Berlin and New York: Walter de Gruyter. Pages 968–1075.

King, Helen. 1998. "Once upon a Text: Hysteria from Hippocrates." In *Hippocrates' Woman. Reading the Female Body in Ancient Greece*. London and New York: Routledge. Pages 205–246.

Koren, Sharon Faye. 2004. "Kabbalistic Physiology: Isaac the Blind, Nahmanides, and Moses de Leon on Menstruation." *AJS Review* 28,2: 317–339.

Muntner, Suessman. 1947. "R. Jacob ha-Qaṭan, the Anonymous Translator." *Tarbiz* 18: 192–199. [In Hebrew]

Pormann, Peter E. and Emilie Savage-Smith. 2007. *Medieval Islamic Medicine*. Edinburgh: Edinburgh University Press.

Richler, Benjamin. 1986. "Manuscripts of Moses ben Maimon's Pirke Moshe in Hebrew Translation." *Koroth* 9,3–4: 345–356.

Ruiz Morell, Olga. 2012. "Niddah: la mujer menstruante de la Ley Escrita a la Ley Oral." *El Olivo* 76: 21–42.

Sela, Shelomo. 2003. *Abraham Ibn Ezra and the Rise of Medieval Hebrew Science*. Leiden: Brill.

Steinschneider, Moritz. 1893. *Die hebraeischen Uebersetzungen des Mittelalters und die Juden als Dolmetscher*. Berlin: Kommissionsverlag des Bibliographischen Bureaus.

Zonta, Mauro. 2011. "Medieval Hebrew Translations of Philosophical and Scientific Texts. A Chronological Table." In *Science in Medieval Jewish Cultures*. Edited by Gad Freudenthal. Cambridge: Cambridge University Press. Pages 17–73.

.

General Index (Names and Subjects)

DOI: 10.13173/9783447108263.375

Notes on Contributors

Carmen Caballero Navas is Senior Lecturer of Hebrew and Jewish Studies at the Department of Semitic Studies at the University of Granada, Spain. Her research focuses on Hebrew texts about women's health care in the medieval Mediterranean West. Other research interests include the transmission and reception of medical ideas among medieval Jews; Jewish debates on sexual difference and the female body; the historical experience of medieval Jewish women, especially as receivers and providers of health care; and Jewish knowledge and practice of magic in the Middle Ages. She currently leads the project "Language and Literature of Rabbinic and Medieval Judaism", funded by the Spanish Government. She has authored four monographs and edited one volume. Among her numerous book chapters and articles are: "The Reception of Galen in Hebrew Medieval Scientific Writings," in *Brill's Companion to the Reception of Galen* (eds. P. Bouras-Vallianatos/B. Zipser; Brill, 2019), pp. 535–558, "Virtuous and Wise: Apprehending Female Medical Practice from Hebrew Texts on Women's Health Care," *Social History of Medicin*, 32/4 (2019): 691–711; "Del árabe al hebreo. El nacimiento de la ginecología hebrea medieval y el *Canon de medicina* de Ibn Sīnā," *Sefarad* 79/1 (2019): 89–122; "Writing in Hebrew in Romance-Speaking Settings. The Sefer Ahavat Našim and the Language of Medieval Hebrew Medical Texts," *eHumanista/IVITRA* 14 (2018): 898–910; "She will give birth immediately. Pregnancy and Childbirth in Medieval Hebrew Medical Texts Produced in the Mediterranean West," *Dynamis* 34/2 (2014): 377–401.

Kenneth Collins worked as a general medical practitioner in Glasgow for over thirty years. He has published several volumes on the Jews and medicine in Scotland and on Scottish Jewish history. He is Chairman of the Scottish Jewish Archives Centre, Senior Research Fellow at the Centre for the History of Medicine and is currently Visiting Professor, History of Medicine, at the Hebrew University of Jerusalem. He was editor of *Vesalius: Journal of the International Society for the History of Medicine* from 2008 to 2017 and is a guest editor of *Korot: Journal of the Israeli Journal for the History of Medicine and Science*. He has co-edited three volumes on famous Jewish physicians including *Moses Maimonides and His Practice of Medicine* (Haifa 2013) and *Isaac Israel: the Philosopher Physician* (Jerusalem 2015).

Federico Dal Bo (b. 1973) holds a PhD in Translation Studies (University of Bologna, 2005) and a PhD in Jewish Studies (Freie Universität Berlin, 2009). He currently is a post-doctoral fellow at the University of Heidelberg / Hochschule für Jüdische Studien in the project "Material Text Cultures". His most recent publications are:

DOI: 10.13173/9783447108263.379

Emanation and Philosophy of Language. An Introduction to Josef ben Abraham Giqa-tilla (Cherub Press, 2019), *Deconstruting the Talmud. The Absolute Book* (Routledge, 2019), and *Qabbalah e traduzione. Un saggio su Paul Celan* (Orthotes, 2019). For more information: www.federicodalbo.eu.

Estēe Dvorjetski is Professor of Ancient History and Archaeology at Oxford Brookes University, UK and at Zinman Institute of Archaeology, University of Haifa, Israel. She has published numerous studies on the Land of Israel in the Hellenistic, Roman and Byzantine periods on diseases and healing, the Dead Sea, leisure-time activities, talmudic literature, baths and bathing, numismatics, art history, and historical geography. She is the author of *Ecology and Values* (2000, Heb.), *Leisure, Pleasure and Healing: Spa Culture and Medicine in Ancient Eastern Mediterranean* (2007), and *The Genesis of Medicine: Handbook for Students* (2008). She is currently writing a book on *Medicine, Ecology and Public Health in the Holy Land from Biblical Times to the Late Roman Period: Historical-Archaeological Perspectives*. She has been a scientific consultant for exhibitions on history of medicine at Rambam Medical Centre in Haifa (2009) and Tower of David Museum in Jerusalem (2014–2015), and a reviewer for the Wellcome Trust Centre and the AHRC. She was laudable for years at the University of Haifa and the Technion for excellence in teaching.

Reuven Kiperwasser received his doctorate from Bar Ilan University, Israel in 2005 (*The Midrashim on Kohelet: Studies in their Formation and Redaction*). Currently, he is teaching at Ariel University and is a research associate at Hebrew University Jerusalem. He was Alexander von Humboldt fellow at the Freie Universität Berlin, Israel Science Foundation fellow, and held a fellowship at the Frankel Institute, University of Michigan, Ann Arbor and the Maimonides Center of Advanced Studies at Hamburg University. Specializing in rabbinic literature, his research interests include interactions between Iranian mythology, Syriac-Christian storytelling, rabbinic narrative, and trans-cultural relationships between traditions in Late Antiquity. Soon he will publish a critical edition and commentary of Kohelet Rabbah 7–12 (Schechter Institute, 2021) as well as a monograph about Babylonian immigrants in the Land of Israel and the acceptance of the Other in rabbinic culture (Brown Judaic Studies). Recent journal articles include "Wives of Commoners and the Masculinity of the Rabbis: Jokes, Serious Matters and Migrating Traditions," *Journal for the Study of Judaism* 48, 418–445; "'Three Partners in a Person', The Metamorphoses of a Tradition and the History of an Idea (edited and updated version)," *Irano-Judaica* 8 (2019), 393–438.

Samuel S. Kottek (b. 1931, Strasbourg) received his MD from the Université de Strasbourg in 1959 and specialized in pediatric medicine. He studied under Prof. Joshua Leibowitz and eventually became the Harry Friedenwald Chair of History of Medicine at the Hebrew University's Hadassah Medical School in 1976 (emeritus since 2000). His main research interest is medicine in ancient Hebrew or Jewish sources and the history of Pediatrics (17th–18th cent.). He is the editor of the journal *Korot* and has published about 200 papers. Among his authored and edited books are: *Medicine* *and Hygiene in the Works of Flavius Josephus* (Leiden 1994); [with M. Waserman, eds.] *Health and Disease in the Holy Land* (Lewiston, 1996); [with M. Horstmanshoff et al., eds.] *From Athens to Jerusalem: Medicine in Hellenized Jewish Lore and in Early Christian Literature* (Rotterdam, 2000); [with Kenneth Collins and Fred Rosner, eds.] *Maimonides and his Practice of Medicine* (Haifa, 2013); [with Kenneth Collins and Helena Paavilainen, eds.] *Isaac Israeli: The Philosopher Physician*, (Jerusalem, 2015).

Y. Tzvi Langermann received his Ph.D. in History of Science from Harvard, where he studied under A.I. Sabra and John Murdoch. For fifteen years he catalogued Hebrew and Judaeo-Arabic texts in philosophy and science at the Institute of Microfilmed Hebrew Manuscripts in Jerusalem, before joining the Department of Arabic at Bar Ilan, from which he recently retired. In collaboration with Gerrit Bos he published *The Alexandrian Summaries of Galen's On Critical Days: Editions and Translations of the Two Versions of the Jawāmiʿ, with an Introduction and Notes* (Brill, 2014) and *Maimonides, On Rules Regarding the Practical Part of the Medical Art. A parallel Arabic-English edition* (Brigham Young University Press, 2014); and, with Robert Morrison, *Texts in Transit in the Medieval Mediterranean* (Pennsylvania State University Press, 2016). Recently, his translation and study of a treatise by Ibn Kammūna, *Subtle Insights Concerning Knowledge and Practice* (Yale University Press, 2019) has been published.

Lennart Lehmhaus is a postdoctoral researcher focusing on premodern rabbinic literature and culture, history of medicine, sciences and knowledge in Jewish traditions and the manifold entanglements between Jews and their various cultural contexts. From 2013 to 2020 he was part of the working group A03 on late antique medicine within the Collaborative Research Center 'Episteme in Motion' (SFB 980) at the Freie Universität Berlin. He received his doctorate in Jewish Studies and rabbinic literature from Martin-Luther University in Halle, Germany. After his studies in Duisburg, Jerusalem, Düsseldorf and Kraków, he held research and teaching appointments at Martin-Luther-University Halle, Harvard University, The Katz Center for Advanced Judaic Studies at the University of Pennsylvania, and Freie Universität Berlin. In addition to several peer-reviewed articles/chapters, he is the author of two books (*Seder Eliyahu Zuta*; *Sourcebook of Talmudic Medicine I*; both Mohr Siebeck, 2021), (co-) edited three volumes (*Collecting Recipes*, De Gruyter 2017; *Defining Jewish Medicine*; *Female Bodies and Female Practitioners*, Mohr Siebeck 2021) and is the founding editor of the series *ASK-Ancient Cultures of Sciences and Knowledge* (Mohr Siebeck).

Tirzah Meacham is an associate professor in Department of Near and Middle Eastern Civilizations at University of Toronto. She received her doctorate in Talmudic and Rabbinic Literature from The Hebrew University, Jerusalem with a critical edition of Mishnah Niddah with chapters in legal history and realia. She published *Sefer haBagrut leRav Shmuel ben Hofni Gaon veSefer haShanim leRav Yehuda ben Yosef Rosh haSeder* with Miriam Frenkel which deals with the boundaries of legal minority and majority. She co-edited with Harry Fox *Introducing Tosefta: Textual, Intratextual* *and Intertextual Studies,* and the Jewish Law Association Studies volume 28 entitled *The Jewish Family.* They co-edited with Daniel Maoz *From Something to Nothing: Jewish Mysticism in Contemporary Canadian Jewish Studies.* She is working on a Feminist Commentary to Babylonian Talmud Niddah and petitionary prayers in Hebrew from Italy and other topics in history of medicine and commentary.

Aviad Recht is a scholar working on the history of medicine, the Babylonian Talmud and late antique Judaism. His doctoral dissertation "Babylonian Talmudic Medicine—A Diachronic Perspective" has been submitted to the Chaim Rosenberg School of Jewish Studies and Archaeology, Tel Aviv University in 2020.

Shulamit Shinnar holds a postdoctoral faculty position as a Core Lecturer for Literature Humanities in the Department of History and the Center for the Core Curriculum at Columbia University, New York City. She received her PhD in History from Columbia University in 2019, where her dissertation explored rabbinic medical culture in late antiquity, focusing on medicine as a site for social encounter and cultural exchange between different ethnic, religious, and gender identities.

Tamás Visi is an Associate Professor at the Kurt and Ursula Schubert Centre for Jewish Studies at Palacky University (Olomouc, Czech Republic). He earned his doctorate with a dissertation on the early Ibn Ezra supercommentaries at the Central European University in Budapest in 2006. In 2012 he was a Fellow of the Institute for Advanced Studies at the Hebrew University of Jerusalem. Since 2016 he has worked for the Averroes Edition Project at the Thomas Institute of the University of Cologne. Recent publications: "Jewish Physicians in Late Medieval Ashkenaz," *Social History of Medicine* 32 (2019): 670–690. "Medieval Hebrew Uroscopic Texts: The Reception of Greek Uroscopic Texts in the Hebrew *Book of Remedies* Attributed to Asaf," in Y. Tzvi Langermann and Robert G. Morrison (eds.), *Texts in Transit in the Medieval Mediterranean* (University Park, Pennsylvania: The Pennsylvania State University Press, 2016), 162–196. "Plague, Persecution, and Philosophy: Avigdor Kara and the Consequences of the Black Death," in Ephraim Shoham-Steiner, (ed.), *Intricate Interfaith Networks: Quotidian Jewish-Christian Contacts,* (Turnhout: Brepols, 2016) 85–118. "Tradition and Innovation: Isaac Israeli's Classification of Colors," in Kenneth Collins, Samuel Kottek, and Helena Paavilainen (eds.), *Isaac Israeli: The Philosopher Physician* (Jerusalem: Muriel and Philip Berman Medical Library, 2015), 39–66. "Berechiah ben Naṭronai ha-Naqdan's *Dodi ve-Neḵdi* and the Transfer of Scientific Knowledge from Latin to Hebrew in the Twelfth Century," *Aleph* 14.2 (2014): 9–73.

Ronit Yoeli-Tlalim is a Reader in the History Department at Goldsmiths, University of London. Her research deals with the transmission of medical knowledge along the so-called 'Silk-Roads'. She is the author of *ReOrienting Histories of Medicine: Encounters along the Silk Roads* (London: Bloomsbury 2021). Her article "Exploring Persian lore in the Hebrew *Book of Asaf*", was published in *Aleph* (18:1, 2018).

Episteme in Bewegung.
Beiträge zu einer transdisziplinären Wissensgeschichte

Herausgegeben von Gyburg Uhlmann im Auftrag des Sonderforschungsbereichs 980
„Episteme in Bewegung. Wissenstransfer von der Alten Welt bis in die Frühe Neuzeit"

18: Nikolas Pissis, Nora Schmidt, Gyburg Uhlmann (Hg.)

Wissensoikonomien

Ordnung und Transgression vormoderner Kulturen

2020. VIII, 324 Seiten, 7 Abb., gb
170x240 mm
ISBN 978-3-447-11510-0   € 68,– (D)
DOI: 10.13173/9783447115100

Der von Nora Schmidt, Nikolas Pissis und Gyburg Uhlmann herausgegebene Band widmet sich der Frage, wie Wissen zwischen verschiedenen Akteuren ausgetauscht wird: wie es den Besitzer wechselt, wie es einen Ort verlässt und von einer Zeit in eine andere wandert. Der Austausch von Wissen hat mit ökonomischen, technischen, materialen und wissenschaftlichen Prozessen zu tun, lässt sich aber auf keinen von ihnen reduzieren.
Die Autorinnen und Autoren des Bandes arbeiten daher mit dem Konzept der *Wissensoikonomien*: Im Zentrum steht die Vielschichtigkeit der Beziehungsgeflechte und Austauschbeziehungen von Menschen und Materialien, Medien, sozialen Praktiken, Traditionen und Institutionen. Ausgehend von der Beobachtung, dass Transfer von Wissen sich in einer Vielzahl von Modalitäten und Geschwindigkeiten, unter sehr unterschiedlichen Bedingungen und teils über sprachliche, geographische und soziale, religiöse und andere identitätsspezifische Grenzen hinweg ereignet, geht das Konzept der *Wissensoikonomien* der Frage nach, wann solche Wissensbewegungen selbst systembildenden Charakter erhalten. Damit beschreiben *Wissensoikonomien* ein Spannungsfeld zwischen Ordnung und Transgression. In sechzehn einzelnen Fachbeiträgen werden komplexe Aushandlungsprozesse von Wissen in unterschiedlichen vormodernen Kulturen vom Alten Ägypten, über die verschiedenen antiken Kulturen des Mittelmeerraums, China und Korea bis in die Frühe Neuzeit aufgezeigt.

19: Melanie Möller, Matthias Grandl (Hg.)

Wissen *en miniature*

Theorie und Epistemologie der Anekdote

2021. X, 316 Seiten, 8 Abb., gb
170x240 mm
ISBN 978-3-447-11540-7
⊙ *E-Book: ISBN 978-3-447-39088-0*   je € 68,– (D)

Wissen *en miniature* erkundet die epistemischen Potentiale des Miniatur-Narrativs Anekdote als Wissensform in Texten und Bildern von der Antike bis in die Moderne. Philosophischen und kunstgeschichtlichen Perspektiven werden komparatistische philologische Lektüren gegenübergestellt, die Beispiele aus der lateinischen, italienischen, französischen, englischen und deutschen Literatur umfassen. Angeregt von den leitenden Fragestellungen und Begrifflichkeiten des Sonderforschungsbereichs 980 an der Freien Universität Berlin „Episteme in Bewegung" wird analysiert, welchen Prozessen der Umstrukturierung, des Wandels, der Selektion oder der Ausblendung Wissen im Zuge der Neukontextualisierung von Anekdoten oder im Akt des Anekdotisierens selbst unterworfen ist. Untersucht wird, welche Machtkonstellationen und Aushandlungsprozesse sich am Transfer von Anekdoten ablesen lassen und wie diese, auch in der materialen und medialen Gestaltung von Anekdoten, dokumentiert werden.

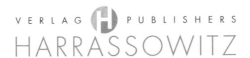

VERLAG PUBLISHERS
HARRASSOWITZ

Episteme in Bewegung.
Beiträge zu einer transdisziplinären Wissensgeschichte

Herausgegeben von Gyburg Uhlmann im Auftrag des Sonderforschungsbereichs 980 „Episteme in Bewegung. Wissenstransfer von der Alten Welt bis in die Frühe Neuzeit"

20: Şirin Dadaş, Christian Vogel (Hg.)

Dynamiken der Negation

(Nicht)Wissen und negativer Transfer
in vormodernen Kulturen

2021. Ca. 450 Seiten, 22 Farbabb.,
10 s/w Abb., gb
170x240 mm
ISBN 978-3-447-11625-1   ca. € 84,– (D)
DOI: 10.13173/9783447116251

Negationen prägen Prozesse des Wissenswandels nicht nur, indem sie zu einem Aussortieren beitragen, Entwicklungen abbrechen und Platz für Neues schaffen, sondern auch durch ihnen innewohnende epistemische Potentiale. Der von Şirin Dadaş und Christian Vogel herausgegebene Band widmet sich in 17 Beiträgen diesen Dynamiken der Negation, die sich als konstitutiv für das vermittelte Wissen erweisen bzw. die Vermittlung von Wissen mitgestalten.

Die Untersuchungen rücken die vielfältigen Impulse der Negation für wissensgeschichtliche Forschungen in den Blick. Es geht weniger um ein Scheitern von Transferprozessen oder um die Absenz von Wissen als um wissensgenerierende Dimensionen der Negation. Das Erkenntnisinteresse der Beiträge, die einen Untersuchungszeitraum von mehr als 2000 Jahren umfassen, richtet sich auf Wissensformen, die sich der Definition entziehen, sich nicht diskursivieren lassen oder Grenzen des Wissbaren anzeigen. Dabei wird den epistemischen Geltungsansprüchen und spezifischen Darstellungsweisen eines solchen ‚(Nicht)Wissens' nachgegangen. Zugleich stehen jene Negationen im Fokus, die als Ausschluss, Auflösung, Schweigen oder Zerstörung zur Wissensvermittlung dazugehören und sich derart als Ausprägungen eines ‚negativen Transfers' beschreiben lassen.

21: Jutta Eming, Volkhard Wels (Hg.)

Darstellung und Geheimnis in Mittelalter und Früher Neuzeit

2021. Ca. 512 Seiten, 15 Abb., gb
170x240 mm
ISBN 978-3-447-11548-3
⊙E-Book: ISBN 978-3-447-39050-7
In Vorbereitung   je ca. € 98,– (D)

Das Mittelalter und die Frühe Neuzeit gelten – teilweise aus unterschiedlichen Gründen – als ‚Zeitalter des Geheimnisses' und werden damit von der Moderne als einer ‚entzauberten' Epoche abgegrenzt. Wissenschaftliche, theologische und literarische Texte bilden die wesentliche Basis für diese Auffassung. Die Gralszene aus Wolfram von Eschenbachs Parzival zum Beispiel stellt für das ‚geheimnisvolle Mittelalter' ein Paradebeispiel dar, ebenso die Gattungen der Mystik, das ‚Mysterienspiel' oder die Alchemie.

In den Mikroanalysen, welche die Beiträge des von Jutta Emig und Volkhard Wels herausgegebenen Bands bieten, geht es nicht darum, diese Paradigmen weiter zu entfalten, sondern um detaillierte Analysen dessen, was auf synchroner und systematischer Ebene konkret unter ‚Geheimnis' und ‚Rätsel' zu verstehen ist. Leitend dafür ist eine wissensgeschichtliche Fragestellung nach den Formen und den Gründen für Darstellungsmodi von Rätsel oder Geheimnis sowie nach den Funktionen, welche diese für Literatur und Kultur der Vormoderne übernehmen. Es geht nicht darum, die große Erzählung vom Geheimnis als einer Epochensignatur fortzuschreiben, sondern um eine Bestimmung von Geheimnis und Rätsel als Wissensformen und ästhetischen Strategien, mit anderen Worten als Formen der Darstellung.

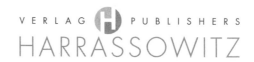

VERLAG PUBLISHERS
HARRASSOWITZ